Essentials in Cytopathology

Volume 30

Series Editor

Momin T. Siddiqui, Department of Pathology and Laboratory Medicine,
Weill-Cornell Medicine, New York Presbyterian Hospital, New York, NY, USA

The subspecialty of Cytopathology is 60 years old and has become established as a solid and reliable discipline in medicine. As expected, cytopathology literature has expanded in a remarkably short period of time, from a few textbooks prior to the 1980's to a current library of texts and journals devoted exclusively to cytomorphology that is substantial. Essentials in Cytopathology does not presume to replace any of the distinguished textbooks in Cytopathology. Instead, the series will publish generously illustrated and user-friendly guides for both pathologists and clinicians.

Ricardo H. Bardales

Editor

The Interventional Cytopathologist

Ultrasound Guided Fine-Needle Aspiration of Superficial Masses with Ultrasound Correlation

Second Edition

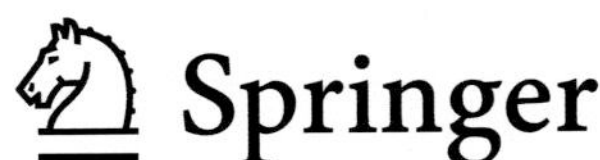

Editor
Ricardo H. Bardales
Precision Pathology
Outpatient Pathology Associates
Sacramento, CA, USA

ISSN 1574-9053 ISSN 1574-9061 (electronic)
Essentials in Cytopathology
ISBN 978-3-031-73701-5 ISBN 978-3-031-73702-2 (eBook)
https://doi.org/10.1007/978-3-031-73702-2

This Springer imprint is published by the registered company Springer Nature Switzerland AG
The registered company address is: Gewerbestrasse 11, 6330 Cham, Switzerland

If disposing of this product, please recycle the paper.

Dedicated to:

My parents Waldetrudis (QEPD) and Ricardo (QEPD).

Angela, Ricky, and Angie for their encouragement, support, and for being my best friends and role models.

My mentors Abel Mejia, Benjamin Koziner, Leopold G. Koss, Klaus Schreiber, Michael W. Stanley, Norwin Becker, and John S. Abele.

My pathology residents and cytology fellows.

Dr. Bardales has reviewed the history of fine needle aspiration, placing this volume at the forefront of this discipline. Before it was applied to current methods, it began as a tool in the hands of our clinical colleagues who sent us specimens for microscopic interpretation. These punctures were directed mostly at palpable lesions. Those active in this field today can imagine the interpretive difficulties that must have arisen in an era when virtually every specimen seemed new. Such difficulties continue to arise and are the subject of our enlarging collective published experience.

In many settings, fine needle aspiration of palpable masses moved into the hands of pathologists. This provided the possibility of immediate interpretation, repeat of inadequate samples, and close correlation of clinical with cytologic findings. Many pathologists made the required pilgrimage to study with the method's masters in Sweden during the 1970s and 1980s. As our diagnostic prowess increased, our enthusiasm and confidence grew as well. Many clinicians welcomed the expanding role of pathologists in specimen acquisition, as improved specimen preparation and concentration of clinical and cytologic assessment were merged into a single pair of hands. Many of us have found that pathologist-performed fine needle aspiration simply works better than asking busy clinicians to be responsible for aspiration, preparation, and triage to special studies without adequate training. In other words, what happens at the microscope is limited by what happened at the bedside. What happens at the bedside is predicated on what is expected to happen at the microscope.

Dr. Bardales has for some years been associated with Outpatient Pathology Associates (OPA) in Sacramento, California, USA. These academically productive inhabitants of private practice cytology have long been leaders in our field. Many will recall his previous book *Practical Urologic Cytopathology* as the definitive source in the field. We cannot review this history here, but many of us will recall having met and learned from other members of this school, including Dr. John Abele and Dr. Ted Miller. It seems only natural that this group should move decisively into practicing the newest methods that patients will perceive as efficient, high-quality, one-stop cytologic diagnosis. Dr. Bardales' new book, *The Interventional Cytopathologist: US Guided FNA of Superficial Masses*, reports on OPA's capabilities and expands Dr. Bardales' experience with many thousands of palpable-lesion biopsies to pathologist-performed ultrasound-guided sampling of more deeply situated or more palpably subtle masses.

Many of us have been intimidated by learning to perform and interpret ultrasound or by the method's seeming complexity or by the instrumentation's cost. As emphasized by Dr. Bardales, the latter two have been ameliorated considerably of late. The former is dealt with early in this book. Issues as basic, but as essential, as concepts of echogenicity are described and illustrated. More traditional issues such as the basics of aspiration technique and specimen preparation remain keys to ultimate diagnostic success and are also considered here.

It is reasonable that the thyroid is addressed extensively. For many of us, this is the most frequent site of needle aspiration biopsies. The thyroid is also one of the sites in which ultrasound imaging is most helpful. Many thyroid lesions are difficult to palpate with confidence. Others are confused by their presence in the setting of multinodular goiter. Called to do a thyroid aspirate in this setting, one is sometimes unsure that his selected target is the same as that for which the aspiration referral was originally made. Diagnostic considerations in thyroid cytology are placed firmly within Bethesda System's terminology, criteria, and follow-up recommendations. The parathyroid glands can be clinical, cytomorphologic, and anatomic cousins to the larger organ. Most such aspirations require ultrasound guidance. One may also perform parathormone chemistry on samples obtained during aspiration to great effect.

Other head and neck sites, as well as lymph nodes in many areas, also benefit from ultrasound-guided aspiration. A portion of this book is dedicated to breast cytology with a much needed update of diagnostic criteria. While OPA and other practices remain very active in breast aspiration, many of us have long since conceded this area to those wielding much larger core biopsy instruments and using guidance by either stereotactic or ultrasound methods. It is tempting to speculate that pathologists' use of ultrasound might regain some of this territory, allowing patients to enjoy more rapid interpretations.

I predict that this book will not only allow but will encourage pathologists to enter the realm of ultrasound-guided fine needle aspiration. The tools are here.

Department of Pathology   Michael W. Stanley
United Hospital
St. Paul, MN, USA

It is with great pleasure that I present the foreword to the second edition of *The Interventional Cytopathologist: Ultrasound-Guided Fine-Needle Aspiration of Superficial Masses with Ultrasound Correlation*. This book remains an invaluable resource in the ever-evolving field of interventional cytopathology, where the integration of advanced imaging techniques, molecular diagnostics, and the latest WHO Reporting Systems for Cytopathology and histological classifications has revolutionized our practice.

Since the first edition, there have been significant advancements in both technology and methodology, which have greatly enhanced our diagnostic capabilities. The second edition reflects these developments and provides a comprehensive guide that covers a broad spectrum of topics essential for practitioners in this field.

This book begins with general considerations on ultrasound in Chap. 1, providing foundational knowledge that is crucial for understanding and applying ultrasound in cytopathology. Chapter 2 discusses the role of the interventional cytopathologist, emphasizing the integration of clinical, imaging, and pathological data in patient management.

Subsequent chapters delve into specific anatomical regions and their related pathologies. Chapter 3 focuses on the thyroid gland, while Chap. 4 explores the parathyroid gland, each providing detailed insights into ultrasound-guided fine-needle aspiration (FNA) and its correlation with cytological findings. Chapter 5 addresses the salivary glands, offering guidelines for the diagnosis and management of lesions in these complex structures.

Chapter 6 covers miscellaneous head and neck lesions, expanding the scope to include a variety of challenging cases. Chapter 7 discusses lymph nodes, an area of critical importance in the diagnosis of both benign and malignant conditions.

The discussion extends to the breast in Chap. 8, where the integration of cytopathology with ultrasound imaging plays a vital role in the early detection and management of breast lesions. This chapter is particularly enriched by the contributions of Dr. Eugenio Leonardo, whose expertise adds depth to the discussion.

Finally, Chap. 9 offers a personal narrative of the experiences and lessons learned by Dr. Ricardo H. Bardales, providing invaluable "pearls" and illustrative cases drawn from his extensive career in performing ultrasound-guided FNA of superficial masses.

The authors have meticulously updated this edition to reflect current best practices, and their dedication to advancing our field is evident throughout. I am confident that this book will continue to guide cytopathologists in honing their skills and integrating new technologies into their practice, ultimately leading to better patient outcomes.

I extend my sincere gratitude to the authors for their hard work and commitment to excellence, and I am honored to introduce this important work to the community of interventional cytopathologists.

Professor of Pathology, Medical Faculty of Porto University   Fernando Schmitt
President of the International Academy of Cytology
Porto, Portugal

Preface: 2nd Edition

The use of ultrasonography (US) has become essential in the evaluation of superficial palpable and nonpalpable lesions. In addition to its diagnostic benefit, US can be used as a tool for needle guidance in diagnostic US-guided fine-needle aspiration (USG-FNA), therapy, e.g., cyst drainage, and administration of agents, e.g., alcohol ablation. These procedures can be done in an outpatient office or in a hospital setting.

This book provides a comprehensive review of the cytology of palpable and/or US-visible superficial neoplastic and non-neoplastic disease processes, as obtained by percutaneous USG-FNA, particularly of the head and neck, including salivary gland, thyroid, parathyroid, breast, lymph nodes, as well as skin and soft tissue. The most salient US features, immuno-profile, and molecular profile for the most common entities are also provided. Selected video clips are included to illustrate the most salient US findings of common entities and the methodology to appropriately harvest adequate material for diagnosis and performance of ancillary tests. The most current World Health Organization classifications of tumors of the thyroid, parathyroid, salivary glands, breast, and lymph nodes are included in the corresponding chapters, and they are followed to complement the cytomorphology and ancillary tests of the described entities.

Sacramento, CA, USA   Ricardo H. Bardales

The original version of this book was inadvertently published without an Acknowledgement and Dedication. The above-listed front matter elements have been included in the revised publication.

Acknowledgements

Special thanks to pathology residents and fellows, who throughout the years have contributed with cases that always occupy special places in the library of my brain and heart. I thank Melanie E. Brink of Outpatient Pathology Associates, who contributed to retrieving archival material, making endless phone calls to inquire about patient follow-up, and consenting to obtain ultrasound images of her normal superficial organs. Also, I thank Mrs. Lillie Mae Gaurano, Editor of Clinical Medicine (books) at Springer, Janani Natarajan, Project Manager (books production) at Springer, and Janakiraman Ganesan, Production Editor at Springer for their constant support and patience. Last but not least, my special gratitude to Mrs. Elisabeth Lanzl, Senior Editor at the University of Chicago for her undaunted effort to improve my English grammar and syntax of my manuscripts and books to transform them into readable documents. I learned so much, and there are still lots of room for improvement.

Ricardo H. Bardales, MD, FIAC, ECNU

Contents

Ricardo H. Bardales

The Ultrasound System

A wide variety of systems is available for US evaluation. The operator should be trained by an experienced sonographer and should be familiar with the basic operation of the US equipment to be used, including patient data entry, proper use of transducers, "basic knobology" (US knobs and system controls to produce a high-quality image), and image storage.

The US equipment should have a linear array transducer probe (for evaluation of superficial lesions) that has a 3.5–5.0 cm footprint and multiple frequency settings ranging from 7.5 to 14 MHz. The system should also have the capacity to do power and color-flow Doppler imaging. We, at Outpatient Pathology Associates (OPA)/Precision Pathology, use a Siemens Acuson X300 ultrasound system featuring a VF 11.5 MHz linear array Acusson X300 transducer probe, a panel of adjustable controls, and a 15′ flat-screen display for routine evaluation of palpable and non-palpable superficial lesions. We also use MyLab50 (Esaote North America, Inc., Indianapolis, IN) (Figs. 1.1, 1.2, 1.3 and 1.4).

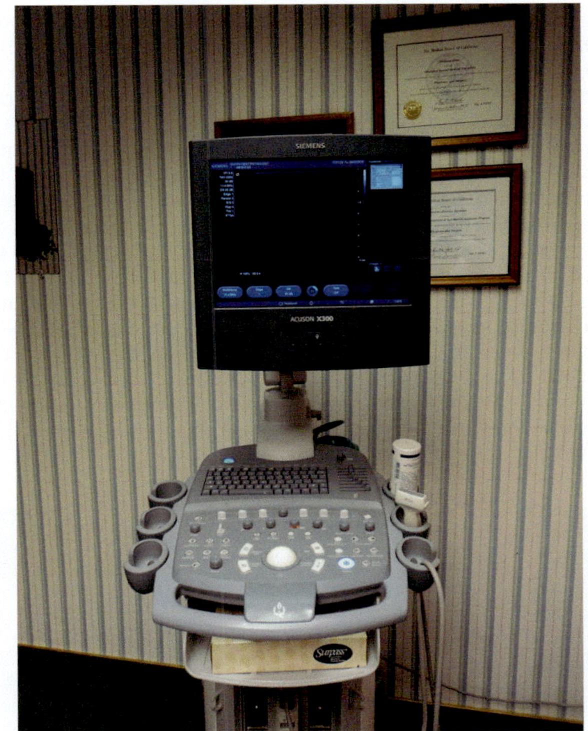

Fig. 1.1 Siemens Acusson X300 ultrasound system

R. H. Bardales (✉)
Precision Pathology, Outpatient Pathology Associates,
Sacramento, CA, USA

© The Author(s), under exclusive license to Springer Nature Switzerland AG 2024
R. H. Bardales (ed.), *The Interventional Cytopathologist*, Essentials in Cytopathology 30,
https://doi.org/10.1007/978-3-031-73702-2_1

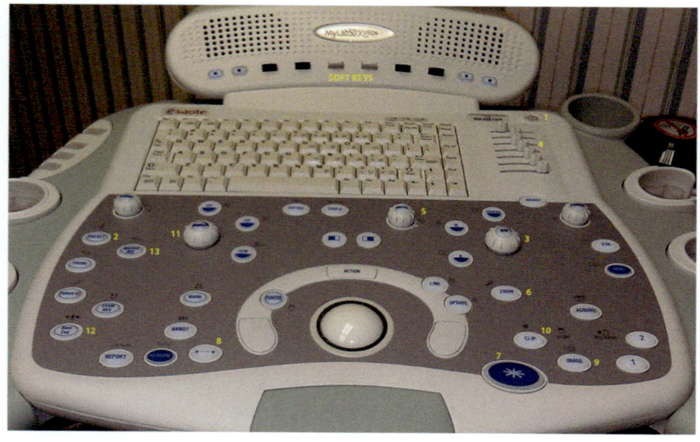

Fig. 1.2 MyLab50. Panel of adjustable controls. (1) System ON/OFF switch; (2) Preset key allows the user to select from various menu items; (3) Gain alters the amplification of the received signals in the image, and by changing of the gain, the image brightness can be increased or decreased; (4) Time-gain compensation and depth-gain compensation manual controls are useful for controlling the amount of amplification at different depths particularly when there is low attenuation of the image; (5) Depth alters the image, and a better view of the surrounding anatomy and fewer artifacts can be viewed in a large-depth image; (6) The zoom function is used for magnifying a region of the image on the screen; (7) The freeze function captures the image on the screen and allows one to focus on, measure, and save the image; (8) The calipers used for marking the area to be measured; (9) The image function saves the image in the system; (10) The clip function allows one to capture a video clip of various durations; (11) Doppler gain; (12) The start/end key saves the patient data and makes the system ready for the next study; (13) The archive review key permits the review of a specific examination and to save the entire session to an external drive, i.e., DVD, USB, etc

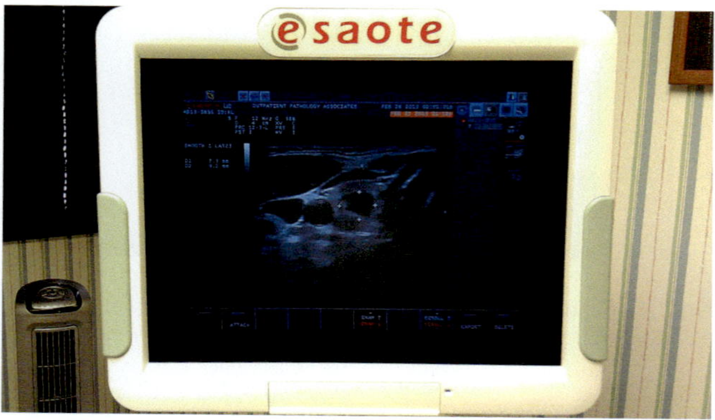

Fig. 1.3 MyLab50. Flat-screen display monitor

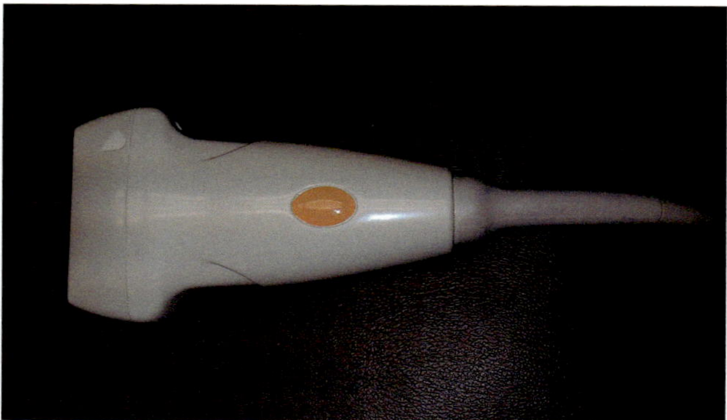

Fig. 1.4 Linear-array transducer probe

Basic Concepts in Ultrasound

The following are a few important basic concepts with which any professional using US should be familiar.

1. Sound is a form of mechanical energy that needs a transmitting material (air, fluid, soft tissue, etc.) to travel. The speed of sound depends on and is constant in a specific material and does not change with frequency or wavelength.
2. Frequency is the number of cycles per time of the vibration of the sound waves and it is measured in Hertz. A Hertz (Hz) is defined as one cycle per second.
3. The frequency of sound waves in the audible spectrum ranges from 30 to 20,000 Hz. The frequency of sound waves used in diagnostic US ranges from five million to 15 million cycles per second (5–15 MHz).
4. Higher frequencies of sound waves are associated with higher image resolution and with greater attenuation (limited ability to penetrate tissue). As a result, tissue penetration is inversely proportional to the US frequency. Superficial organs such as the breast and thyroid can be scanned at high frequencies (10–15 MHz) (less tissue penetration, high image resolution); the abdomen and pelvis are typically scanned at 2.5 MHz (more tissue penetration, less image resolution).

5. The transducer has a linear array of piezoelectric crystals that, when the electricity produced by the US machine is applied to the crystals, vibrate, and produce sound that penetrates the tissue. Conversely, when the transducer captures US waves (reflected back from the tissues) it converts them into electrical signals. This process repeats many times per second. The result is the creation of a two-dimensional gray-scale image in the screen monitor. The upper edge of the image corresponds to the surface of the skin (Fig. 1.5).

6. The type/design of the transducer determines the shape of the image seen in the screen monitor: linear array produces a rectangular image and curved array, a "piece-of-pie" shaped image. Linear array transducers with high frequencies are normally used for evaluation of superficial organs. Curved array transducers with low frequencies are commonly used for evaluation of abdominal and pelvic organs.

7. The speed of sound in all of the soft tissues of the body (excluding fat) is within 5% of the average value of 1540 m/s. The US equipment uses this average speed of the sound. The coupling gel applied to the skin transmits the US waves at the value of 1540 m/s and removes the air pockets between the transducer footprint and the patient's skin.

8. Acoustic impedance is the inverse of the capacity of a material to transmit sound (resistance to passage of the US waves) and depends on the density (concentration of matter) and stiffness (capacity to change shape) of the material and the speed of sound.

9. The soft tissues of a given anatomic region have differences (heterogeneity) in acoustic impedance with different amounts of reflection of the sound waves, leading to the generation of a characteristic US pattern. The mass of a given organ may have a characteristic pattern as well.

10. A cyst containing serous clear fluid has uniformly low impedance with high sound transmission and no reflected sound and will appear *anechoic*. The echogenicity of a nodule or mass is compared with the brightness of the adjacent tissue (adipose or muscle). When masses have uniform echoes, they can be *hypoechoic* (slightly darker than fat or muscle), *isoechoic* (light gray like fat or muscle), or *hyperechoic* (slightly brighter than fat or muscle) (Figs. 1.6, 1.7 and 1.8).

11. Benign lesions usually have smooth, lobulated, and well-defined pushing rather than infiltrating margins (Fig. 1.9). A malignant tumor is usually hypoechoic and heterogeneous, with ill-defined, irregular, and angulated borders due to infiltration of the malignant growth into the surrounding tissue (Fig. 1.10).

12. *Acoustic shadowing* is an artifact that refers to a dark shadow seen behind a calcified nodule due to near or total lack of sound transmission, e.g., an eggshell calcification in a thyroid nodule (Fig. 1.11).

13. *Acoustic enhancement* is an artifact that refers to a bright shadow seen behind a nodule with little attenuation due to great intensity of sound waves behind the nodule, e.g., cystic lesions, colloid-rich thyroid nodules, or even homogeneous solid nodules, e.g., lipid-rich nodules

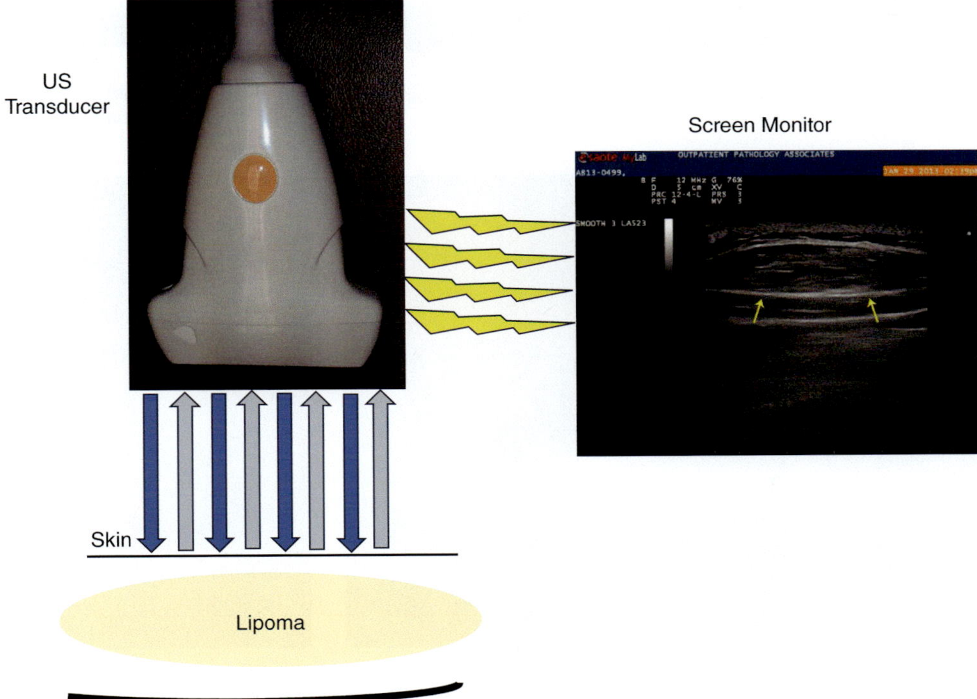

Fig. 1.5 Sound waves (arrows) produced by the transducer penetrate the tissue and are reflected from the target mass (lipoma) to be converted by the transducer into electrical signals (yellow signals) to create a gray-scale image in the screen monitor. Lipoma is seen as oval-shaped image horizontally below the skin (arrows)

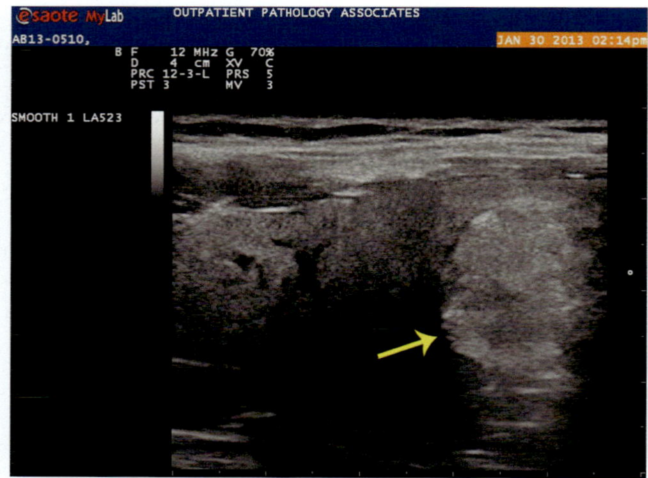

Fig. 1.6 Hyperechoic mass (arrow). The echogenicity of the mass is brighter than that of the surrounding thyroid tissue

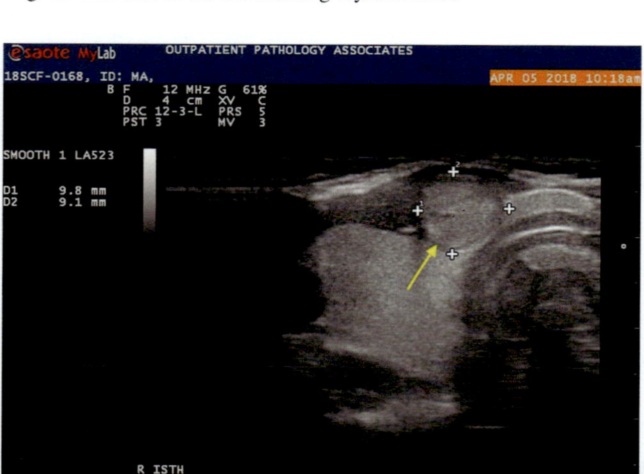

Fig. 1.7 Isoechoic nodule (arrow). The echogenicity is similar to that of surrounding thyroid tissue

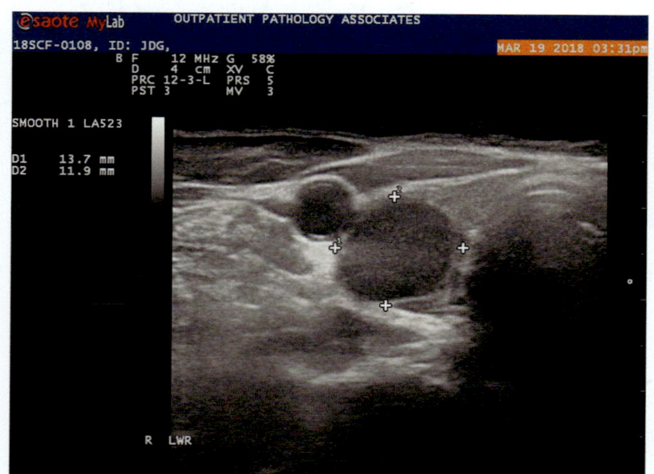

Fig. 1.8 Hypoechoic nodule. The echogenicity is darker than that of the surrounding tissue

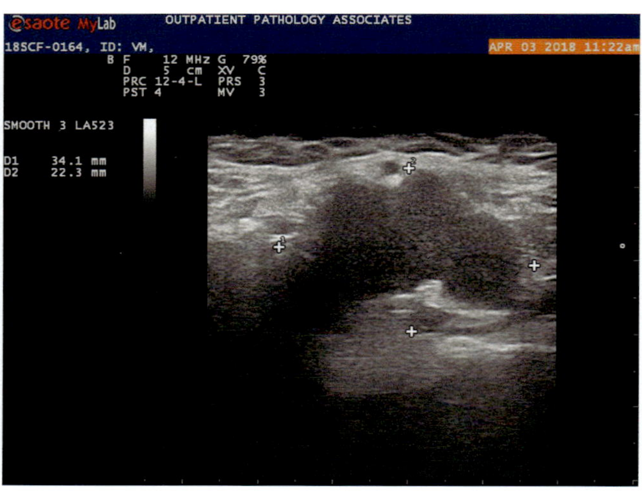

Fig. 1.9 Hypoechoic nodule with lobulated and pushing borders (parotid gland benign mixed tumor)

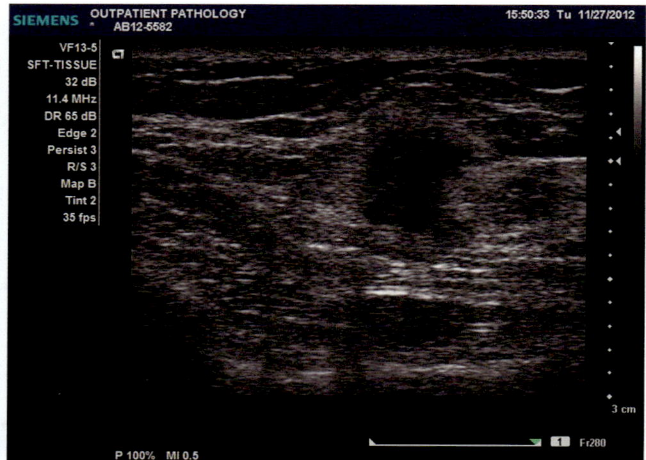

Fig. 1.10 Hypoechoic mass with ill-defined borders and irregular, angulated, and infiltrating margins (mammary carcinoma)

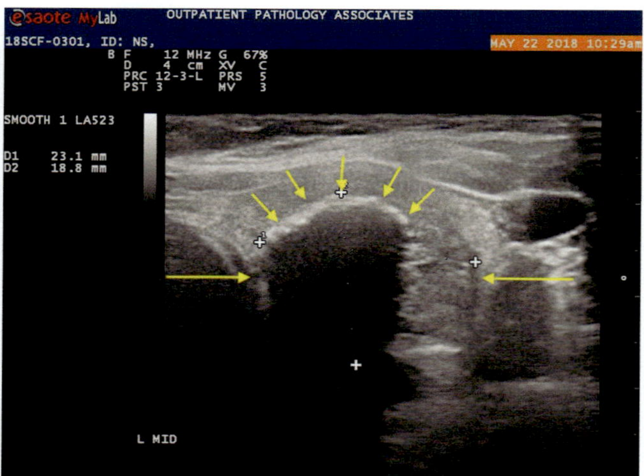

Fig. 1.11 Posterior acoustic shadowing. The thyroid nodule is demarcated by large arrows. The small arrows point the calcified rim that projects a dark shadow due to lack of sound transmission

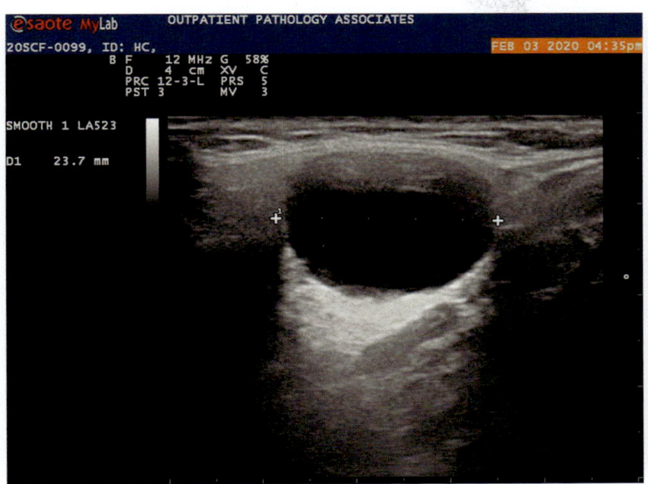

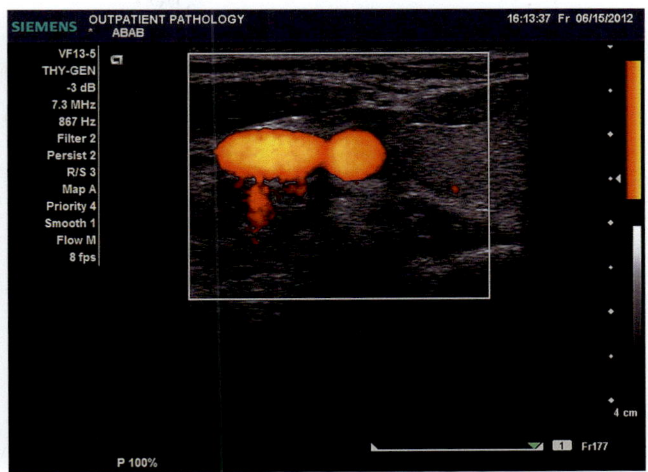

Fig. 1.12 Posterior acoustic enhancement. A uniform bright shadow is projected posterior to this cystic lesion

Fig. 1.14 Power Doppler provides information on the total amount of blood flow present and is generally the preferred modality for evaluating tissue vascularity

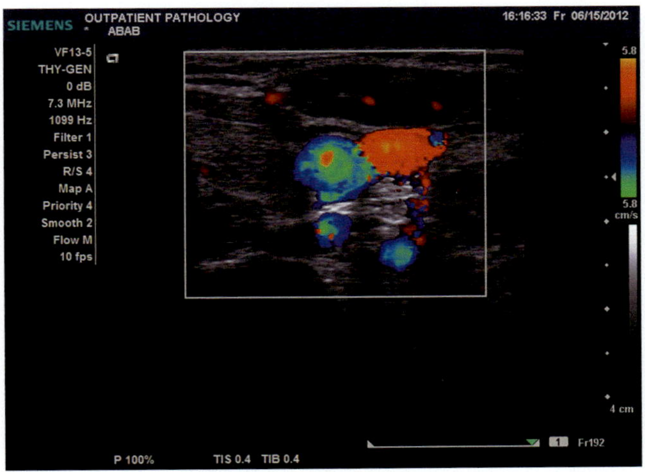

Fig. 1.13 Color-flow Doppler provides information regarding the direction and speed of blood flow within the tissue

The Ultrasound (US) Examination

The US examination of a patient starts with the selection of a particular default setting which the US system may have, i.e., breast or small body parts; selection of the appropriate transducer; and entering of the patient's demographics. Familiarity with the scanning technique and with a reduced list of system controls (*depth* of view of the US image, *gain* that is the term for image amplification, *time-gain-compensation*, *calipers* for measurement, and *freeze and store*) are paramount for obtaining interpretable US images (Fig. 1.2).

(Fig. 1.12). Both acoustic shadowing and enhancement are artifacts due to attenuation and occur when sound travels between two extreme interfaces.

14. Doppler US is used for evaluation of the vascularity of tissues and plays an important role in thyroid imaging. *Color-flow Doppler* provides information regarding the direction and speed of blood flow within the tissue and is particularly useful in vascular studies (Fig. 1.13). *Power Doppler* provides information on the total amount of blood flow present, independent of the direction or speed, and is generally the preferred modality for evaluating tissue vascularity (Fig. 1.14).

1. The operator holds the transducer with warmed coupling gel in contact with the skin surface of the patient.
2. The transducer produces short pulses of US, which travel through the patient's skin and underlying tissue planes/organs. The depth of US penetration depends on the US frequency.
3. The pulses of US are reflected and/or transmitted from the tissue planes back to the transducer in a repetitive manner.
4. The transducer converts the different amounts of reflected US echoes into electrical signals.
5. The electrical signals lead to the generation of a characteristic US pattern that corresponds to the echoes reflected from the underlying tissue planes.
6. The system processor forms an image of the anatomic structure based on the information received, i.e., the direction of the US pulses and the speed of reflection. The

result is the creation of a two-dimensional gray-scale B-mode image (B for brightness) in the screen monitor, which can be stored as a static image or video clip.

Further Reading

Bardales R. The invasive cytopathologist. In: Ultrasound guided fine-needle aspiration of superficial masses. New York: Springer; 2014.

Baskin HJ, Duick DS, et al. Thyroid ultrasound and ultrasound-guided fine-needle aspiration. 3rd ed. New York: Springer; 2013.

Lieu D. Ultrasound physics and instrumentation for pathologists. Arch Pathol Lab Med. 2010;134(10):1541–56.

Lieu D. Breast imaging for interventional pathologists. Arch Pathol Lab Med. 2013;137(1):100–19.

Martin K. Basic equipment, components, and image production. In: Allan PL, Baxter GM, Weston MJ, editors. Clinical ultrasound, vol. 1. London: Churchill Livingstone Elsevier; 2011. p. 16–30.

McDicken WN, Anderson T. Basic physics of medical ultrasound. In: Allan PL, Baxter GM, Weston MJ, editors. Clinical ultrasound, vol. 1. London: Churchill Livingstone Elsevier; 2011. p. 3–15.

Ricardo H. Bardales

The role of the interventional cytopathologist evolved parallel to the evolution of the cytopathology and the fine needle aspiration (FNA) technique. One of the first manuscripts on the subject was published in 1904 by Grieg and Gray, who described the aspiration of lymph nodes with a needle of unstated caliber for identification of trypanosomes in patients who had sleeping sickness in Uganda. Years later, Martin and Ellis in 1930 and Fred Stewart in 1933 wrote seminal articles describing the use of 18-gauge needles for sampling of palpable tumors, predominantly from the head and neck. The latter article details the needle aspiration technique and the use of local anesthesia. Whereas cytopathology remained dormant in the USA for the next four decades, it became a strong diagnostic modality in Europe, pioneered by the Karolinska Institute in Stockholm, Sweden.

Ultrasound (US) imaging is a technology that allows the transmission of sound waves to a computer screen as images. In the 1940s, US was used in medicine mainly for research and therapeutic purposes. In the 1950s, US technology made it possible to visualize and measure breast nodules with 90% accuracy. US evaluation of thyroid nodules started in the late 1960s in the hope that, with this technology, one could distinguish benign from malignant processes. Currently, US gives accurate results in demonstrating the characteristics of a nodule or mass, but is less accurate for the diagnosis of malignancy. The combination of FNA and US to improve the accuracy of the cytologic diagnosis of thyroid nodules was first described in the 1970s. Doppler US was developed in the 1980s, allowing for the detection of blood flow within a lesion, which is important for assessment of the likelihood of malignancy and for minimizing blood contamination during FNA sampling.

The use of bedside US for better placement, visualization, and guidance (G) of the needle and improvement in the diagnostic accuracy of USG-FNA has become indispensable for the evaluation of palpable or US-visible masses. Currently, USG-FNA is universally accepted as a simple, inexpensive, accurate, safe, and rapid technique that, when properly used, yields valuable information for adequate clinical management.

The USG-FNA technique, simplistically outlined as "insert the needle in the target, obtain the sample, prepare and stain smears, and read them in the microscope," must be practiced by well-trained professionals who have a full understanding of the pitfalls in every step of the procedure. All steps are strongly linked to one another, and a successful microscopic evaluation depends on and is directly related to the other steps. It is accepted that the FNA accuracy is highest when the same professional examines the patient, performs the US examination, interprets the US features of the target mass, performs the USG-FNA procedure, prepares the smears, and renders a cytologic diagnosis. Also, the cytopathologist who performs several FNAs a day is probably the person with more experience in assessing superficial palpable masses and performing USG-FNAs than are persons who seldom do them.

Following along these lines, I will describe our experience in performing USG-FNA. Table 2.1 shows the numbers and types of FNAs evaluated at our Interventional Cytology Clinic, including "clinic cases" and "sent-ins." The outpatient FNA biopsy clinic was founded 1986 by Drs. John S. Abele and Anthony J. Mathios (QEPD); both introduced USG-FNA in 2003. Currently, we see eight patients a day and perform an average of 10–12 USG-FNAs a day. All patients referred to our clinic have palpable or non-palpable, but US-visible lesions, and the US evaluation of the lesion is a routine component of the brief, but thorough focused physical examination. In our clinic, we see approximately 2000 patients a year, and more than 70% of them undergo thyroid USG-FNA, which is often performed in more than one nod-

Supplementary Information The online version contains supplementary material available at https://doi.org/10.1007/978-3-031-73702-2_2.

R. H. Bardales (✉)
Precision Pathology, Outpatient Pathology Associates,
Sacramento, CA, USA

Table 2.1 Interventional Cytology Statistics for cases from 1984 to 2022

Site/Cases	1984–2013 (%)[a]	2014 (%)[a]	2015–2022 (%)[b]
Thyroid	81,073 (53)	4884 (82)	7507 (79)
Breast	32,540 (21)	142 (2)	110 (1)
Soft tissue and lymph node	28,916 (19)	721 (12)	1098 (12)
Salivary gland	5757 (4)	214 (4)	427 (5)
Prostate	2980 (2)	0	0
Miscellaneous	1167 (1)	0 (0)	311 (3)
	152,433 (100)	5962 (100)	9453 (100)

[a]Includes "clinic" and "sent-in" cases

[b]Includes "clinic" cases only. USG-FNA was performed by 1 cytopathologist 3 days per week (2015–2017)

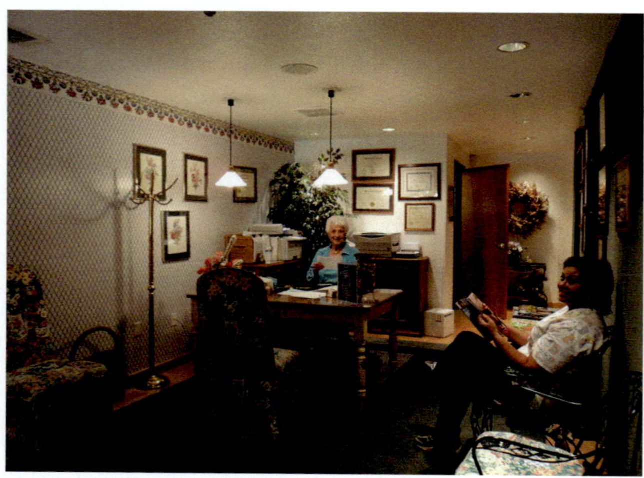

Fig. 2.1 Outpatient Pathology Associates FNA clinic, reception room

ule (Fig. 2.1). In 2012, we accessioned more than 6500 "clinic USG-FNA cases" and referral "sent-in" FNA cases from more than 200 physicians in more than 20 states within the USA. Details for setting up an USG-FNA outpatient clinic have been reviewed by Drs. John S. Abele and Theodore Miller (Cytopathology Annual, 1993).

In our experience, USG-FNA accuracy, sensitivity, and specificity in the evaluation of superficial palpable or US-visible masses are well above 95%, and diagnostic material has been obtained in >99% of samples (data not published).

Clinical Evaluation

The clinical evaluation is of paramount importance for an accurate FNA diagnosis. In our practice, the referring clinical team submits the pertinent clinical information and imaging study reports to us prior to a patient's appointment. This information is reviewed by the cytopathologist before he sees the patient.

An information brochure mailed to the patient in advance and available at our clinic reception desk is helpful for having the patient informed about the visit and what to expect. The brochure briefly answers common questions, such as "What is FNA?," "What is the history of FNA?," "What is the purpose of performing an FNA?," "What is involved in the FNA procedure?," "What are the possible complications?," "Will the FNA make the tumor spread?," "How are the FNA results obtained?," "What are the goals and limits of FNA," "Are you thinking of not coming in?," "Who will perform the FNA?"

The following are sequential steps prior to performance of the USG-FNA.

1. *Anamnesis*
   (a) The interview helps the cytopathologist take a concise, complete history of the lesion and other significant medical problems, explain the procedure step by step, and provide reassurance to the patient.
   (b) The anamnesis is often more accurate and pertinent to the mass or lesion diagnosis when the cytopathologist directly obtains it from the patient than when it is read from the data provided by the clinical team.
   (c) The patient should be given the option to ask questions, particularly at the end of the anamnesis.
2. *Physical examination*
   (a) Findings of a careful and focused physical examination provide valuable information about the mass or lesion and narrow the differential diagnosis.
   (b) Initial findings may trigger the cytopathologist to perform a more extensive and pertinent physical examination looking for additional information to narrow the clinical impression, e.g., lower-extremity examination of a patient with inguinal lymphadenopathy.
3. *Ultrasound evaluation*
   (a) The US is part of the clinical examination and complements the anamnesis and tactile physical examination, helping the cytopathologist to plan the FNA procedure.
   (b) The patient is positioned appropriately in an adjustable examination table or chair (Fig. 2.2). Occasionally, the procedure is performed while the patient is in the sitting position or in a wheelchair.
   (c) An explanation is given to the patient about the details of the US examination and how it will be done.
   (d) US is done in the transverse (axial) and longitudinal (sagittal) planes. The linear-array US transducer is the most suitable for the examination of superficially seated masses.
   (e) The transducer is used by the right hand (right-handed examiner), and the US control knobs is operated with the left hand. The opposite is adopted if the examiner is left-handed.

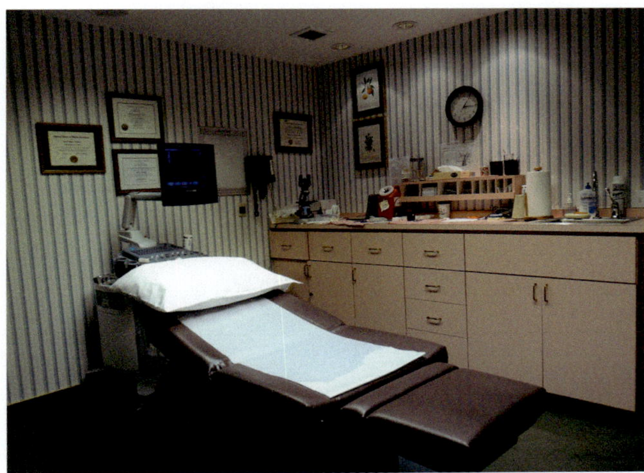

Fig. 2.2 Interventional Cytology Clinic brochure. Answers to frequently asked questions

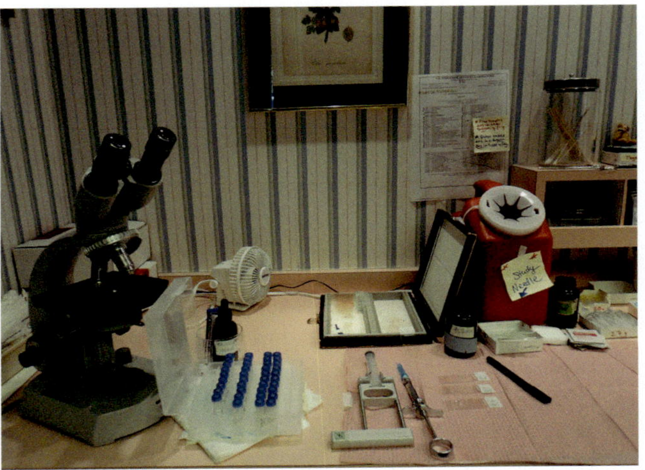

Fig. 2.3 Immediate FNA evaluation and specimen triage section

(f) The examiner should adjust the US settings based on the location of the mass (deep or superficial) and the anatomy of the region where the target is located., e.g., short, thick, or obese neck.

(g) The US evaluation should be systematic and extend from surface to deep-tissue planes, focused first on the finding of normal anatomic landmarks. This will be helpful for the identification of the mass/lesion and recognition of its US features.

4. *Sample triage*

(a) The prior considerations, supported by a rapid on-site cytology evaluation (ROSE) in selected cases, will prompt the cytopathologist to allocate material for special studies, e.g., bacterial, or fungal cultures, flow cytometry, cytogenetics, molecular tests, cell block for immunohistochemistry, and rinse of the contents of USG-FNA needles for measurement of

thyroglobulin, parathyroid hormone, calcitonin levels, etc. ROSE will prompt the cytopathologist to perform a USG-core needle biopsy (CNB) for tissue confirmation in soft tissue or breast tumors to assess invasion and perform hormonal studies and Her-2 in breast cancer (Fig. 2.3). Lymph node and thyroid CNB may be performed in exceedingly rare cases; I have not done any in my personal 17 years of experience.

The USG-FNA Aspiration Procedure

The operator must be familiar with the materials needed and the step-by-step procedures for performing FNA of the palpable lesions described in various cytology treatises, including the textbook "Fine Needle Aspiration of Palpable Masses," skillfully written by Michael W. Stanley, M.D., and Torsten Löwhagen, M.D.

In the next paragraphs, I describe our experience performing USG-FNA. As a rule, patient positioning should provide patient comfort, a good US evaluation, and good sampling of the mass.

We perform the USG-FNA by using the Zajdela technique "without aspiration or by capillarity" (Zagdela A, 1986, Diagn Cytopathology). In our experience, this technique offers sensitivity, specificity, and diagnostic accuracy, which are very similar to, if not better than the conventional FNA (with aspiration) for evaluating superficial lesions, especially of the head and neck, and in particular for evaluating thyroid nodules. For thyroid nodules and lymph node sampling, we use 27- and 25-gauge needles respectively, with >99% sample adequacy.

Contraindications for USG-FNA

There are few, if any, instances that may preclude doing the procedure. The only absolute contraindication may be a severe bleeding disorder or coagulopathy. In some cases, stopping anticoagulant or antiplatelet therapy for 24 h may be necessary. Relative contraindications include the use of warfarin products or heparin; however, local bleeding can be controlled with manual pressure at the site of puncture. Mild sedation may be given to the anxious patient.

Approaches Used in USG-FNA Sampling

1. *Perpendicular approach*. The needle placed in the center of the upper lateral border of the US probe intersects the US beam perpendicularly and travels through the tissue in a non-continuous fashion, resulting in visualization of the needle tip only in the screen display (Fig. 2.4).

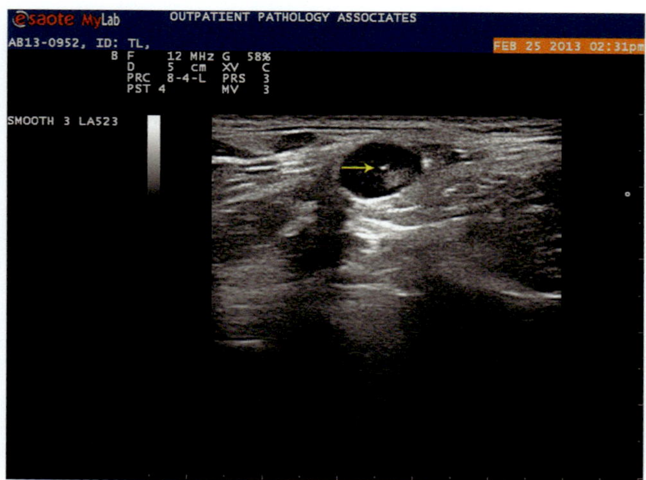

Fig. 2.4 Perpendicular approach. The needle tip is seen as a bright spot (arrow)

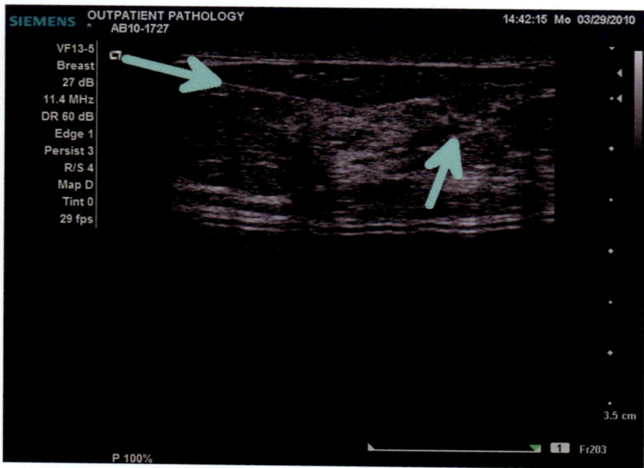

Fig. 2.5 Parallel approach. The entire needle length is visualized (arrows). (Courtesy, Dr. John S. Abele, Pathologist. Sacramento, California)

2. *Parallel approach.* The needle placed in the center of one of the tips of the US probe travels parallel to the US beam in a continuous fashion, allowing the visualization of the entire needle length, emerging from the right upper corner in the screen display if the procedure is done with the right hand. The needle plane must coincide with the US beam for the needle length to be visualized (Fig. 2.5).

We often use the perpendicular approach for USG-FNA sampling and the parallel approach for USG-NCB and occasionally for USG-FNA. Of note, because any needle is visualized with modern high-resolution US equipment, there is no need to use echogenic needles for routine USG-FNA. Likewise, use of heparinized needles is not necessary.

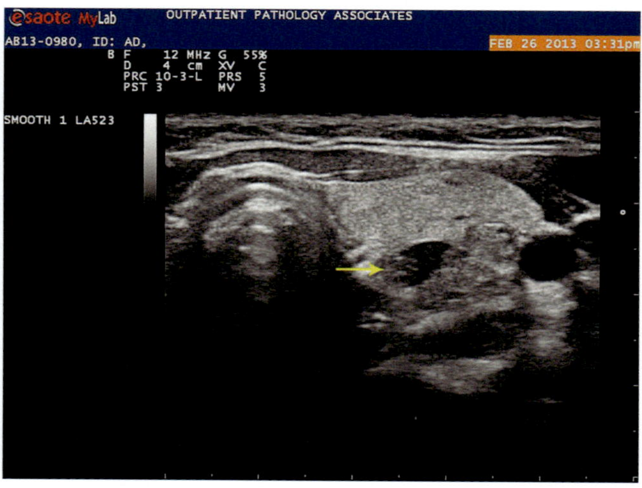

Fig. 2.6 The target is positioned in the center of the screen (arrow)

Steps Prior to USG-FNA (Perpendicular Approach)

The following steps should be followed sequentially:

1. Patient in supine position. For thyroid nodules, apply a soft pillow beneath the neck and shoulders. A semi-sitting position may be recommended for patients having limitations to adopting a supine position.
2. Wear gloves for all US examinations and USG-FNA procedures.
3. Apply a warm sterile coupling gel to the transducer face.
4. Hold the transducer firm and look for the transducer orientation marker (ridge, groove, or light). The marker should always be directed to the patient's right for a transverse evaluation of the lesion, or to the patient's head for a longitudinal evaluation.
5. Find the target lesion with the US probe. The transducer should be held at a 90-degree angle to the target lesion.
6. Move the transducer gently and slowly. Document US characteristics of the lesion, include a power Doppler evaluation.
7. Center the intended biopsy site of the lesion in the screen display (Fig. 2.6).
8. Use a pen or pencil and make its tip shadow coincide with the intended biopsy site of the lesion (Fig. 2.7).
9. Withdraw the US probe and keep the pen or pencil tip on the skin surface.
10. Dot the skin surface 1–2 mm above the tip of the pen or pencil with an erasable cutaneous marker (Fig. 2.8).
11. Re-position the US probe over the marked skin to make sure that the biopsy site is centered in the screen display.

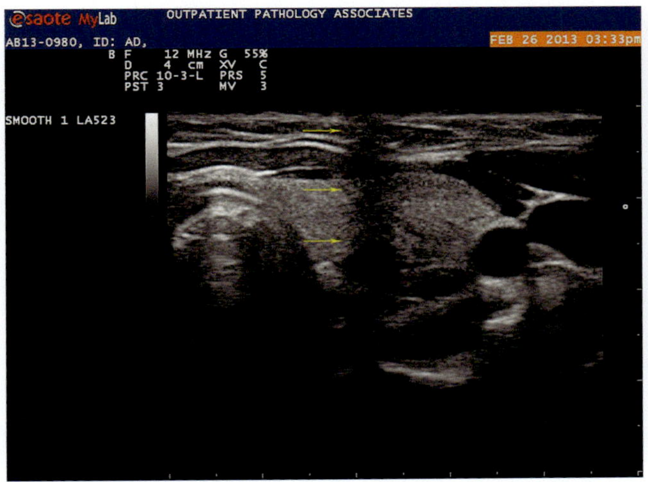

Fig. 2.7 Shadow of the tip of the pen coinciding with the target to be sampled (arrows)

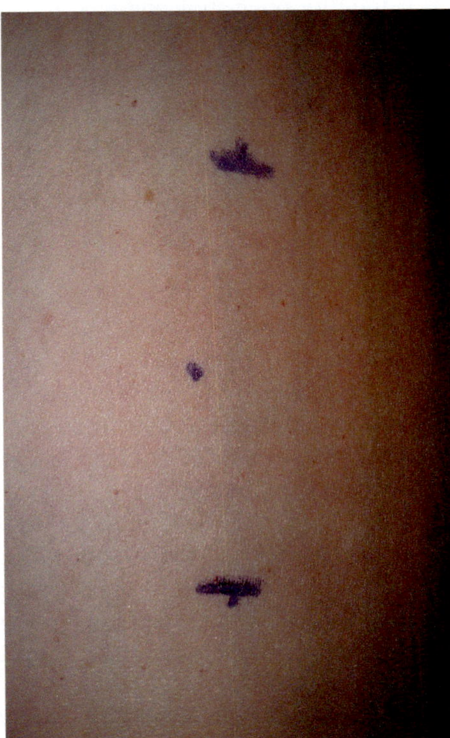

Fig. 2.8 Marking of the skin. The central blue dot corresponds to the underlying target lesion. The lateral short blue lines coincide with the lateral edges of the linear US transducer

12. Clean <u>all</u> US gel from the skin.
13. Thoroughly disinfect the skin with alcohol.
14. Apply local 2% lidocaine hydrochloride with epinephrine or epinephrine-free 3% carbocaine, using equipment available from dental supply stores. The syringe uses a 30-gauge disposable needle, a tubular 2 mL disposable cartridge of lidocaine or carbocaine, and a reusable

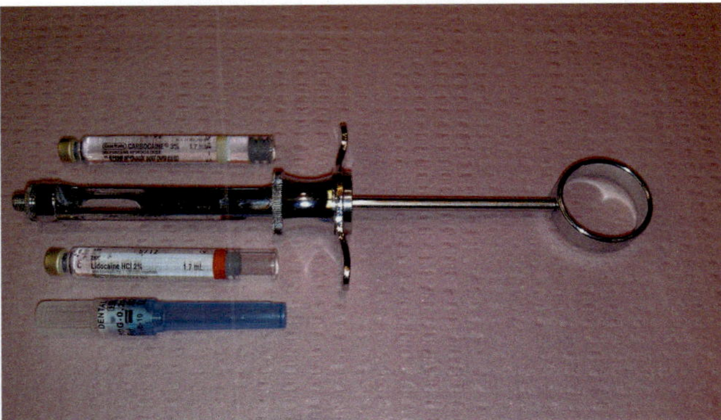

Fig. 2.9 Local anesthesia supplies

metallic injection handle. This step may be considered optional; however, it is always welcomed by our patients. In the neck, make sure that the muscles overlying the target lesion are properly anesthetized. Carbocaine <u>must</u> be used for sampling of lesions of the breast areola or nipple, tips of fingers or toes, and penis (Fig. 2.9).
15. Wait for 1 or 2 min before the USG-FNA is performed.

USG-FNA (Perpendicular Approach)

1. Disinfect skin with alcohol.
2. First, insert the 25- or 27-gauge needle through the marked skin. We use a 1 1/2″ (3.8 cm) long needle for most USG-FNAs (Fig. 2.10). Needles thicker than 23-gauge often causes more bleeding rather than better specimens.
3. Next, apply the US probe with a small amount of warm gel on the skin.
4. Identify the bright image of the needle tip on the screen. Orienting the bevel of the needle tip toward the transducer improves its visualization.
5. Advance and/or redirect the needle tip into the target lesion (i.e., the solid component of a cystic and solid lesion) as shown in Fig. 2.4.
6. Perform the FNA using the Zajdela technique, making the needle travel repeatedly back and forth (thrusts) inside the lesion or mass and in the same direction.
    (a) We perform 3–4 passes or FNAs.
    (b) All thyroid nodules can be sampled best with 27-gauge (0.4 mm diameter) needles. Each FNA pass lasts no more than 3 s, with a cadence of 2–3 thrusts per second. Doppler findings must be kept in mind to minimize the amount of blood present in the sample that may prevent an adequate cytological interpretation of the smears.
    (c) Cyst drainage can be done with a 25- or 23-gauge needle attached to an I.V. 4 mL extension 34″ long male

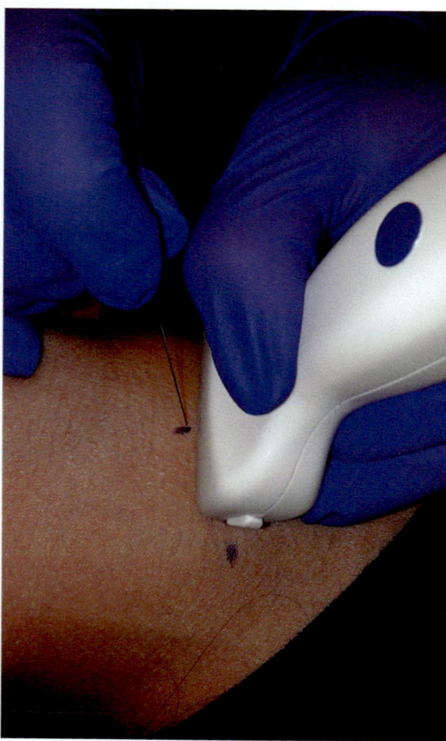

Fig. 2.10 Perpendicular approach. Apply a small amount of coupling gel to the US transducer. First, insert the needle in the marked skin (center dot) overlying the target lesion, and then position the US transducer to avoid gel contamination. Orient and advance the needle perpendicularly towards the lesion until the bright needle tip is identified within it (Videos 2.1, 2.2 and 2.3)

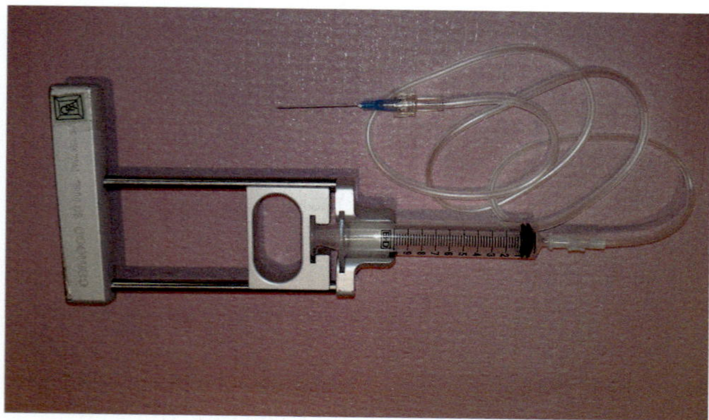

Fig. 2.11 Cyst drainage supplies

Luer (Baxter) and to a 10-cc or 20-cc size syringe in a FNA pistol. A second person is needed who maneuvers the pistol and aspirates the fluid (Fig. 2.11).

(d) Sampling of stroma-rich nodules can be performed by use of a 25-gauge (0.5 mm diameter) needle and the same I.V. extension to apply suction while the operator gently moves the needle within the target. A 23-gauge (0.6 mm diameter) needle can be used particularly for soft tissue stromal nodules.

7. Release suction, if it has been applied, before withdrawing the needle from the target lesion.
8. Remove the needle from the patient. Apply pressure to the puncture site with sterile gauze after each pass.
9. Apply a band aid when the procedure has been finished.

Steps Prior to USG-FNA (Parallel Approach)

Follow all steps listed for "prior to USG-FNA (perpendicular approach)."

For step 7, position the intended biopsy site in the lateral 1/3 of the screen close to the needle entry site on the skin, which will be visualized in the right or left upper corner of the screen.

For step 10, dot the skin surface under the tip of the pen or pencil <u>as well as</u> the mid-portion of each of the two lateral ends of the US probe with an erasable cutaneous marker. This step is helpful for orientation and repositioning of the US probe.

The skin entry site is the dotted selected lateral one closest to the intended biopsy site (Fig. 2.12).

USG-FNA and USG-NCB (Parallel Approach)

For USG-FNA:
1. First, insert the 25- or 27-gauge needle through the dotted skin in the mid-portion of the selected lateral end of the US probe (Fig. 2.13).
2. Then, apply the US probe to the skin. The transducer should be held at a 90-degree angle to the target tissue.
3. Make certain that the border of the target lesion is in the 1/3 close to the needle insertion site.
4. Advance and guide the needle into the biopsy site. The needle will travel parallel to the mid-plane (azimuthal) of the transducer probe length at an angle that can range from 30 to 70° depending on the depth of the target lesion (usually at a 45-degree angle) and will be visualized in its entirety, as shown in Fig. 2.5.
5. Perform the USG-FNA as described in step 6 of the USG-FNA (perpendicular approach).

For USG-NCB:
The steps are like those listed for "steps prior to USG-FNA and USG-FNA by parallel approach."
1. Using an 18-gauge needle tip edge, gently open a 1.5 mm entry site in the dotted skin corresponding to the lateral tip of the US probe closest to the target lesion.
2. Under US guidance, the core needle is carefully guided to the periphery of the target lesion.
3. We use a Bard®Monopty® disposable core biopsy instrument (20-gauge × 9 cm) with a penetration depth of 11 mm (Fig. 2.14).

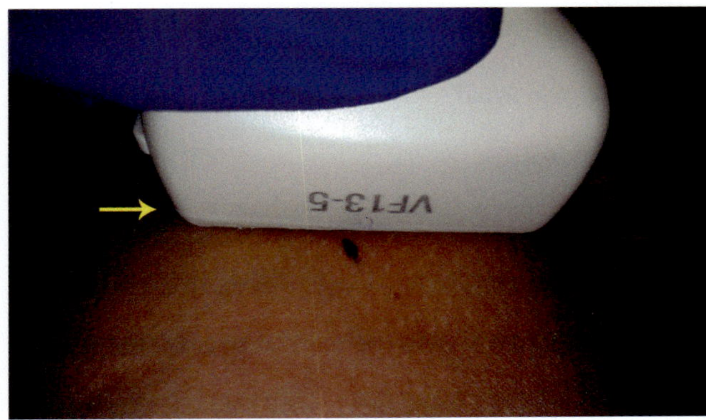

Fig. 2.12 Parallel approach. The dot placed in the skin at the edge of the US transducer lateral to the target lesion is the entry site (arrow)

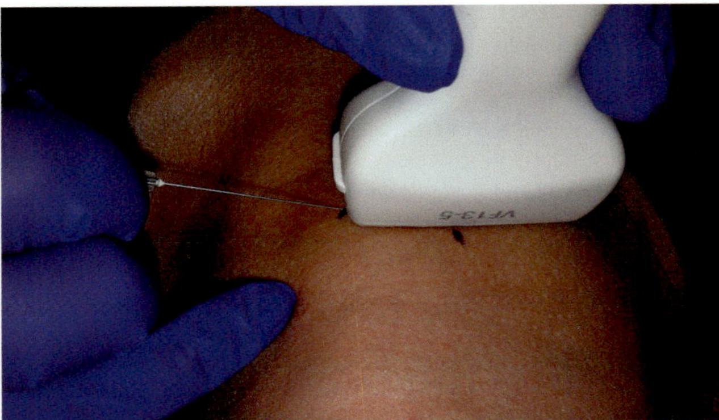

Fig. 2.13 Parallel approach. Apply a small amount of coupling gel to the US transducer. First, insert the needle in the marked skin (lateral dot), and then place the US probe to avoid gel contamination. Orient, advance, and guide the needle diagonally towards the target lesion, always visualizing the entire needle length (Video 2.4)

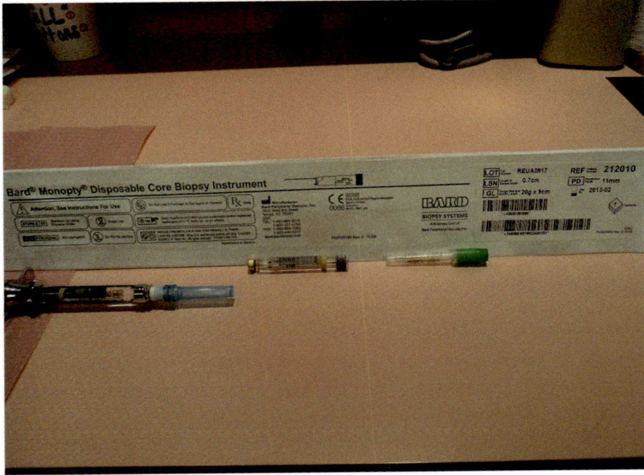

Fig. 2.14 Core needle biopsy supplies

4. Three USG-NCB tissue samples are usually obtained. Follow the instructions of the manufacturer to retrieve the tissue.
5. The biopsy site is carefully evaluated, and local pressure with sterile gauze is applied after each USG-NCB.
6. Place the tissue in formalin or another tissue fixative as needed.

USG-FNA Specimen Handling

The selection of the smearing technique depends on the type of FNA material obtained, and on the operator's skill and preference. In general, we use the one-step method for small-volume specimens as it allows better control of the pressure applied to the specimen and yields excellent smears; and the two-slide-pull method for larger volume specimens, the two-step method for liquid specimens, or the modified two-step method for larger volumes of blood or fluid.

We encourage the reader to consult textbooks and Internet sources such as the Papanicolaou Society of Cytopathology (www.papsociety.org) for details on how to handle FNA specimens. All steps are crucial and should be mastered by the operator so that he or she obtains a smear with well-preserved cells, thinly spread to allow for adequate staining and light-microscopy interpretation. In the following text, we summarize how we handle the material obtained by USG-FNA with the one-step method.

(The material is in the needle cylinder and hub)

1. Fill a 10-cc slip tip syringe with air.
2. Attach the needle with the harvested FNA material to the tip of a slip tip syringe that has been previously filled with air.
3. Keep the needle tip in contact with the slide surface with the bevel facing down at a 45° angle. This maneuver will prevent specimen dispersion and desiccation.
4. Gently express the specimen onto the surface of a non-frosted glass slide.
5. Place the spreader slide onto the droplet, applying gentle pressure without crushing the droplet.
6. Draw the spreader slide along the length of the lower slide in a constant and steady manner. It is important to remember that the long axes of both glass slides must be perpendicular, but the flat surfaces parallel. When smearing is properly done, no residual material is left in the spreader glass slide (Fig. 2.15).
7. Gently wave the smear in the air for a few seconds or place the smear in front of a small battery-powered

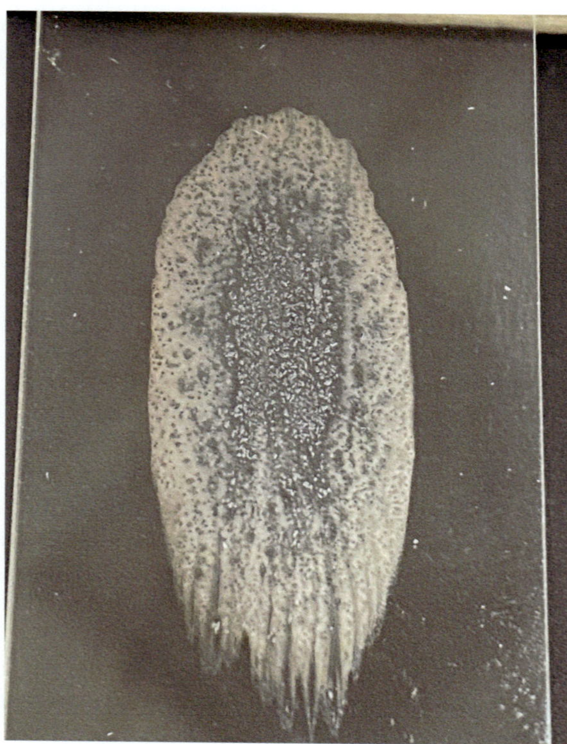

Fig. 2.15 Non-stained, air-dried smear prepared by use of the one-step technique

electric fan for quick drying and then staining with May-Grunwald-Giemsa (MGG) stain. Alternatively, immerse the smear in 96% ethyl alcohol for subsequent Papanicolaou or H&E stain. In general, both types of smears should be prepared; however, we prefer air-dried smears in most thyroid and lymph node USG-FNAs.

8. Immediate interpretation of the smear can be done with Toluidine Blue stain after 1 min of 96% ethyl alcohol fixation. The stain also is effective on air-dried smears previously fixed by 96% ethyl alcohol fixation. After rapid interpretation, the smear can be placed back into and left in 96% ethyl alcohol for conventional Papanicolaou or H&E stain or left air-drying for subsequent MGG stain. It is our experience that having the cytopathologist perform both the US evaluation and USG-FNA, and doing 3–4 passes, reduces the number of unsatisfactory/nondiagnostic specimens. I can count less than five unsatisfactory specimens after performing over 5000 USG-FNAs of nodules in superficial organs, predominantly thyroid.

9. Clotted blood or fluid with minute fragments of tissue is placed in 10% formalin for cell block embedding as histologic specimen.

10. Cyst fluid may be processed by centrifugation or liquid-based techniques following the manufacturer's specifications. We avoid the use of the latter to evaluate FNAs from solid lesions and prefer the use of conventional smearing techniques instead.

Further Reading

Abele JS. The case for pathologist ultrasound-guided fine-needle aspiration biopsy. Cancer. 2008;114(6):463–8.

Abele JS. Putting aspiration back into thyroid fine-needle biopsy-the re-emerging role of vacuum assistance. Cancer Cytopathol. 2012;120(6):366–72.

Abele JS. Building an USGFNA clinic from scratch: a recipe from the USGFNA cookbook for successes. Semin Diagn Pathol. 2022;39(6):421–5.

Abele JS, Miller TR. Implementation of an outpatient needle aspiration biopsy service and clinic: a personal perspective. In: Schmidt WA, editor. Cytopathology annual. Baltimore, MD: Williams & Wilkins; 1993. p. 43–71.

Ammanagi AS, Dombale VD, et al. On-site toluidine blue staining and screening improves efficiency of fine-needle aspiration cytology reporting. Acta Cytol. 2012;56(4):347–51.

Bardales R. The invasive cytopathologist. In: Ultrasound-guided fine needle aspiration of superficial masses. New York: Springer; 2014.

Baskin HJ, Duick DS, et al. Thyroid ultrasound and ultrasound-guided fine-needle aspiration. New York: Springer-Verlag; 2008.

Cibas ES, Alexander EK, et al. Indications for thyroid FNA and pre-FNA requirements: a synopsis of the National Cancer Institute thyroid fine-needle aspiration state of the science conference. Diagn Cytopathol. 2008;36(6):390–9.

de Carvalho GA, Paz-Filho G, et al. Adequacy and diagnostic accuracy of aspiration vs. capillary fine needle thyroid biopsies. Endocr Pathol. 2009;20(4):204–8.

Lieu D. Cytopathologist-performed ultrasound-guided fine-needle aspiration and core-needle biopsy: a prospective study of 500 consecutive cases. Diagn Cytopathol. 2008;36(5):317–24.

Lieu D. Value of cytopathologist-performed ultrasound-guided fine-needle aspiration as a screening test for ultrasound-guided core-needle biopsy in nonpalpable breast masses. Diagn Cytopathol. 2009;37(4):262–9.

Lieu D. Ultrasound physics and instrumentation for pathologists. Arch Pathol Lab Med. 2010;134(10):1541–56.

Lieu D. Breast imaging for interventional pathologists. Arch Pathol Lab Med. 2013;137(1):100–19.

Ljung BM, Langer J, et al. Training, credentialing and re-credentialing for the performance of a thyroid FNA: a synopsis of the National Cancer Institute thyroid fine-needle aspiration state of the science conference. Diagn Cytopathol. 2008;36(6):400–6.

Martin K. Basic equipment, components, and image production. In: Allan PL, Baxter GM, Weston MJ, editors. Clinical ultrasound. London: Elsevier; 2011. p. 16–30.

McDicken WN, Anderson T. Basic physics of medical ultrasound. In: Allan PL, Baxter GM, Weston MJ, editors. Clinical ultrasound. London: Elsevier; 2011. p. 3–15.

Oertel YC. Emerging role of the interventional pathologist. Diagn Cytopathol. 2004;30(5):295–6.

Pitman MB, Abele J, et al. Techniques for thyroid FNA: a synopsis of the National Cancer Institute thyroid fine-needle aspiration state of the science conference. Diagn Cytopathol. 2008;36(6):407–24.

Stanley MW, Löwhagen T. Equipment, basic techniques, and staining procedures. In: Fine needle aspiration of palpable masses. Boston: Butterworth-Heinemann; 1993a. p. 1–58.

Stanley MW, Löwhagen T. The patient: clinical techniques and results reporting. In: Fine needle aspiration of palpable masses. Boston: Butterworth-Heinemann; 1993b. p. 58–118.

Wu M. A comparative study of 200 head and neck FNAs performed by a cytopathologist with versus without ultrasound guidance: evidence for improved diagnostic value with ultrasound guidance. Diagn Cytopathol. 2011;39(10):743–51.

Zajdela A, de Maublanc MA, et al. Cytologic diagnosis of orbital and periorbital palpable tumors using fine-needle sampling without aspiration. Diagn Cytopathol. 1986;2(1):17–20.

The Thyroid Gland

Ricardo H. Bardales

The Normal Thyroid Gland by US (Fig. 3.1a, b)

The thyroid lobes have a pear shape and a bright homogeneous echotexture. The thyroid gland measures 4.5–5.5 cm in length (longitudinal), 2–3 cm in width (transverse), and ≤2 cm in depth (antero-posterior), and the isthmus measures ≤0.5 cm in thickness. The right lobe is slightly larger than the left lobe. The gland has the following boundaries:

- Anterior: platysma and strap neck muscles (sternohyoid, sternothyroid, and omohyoid).
- Lateral: sternocleidomastoid muscle, carotid artery, and the internal jugular vein.
- Posterior: *longus colli* muscle.
- Medial: trachea.
- The esophagus may be seen in the left lateral border. The parathyroid glands are not visible unless they are enlarged.

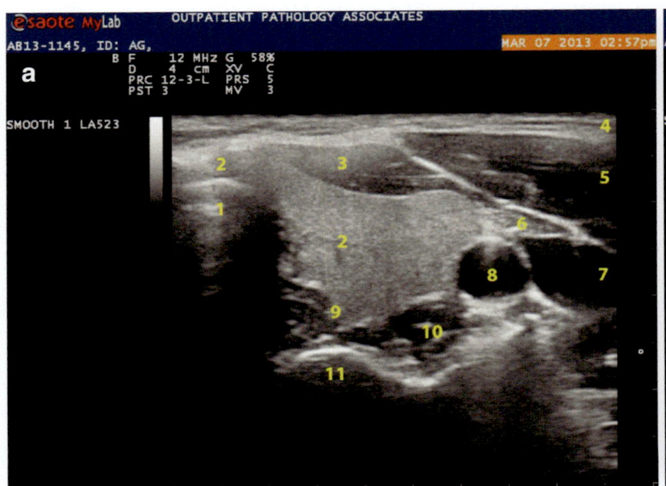
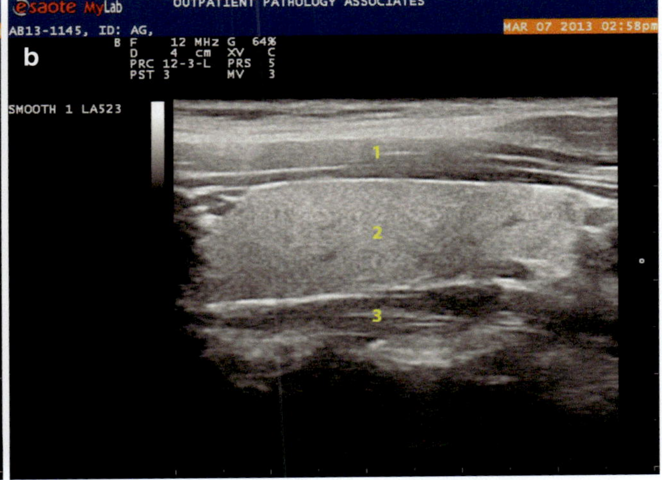

Fig. 3.1 (**a**) Normal thyroid gland. Axial or transverse ultrasound of the left lobe. (1) trachea, (2) thyroid, (3) strap muscles (sternohyoid and sternothyroid), (4) platysma muscle, (5) sternocleidomastoid muscle, (6) omohyoid muscle, (7) internal jugular vein, (8) common carotid artery, (9) esophagus, (10) longus colli, (11) C6 vertebral body. (**b**) Normal right thyroid, longitudinal ultrasound. (1) strap muscles, (2) thyroid, (3) *longus colli* muscle

Supplementary Information The online version contains supplementary material available at https://doi.org/10.1007/978-3-031-73702-2_3.

R. H. Bardales (✉)
Precision Pathology, Outpatient Pathology Associates, Sacramento, CA, USA

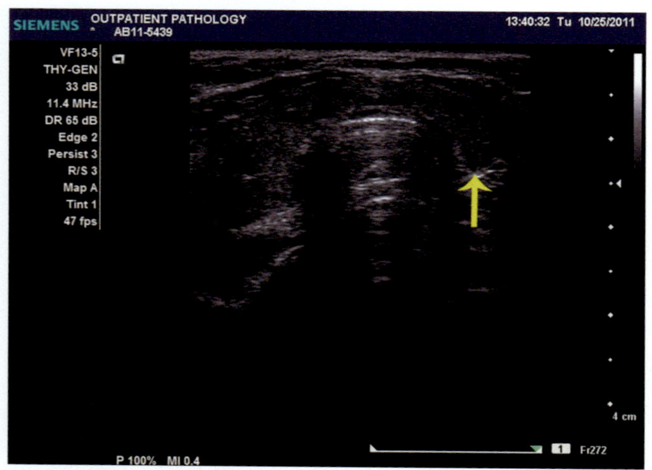

Fig. 3.2 Agenesis of the left thyroid lobe (arrow). Background of chronic thyroiditis. The right thyroid lobe shows a small hypoechoic nodule with lobulated borders

Thyroid and Nonthyroidal Anomalies Seen by US

Hemiagenesis of the thyroid gland has an incidence of 1 in 2500, is more common in girls, and affects predominantly the left lobe (Fig. 3.2). The isthmus is usually present. These patients have a slightly high incidence of thyroid pathology, including carcinoma.

Aberrant or ectopic thyroid tissue can be seen anywhere in the neck from the base of tongue to above the larynx in the midline and is undivided and of variable size and shape. Occasionally, it can be identified in the lateral neck. Ultrasound shows a homogeneous mass with smooth borders and echogenicity similar to that of the thyroid gland. The thyroid bed may show a small or no thyroid tissue. The FNA shows benign follicular cells and colloid (Fig. 3.3a–d).

Esophageal diverticulum is visualized as an outpouching of various sizes, usually adjacent to the left posterior thyroid lobe. The wall shows concentric hyperechoic and hypoechoic layers, and moving contents are visualized in the center of the diverticulum when the patient swallows. The importance of recognizing this anomaly is to avoid mistaking it for a thyroid nodule; however, a FNA is performed on rare occasions and shows benign squamous cells (Fig. 3.4a, b) (Video 3.1).

Epidermal inclusion cysts are commonly seen in children and may be palpable. The exact origin is unknown; however, it is considered to be derived from foci of squamous metaplasia. They are well circumscribed, avascular, and have similar echotexture to that of the thyroid gland by US. FNA smears show benign anucleated and nucleated squamous cells (Fig. 3.5a, b).

Undescended thymus is seen inferior to the thyroid gland, and a thyrothymus ligament may be visualized, allowing for the movement of the thymus along with the thyroid gland while the patient swallows. Compared with the thyroid gland, the thymus is less well-defined, has an abnormal shape, and shows fine internal linear septations.

Ectopic intrathyroidal thymic and parathyroid tissues are congenital anomalies that, on imaging studies, may be mistaken for a thyroid nodule. Ultrasound features of ectopic thymus recapitulate the gross anatomy including a well-circumscribed hypoechoic fusiform lesion with well-defined margins or linear microreflectors that mimic microcalcifications; however, they show no posterior acoustic shadowing. The smears of ectopic thymic tissue show single and aggregated benign predominantly small lymphocytes and bland-appearing thymic epithelium showing large cells with abundant clear cytoplasm and round nuclei; the epithelial elements are obscured by lymphocytes (Fig. 3.6a–d).

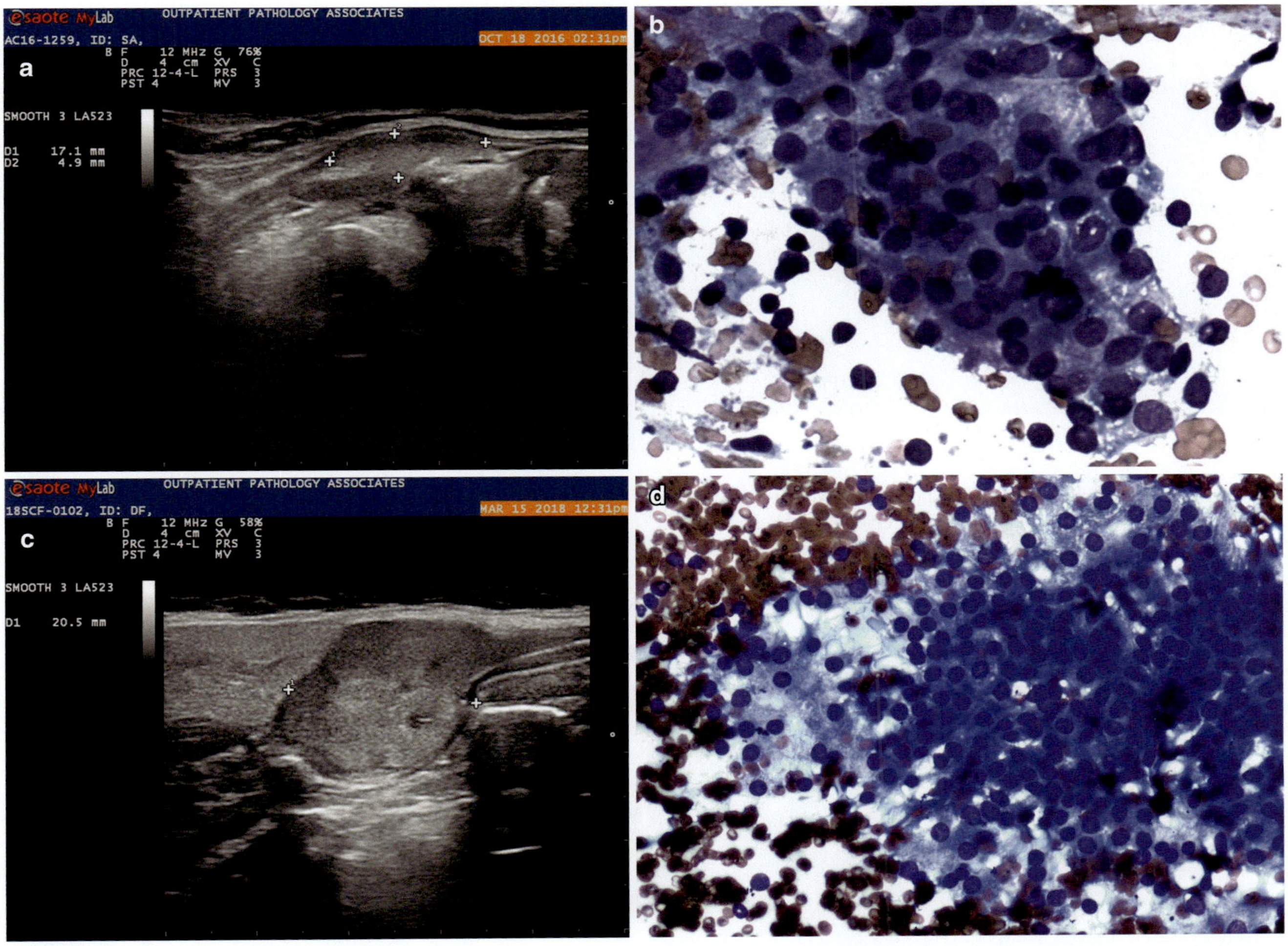

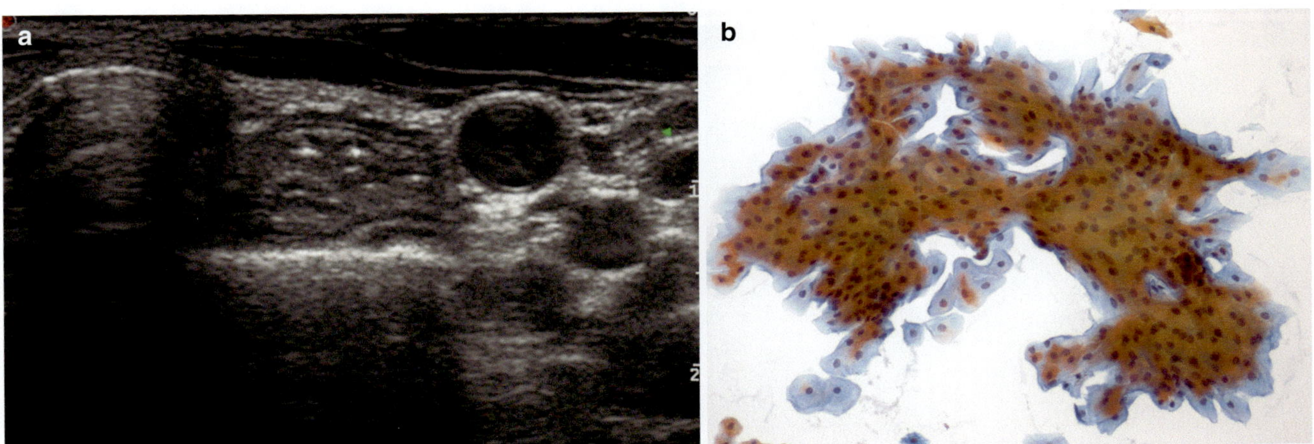

Fig. 3.3 Ectopic thyroid tissue present in the midline of neck above the larynx (**a**) and right neck medial to the submandibular gland (**c**). FNA shows benign follicular cells and colloid (**b**, **d**)

Fig. 3.4 Esophageal diverticulum. This case was submitted in consultation as FNA of a left neck lymph node. US shows concentric bright and dark layers (arrow) with punctate bright luminal esophageal contents (**a**). Smears show sheets of benign squamous cells (**b**). (**b**, Papanicolaou stain, low magnification)

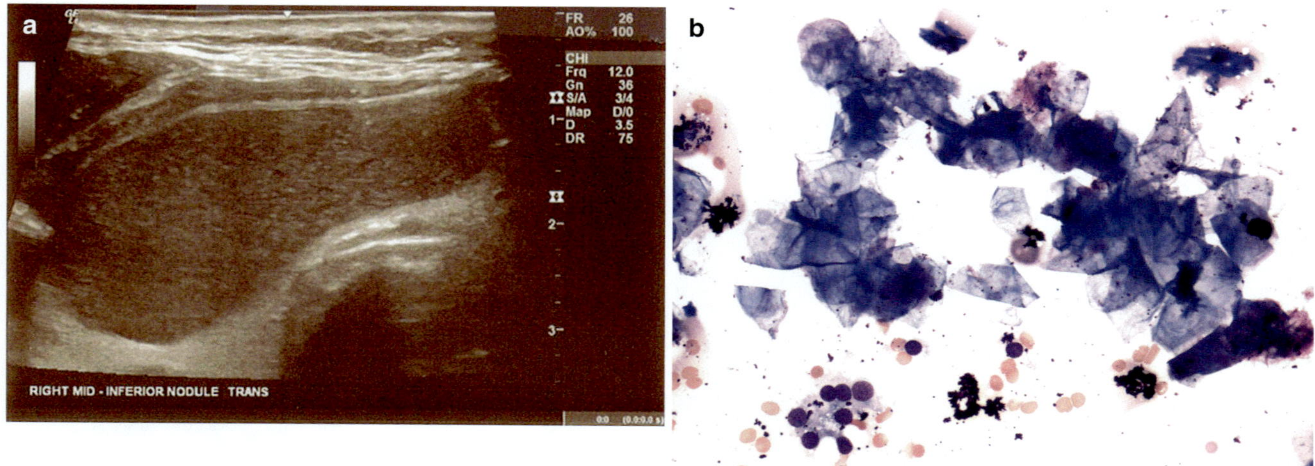

Fig. 3.5 Epidermal inclusion cyst. The clinical diagnosis was right thyroid nodule. US shows a large thyroid mass that occupies the right upper thyroid lobe and extends to the isthmus. The mass is hypoechoic, uniform, and granular with smooth borders (**a**). USG-FNA shows benign predominantly anucleated squamous cells and rare atrophic-type benign follicular epithelial cells (left lower area) (**b**). (**b**, MGG stain, medium magnification)

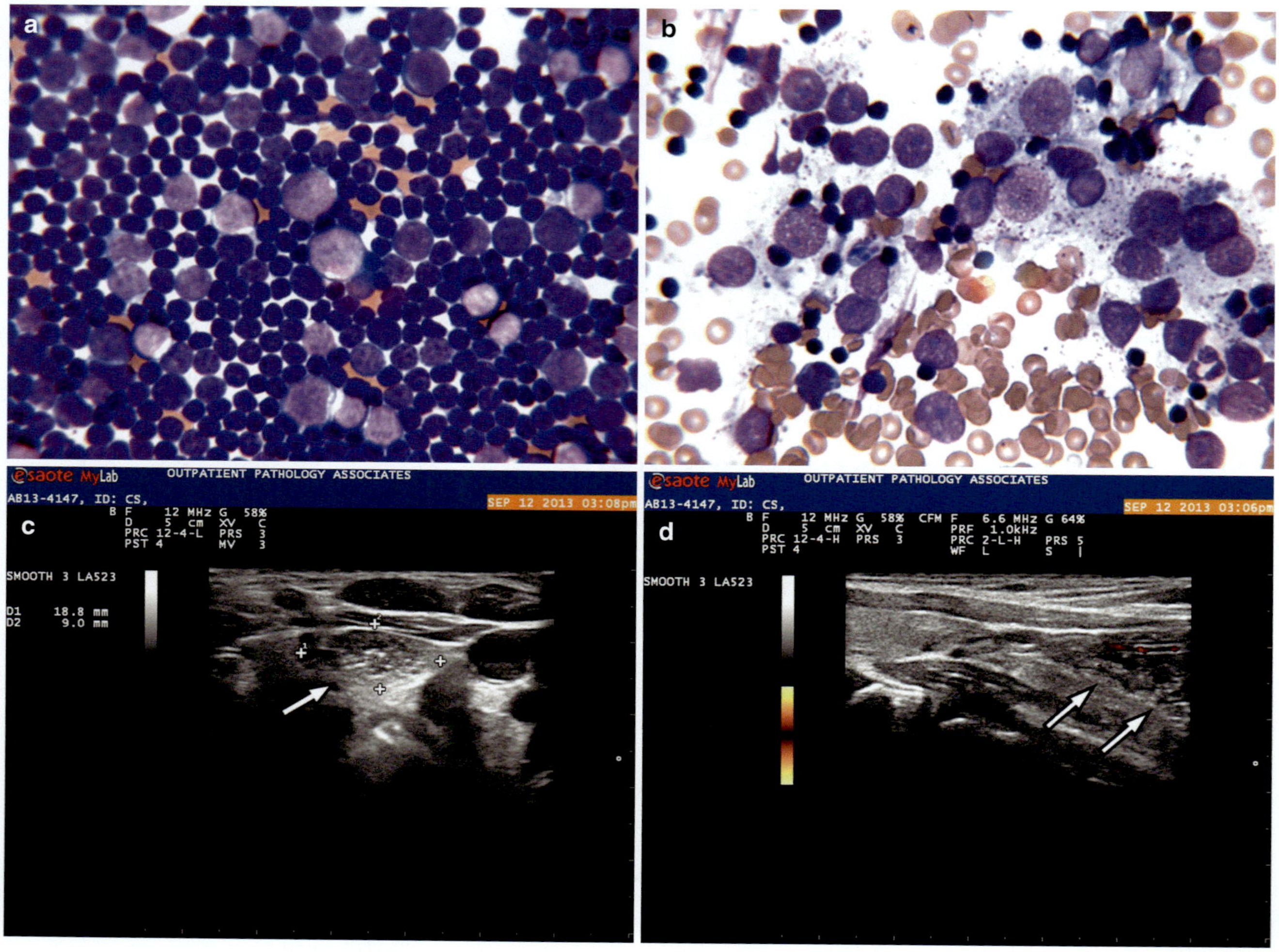

Fig. 3.6 Ectopic thymic tissue. (**a**) Population of predominantly small lymphocytes along with scattered larger lymphocytes. (**b**) Sheet of thymic epithelial cells showing ample clear cytoplasm, red cytoplasmic granules, and round nuclei; the cells are obscured by overlapping lymphoid elements. (**c**) Ultrasound exam shows a fusiform lesion with well-defined margins, marked hypoechogenicity, and numerous internal punctate and linear echogenic foci (*arrow*). (**d**) Doppler examination shows no increased internal vascularity (*arrows*). (**a, b**, MGG stain, high magnification)

The Patient with Thyroid Nodules

Patients with thyroid nodules are candidates for USG-FNA. However, palpable "nodules" are not always true nodules by US in up to 30% of patients, and a palpable "not nodular" thyroid gland may hide a small and/or posterior nodule that may not be palpable, but may be amenable to USG-FNA. Because US alters the clinical management, patients with suspected thyroid nodules, goiter, and palpable thyroid nodule(s), or having risk factors for malignancy should undergo US examination of the thyroid gland and soft tissue of the neck, in addition to a complete clinical history, physical examination mainly of the head and neck, and serum levels of thyroid-stimulating hormone (TSH).

Patients with normal or high TSH levels and US-visible nodule(s) may be candidates for USG-FNA. Patients with low TSH levels and US-visible nodule(s) should have a radionuclide thyroid scan to exclude a "hot" or functioning nodule. A functioning nodule often does not need to undergo FNA, because the possibilities of malignancy are extremely low. When abnormal lymph nodes are present, USG-FNA of the lymph node for cytology and thyroglobulin (TG) levels in needle rinses should be performed at the time of USG-FNA of the thyroid nodule.

Clinical Evaluation

The clinical evaluation identifies pertinent risk factors predicting malignancy in a thyroid nodule, such as:

- Male gender.
- Patient's age <14 years or >70 years.
- History of head and neck irradiation for thymic and tonsilar hypertrophy, acne, etc., or radiotherapy of any kind.
- Family history of thyroid cancer. Papillary thyroid carcinoma (PTC) can be familial in up to 10% of cases. There is an eightfold-increased risk of developing thyroid cancer when there is such a history in a first-degree relative.
- Personal history of syndromes or malignancy associated with thyroid cancer in a first-degree relative, i.e., Cowden syndrome (multiple hamartomas), MEN type 1 (Wermer syndrome that causes tumors in the parathyroid glands, pituitary, and pancreas), MEN type 2, [Sipple syndrome that causes benign oral and submucosal tumors and endocrine malignancies including medullary thyroid carcinoma (MTC)], familial polyposis, Carney complex (skin pigmentary abnormalities, myxomas, endocrine tumors). PTC can occur in association with acromegaly, papillary renal cell carcinoma, parathyroid tumors, paragangliomas, and ataxia-telangiectasia.
- Rapid nodule growth, firm, fixed to adjacent tissues.

- Hoarseness, vocal cord paralysis, dysphonia, dysphagia, and dyspnea.
- Enlarged ipsilateral neck lymph nodes.

Epidemiologic and Clinical Aspects of Thyroid Nodules and Thyroid Cancer

Thyroid nodules in adults are found by palpation in 4–8%, by US in 10–40%, and in post-mortem exam in 50%. The prevalence is higher in women and increases with age, and in individuals with iodine deficiency and a history of radiation exposure.

The overall incidence of malignancy in thyroid nodules undergoing FNA is the same (10–13%) regardless of the number of nodules identified by US, or if the nodules were incidentally identified or non-palpable.

In patients with multiple thyroid nodules, cancer is found in two-thirds of cases in the dominant nodule and in one-third of cases in a non-dominant nodule. US characteristics of the nodule influence FNA sampling of the nodule, regardless of size.

Thyroid nodules occur less frequently in children than in adults, account for less than 2% of thyroid diseases, and the diagnostic approach and management should be the same as that of adults. The frequency of thyroid cancer in children varies and has been reported as being higher than or similar to that of adults, PTC the most common. Of note, PTC tends to be more aggressive than in adults with a high incidence of locally advanced disease.

There is an increase in the incidence of thyroid cancer, predominantly PTC (with *RET/PTC* rearrangement), in patients exposed to low-dose (therapy for acne and thymic or tonsilar hypertrophy) and high-dose (i.e., therapy for Hodgkin lymphoma) radiation. A well-known example is the Chernobyl nuclear accident, where the population is at increased risk for thyroid cancer.

Ultrasound Characteristics of Thyroid Nodules

The Society of Radiologists in Ultrasound issued a consensus statement in 2004 to determine which thyroid nodules should or should not undergo USG-FNA based on US characteristics. It was concluded that (1) the various US features studied are not specific in separating benign from malignant thyroid nodules due to overlapping characteristics, and (2) FNA diagnosis is required before the patient undergoes thyroid surgery for a possible thyroid malignancy.

The US evaluation of a thyroid nodule includes size, echogenicity (isoechoic, hypoechoic, or hyperechoic), composition (cystic, solid, mixed), calcifications (fine, coarse, interrupted eggshell calcification), halo, margins (regular, irregular, spiculated, lobulated), and vascularity determined by Doppler. The value of these features to predict malignancy is highly variable. A single abnormal US finding is seen approximately 70% of benign thyroid nodules. Thus, a combination of features such as marked hypoechogenicity, solid echotexture, irregular borders, microcalcifications, interrupted eggshell calcification, and central intranodular blood flow increases the likelihood of thyroid cancer.

1. *Echotexture or composition.* A purely cystic nodule (Fig. 3.7 and Video 3.2), a spongiform-appearing nodule (multiple microcystic components in >50% of the volume) (Fig. 3.8), or a complex nodule (more than 50% cystic) (Fig. 3.9) are highly predictive for being benign. However, malignancy should be considered in complex cysts with an irregular/thick wall, microcalcifications, or when a mural nodule has an increased vascularity or has an acute angle with the wall of the nodule (Fig. 3.10a–c). Of note, a macrofollicular subtype of PTC may show a spongiform pattern. A solid echotexture (Fig. 3.11) has high sensitivity but low specificity and a low positive predictive value.

2. *Echogenicity.* Marked hypoechogenicity (echogenicity darker than the neck strap muscles) is very suggestive of malignancy. Iso- and hyperechogenicity are more commonly seen in benign thyroid nodules. Follicular neoplasms, particularly oncocytic adenoma and carcinoma, and rarely PTC may be hyperechogenic (Fig. 3.12a–d).

3. *Calcifications.* Any calcification increases the likelihood of malignancy. Calcifications are present in approximately 30% of nodules and are classified as micro, coarse, and eggshell calcifications.

   (a) Microcalcifications or microreflectors are less than 1 mm in size and do not produce posterior acoustic shadowing, are associated with a threefold increase in cancer risk in a solid nodule, and may represent aggregated psammoma bodies. (Fig. 3.13a) They are much less common in benign nodules and Hashimoto's thyroiditis.

   (b) Macrocalcifications are larger than 2 mm and produce posterior acoustic shadowing, are associated with a twofold increase in cancer risk in solid nodules, and represent dystrophic calcification in areas of fibrosis and degeneration; however, a central location within the nodule and association with microcalcifications raise the suspicion for malignancy. (Fig. 3.13b).

   (c) Eggshell calcifications with smooth, thin, and regular contours are more associated with benign and less commonly with malignant thyroid nodules; however, eggshell with interrupted rim is suggestive of thyroid cancer permeating through the defect to invade the surrounding tissue (Fig. 3.13c–f).

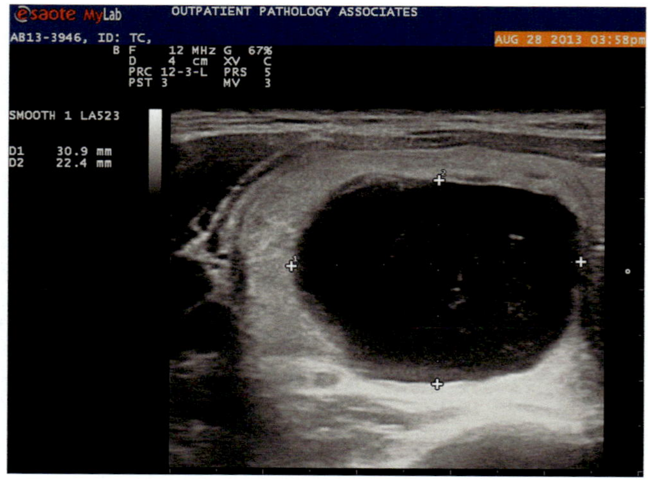

Fig. 3.7 Cystic nodule. USG-FNA showed thin colloid and scattered macrophages

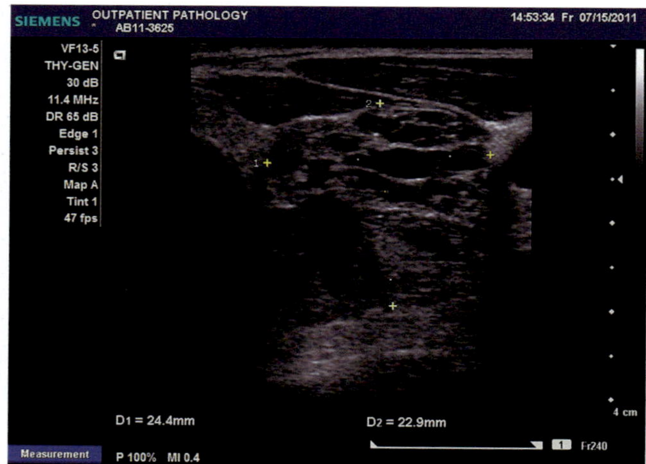

Fig. 3.8 Spongiform nodule. USG-FNA diagnosis was benign thyroid nodule

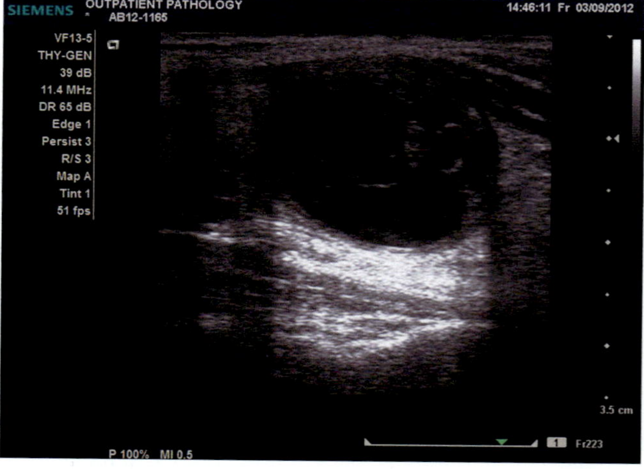

Fig. 3.9 Complex nodule, more than 50% cystic. USG-FNA diagnosis was benign thyroid nodule

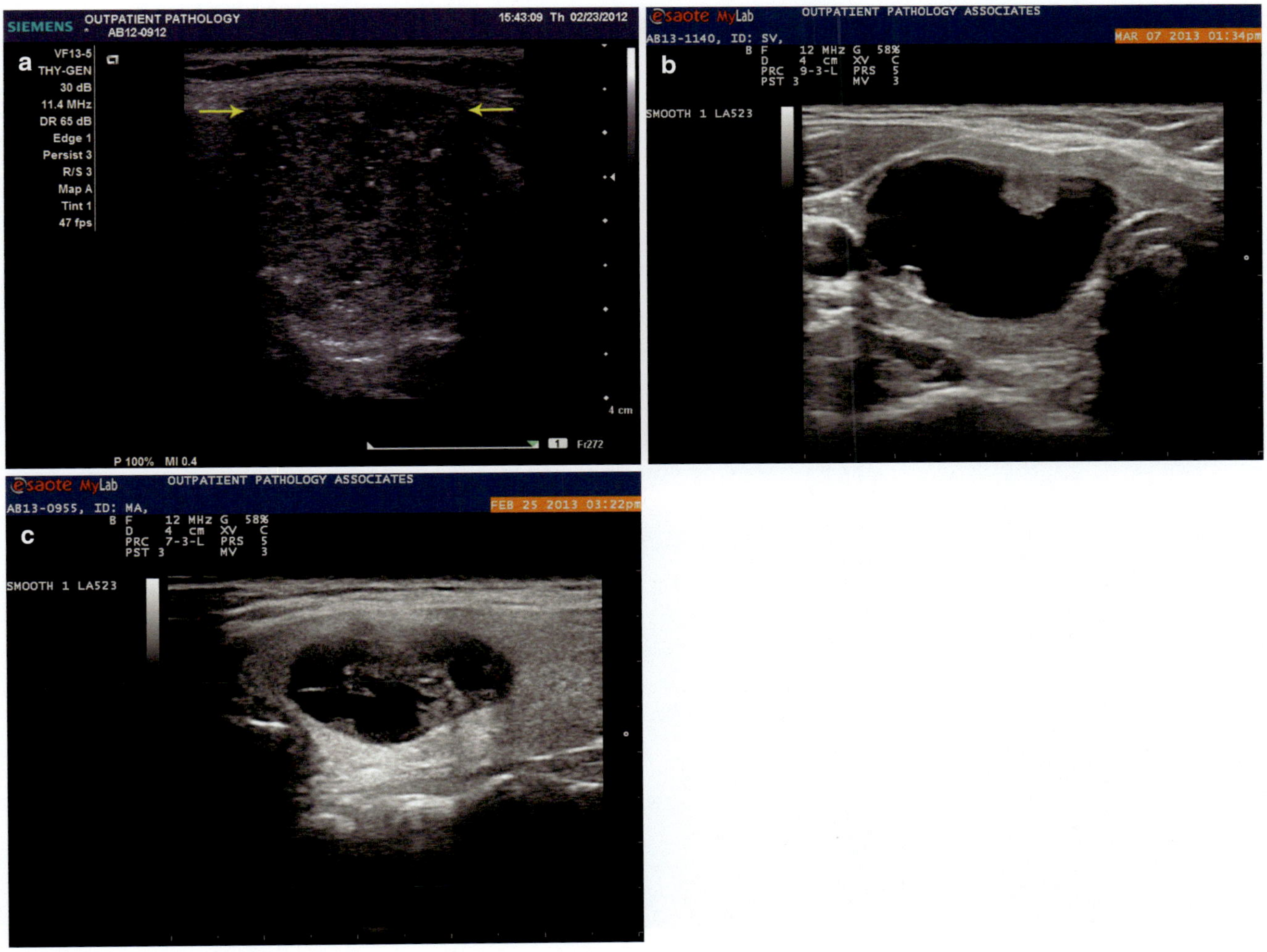

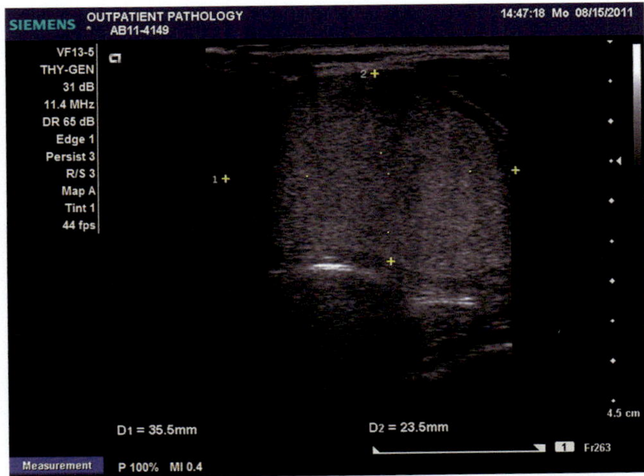

Fig. 3.10 (**a**) Predominantly solid nodule with irregular thick wall (arrows), microcalcifications, and ill-defined margins. USG-FNA diagnosis was papillary thyroid carcinoma. (**b**) Predominantly cystic nodule with mural solid component, vascular by Doppler examination (not shown). USG-FNA diagnosis was benign thyroid nodule. (**c**) Predominantly cystic complex nodule with solid central component, vascular by Doppler examination (not shown). USG-FNA diagnosis was cystic papillary thyroid carcinoma

Fig. 3.11 Solid homogeneous isoechoic thyroid nodule. USG-FNA diagnosis was benign thyroid nodule

4. *Margins*. The margins of a benign thyroid nodule are usually regular and well-defined, usually with a smooth, thin surface (Fig. 3.14a). Infiltrative, irregular, spiculated, and lobulated borders are worrisome for an invasive malignancy (Fig. 3.14b).

5. *Halo*. The halo is a hypoechoic ring that surrounds an iso- or hyperechoic nodule, and probably represents compressed peripheral thyroid tissue and vessels, usually associated with benignity (Fig. 3.15a). A thick, irregular, and avascular capsule or halo may indicate the presence of a fibrous capsule surrounding a thyroid neoplasm i.e., follicular or oncocytic. Fuzzy, ill-defined, and indistinct borders are not considered to be a sign of malignancy. A thick halo produces an "edge" artifact (Fig. 3.15b). Both margins and halo may not be as helpful as originally thought for the differentiation of benign from malignant thyroid nodules, except when there is loss of halo or cap-

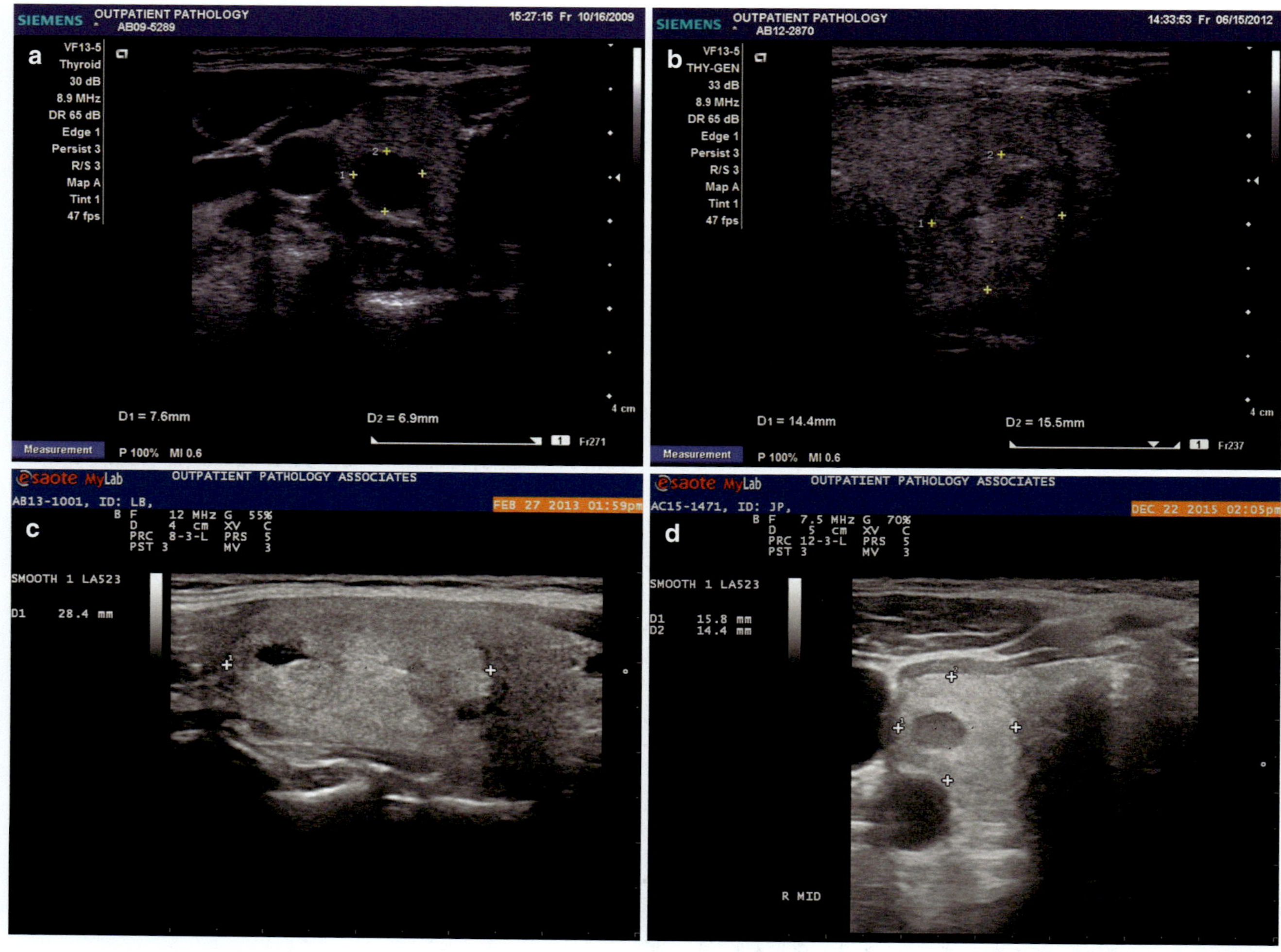

Fig. 3.12 (**a**) Hypoechoic sub-centimeter thyroid nodule. USG-FNA diagnosis was suspicious for papillary thyroid carcinoma. (**b**) Isoechoic nodule. USG-FNA diagnosis was benign thyroid nodule. (**c**) Hyperechogenic thyroid nodule. USG-FNA diagnosis was benign thyroid nodule with oncocytic features. (**d**) Hyperechogenic nodule with a hypoechoic central area. USG-FNA diagnosis was papillary thyroid carcinoma

sule due to invasion into surrounding tissue. The combination of a peripheral halo and interrupted eggshell-type calcification may be a high predictor for malignancy (Fig. 3.15c). The distinction between all these features has a high interobserver variability.

6. *Color and power Doppler.* Most benign nodules lack intranodular flow on power Doppler analysis, and most malignancies have central blood flow. Also, peripheral blood flow suggests a benign nodule. However, lack of extensive vascularity cannot be used to exclude malignancy. Of note, functioning nodules are highly vascular. Vascularity in a thyroid nodule can be categorized as follows:
   (a) Type 1. Absent. No flow detectable (Fig. 3.16a).
   (b) Type 2. Perinodular. Peripheral flow only (Fig. 3.16b).
   (c) Type 3. Perinodular and intranodular. Peripheral blood flow and scant central flow (Fig. 3.16c).
   (d) Type 4. Intranodular. High-intensity central flow (Fig. 3.16d).
7. *Shape.* The nodule shape may help to predict malignancy and prompt one to perform a USG-FNA. Spherical shape and nodules that are taller (antero-posterior diameter) than wide (transverse diameter) in the transverse view statistically may be associated with a malignant diagnosis (Fig. 3.17a, b).
8. *Comet tail sign.* Comet tails are reverberation ("echo") artifacts that result from the reflection of sound waves off of the crystals present in the desiccated thick colloid, resulting in a bright signal; the crystals vibrate under the sound energy, producing the comet tail. This sign is reported to be almost pathognomonic for a benign thyroid nodule, particularly if present at the periphery of cystic nodules (Fig. 3.18a). However, often it is difficult to state conclusively its presence in a given thyroid nodule.

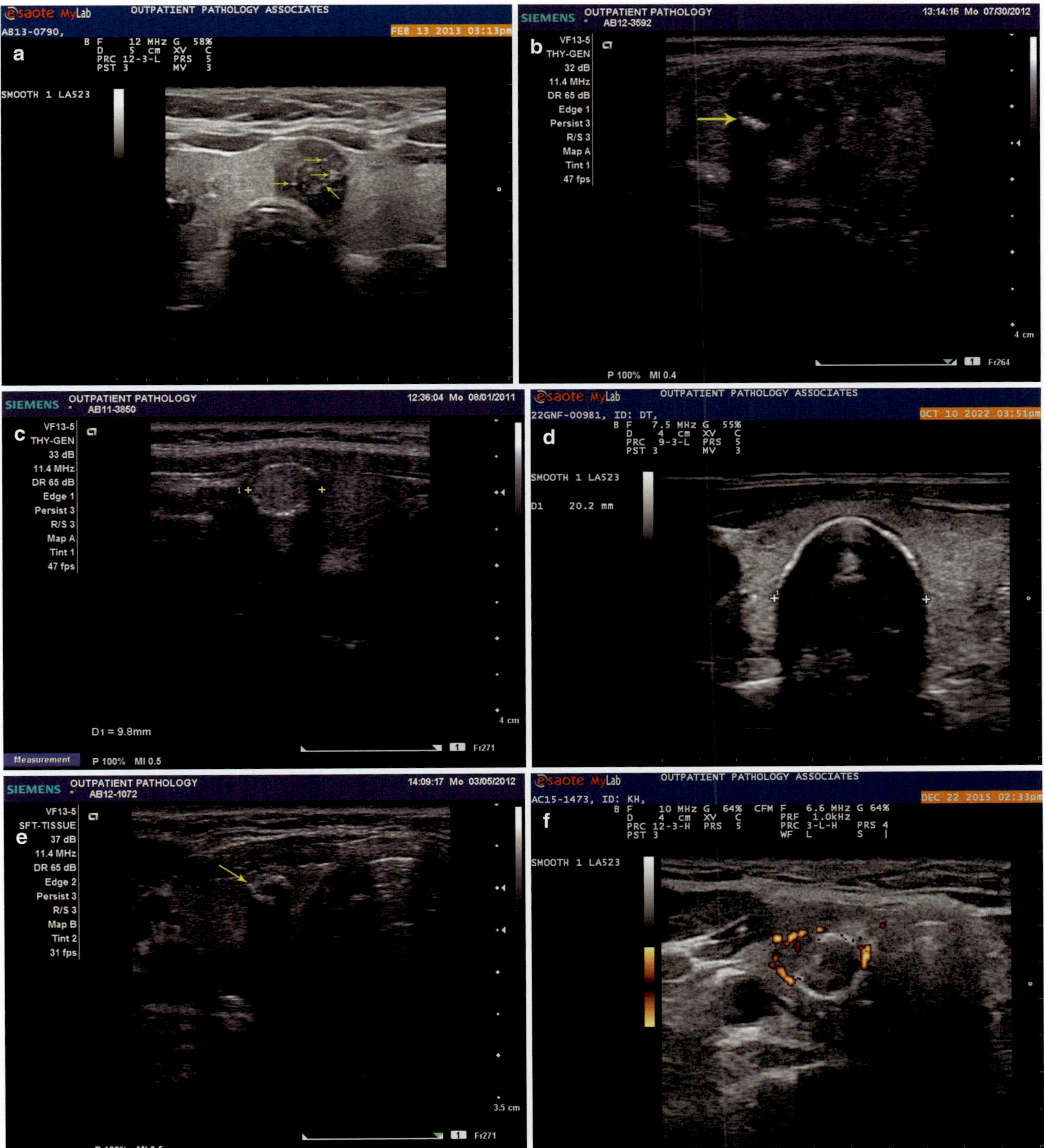

Fig. 3.13 (**a**) Microcalcifications in a hypoechoic nodule. USG-FNA diagnosis was papillary thyroid carcinoma. (**b**) Macrocalcifications with posterior acoustic shadow. USG-FNA diagnosis was chronic thyroiditis. (**c**) Eggshell calcification. USG-FNA diagnosis was benign thyroid nodule. (**d**) Eggshell calcification. USG-FNA was non-diagnostic; unable to penetrate needle through the wall of the calcified nodule. (**e**) Small nodule with interrupted (arrow) eggshell calcification. USG-FNA diagnosis was papillary thyroid carcinoma. (**f**) Interrupted eggshell calcification with thyroid tissue permeating through the defect and invading the surrounding thyroid tissue (Doppler examination). USG-FNA was papillary thyroid carcinoma

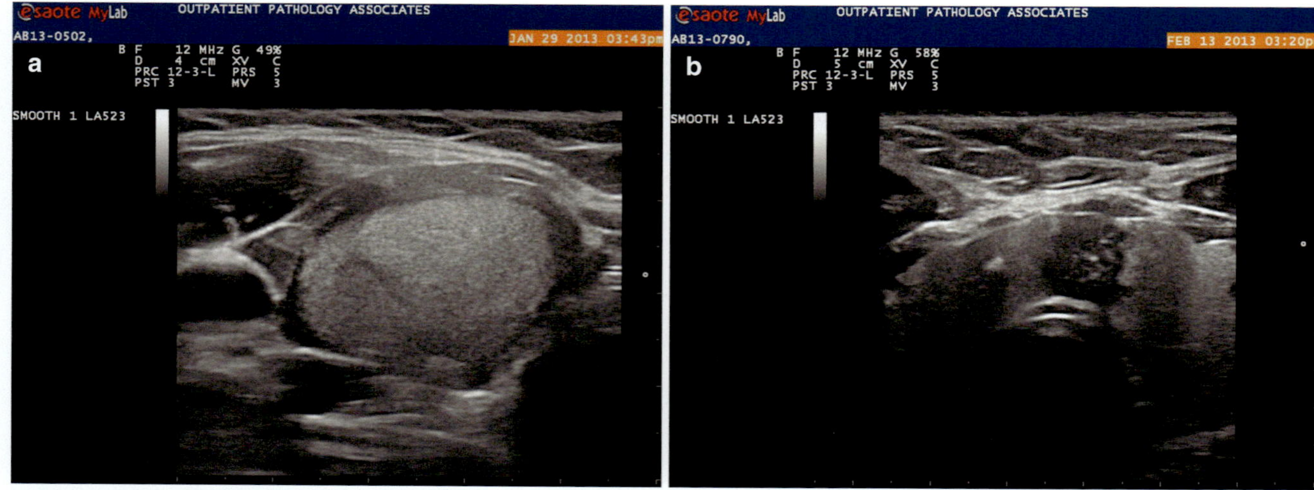

Fig. 3.14 (**a**) Smooth, thin, and well-defined margins. USG-FNA diagnosis was benign thyroid nodule. (**b**) Lobulated and spiculated margins. USG-FNA diagnosis was papillary thyroid carcinoma

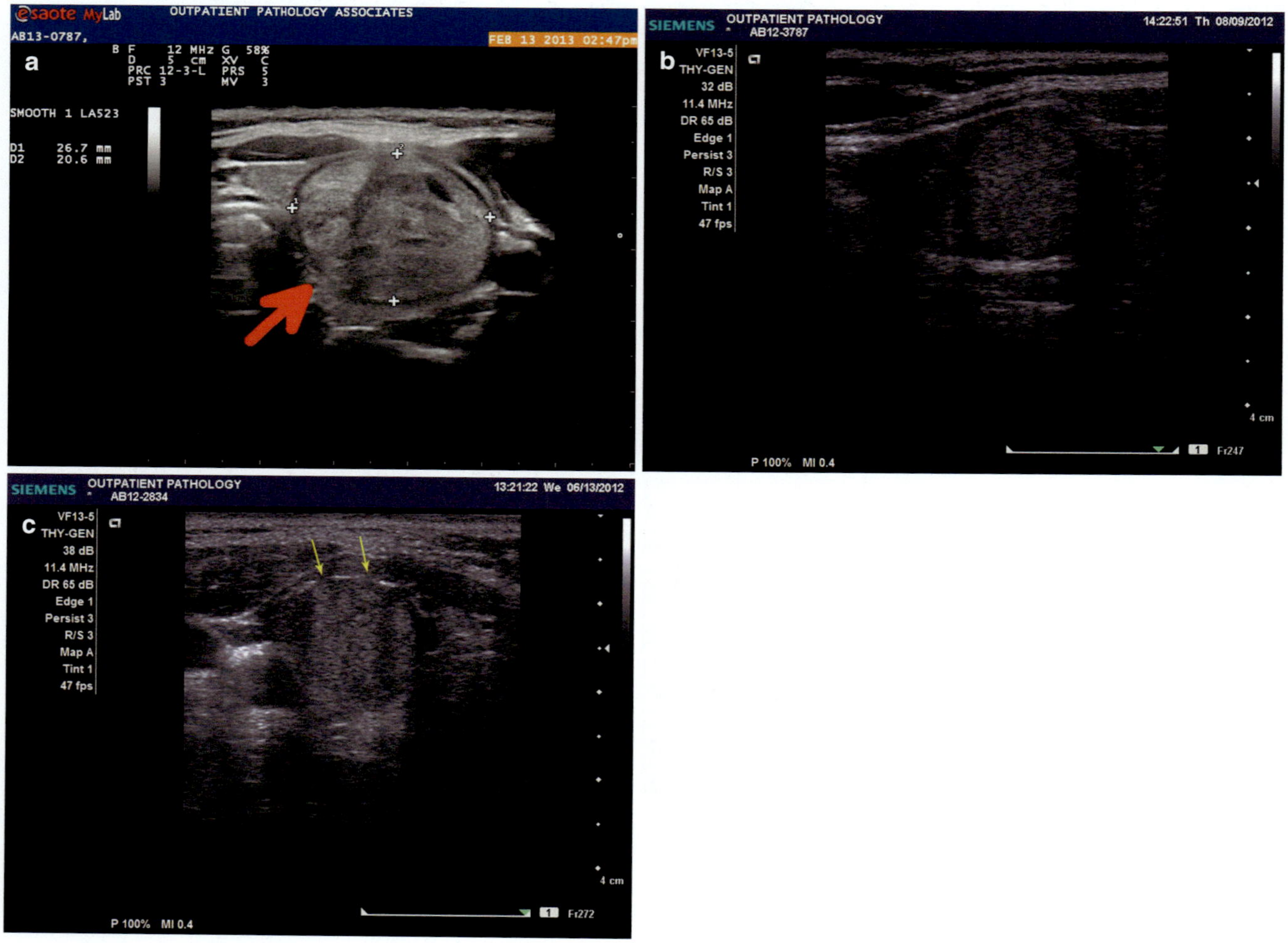

Fig. 3.15 (**a**) Halo. Isoechoic nodule (arrow) with a smooth uniform halo. USG-FNA diagnosis was benign thyroid nodule. (**b**) Edge shadows from a thick halo. USG-FNA diagnosis was benign thyroid nodule. (**c**) Thin, irregular, inconspicuous halo and interrupted eggshell calcification. USG-FNA diagnosis was papillary thyroid carcinoma

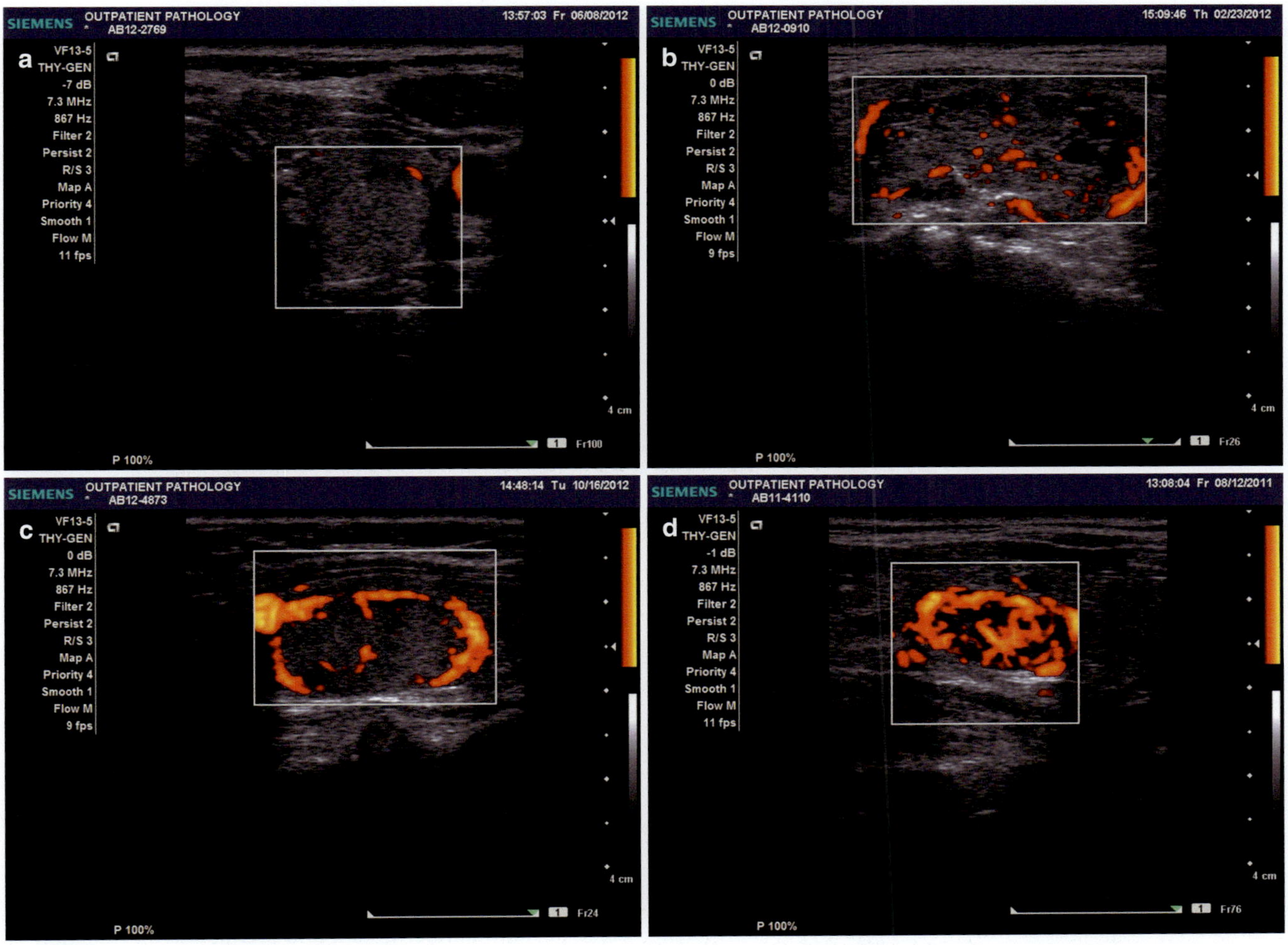

Fig. 3.16 (**a**) Nodule vascularity. Type 1. There is no blood flow. USG-FNA diagnosis was benign thyroid nodule. (**b**) Type 2. There is peripheral blood flow and incipient central blood flow. USG-FNA diagnosis was benign thyroid nodule with cystic change. (**c**) Type 3. There is marked peripheral and less prominent central blood flow. USG-FNA diagnosis was mixed pattern of benign thyroid nodule and chronic thyroiditis. (**d**) Type 4. There is prominent peripheral and central blood flow. USG-FNA diagnosis was microfollicular tumor

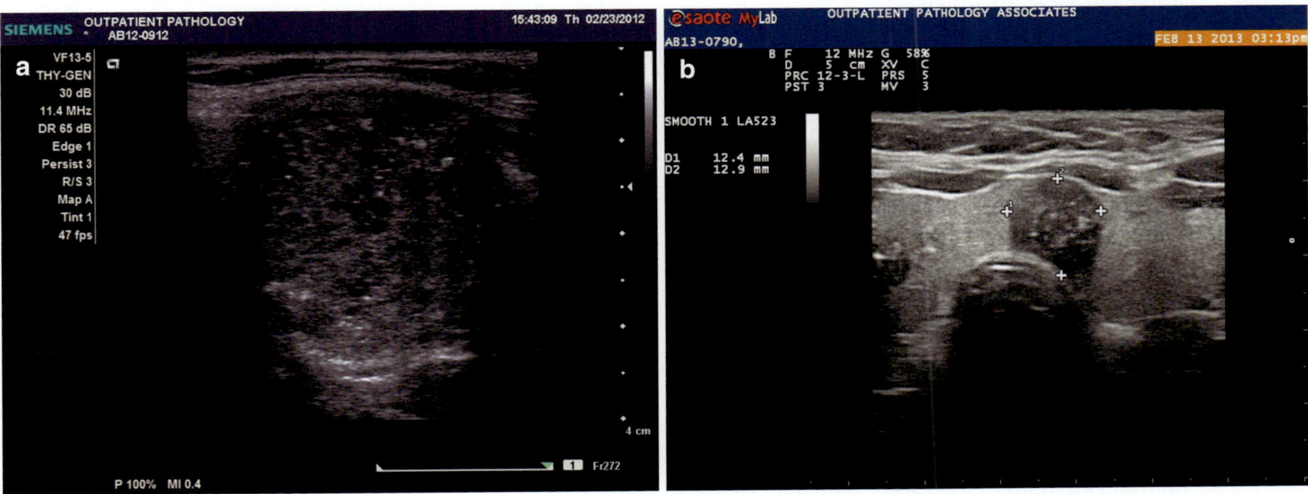

Fig. 3.17 (**a**) Taller than wide with microcalcifications. USG-FNA diagnosis was papillary thyroid carcinoma. (**b**) Taller than wide with microcalcifications. USG-FNA diagnosis was papillary thyroid carcinoma

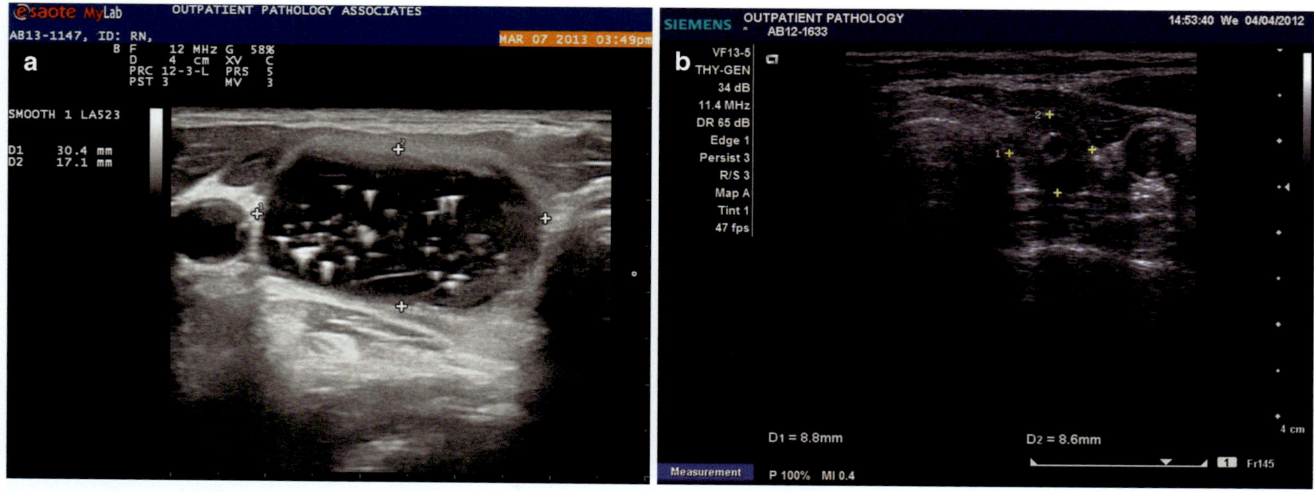

Fig. 3.18 (**a**) Comet tail artifact. USG-FNA diagnosis was colloid-rich benign thyroid nodule. (**b**) Fishs eye artifact. USG-FNA diagnosis was benign thyroid nodule

Comet tails have also been described in PTC, particularly in the cystic subtype. Condensed colloid in a hypoechoic nodule ("cat's eye") correlates with a benign thyroid nodule (Fig. 3.18b).

Documentation of the following US features must be included in the USG-FNA report:

1. Nodule echogenicity with respect of the background thyroid, i.e., hyper-, hypo-, isoechoic. A nodule is classified as deeply hypoechoic when it is more hypoechoic than the echogenicity of the strap muscles.
2. Nodule echotexture, i.e., heterogeneous, homogeneous, spongiform, complex.
3. Nodule margins, i.e., well- or poorly circumscribed, interrupted, irregular, spiculated, lobulated, halo (thick, thin, irregular, vascular, avascular).
4. Calcifications, i.e., micro, coarse, eggshell (interrupted, continuous, displaced).
5. Intranodular blood flow pattern on Doppler exam (peripheral and/or central, mild or marked, uniform or chaotic).
6. Other intranodular features, i.e., cystic, comet tails.
7. Echotexture of the surrounding thyroid.
8. Presence or absence of regional neck lymph nodes, i.e., normal or abnormal US features.

The standard US evaluation of thyroid nodules must include a sonographic evaluation of regional cervical lymph nodes. Metastasis to cervical lymph nodes, usually pre- and paratracheal and anterior cervical (neck compartment VI) is the first manifestation of the disease in an average of 20% of adults with thyroid carcinoma, often PTC. This presentation is much higher in patients younger than 20 years. Other aggressive malignancies including lymphoma have lymph node involvement at initial diagnosis. Lymph nodes with cystic change, microcalcifications, round shape, abnormal echogenic pattern including deep hypoechogenicity, irregular cortex, lack of hilum, and abnormal vascular blood flow must be evaluated by USG-FNA to exclude a metastatic disease.

We should emphasize that (1) according to the American Thyroid Association (ATA), American Association of Clinical Endocrinologists (AACE), American College of Endocrinology (ACE), and Associazione Medici Endocrinologi (AME) guidelines, US is the imaging modality of choice in the evaluation of thyroid nodules, surveillance of multinodular goiter, and preoperative evaluation of patients with known differentiated thyroid cancer (DTC), (2) since the indications for an USG-FNA of a given thyroid nodule are determined mainly by the US characteristics of the nodule and less by the number of nodules or the nodule size, it is currently accepted that the sonographic patterns (combination of individual US features) are more accurate to predict thyroid cancer risk, 3) the US features of a thyroid nodule are helpful in predicting malignancy or benignity, but they do not replace the need to perform USG-FNA.

Ultrasound Patterns of Thyroid Nodules

The appearance of some US features that are present in low-risk, intermediate-risk, and high-risk for malignancy lesions are usually identified together in each risk category. The following list summarizes the US patterns and risk of malignancy (ROM) as classified by the AACE, ACE, AME, and ATA.

Low-risk lesion (AACE/ACE/AME): ROM <1%

– Cysts (more than 80% fluid).
– Mostly cystic nodules with comet tail artifacts.
– Isoechoic spongiform nodules.

Benign (ATA): ROM 0%

– Purely cystic nodules.

Very low suspicion (ATA): ROM <3%

– Spongiform or partially cystic nodules without low-, intermediate-, or high-suspicious US features.

Low suspicion (ATA): ROM 5–10%

– Isoechoic or hyperechoic solid nodule or partially cystic nodule with eccentric solid component without microcalcifications, irregular margin, extrathyroidal extension, or taller than wide shape.

Intermediate-risk thyroid lesion (AACE/ACE/AME): ROM 5–15%

– Slightly hypoechoic or isoechoic nodules with ovoid to round shape, smooth to ill-defined margins.
– May be present: intranodular hypervascularity, elevated stiffness at elastography, macrocalcifications, continuous eggshell calcification, indeterminate hyperechoic spots.

Intermediate suspicion (ATA): ROM 10–20%

– Hypoechoic solid nodule with smooth margins without microcalcifications, extrathyroidal extension, or taller than wide shape.

High-risk thyroid lesion: (AACE/ACE/AME): ROM 50–90%

– Nodules with at least one of the following features: marked hypoechogenicity compared with peri thyroid muscles, spiculated or lobulated margins, microcalcifications, taller than wide shape, extrathyroidal growth, pathologic regional adenopathy.

High suspicion (ATA): ROM >70–90%

– Solid hypoechoic nodule o solid hypoechoic component of a partially cystic nodule with one or more of the following features: irregular margins (infiltrative or microlobulated), microcalcifications, taller than wide shape, eggshell calcification with small extrusive soft tissue component, extrathyroidal extension.

Indications for USG-FNA of Thyroid Nodules

The indications are summarized in Table 3.1. USG-core needle biopsies are not recommended for thyroid nodules due to lack of appropriate sampling, particularly in follicular neoplasms or lesions, and serious complications such as bleeding and pain, nerve injury, tracheal perforation, and architectural distortion that preclude accurate histologic interpretation in subsequently excised specimens. However, USG-core needle biopsies may be complementary to FNA in selected cases such as diffuse Hashimoto's thyroiditis and perhaps an advanced malignant neoplasm.

Table 3.1 Recommendations for USG-FNA: Various Societies[a]

A. Thyroid nodules that are ≥1.0 cm

1.	All societies except the SRUS recommend USG-FNA of all nodules ≥1.0 cm
2.	Solitary nodule with microcalcifications if ≥1 cm (SRUS)
3.	Solitary nodule with coarse calcifications or solid nodule if ≥1.5 cm (SRUS)
4.	Solitary nodule with high- or intermediate suspicion (ATA) or high-risk (AACE) if ≥1 cm
5.	Solitary predominantly cystic with a solid mural component or mixed solid and cystic nodule if ≥2 cm (SRUS)
6.	Solitary nodule with low or intermediate risk (AACE) if ≥2 cm
7.	Solitary nodule having a substantial growth since prior US examination. The ATA considers 20% increase in 2 of the 3 diameters (≥ 2 mm each) as reasonable nodule growth
8.	Solitary nodule with benign US pattern (ATA) no USG-FNA
9.	If multiple nodules are present, select the one(s) for USG-FNA, applying the previous 2–7 criteria for solitary nodules (in that order)
10.	If cervical lymph node(s) is/are present, USG-FNA of the lymph node and or any ipsilateral thyroid nodule should be done regardless of the US characteristics.
(a)	The US features associated with cancer in a lymph node include loss of fatty hilum, round shape, well-defined edges, taller than wide, calcifications, cystic areas, and increased peripheral vascularity regardless of size (Fig. 3.19)
(b)	Thyroid cancer most commonly metastasizes to neck levels III, IV, and VI. Malignancy is confirmed by cytologic evaluation and/or thyroglobulin (TG) measurement in needle rinses
11.	If the nodule is entirely cystic, or stable in size, or none of the above listed features is seen, then probably USG-FNA is unnecessary
12.	For a diffusely enlarged thyroid gland with no US-visible nodules, USG-FNA is probably unnecessary

(continued)

Table 3.1 (continued)

B. Special considerations for USG-FNA of nodules < 1 cm.
1. Ultrasound features suggestive of malignancy (calcifications, solid, increased intranodular blood flow on power Doppler, or taller than wide in the transverse view on US). Nodules can be accurately aspirated by USG-FNA with a 90% diagnostic rate (Fig. 3.20)
2. Abnormal neck lymphadenopathy. US criteria as described in the prior section
3. History of head and neck irradiation in childhood or adolescence
4. History of thyroid cancer in one or more first-degree relatives
5. History of heritable syndromes associated with thyroid cancer
6. History of prior hemithyroidectomy with incidentally found thyroid cancer
7. Nodule incidentally found by 2-deoxy-2[^{18}F]fluoro-D-glucose positron emission tomography (^{18}FDG-PET) imaging for other reasons. The risk of malignancy in these nodules is 15%– 50%, and cancers may be more aggressive. Most are PTC and others are follicular or oncocytic cell neoplasms
8. Nodule incidentally found by sestamibi scan, a nuclear medicine scan for parathyroid gland disorders and confirmed by thyroid US, has a high incidence of malignancy (22%–66%) and should be sampled

[a]*ACT* Academy of Clinical Thyroidologists, *ATA* American Thyroid Association, *ACE* American College of Endocrinology, *AACE* American Association of Clinical Endocrinologists, *SRUS* Society of Radiologists in Ultrasound, *AME* Associazione Medici Endocrinologi

The Thyroid Imaging Reporting and Data System (TI-RADS)

The TI-RADS, proposed by the American College of Radiologists in 2017, is a score system for reporting US characteristics of thyroid nodules based on five features (composition, echogenicity, shape, margin, and echogenic foci). The system provides scoring, classification, and recommendations for FNA based on the risk of malignancy. The highest the score level of the nodule, the highest the likelihood of malignancy. TI-RADS system has 75–97% sensitivity and 53–67% specificity that result in low rates of unnecessary FNA.

One score is assigned from each category:

- Composition (chose one).
  - Cystic or completely cystic: 0 points.
  - Spongiform: 0 points.
  - Mixed cystic and solid: 1 point.
  - Solid or almost completely solid: 2 points.
- Echogenicity (chose one).
  - Anechoic: 0 points.
  - Hyper- or isoechoic: 1 point.
  - Hypoechoic: 2 points.
  - Very hypoechoic: 3 points.
- Shape assessed on the transverse plane (chose one).
  - Wider than tall: 0 points.
  - Taller than wide: 3 points.
- Margin (chose one).
  - Smooth: 0 points.
  - Ill-defined: 0 points.
  - Lobulated/irregular: 2 points.
  - Extrathyroidal extension: 3 points.
- Echogenic foci (*chose one or more*).
  - None: 0 points.
  - Large comet tail artifact: 0 points.
  - Macrocalcifications: 1 point.
  - Peripheral/rim calcifications: 2 points.
  - Punctate echogenic foci: 3 points.

TI-RADS scoring (TR), classification, and recommendations:

- TR1: 0 points. Benign. Risk of malignancy 0.3%. No FNA required.
- TR2: 2 points. Not suspicious. Risk of malignancy 1.5%. No FNA required.
- TR3: 3 points. Mildly suspicious. Risk of malignancy 4.8%. ≥1.5 cm follow-up, ≥2.5 cm FNA. Follow-up: 1, 3, 5 years.
- TR4: 4–6 points. Moderately suspicious. Risk of malignancy 9.1%. ≥1 cm follow-up, ≥1.5 cm FNA. Follow-up: 1, 2, 3, 5 years.
- TR5: >7 points. Highly suspicious. Risk of malignancy 35%. ≥0.5 cm follow-up. ≥1 cm FNA. Annual follow-up for up to 5 years.

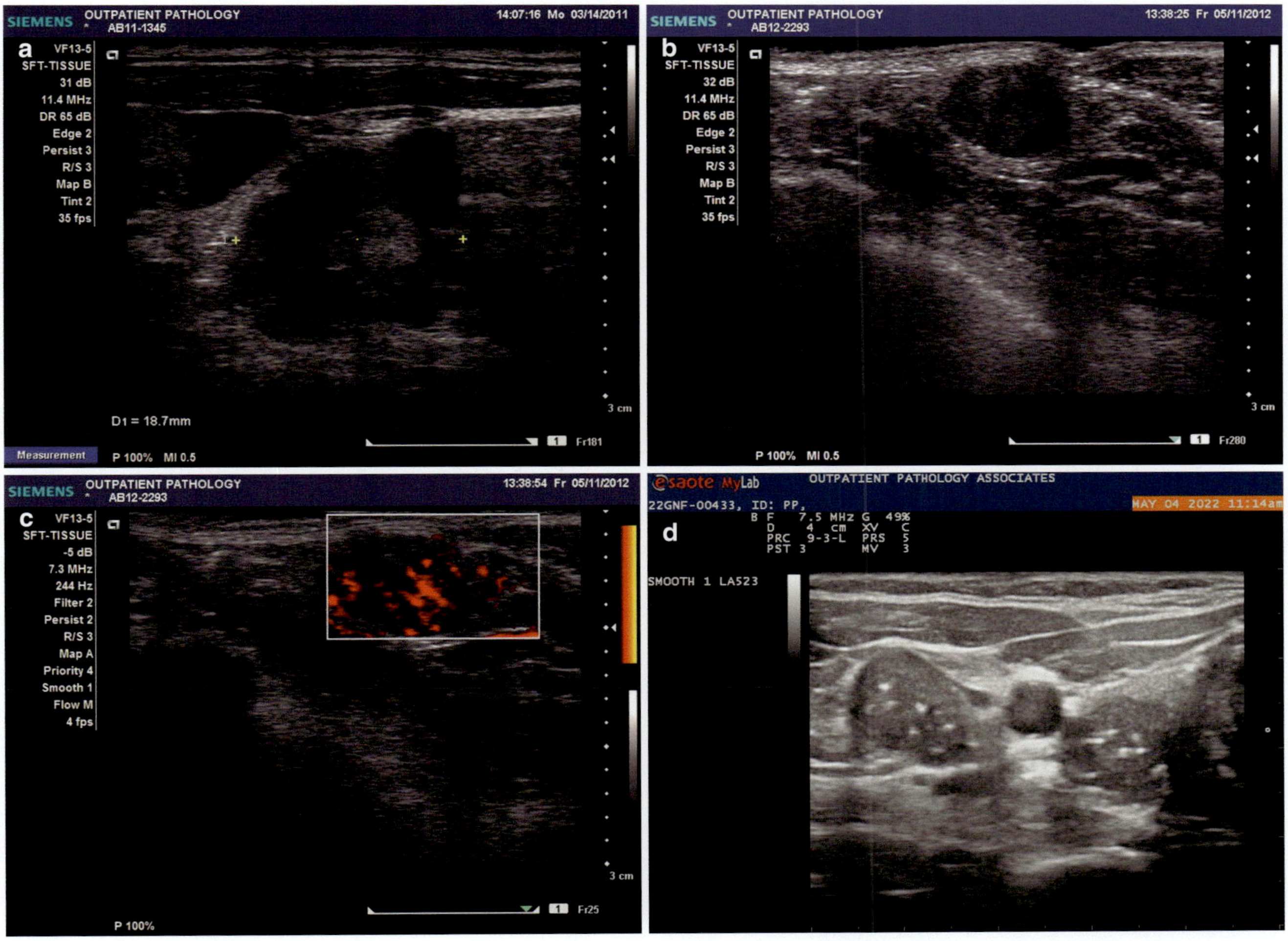

Fig. 3.19 (**a**) Large cervical lymph node with irregular lobulated borders, complex echotexture, and loss of fatty hilum. USG-FNA diagnosis was metastatic papillary carcinoma. (**b**) Left cervical lymph node with abnormal US features (heterogenous echotexture, lack of hilum, marked hypoechogenicity, round shape, and irregular borders invading the deep subcutaneous tissue and puckering the skin). USG-FNA diagnosis was metastatic papillary carcinoma. (**c**) Left cervical lymph node (**b**) with diffuse chaotic vascularity by Doppler examination. (**d**) Right cervical lymph node with abnormal features and microcalcifications (right from the carotid artery); notice a right thyroid mass with microcalcifications (left from the carotid artery). USG-FNA diagnosis was metastatic medullary thyroid carcinoma

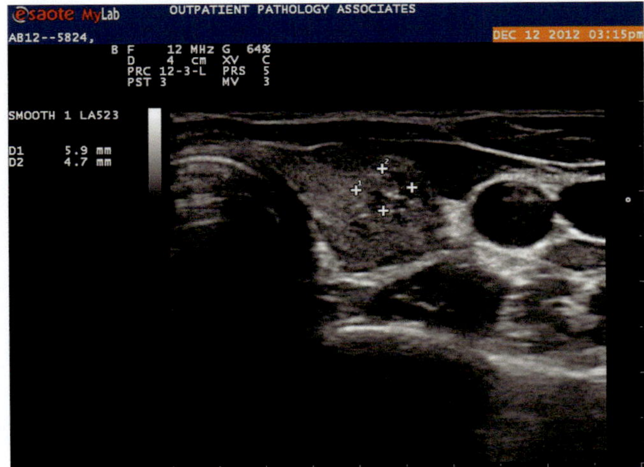

Fig. 3.20 Subcentimeter thyroid nodule with microcalcifications and ill-defined fuzzy margins. USG-FNA diagnosis was papillary thyroid carcinoma

Thyroid USG-FNA Approach

The superficial location of the thyroid gland facilitates tactile examination, US evaluation, and FNA Adequate patient positioning is crucial for achieving success. With the patient in the supine position, a pillow should be placed under the shoulders to produce slight overextension of the neck (Fig. 3.21). Then, US evaluation of both lobes in the transverse and longitudinal planes is performed (Fig. 3.22a, b). Of note, the US evaluation should include the entire neck, looking for abnormal lymph nodes, enlarged parathyroid glands, and other masses. Once a nodule is identified, USG-FNA is performed as described in Chap. 2 (Video 3.3).

USG-FNA is the gold-standard technique for screening and diagnosis of thyroid nodules. USG-FNA is recommended particularly for non-palpable, predominantly cystic, or posteriorly located nodules; however, USG-FNA should be used for sampling of *all* types of thyroid nodules. It is highly accurate in experienced hands and is quick, safe, and cost-effective and can be performed in an outpatient clinic. Contraindications to thyroid USG-FNA are perhaps limited to uncooperative patients and those with a severe bleeding diathesis. Complications are extremely rare and include local hematoma, and nodule infarction particularly in oncocytic neoplasms; we have observed one instance of each case. Needle track seeding of a thyroid malignancy has been reported anecdotally. Of note, the operator should try to avoid possible injury of neck organs, particularly in patients with non-palpable or distorted anatomic landmarks.

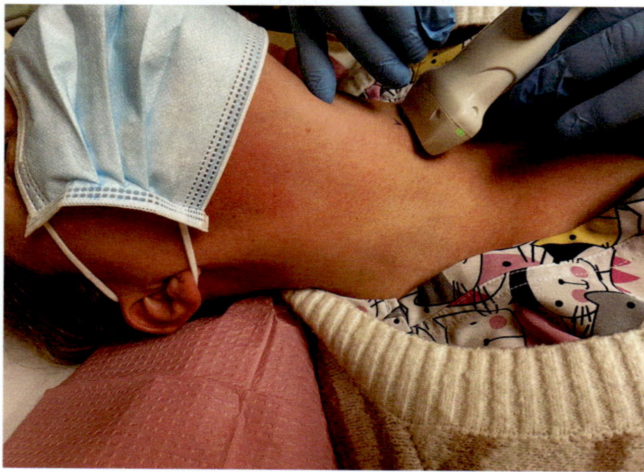

Fig. 3.21 USG-FNA of thyroid by perpendicular approach. There is slight overextension of the neck, which is supported by a pillow placed in the posterior neck/shoulders. The transducer is placed transverse to the midline of the neck and the procedure is performed using a 27-gauge needle (perpendicular approach) without suction (Zajdela Technique)

Advantages of US and USG-FNA

1. The US test is cost-effective, relatively available, and does not involve ionizing radiation.
2. The US test provides the characteristics of the thyroid gland and is of particular use in thyroiditis and hyperthyroidism.
3. The US test identifies and characterizes US features for selecting of the most dominant or the most suspicious nodule to be sampled by USG-FNA.
4. US provides precise needle placement for nodule sampling in obese patients or muscular patients.
5. US provides visualization and sampling of non-palpable or small nodules with high accuracy, making sure the needle tip is within the nodule.
6. *Drainage of fluid in cystic lesions*. Careful needle guidance to the cystic component for drainage of the fluid will allow better visualization and sampling of the residual solid-phase component after drainage (Fig. 3.23a, b and Video 3.4). Initial avoidance of the solid component is important to avoid intra-lesional bleeding in highly vascular lesions; fluid should be drained first (Fig. 3.24 and Video 3.5). The cyst fluid should be processed by centrifugation followed by smear preparations of the sedimented pellet or by liquid-based techniques aimed mainly at ruling out a cystic subtype of PTC.
7. *Sampling of highly vascular lesions*. Nodules with central vascularity by Doppler US usually yield bloody aspirates. The amount of blood present in the smears is directly proportional to the needle caliber, syringe suction, and dwelling time. Excellent samples can be obtained by performing the Zajdela technique (no syringe suction) with 27-gauge (0.4 mm diameter) needles, and monitoring of intranodular needle motion as mentioned in Chap. 2. These steps minimize blood contamination and increase the likelihood of a diagnostic aspirate (Fig. 3.25a–d and Video 3.6).

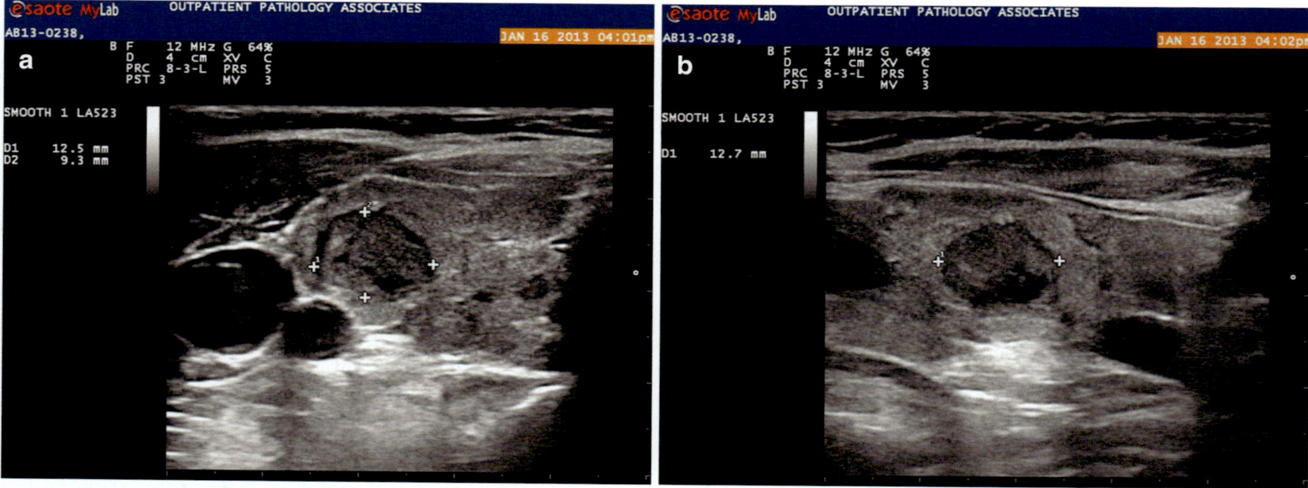

Fig. 3.22 Transverse (**a**) and longitudinal (**b**) views of a right thyroid nodule. The USG-FNA diagnosis was benign thyroid nodule

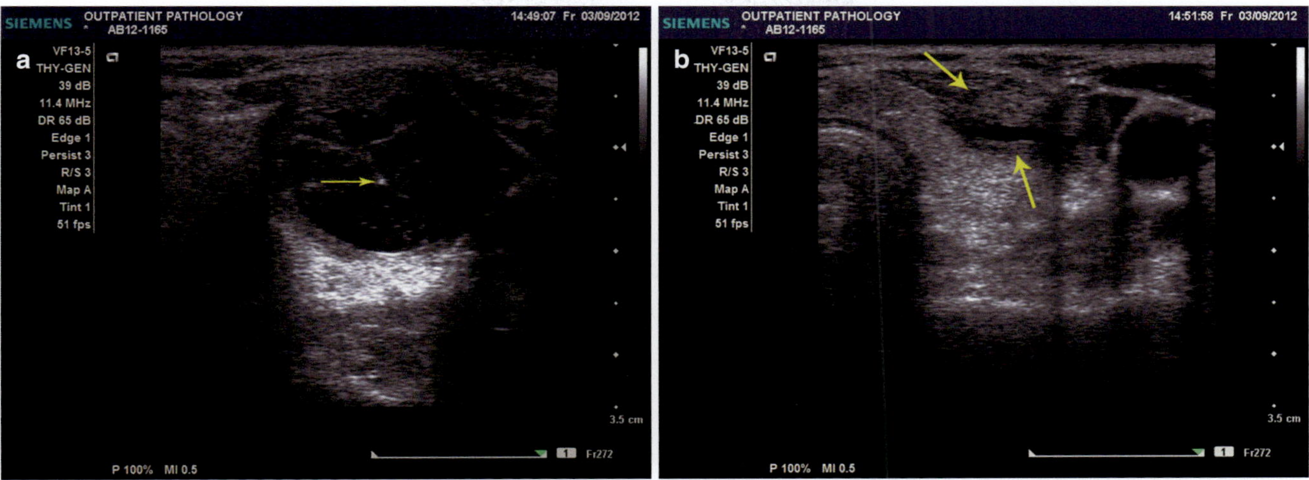

Fig. 3.23 (**a**) Cystic nodule with posterior acoustic enhancement. Tip of needle (arrow) is visualized in the transverse plane. (**b**) Almost totally collapsed cystic nodule after fluid drainage. USG-FNA diagnosis of the solid component was benign

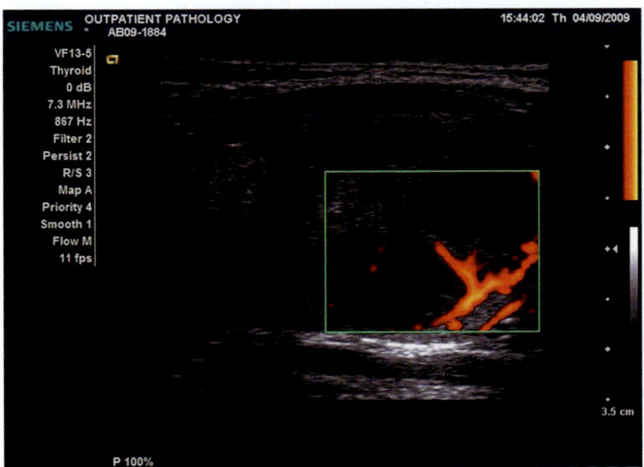

Fig. 3.24 Cyst drainage is needed to accurately sample the posterior vascular solid component and avoid smear dilution with blood and cyst contents. USG-FNA diagnosis was papillary thyroid carcinoma

8. Sampling of hypoechoic areas or suspicious features in heterogeneous nodules, i.e., microcalcifications, high vascular flow, etc. (Fig. 3.26a–d and Videos 3.7, 3.8, 3.9 and 3.10).
9. USG-FNA increases the diagnostic accuracy, sensitivity, and specificity of palpation guided-FNA in the diagnosis of thyroid nodules. For thyroid nodules with a benign FNA diagnosis, the false-negative rate is higher with palpation FNA (2%–5%) than with USG-FNA (0.6% in my experience).

The use of the Zajdela technique is most useful particularly for evaluating small thyroid nodules. The needle grip provides an excellent control for sampling of the lesion and adds an exquisite degree of sensitivity to perceiving the tissue texture changes along the path the needle travels, to the point that the operator is able to "feel" when the periphery of the target is penetrated.

Important Concepts in Thyroid FNA

- All FNA samples must be well-preserved and well-prepared for interpretation.
- The size of normal follicular epithelial cell nuclei is about the size of a red blood cell or lymphocyte (8–10 μm in diameter). The diameter of a normal three-dimensional follicle averages 200 μm (Fig. 3.27a–d). Thus, the inner diameter of a 27-gauge needle allows for the passage of such structures or even small stromal-epithelial fragments.
- The adequacy of an FNA specimen is dictated by the presence of a minimum of six groups of at least ten follicular epithelial cells each, preferably in each smear.
- Cyst fluid with less than six groups of ten follicular cells may be considered nondiagnostic.
- The presence of *thick colloid* reliably identifies most benign processes and overrules the absence or paucity of follicular epithelial cells, and the specimen is considered adequate (Fig. 3.28).
- Inflammatory entities such as thyroiditis or a thyroid abscess do not require the presence of follicular elements for specimen adequacy.
- If cytologic atypia is seen, it must be reported regardless of specimen adequacy, including cell count.
- Poorly prepared, poorly stained, or obscured follicular cells are considered nondiagnostic specimens (Fig. 3.29a–c).
- The numbers of follicular cell clusters or sheets may not be important for specimen adequacy in liquid-based smears. A total individual count of 180–320 cells has been proposed as sufficient. Further validation of these findings is needed. We discourage the use of liquid-based cytology in thyroid nodules, except for evaluating cyst fluid.

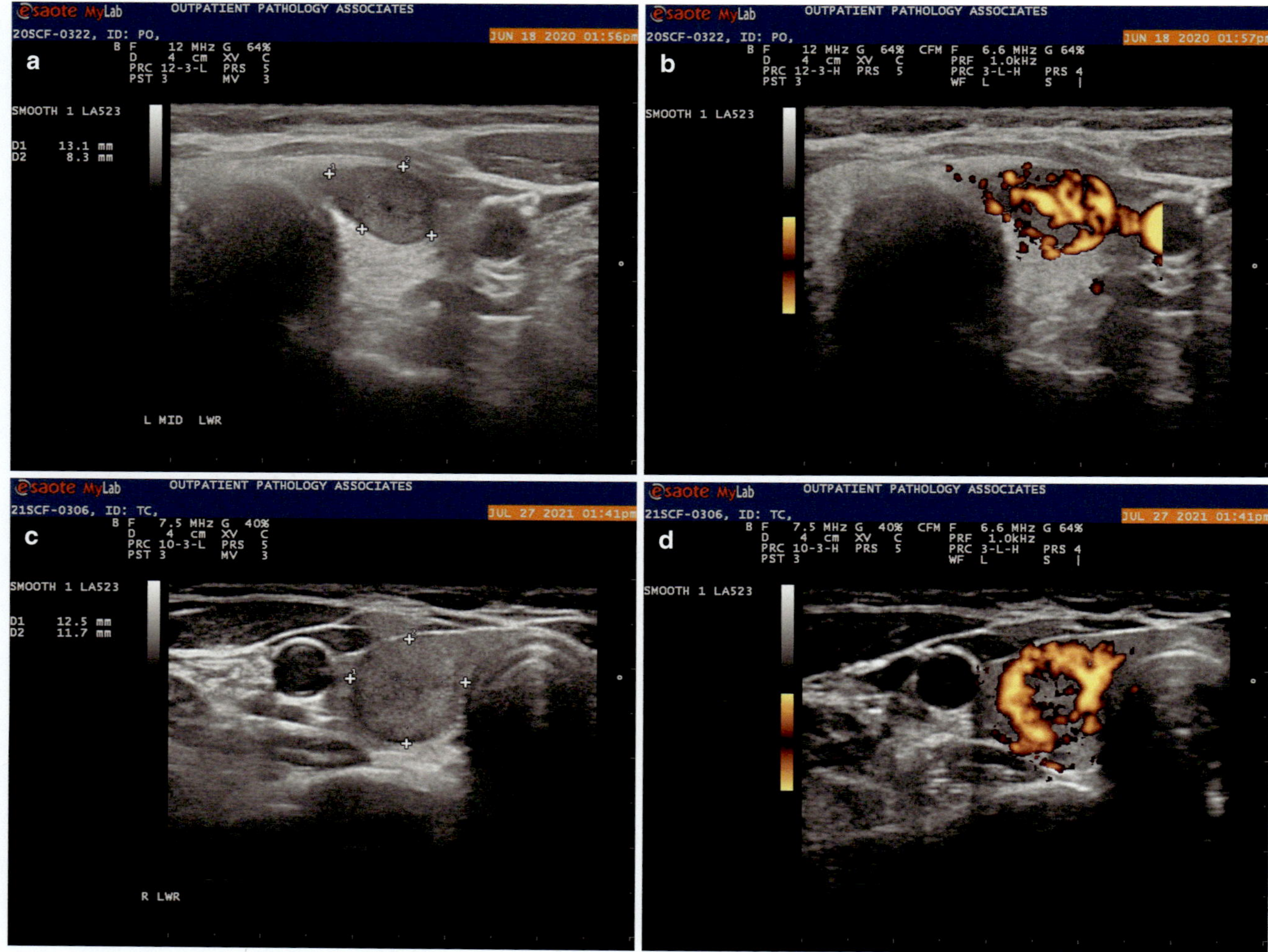

Fig. 3.25 (**a**–**d**) Two solid vascular hypoechoic nodules with smooth margins. USG-FNA was Bethesda category 4 (follicular neoplasm)

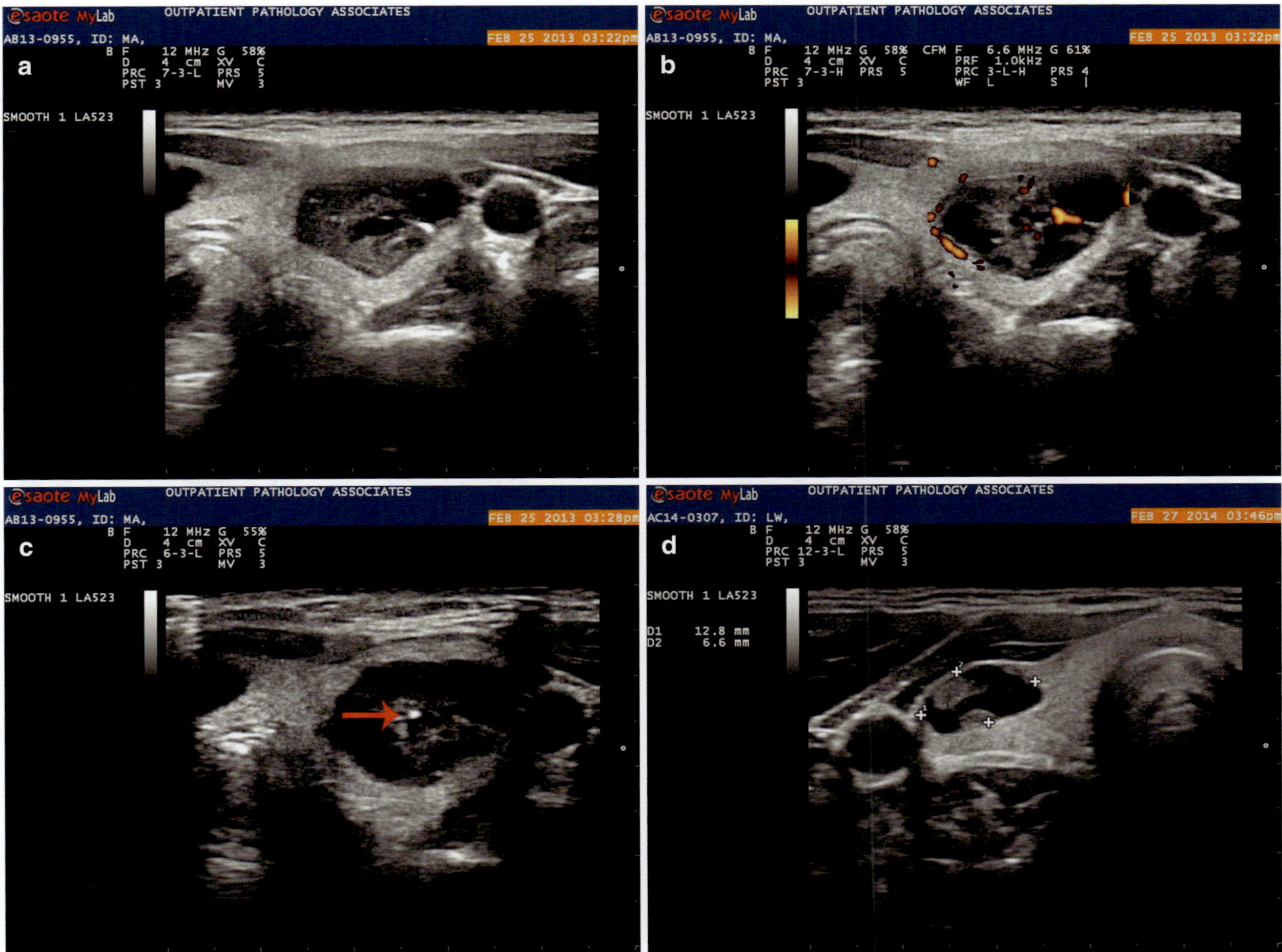

Fig. 3.26 (**a**) Complex solid and cystic left thyroid nodule. (**b**) The central solid component has increased vascular blood flow by Doppler examination. (**c**) Needle tip (arrow) samples the solid component. USG-FNA diagnosis was papillary thyroid carcinoma with prominent cystic change. (**d**) Small complex nodule with slightly hypoechoic mural solid component. USG-FNA diagnosis was benign

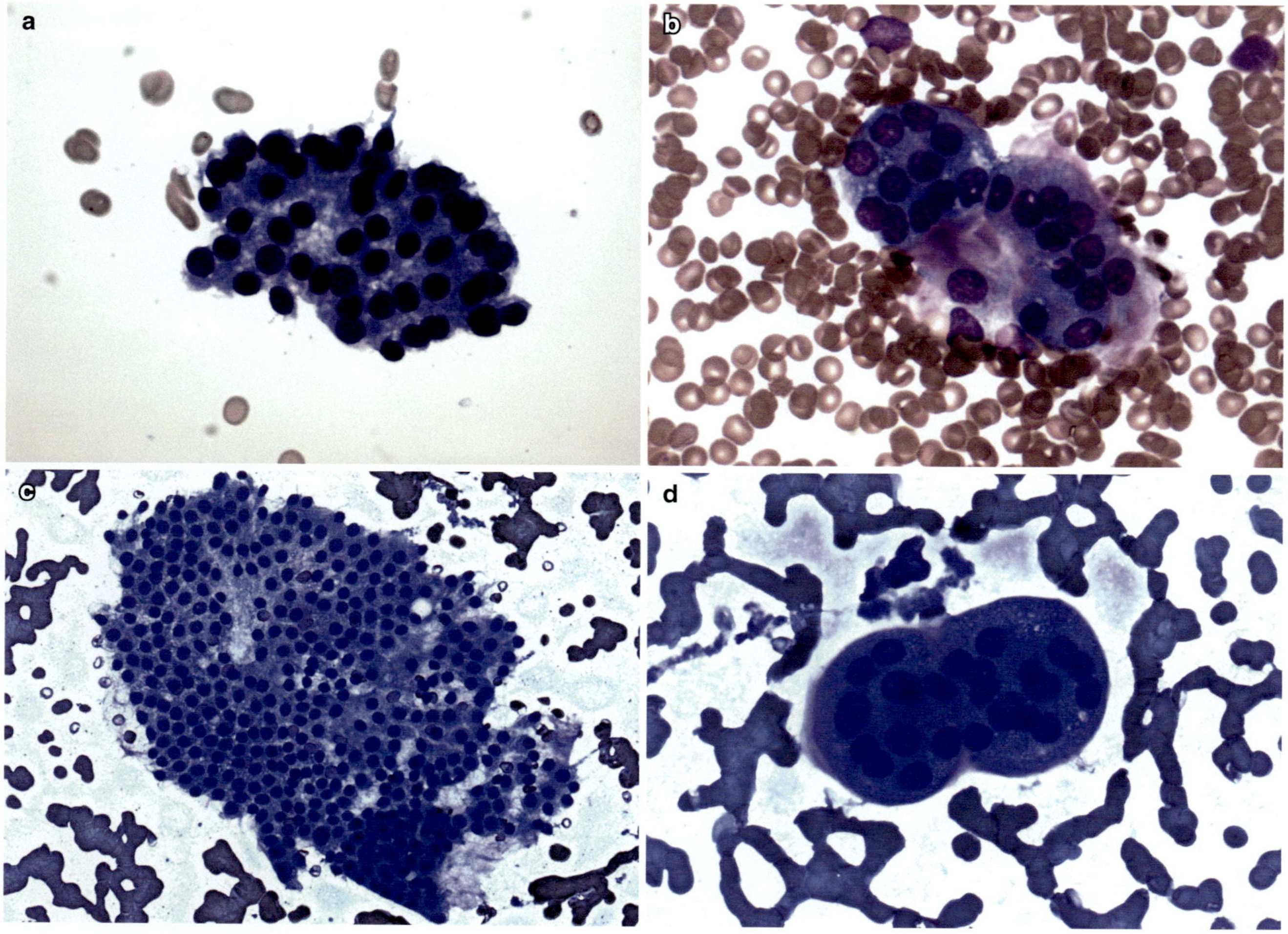

Fig. 3.27 Benign follicular cell sheet (**a**) and partially ruptured benign atrophic thyroid follicle (**b**). Large cell sheet that corresponds to a macrofollicle (**c**). Two intact small thyroid follicles (**d**). The nuclear sizes of the follicular cells are similar or slightly larger than those of red blood cells. (**a**, **b**, **d**, MGG stain, high power; **c**, MGG stain medium power)

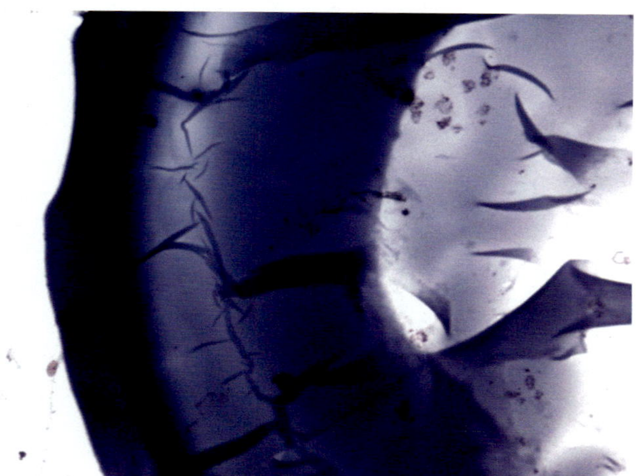

Fig. 3.28 Thick colloid. (MGG stain, low power)

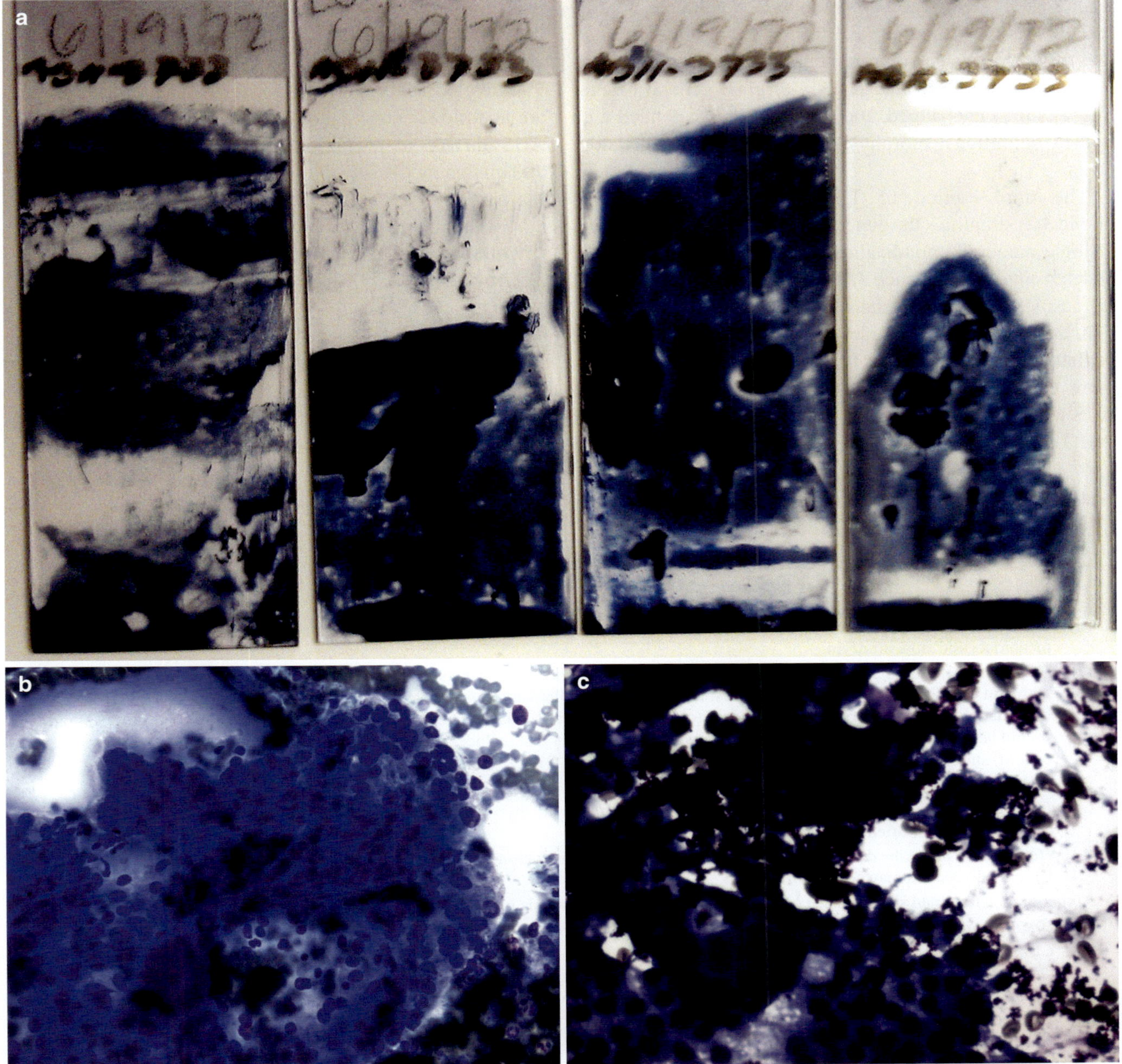

Fig. 3.29 (**a**) Non-diagnostic smear with extensive clotting. (**b**) Obscuring blood clot and fibrin strands. (**c**) Obscuring ultrasound gel. (**b, c**, MGG stain medium power)

USG-FNA and the Bethesda System for Reporting Thyroid FNA Cytology (TBSRTC)

The National Cancer Institute (NCI) sponsored the NCI Thyroid Fine Needle Aspiration (FNA) State of the Science Conference on October of 2007 in Bethesda, MD. Six committees were formed to review (1) indications/pre-FNA requirements, (2) training and credentialing, (3) technique, (4) terminology and morphologic criteria, (5) ancillary studies, and (6) post-FNA options for testing and treatment. Results were included in the first edition of TBSRTC that included six general categories: (1) nondiagnostic, (2) benign, (3) atypia of undetermined significance or follicular lesion of undetermined significance, (4) follicular neoplasm or suspicious for a follicular neoplasm, (5) suspicious for malignancy, and (6) malignant.

The second edition of TBSRTC, published in 2017 included revised clinical guidelines for the management of patients with thyroid nodules, the introduction of molecular testing as an adjunct to cytopathologic evaluation, and the reclassification of noninvasive follicular variant of PTC as noninvasive follicular thyroid neoplasm with papillary-like nuclear features (NIFTP). The six original general categories remained unchanged, and chapters were expanded with refined definitions, morphologic criteria, and explanatory notes.

The third edition of TBSRTC, published in 2023 (Table 3.2) simplifies the general diagnostic categories under a single name: (1) nondiagnostic, (2) benign, (3) atypia of undetermined significance (AUS), (4) follicular neoplasm, (5) suspicious for malignancy, and (6) malignant. In addition, the third edition provides data of using TBSRTC in the pediatric population, refines the risk of malignancy based on more extensive published data, subcategorizes AUS into AUS with nuclear atypia versus AUS-other, follows the 2022 WHO classification of thyroid neoplasms, incorporates high-grade follicular-derived carcinomas, and covers imaging studies and the use of ancillary tests including molecular studies.

Reported statistics for the various diagnostic categories are as follows: nondiagnostic (10–15%), benign (60–80%), AUS and follicular neoplasm (10–20%), suspicious (3–10%), and malignant (4–10%).

Impact of FNA Diagnosis on Clinical Management

The FNA diagnosis dictates the management modality for patients, including the selection for surgery, with a positive impact on the cancer diagnoses and a negative impact on the number of unnecessary surgeries for benign conditions (Table 3.3).

Table 3.2 TBSRTC (2023) diagnostic categories: significance, common underlying disease processes, and helpful tips for diagnosis

1. Nondiagnostic	
(a)	*Underlying causes.* Virtually acellular specimen, obscuring blood, clotting artifact, drying artifact, etc. Few or no follicular epithelial cells seen in a pure cyst (not colloid cyst), thick or calcified capsule, hypervascular or necrotic lesion, and benign or malignant sclerotic lesions
(b)	*Preventable cause.* Poor technique includes a missed target, obscuring blood, clot artifact, mechanical distortion due to poor smearing technique, and slow-air drying
(c)	*Helpful tips.* Look for stripped atrophic nuclei in the smear edges; look for inconspicuous sheets of atrophic cells in bloody smears with thin colloid; correlate with US features, because simple colloid cysts may yield only colloid and macrophages with no or limited follicular elements. Smears with colloid only (easily identified) are considered benign. Smears with acellular cyst fluid (not colloid) should be interpreted as "cyst fluid only" followed by a comment that includes correlation with US features. If a cyst fluid (not colloid) smear shows atypical cells, the category is AUS
2. Benign thyroid nodule	
(a)	*Underlying causes.* Follicular nodular disease, chronic lymphocytic thyroiditis, subacute thyroiditis, thyroid nodule with cystic change, and colloid-rich benign thyroid nodule
(b)	*Helpful tips.* Make the diagnosis only if there is good cell representation and preservation. PTC may have a prominent cystic change. Chronic thyroiditis may coexist with PTC
3. Atypia of undetermined significance (AUS): Specify if AUS-nuclear atypia or AUS-other (non-nuclear)	
(a)	*Underlying causes.* Follicular nodular disease, lymphocytic thyroiditis, NIFTP, thyroid cancer
(b)	*Cytologic findings.* Nuclear and/or architectural atypia. Microfollicular pattern and/or oncocytic cell pattern in variable proportions. Oncocytic cells forming microfollicles are seen in lymphocytic thyroiditis. Metaplastic cells with squamoid features (may be the cyst lining cells). "Histiocytoid" cells (large cells with abundant multivacuolated cytoplasm and pleomorphic nuclei). Atypical lymphoid cells
(c)	*Helpful tips.* Look for follicular cell sheets (from macrofollicles) comprising >50%–75% of smear cellularity that may indicate a mixed macro- and microfollicular pattern nodule. Look for intact or entangled lymphocytes to exclude lymphocytic thyroiditis. If needed, repeat or perform USG-FNA in not less than 3 months. Consider doing molecular testing; a split sample for cytology and molecular testing should be obtained
4. Follicular neoplasm (specify if oncocytic)	
(a)	*Underlying causes.* Follicular and oncocytic cell neoplasms. Histologic diagnoses include follicular nodular disease, follicular adenoma, NIFTP, follicular subtype of PTC, invasive encapsulated follicular variant (IEFV)-PTC, and follicular thyroid carcinoma (FTC). Rare lesions (paraganglioma, hyalinizing trabecular tumor (HTT), metastatic low-grade carcinomas, and parathyroid neoplasms) have a microfollicular pattern present in variable proportions and must be considered in the differential diagnosis.
(b)	*Cytologic findings.* Hypercellular smears, cell monotony, microfollicular arrangements, significant cell crowding, trabeculae, or dispersed single cells, minimal or absent colloid, subtle nuclear features of PTC, and absent lymphoid cells
(c)	*Helpful tips.* Look for lymphoid cells to exclude chronic thyroiditis. Atrophy mimics microfollicles. Presence of colloid, follicular cell sheets, and oncocytic cells is more in favor of a follicular nodular disease. Most cases show no cellular or nuclear atypia, normal size round nuclei, absent or inconspicuous nucleoli. True papillae, psammoma bodies, and distinct nuclear features of PTC are absent; consider NIFTP, follicular subtype of PTC, or IEFV-PTC if rare nuclear features of PTC are present. Consider the category of oncocytic follicular neoplasm (OFN) if oncocytic cells are present to any significant degree. Oncocytes with nuclear features of PTC are excluded from this category. Make the diagnosis of follicular neoplasm only if there is good cell representation and preservation; otherwise, repeat USG-FNA in not less than 3 months

(continued)

Table 3.2 (continued)

5. Suspicious for malignancy
(a) *Underlying cause*. Usually thyroid malignancy. Except for follicular thyroid carcinoma (FTC) and oncocytic thyroid carcinoma (OTC), most primary thyroid malignancies have features that are easily diagnosed on FNA. Unusual subtypes of PTC or MTC, overlapping cytologic features with other thyroid lesions, NIFTP, HTT, or inability to perform ancillary tests for PTC, MTC, or lymphoproliferative processes are common causes for a suspicious FNA diagnosis
(b) *Cytologic findings*. Cytologic criteria are short for making a malignant diagnosis. Suspicious for PTC (presence of patchy or incomplete nuclear changes, limited cellularity, cystic change). Suspicious for MTC (monomorphic population of small to medium size cells with high N/C ratio, eccentric nuclei, no distinct cytoplasmic granules, scant amyloid that mimics colloid, limited cellularity, inability to perform ancillary tests). Suspicious for lymphoma (limited cellularity, obscuring blood, dissociated atypical lymphoid cells, inability to perform ancillary tests)
(c) *Helpful tips*. Presence of lymphocytes does not exclude PTC. Make the diagnosis only if there is good cell representation and preservation; otherwise, repeat USG-FNA in not less than 3 months for cytomorphology only, or sooner to harvest material for ancillary tests
6. Malignant
(a) *Underlying causes*. Well-differentiated thyroid carcinoma (WDTC) (includes PTC, MTC, and OTC), follicular cell-derived non-anaplastic carcinomas, high grade [includes poorly differentiated thyroid carcinoma (PDTC) and differentiated high-grade thyroid carcinoma (DHGTC)], undifferentiated (anaplastic) carcinoma (ATC), squamous cell carcinoma (SCC), lymphoma, miscellaneous thyroid malignancies, and metastasis
(b) *Cytologic findings*. Cytologic criteria fulfill the diagnosis of malignancy. PDTC commonly shows tumor necrosis, high mitotic activity, solid, insular, and trabecular features, convoluted nuclei, and rare or absent nuclear features for PTC. Prominent oncocytic features are seen in some PDTC. In contrast to PDTC, DHGTC are carcinomas with papillary or microfolllicular features, high mitotic activity, necrosis, nuclear pleomorphism with features of PTC, and lack solid, insular, and trabecular features
(c) *Helpful tips*. Consider PDTC and DHGTC in the presence of necrosis and high mitotic activity. Correlation with US features (PDTC and DHGTC are large tumors with extrathyroidal extension). PDTC and DHGTC can resemble oncocytic neoplasms. PDTC has overlapping features with follicular neoplasms, and in contrast to ATC it lacks marked nuclear pleomorphism, high-grade features, and sarcomatoid features. PDTC with prominent cell dissociation and absent nucleoli resembles MTC. Plasmacytoid features and high cell dissociation may be seen in PDTC suggesting a lymphoproliferative disorder. DHGTC has overlapping features with PTC. PTC has overlapping features mainly with HTT. Degenerative changes, inadequate specimen, and lack of cytopathologist's experience are main causes for a *false-positive* diagnosis

AUS atypia of undetermined significance, *DHGTC* differentiated high-grade thyroid carcinoma, *FVPTC* follicular variant of PTC, *HTT* hyalinizing trabecular tumor, *MTC* medullary thyroid carcinoma, *N/C* nuclear/cytoplasm, *NIFTP* noninvasive follicular thyroid neoplasm with papillary-like nuclear features, *PDTC* poorly differentiated thyroid carcinoma, *PTC* papillary thyroid carcinoma, *TBS* The Bethesda System, *US* ultrasound, *USG-FNA* ultrasound-guided fine needle aspiration

Table 3.3 Clinical Management of Thyroid Nodules Based on the FNA Diagnosis

Diagnosis	Risk of malignancy and management
Nondiagnostic	The risk of malignancy is probably 10%–13%. Repeat FNA under US guidance (unless nodule is purely cystic) in not less than 3 months, perform rapid cytology evaluation, use liquid base cytology, and prepare a cell block in cyst fluid, if available. If again nondiagnostic, close follow-up or surgery may be considered, particularly in the case of solid nodules. Correlation with US and clinical findings is mandatory
Benign	Carries <4% risk of malignancy. The false-negative rate is <3% (<2% by USG-FNA). Clinical follow-up including US in 6–18 months and repeat FNA if nodule volume grows >50% (20% increase in at least 2 dimensions with a minimal increase of 2 mm) or develops US abnormalities
AUS	Carries 36–44% and 15–23% risk of malignancy for AUS with nuclear atypia and AUS with other patterns respectively. Submit smears for thyroid molecular testing by microdissection, if available. Otherwise, repeat USG-FNA in 3 months and perform molecular markers if available
Follicular neoplasm	Carries 70% risk of neoplasm, 20%–50% risk of malignancy (average 30%), and up to 30% risk of non-neoplasm. Thyroid molecular testing results provide management guidance. Lobectomy or total thyroidectomy if the overall evaluation shows a high- or low-risk for malignancy, respectively
Oncocytic follicular neoplasm	Carries 25–50% risk of malignancy. Most nodules are benign. OTCs represent 15–20% of all FTCs. Thyroid molecular testing can provide management guidance. Lobectomy is indicated for precise histologic classification
Suspicious for PTC	Carries 60–75% risk of malignancy. Accounts for approximately 3% of all thyroid FNAs. Thyroid molecular testing results provide management guidance. Lobectomy or total thyroidectomy
Malignant	Carries <1% false-positive diagnosis. Near total or total thyroidectomy. Further diagnostic workup is recommended for anaplastic carcinoma, lymphoma, and metastasis before surgery

US ultrasound, *FNA* fine needle aspiration, *USG* ultrasound guided, *AUS* atypia of undetermined significance, *OTC* oncocytic thyroid carcinoma, *FTC* follicular thyroid carcinoma, *PTC* papillary thyroid carcinoma

The 2022 WHO Classification of Thyroid Tumors

The TBSRTC categories and the thyroid entities described must be correlated with current terminology as described in the 2022 classification of thyroid tumors. Several tumor entities have been renamed. The following are novel histopathologic concepts in the nomenclature, grading, and prognosis of thyroid neoplasms based on pathologic features and molecular profile.

- Benign follicular cell-derived thyroid tumors.
  - Thyroid follicular nodular disease (TFND): it is defined as multifocal benign proliferation with nodular hyperplasia. The term has been coined since it is impossible to distinguish between non-neoplastic and benign neoplastic follicular neoplasms by morphology alone. It comprises nonclonal/hyperplastic and clonal/neoplastic proliferations.
  - Follicular thyroid adenoma (FTA): it is surrounded by a thin capsule that is grossly and histologically complete, lacking capsular, vascular, or thyroid invasion. It is a clonal expansion with *RAS* mutations that are related to its follicular architecture. The pattern may be microfollicular, normofollicular, macrofollicular, trabecular, solid, and/or papillary. No molecular test can differentiate between FTA and follicular thyroid carcinoma (FTC).
  - FTA with papillary architecture (previously named as papillary adenomatous/hyperplastic nodule). These tumors show *TSHR*, *GNAS*, or *EZH1* mutations that distinguish them from FTAs. Other gene alterations may occur in association with DICER1, McCune-Albright, and Carney complex syndromes.
  - Oncocytic thyroid adenoma (OTA): it requires 75% of oncocytic cells present. These tumors show specific genetic alterations including mitochondrial DNA mutations and increased copy number alterations (35% of cases).
- Low-risk follicular cell-derived neoplasms: These tumors have an excellent prognosis with low-risk for recurrences or metastasis. Except for hyalinizing trabecular tumor (HTT), these tumors are mostly *RAS*-driven.
  - NIFTP: this tumor has a microfollicular pattern, PTC-related nuclear atypia, absent BRAF-V600E mutation, and lacks high-grade features (mitoses, necrosis, convoluted nuclei). A subset may harbor *THADA* or *PAX8::PPARG* gene fusions.
  - Follicular thyroid tumor of uncertain malignant potential (FT-UMP): confirmation of vascular and/or capsular invasion is equivocal.
  - Well-differentiated thyroid tumor of uncertain malignant potential (WD-UMP).
  - HTT: it has PTC-related nuclear atypia, trabecular growth pattern, extracellular fibrillary matrix, and specific *PAX8::GLIS1* and *PAX8::GLIS3* fusions.
- Malignant thyroid neoplasms.
  - PTC: *BRAF* mutations are required for the diagnosis, particularly in the columnar cell, tall cell, and hobnail subtypes, which have high risk of lymph node and distant metastasis, local recurrence, and poor outcome. PTCs with high-grade features (mitoses ≥5/10 high power fields and/or necrosis) are diagnosed as DHGTCs. The tumor formerly call cribriform-morular is no longer categorized as a PTC subtype (currently listed as a tumor of uncertain histogenesis). The macrofollicular variant is no longer a subtype of PTC (included in the infiltrative follicular PTC subtype). For "microcarcinomas," it is recommended to include the measurement and subtype.

    Subtypes of PTC (previously called "variants"): infiltrative follicular, tall cell (≥3 times taller than wide in ≥30% of the tumor), columnar cell, hobnail (≥30% hobnail pattern), solid, diffuse sclerosing (no longer considered an aggressive PTC), Warthin-like, oncocytic.
  - Invasive encapsulated follicular variant (IEFV-) PTC: this tumor is no longer a subtype of PTC. It is RAS-driven, has a follicular pattern, and exhibits subtle nuclear features of PTC.

    Minimally invasive (capsular invasion only).

    Encapsulated angioinvasive.

    Widely invasive.
  - Follicular thyroid carcinoma (FTC): this tumor is mostly *RAS*-driven, has a follicular pattern, and lacks nuclear features of PTC. FTCs with high-grade features (mitoses ≥5/10 high power fields and/or necrosis) are diagnosed as DHGTC.

    Minimally invasive (capsular invasion only).

    Encapsulated angioinvasive.

    Widely invasive.
  - Oncocytic thyroid carcinoma (OTC): it requires capsular or vascular invasion and absence of high-grade features (mitoses ≥5/10 high-power fields and/or necrosis). Poorly differentiated OTC carries a poor prognosis. Like OTAs, these tumors show specific genetic alterations including mitochondrial DNA mutations and increased copy number alterations.

    Minimally invasive (capsular invasion only).

    Encapsulated angioinvasive.

    Widely invasive.
  - Differentiated high-grade thyroid carcinoma (DHGTC): term assigned to PTCs and FTCs including OTC with high-grade features. Tumors may be *BRAF*- or *RAS*-driven indicating that the preceding tumor was PTC or FTC, respectively; however, most develop

from aggressive PTCs. Additional genetic abnormalities including *TERT* promoter and *TP53* gene mutations may be present. If a FTC (*RAS*-driven) with solid and trabecular growth, mitoses ≥3/10 high-power fields, and/or necrosis (focal or large comedo-like) it must be diagnosed as poorly differentiated thyroid carcinoma.

> Criteria: (1) Papillary, follicular, or solid growth; (2) Invasive features; (3) Any nuclear cytology; (4) Mitoses ≥5/10 high-power fields and/or necrosis (focal, comedo-like, or large).

- Poorly differentiated thyroid carcinoma (PDTC): Tumors may be *BRAF-* or *RAS*-driven indicating that the preceding tumor was PTC or FTC, respectively; however, they are often derived from *RAS*-driven FTCs and IEFV-PTCs. Mutations in the microRNA master regulator *DICER1* may be seen in these tumors from adolescents. Additional genetic abnormalities including *TERT* promoter and *TP53* gene mutations (aggressive tumor markers) may be present.

  > Criteria: (1) Solid, trabecular, or insular growth; (2) Invasive features; (3) Mitoses ≥3/10 high-power fields, and/or necrosis (focal, comedo-like, or large), and/or convoluted nuclei; (4) No papillary thyroid carcinoma nuclear features; 5) No anaplastic foci.

- Anaplastic thyroid carcinoma (ATC): This tumor is composed of undifferentiated cells. Molecular testing is recommended in all cases to look for *BRAF*-V600E mutation; patients benefit of targeted therapy with BRAF and MEK inhibitors.

  > Squamous cell carcinoma (SCC) of thyroid; currently classified as a subtype of ATC; most tumors show *BRAF*-V600E mutation.
  >
  > ATC with anaplastic features.
  >
  > ATC, undifferentiated phenotype.

- Thyroid C cell-derived carcinoma: Medullary thyroid carcinoma (MTC) is driven predominantly by *RET* and *RAS* mutational alterations. The grading (low-grade and high-grade) is based on surgically excised specimens and includes elevated mitotic count, tumor necrosis, and Ki67 proliferation index.

  > High-grade MTC: It must show at least one of mitotic count ≥5/10 high-power fields, tumor necrosis, and Ki67 proliferation index >5%. It comprises 10–20% of cases.
  >
  > Low grade MTC: lacks elevated mitotic count, tumor necrosis, and high Ki67.

- Salivary gland-type tumors of the thyroid: both have specific gene fusions.

  > Mucoepidermoid thyroid carcinoma (METC): it has a specific *CRTC1::MAML2* gene fusion and is positive for p63 and CK5.

> Secretory carcinoma: it has a specific *ETV6::NTRK3* gene fusion and is positive for GATA3, mammaglobin, GCDFP15, and S100 protein; TTF1 and TG are negative.

- Intrathyroidal thymic tumors.
  - Intrathyroid thymoma.
  - Intrathyroid thymic carcinoma: this term designates the formerly known as "thyroid carcinoma showing thymic-like differentiation." It may display *TERT* promoter mutations (absent in mediastinal thymic carcinomas).
- Tumors of uncertain histogenesis.
  - Cribriform-morular thyroid carcinoma (CMTC): it is no longer considered as a subtype of PTC (it lacks the *BRAF-V600E* mutation). Tumor shows *APC* and *CTNNB1* gene mutations (Wnt/beta-catenin pathway) and shows nuclear positivity for beta-catenin, estrogen receptor, and progesterone receptor. TG and TTF1 (follicular differentiation markers) are negative. The cribriform component is focally TTF1 positive, but the morular component is negative.
  - Sclerosing mucoepidermoid carcinoma with eosinophilia: it is presumed to arise from the ultimobranchial body remnant or squamous metaplasia. TG and PAX8 are negative.; TTF1 may be seen focally. Genetic alterations include *MET* hyperploidy and *APC*, *NTRK3*, and *NF1* mutations.
- Other tumors.
  - Thyroblastoma: include teratomas or carcinosarcomas with *DICER1* mutations.
  - Extra-nodal marginal zone lymphoma (E-MZL): preferred term for (mucosa associated lymphoid tissue) MALT lymphoma.

TERT promoter, *TP53*, cell cycle genes, chromatin remodeling genes, and mismatch genes increase the risk of developing aggressive thyroid cancer.

FNA Diagnosis of Benign Thyroid Nodule

A benign thyroid nodule is the most common (70%) condition of the thyroid gland in adults and children. The diagnosis of the specific entity cannot be made on FNA cytology only, but needs clinical correlation, and the patient is followed up conservatively.

Thyroid Follicular Nodular Disease

The term "thyroid follicular nodular disease" (TFND) has been recommended by the 2022 WHO classification of thyroid neoplasms to refer to the spectrum of changes formerly designated as colloid nodule, hyperplastic nodule, adenomatous nodule, benign follicular nodule, and adenomatous hyperplasia. It can be endemic (related to iodine deficiency in the diet) or sporadic (unknown cause). Incidental carcinoma is seen in 5%, usually invasive encapsulated follicular variant (IEFV)-PTC and in 15% papillary microcarcinoma.

Clinical Findings Patients, usually women are euthyroid and have a visible goiter.

Histopathology The nodules may have macrofollicles, microfollicles, and areas of follicles with oncocytic cell changes and even a papillary architecture ["follicular thyroid adenoma (FTA) with papillary architecture"]. Rupture of the follicles may produce a foreign body-type granulomatous reaction to the colloid). Calcification and fresh and old hemorrhage can be seen. Chronic inflammation is variably seen and is usually related to the development of hypothyroidism.

Molecular Profile Monoclonality, cytogenetic abnormalities, aneuploidy, and oncogenic mutations have been seen in some hyperplastic nodules. *DICER1* and *PTEN* mutations may be present. Thus, these nodules may or may not be clonal and there is debate whether hyperplastic nodules are in fact neoplastic.

FNA Findings Common findings include colloid of variable quantity and/or quality, and variable numbers of benign follicular epithelial cells, oncocytic cells, macrophages, and lymphocytes. Abundant colloid and scant cellularity are seen in the so-called colloid nodule; scant colloid and moderate cellularity are seen in the so-called adenomatoid/hyperplastic nodule. Follicular cells may be arranged in monolayer sheets, spheres, intact follicles, or singly. Follicular cell nuclei are the size of a red blood cell or small lymphocyte and have a uniform granular chromatin. The amount of cytoplasm is variable and may range from hyperplastic to atrophic, commonly seen as stripped small nuclei. The nucleolus is small or inconspicuous. Nuclear changes below the level of atypia may be seen as a hyperplastic change and following radioiodine treatment. Green-black cytoplasmic lipofuscin and/or hemosiderin pigment granules may be identified. Occasional microfollicles may be seen, usually comprising less than 10% of the cell representation. Papillary fragments with no cellular features of PTC (hyperplastic nodule) are seen in occasional cases and the possibility of FTA with papillary architecture must be suggested. Cyst lining cells with reparative and metaplastic features may be present in cystic nodules; the recognition is important to avoid a misdiagnosis of cystic subtype of PTC (Fig. 3.30a–d). An oncocytic thyroid (OT) neoplasm [adenoma (OTA) and carcinoma (OTC)] should be considered in cellular specimens, absent colloid, and the exclusive or almost exclusive presence of oncocytic

cells; large cell dysplasia and transgressing blood vessels do not distinguish between OTA or OTC (Fig. 3.31a–d). Consider FTA, FTC, follicular subtype of PTC, IEFV-PTC, and NIFTP in the presence of a microfollicular pattern; search for nuclear features of PTC must be conducted. Colloid should be distinguished from amyloid (MTC and amyloid goiter that is seen in primary or secondary amyloidosis).

US Features (Fig. 3.32a–d and Video 3.11)
- Solid, usually isoechoic nodules with well-defined margins.
- Presence of comet tails, the result of crystals of desiccated colloid.
- Cystic degeneration is common.
- Heterogenous echogenicity. Spongiform pattern.
- Calcifications are coarse or curved, peripheral, or dysmorphic.
- Rare microcalcifications can occur in 5% of nodules.
- Variable vascularity, often absent or perinodular.
- TFND has no distinct US features.

Graves' Disease

Graves' disease (diffuse toxic goiter) is an autoimmune process that targets the thyroid follicles. Thyroid-stimulating immunoglobulin (TSI) and thyrotropin-binding inhibitor immunoglobulin (TBII) are involved in the pathogenesis of this disease. Patients develop autoantibodies to thyroid peroxidase, TG, and TSH receptor; this stimulates the TSH receptor and increases the production of thyroid hormone. Thymic hyperplasia may be seen.

Clinical Findings Diffuse toxic goiter occurs more frequently in young females and is accompanied by hyperthyroidism, exophthalmos in 25–50% of cases, and dermopathy including pretibial myxedema. Men are usually older. It can also occur in children. The gland shows mild to moderate symmetric, diffuse enlargement; however, large and/or cold thyroid nodules may be present and may be targeted by USG-FNA. Other causes of hyperthyroidism include "toxic" follicular adenoma, "toxic" sporadic nodular goiter, various thyroiditides, and iatrogenic causes such as amiodarone.

Histopathology There is follicular hyperplasia with small follicles with scant thin colloid and occasional papillary fronds. When colloid is present, it shows peripheral scalloping. The lining epithelium is columnar with nuclear hyperchromasia and usually clear cytoplasm. Lymphoid follicles are present in the stroma, which has prominent vascularity. In late stages, the gland is nodular with oncocytic changes, fibrosis, and follicular atrophy. Incidental microcarcinomas

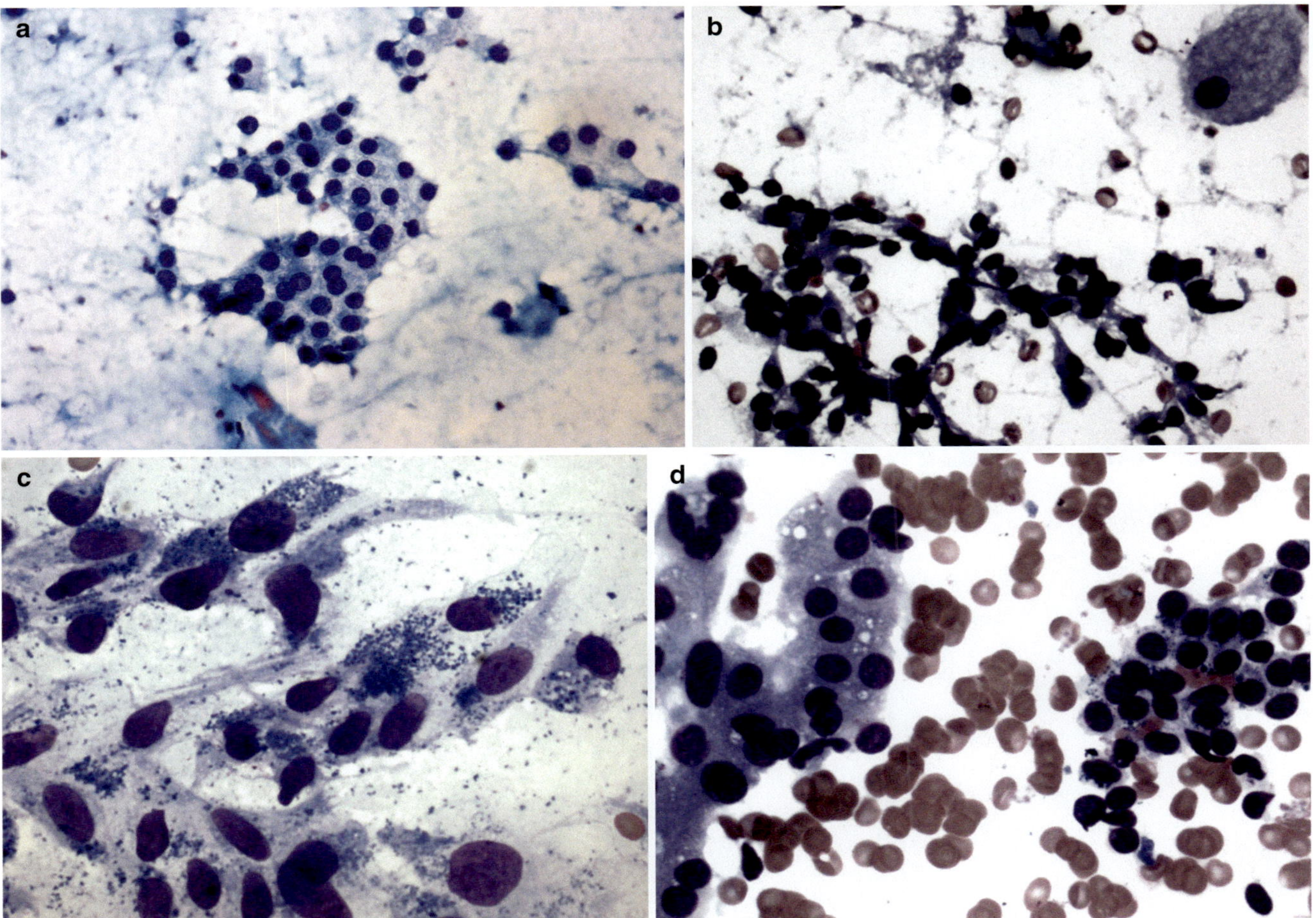

Fig. 3.30 Thyroid follicular nodular disease (benign thyroid nodule) (a) Sheets of follicular epithelial cells and colloid. (b) Atrophic follicular cells, colloid, and macrophages indicating cystic change. (c) Cohesive cyst lining cells with elongated and "reparative" appearance and cytoplasmic lipochrome granules. (d) Sheets of cells with oxyphilic (left) and atrophic (right) changes. (a, Papanicolaou stain, high power; b–d, MGG stain, high power)

of papillary type have been found in Graves' disease with an incidence equal to that found in normal glands.

Molecular Profile Genes associated are *HLA, CD40, CTLA-4, thyroglobulin, TSH receptor*, and *PTPN22*.

FNA Findings Cytologic features are similar to those of TFND. Smears are usually cellular, showing sheets of cohesive cuboidal or columnar cells with abundant slightly clear cytoplasm, a round nucleus, and conspicuous nucleoli. A few microfollicular aggregates, lymphocytes, and oncocytes may be seen. Romanowsky stained smears may show follicular cells with microlobulated cytoplasmic borders/microvacuoles exhibiting accentuated red-pink edges; however, they are not specific for Graves' disease and may be seen in other benign and malignant thyroid conditions. Smears from patients treated with radioactive therapy may have significant architectural and cytologic reactive changes (Fig. 3.33a, b).

US Features (Fig. 3.33c, d)

- The gland is enlarged and may show normal echotexture, but it is usually hypoechogenic, corresponding to the lymphoid infiltrates and decreased amounts of colloid seen histologically. Occasionally, the parenchyma shows small 2–3 mm hypoechoic foci.
- Blood flow is increased (thyroid "inferno") on Doppler examination.
- The incidence of benign thyroid nodules and thyroid cancer in Graves' disease equals that seen in the general population.

Dyshormonogenetic Goiter

This type of goiter (clinical diagnosis) is caused by genetically determined errors in thyroid hormone synthesis and metabolism, in part due to loss-of-function mutation genes.

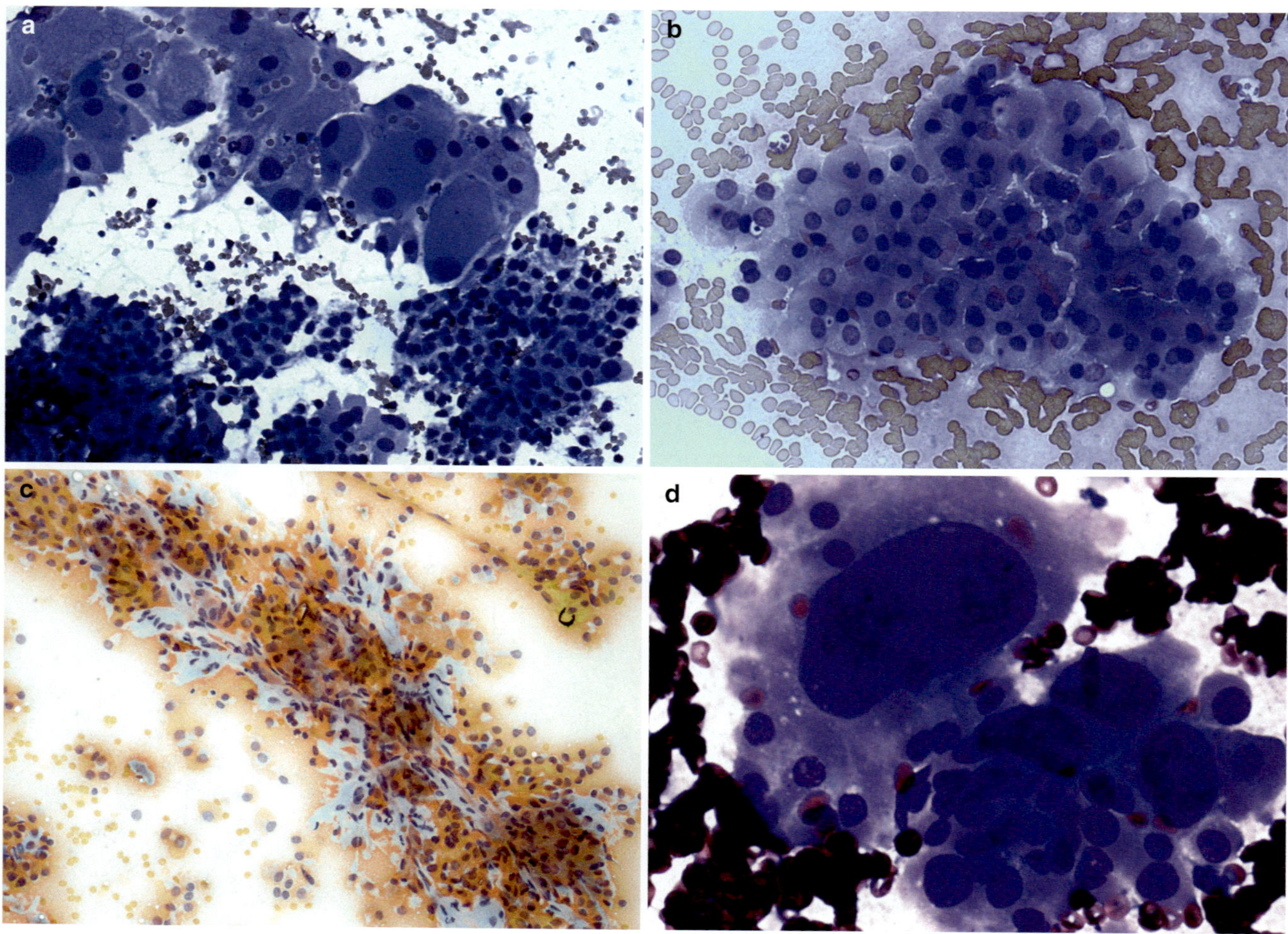

Fig. 3.31 Oncocytic cells, colloid, and sheets of benign follicular cells are seen in these two different cases of thyroid follicular nodular disease (benign thyroid nodules) with oncocytic features (**a**, **b**). Transgressing capillaries (**c**) are present and diagnosed "follicular neoplasm, oncocytic." Similarly, this other nodule measured 1.1 cm that showed large atypical oncocytic cells (**d**) was diagnosed "follicular neoplasm, oncocytic." Final histopathology diagnoses were "oncocytic adenoma" in both (**c** and **d**). (**a**, MGG stain, low power; **b**, MGG stain, medium power; **c**, Papanicolaou stain, medium power; **d**, MGG stain, high power)

Histopathology The thyroid gland is large and nodular and histologically shows a solid and microfollicular pattern with mild cytologic atypia, rare mitoses, and a scant amount of colloid. Rare cases of FTA and FTC, and even rarer cases of PTC have been reported in patients with dyshormonogenetic goiter.

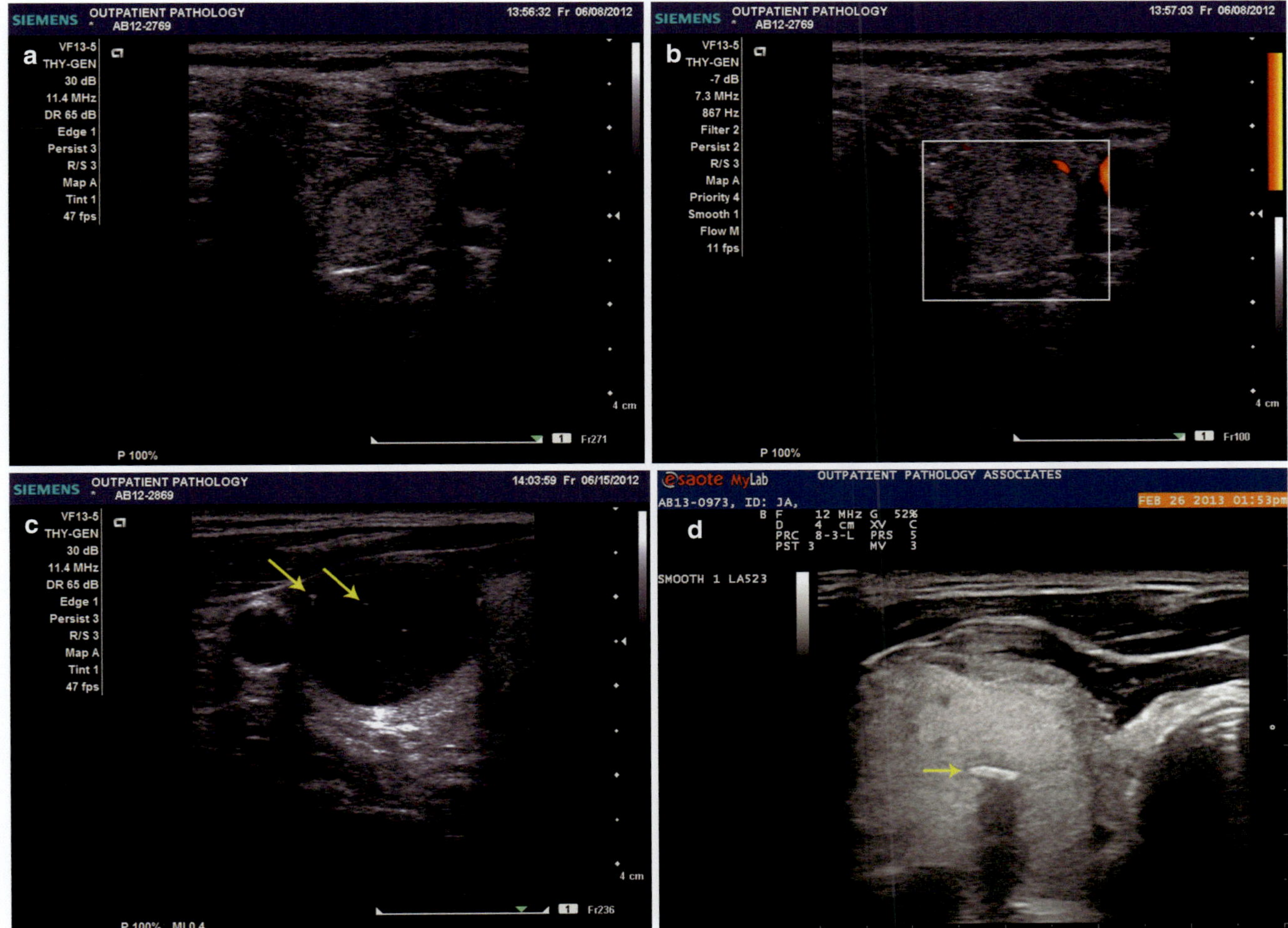

Fig. 3.32 Ultrasound features of thyroid follicular nodular disease (benign thyroid nodules). (**a, b**) Isoechoic nodule with well-defined margins, thick halo, and minimal focal peripheral vascular blood flow by Doppler examination. (**c**) Hypoechoic predominantly cystic nodule with comet tails (arrows). (**d**) Coarse curve-shaped calcification (arrow) with posterior shadow in a hyperechoic nodule

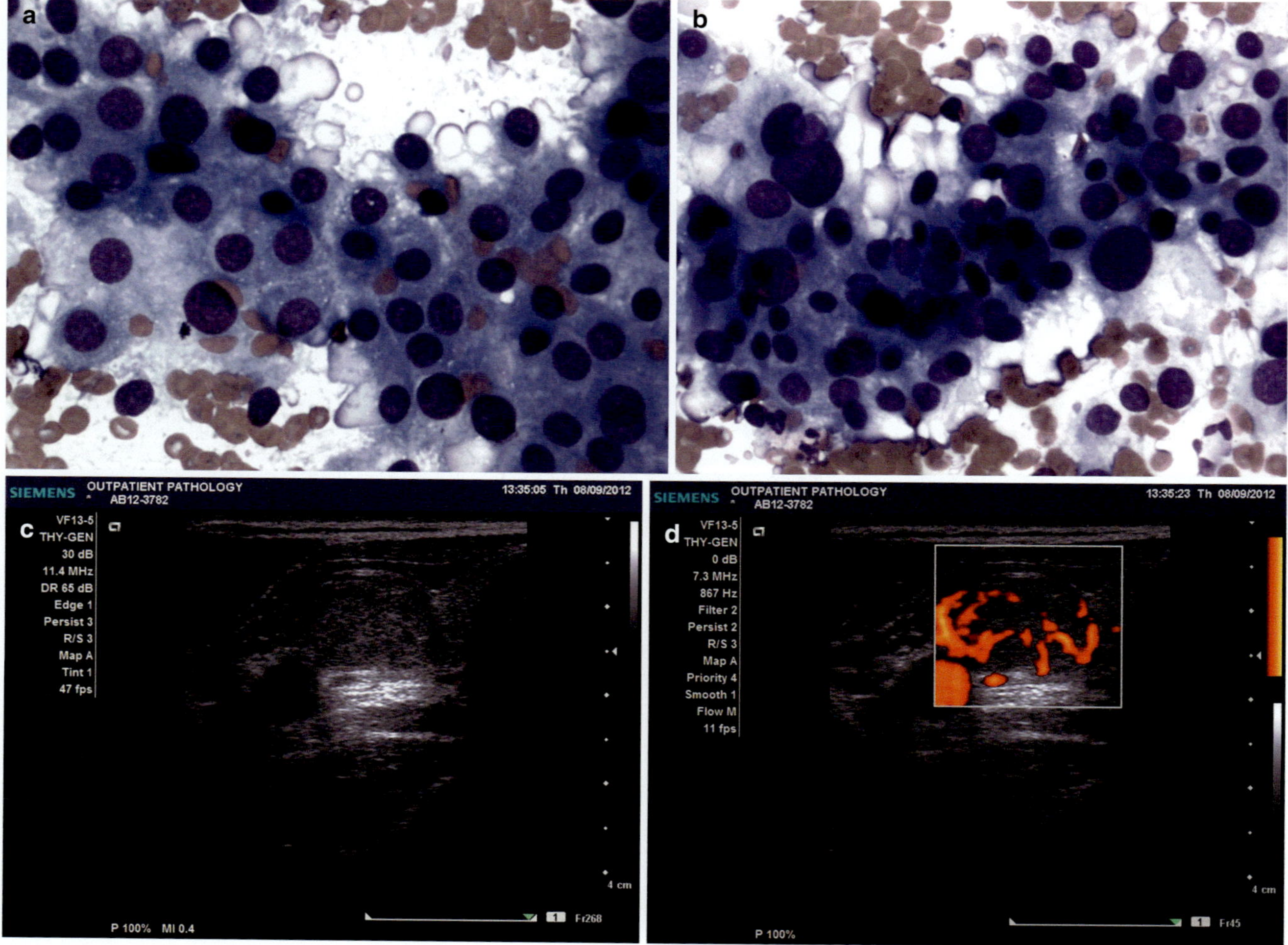

Fig. 3.33 Treated Graves' disease. (**a**, **b**) Slightly complex sheets of large cells with slightly granular cytoplasm, prominent anisocytosis and anisonucleosis, and microlobulated cytoplasmic borders/microvacuoles exhibiting accentuated red-pink edges. (MGG stain, high power). (**c**, **d**) There is an ill-defined slightly hypoechogenic nodule in the right thyroid lobe with increased vascular blood flow by Doppler examination

FNA Diagnosis of Thyroiditis

All forms of thyroiditis are more common in women than in men. They can be classified as autoimmune (chronic lymphocytic or Hashimoto's), subacute granulomatous (De Quervain's), subacute lymphocytic, acute suppurative, and chronic fibrous (Riedel's) thyroiditides. Rare causes of granulomatous thyroiditides include tuberculosis, localized or systemic sarcoidosis, Wegener's granulomatosis, Langerhans cell histiocytosis, foreign-body reactions, and "palpation" thyroiditis.

Ultrasonography is helpful in evaluation of the echotexture of the gland and the presence of nodules. The US characteristics of thyroiditis are variable along the course of the disease and may show focal or diffuse hypoechogenicity. If diffuse, the parenchyma also looks heterogeneous, with hyperechoic streaks representing fibrosis. Likewise, once the inflammatory process improves or resolves, the US appearance of the thyroid gland is also variable, ranging from normal to hypoechoic nodular or atrophic.

Thyroiditides have distinct cytologic findings allowing for a specific FNA diagnosis in most cases.

Autoimmune (Chronic Lymphocytic and Hashimoto's) Thyroiditis

Clinical Findings Autoimmune thyroiditis is a clinicopathologic and serologic entity that shows varying degrees of thyroid dysfunction, diffuse lymphocytic infiltration of thyroid tissue, and positive serum thyroid autoantibodies to thyroid peroxidase (TPO), TG, and TSH receptors. However, serology may be negative in rare cases.

Hashimoto's thyroiditis commonly affects women over the age of 40 years as well as children and adolescents who present with diffuse symmetric, slightly asymmetric, or multinodular goiter. Mild hyperthyroidism usually occurs in the initial phases of the disease process, and hypothyroidism in late stage. Hashimoto's thyroiditis is the leading cause of hypothyroidism in areas with no iodine-deficient diet. It is commonly associated with autoimmune processes in other organs (Addison disease, type 1 diabetes mellitus, Sjogren syndrome, systemic lupus erythematosus, pernicious anemia, myasthenia gravis, vitiligo, celiac disease) and it predisposes to the development of lymphoma. The rate of epithelial malignancy in thyroid nodules in a background of Hashimoto's thyroiditis is higher than that in the general population.

Clinicopathologic forms of Hashimoto thyroiditis include classic, fibrous variant, IgG4 form related variant, juvenile form, Hashitoxicosis, and silent (sporadic or postpartum) thyroiditis. Of note, the IgG4 related variant show no systemic manifestations and is confined to the thyroid gland.

Histopathology Presence of diffuse lymphoid infiltration with germinal center formation is characteristic of autoimmune thyroiditis (chronic lymphocytic and Hashimoto's). Small colloid-depleted thyroid follicles lined with "normal" epithelium are seen in lymphocytic thyroiditis, and with "oncocytic" epithelium in Hashimoto's thyroiditis. Hashimoto's thyroiditis also shows plasma cells, histiocytes, and multinucleated giant cells as well as squamous metaplasia and extensive fibrosis. Large cysts lined with metaplastic squamous epithelium and surrounded by hyperplastic lymphoid follicles may be seen. Hyperplastic nodules may be present, particularly in multinodular Hashimoto's thyroiditis; also, a follicular or oncocytic cell adenoma can occur in the same setting. While diffuse reactive cellular changes are commonly seen in autoimmune thyroiditis, microscopic foci of cells showing pronounced architectural and cytologic atypia (lack papillary architecture or intranuclear cytoplasmic invaginations) are not uncommonly seen and are called "follicular epithelial dysplasia," and may be the precursors of PTC.

Immuno-Profile The immunophenotype of oncocytic cells in Hashimoto's thyroiditis and PTC is similar. Thus, these findings may provide an indication that patients with Hashimoto's thyroiditis have a small, but real risk of developing PTC. Medullary thyroid carcinoma is exceedingly rare to occur in a background of autoimmune thyroiditis. In contrast to reactive cellular changes that are negative or weak and focal for HMBE-1, CK19, and galectin-3, "follicular epithelial dysplasia" are positive in 86%, 96%, and 40%, respectively, and support the concept that these lesions are precursors of PTC that shows similar immunoreactivity.

Molecular Profile It is suggested that multiple genes with variable penetrance are involved in the development of autoimmune thyroiditis. Patients who developed PTC in the Chernobyl accident developed associated chronic autoimmune thyroiditis.

FNA Findings Smears are usually cellular, although the presence of follicular or oncocytic cells is not required for specimen adequacy. The background shows a polymorphous population of benign reactive lymphocytes and plasma cells. Lymphoid elements may be entangled with the epithelial cells. Of note, oncocytic cells may have prominent anisonucleosis, which may be a source for an erroneous diagnosis of atypia, oncocytic neoplasm, or even PTC. Lymphoma should be considered in the presence of monomorphic lymphoid cells. The IgG4 related variant shows plasma cells, eosinophiles, and variable fibrosis; high IgG4 serum levels are necessary to confirm the diagnosis (Fig. 3.34a–f).

US Features (Fig. 3.34g–n)

- The US appearance is highly variable and correlates with the progression of histopathologic changes along the course of the disease. The lymphoid and oncocytic cell components appear homogeneous on US, and fibrous tissue elements as hyperechoic septae.
- Early in the course of the disease, the gland appears diffusely enlarged and profoundly hypoechoic, which correlates with lymphocytic infiltration and colloid depletion without fibrosis. Subclinical thyroid dysfunction is common at this stage.
- As the disease progresses, there is mild hyperechogenicity, heterogeneity, and pseudo-micronodularity ("moth-eaten" or cotton weave) that is the result of destruction of thyroid tissue.
- Poorly outlined hypoechoic pseudonodules may be variably present, often transient, and may represent coalescent aggregates of lymphoid cell-rich tissue, which may be surrounded by echogenic septae. A "Swiss-cheese" appearance on US, the result of small cystic lesions, may be seen in the course of the disease.
- Hyperechogenic pseudonodules may be seen in "regenerative" nodules or as a result of aggregated fibrous tissue ("white knight").
- "Detached" nodules of thyroid tissue may be seen in chronic stages (Fig. 3.34, Video 3.12).
- Blood flow is variable; it ranges from absent to normal to increase on Doppler examination.
- The gland is small, atrophic, hypoechoic, and heterogeneous in end-stage disease.
- True distinct hypoechogenic thyroid nodules with or with calcifications may be seen and need USG-FNA sampling to rule out PTC or lymphoma. Cytologic material for confirmatory flow cytometry studies can be easily obtained by this means.
- A "speckled" pattern is occasionally seen and probably needs a USG-FNA, because occasionally the numerous

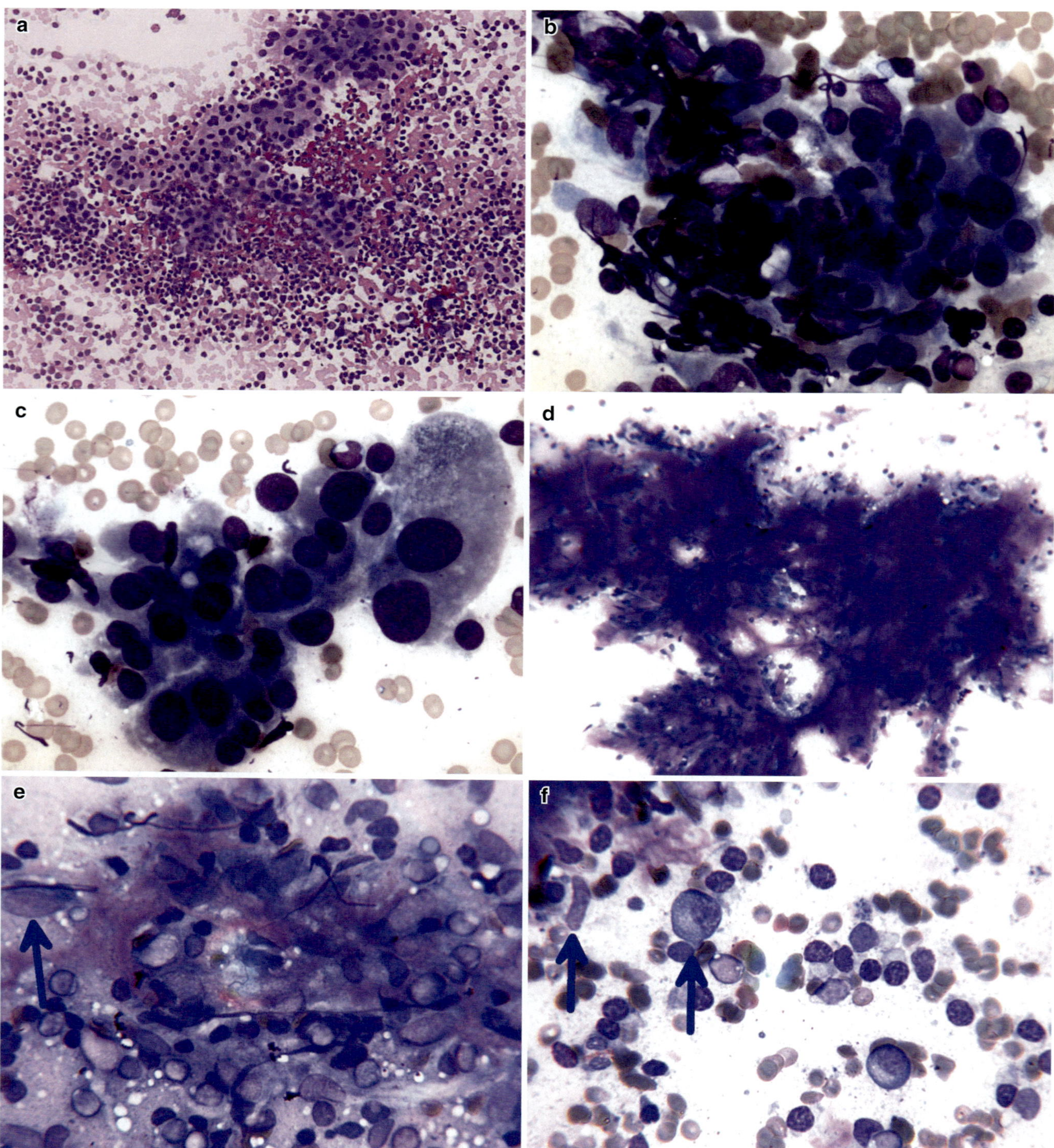

Fig. 3.34 Autoimmune thyroiditis. The smear shows sheets of oncocytic cells and lymphocytes (**a**). The oncocytic cells are both single and clustered, the lymphocytes are both single and entangled with oncocytic cells, and there is lack of colloid (**b**, **c**). Oncocytes, variable fibrosis, and inflammatory cells including plasma cells, lymphocytes and occasional eosinophils are seen in the case of IgG4 variant (**d**–**f**). Ultrasound features show a diffusely enlarged slightly hypoechoic thyroid gland (**g**) and increased blood flow by Doppler examination (**h**). Progressively the gland develops a "moth-eaten" pseudomicronodularity (**i**), echogenic septae surrounding hypoechogenic pseudonodules (**j**), hyperechoic regenerative pseudonodules ("white knight", arrow) (**k**), cobblestone appearance ("giraffe skin") (**l**), and detached pseudonodules (**m**, calipers). Predominantly hyperechoic right thyroid mass with ill-defined margins (**n**) (center arrow indicates the nsampling needle tip, upper arrow indicated the superior border of the mas, and the right arrow shows US features of chronic thyroiditis). (**a**, DiffQuik stain, low power; **b**, **c**, **e**, **f**, MGG stain, high power; **d**, MGG stain, medium power)

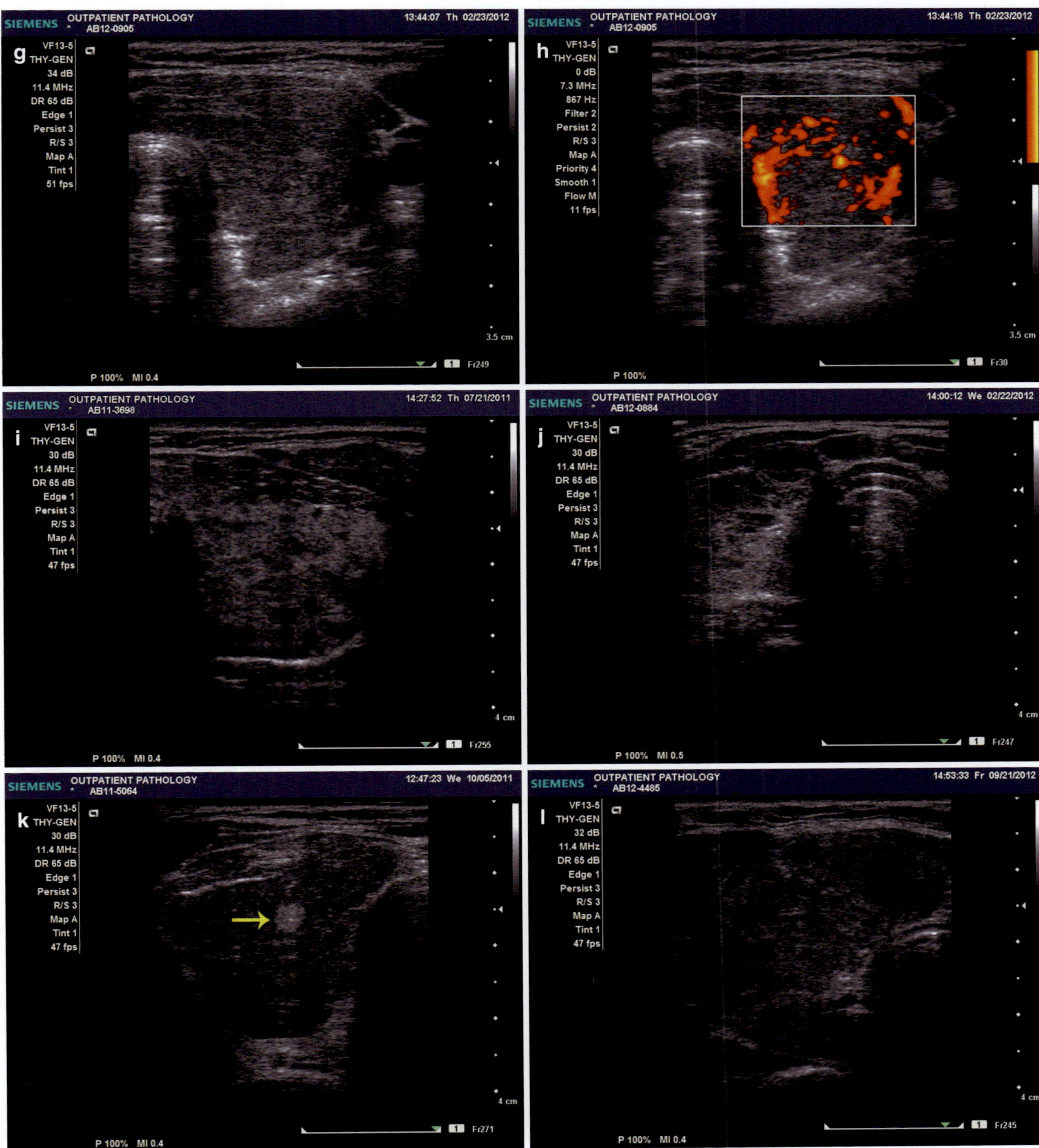

Fig. 3.34 (continued)

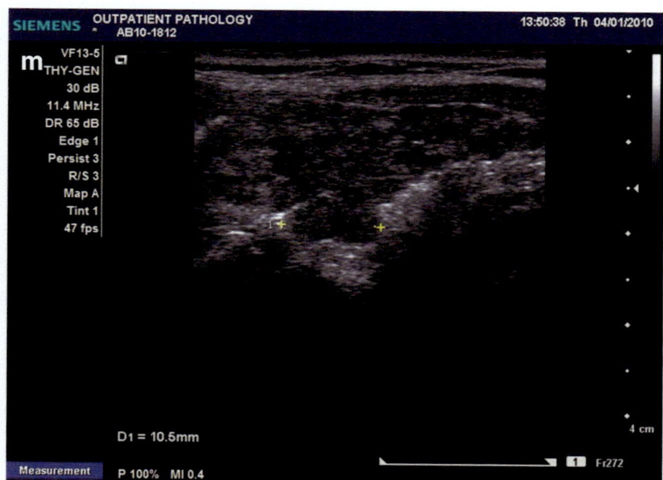
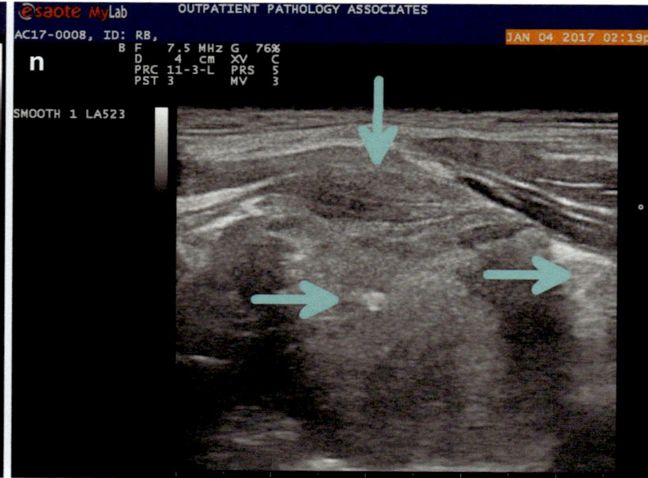

Fig. 3.34 (continued)

"colloid bodies" are difficult to distinguish from the numerous psammoma bodies present in the diffuse sclerosing subtype of PTC.
- Multiple prominent lymph nodes in the central and lateral neck are almost always present.

Subacute Granulomatous (De Quervain's) Thyroiditis

Subacute thyroiditis is a transient self-limited inflammatory process. The etiology is unknown but is generally believed to be of viral origin (mumps, measles, influenza, Coxsackie, Epstein–Barr, and adenovirus). It has been associated with COVID-19 infection. It may also be drug induced.

Clinical Findings Middle-aged women are usually affected and develop a sore throat and anterior lower neck tenderness of rapid onset, accompanied by low-grade fever, myalgias, and malaise. The process commonly follows a viral illness, usually in patients with HLA-Bw35 antigen. The acute phase lasts approximately 1 month with a hyperthyroid stage, followed by several months of hypothyroidism before the patient returns to a euthyroid stage. Thyroid autoantibodies are negative. The glandular involvement is usually asymmetric, and the affected areas are firm.

Histopathology There is a granulomatous inflammatory reaction with multinucleated cells of the giant cell type. Colloid is often seen within the giant cells.

FNA Findings The FNA procedure may be painful, which limits adequate sampling of the nodule. Smears show vari-

able cellularity, multinucleated giant cells with numerous nuclei (usually >100), isolated histiocytes, granulomas, chronic inflammation, and neutrophils, particularly in the early phase of the disease process. Fibrosis and scant cellularity are seen in late phases of the process (Fig. 3.35a–c). Differential diagnosis includes mainly palpation thyroiditis (multinucleated giant cells but no neutrophiles), sarcoidosis, and tuberculosis.

US Features
- The US shows diffuse or localized hypoechogenicity in the affected painful or tender areas. When localized, the US features mimic those of carcinoma or lymphoma (Fig. 3.35d, e).
- No increased vascularity is seen in the affected areas; however, vascularity may be increased in the recovery phase.
- The US appearance usually returns to normal in the recovery phase.

Subacute Lymphocytic (Sporadic or Postpartum) Thyroiditis

This type of thyroiditis (also called "silent" thyroiditis) occurs at any age but is more common in women (5% of postpartum). It is an autoimmune process with positive anti thyroid antibodies (TG and TPO) that develops in the first year after the delivery or spontaneously in patients with family history of autoimmune disorders. It appears to be a variant of Hashimoto's. Patients initially have transient hyperthyroidism and a non-tender thyroid gland, followed by lymphocytic thyroiditis.

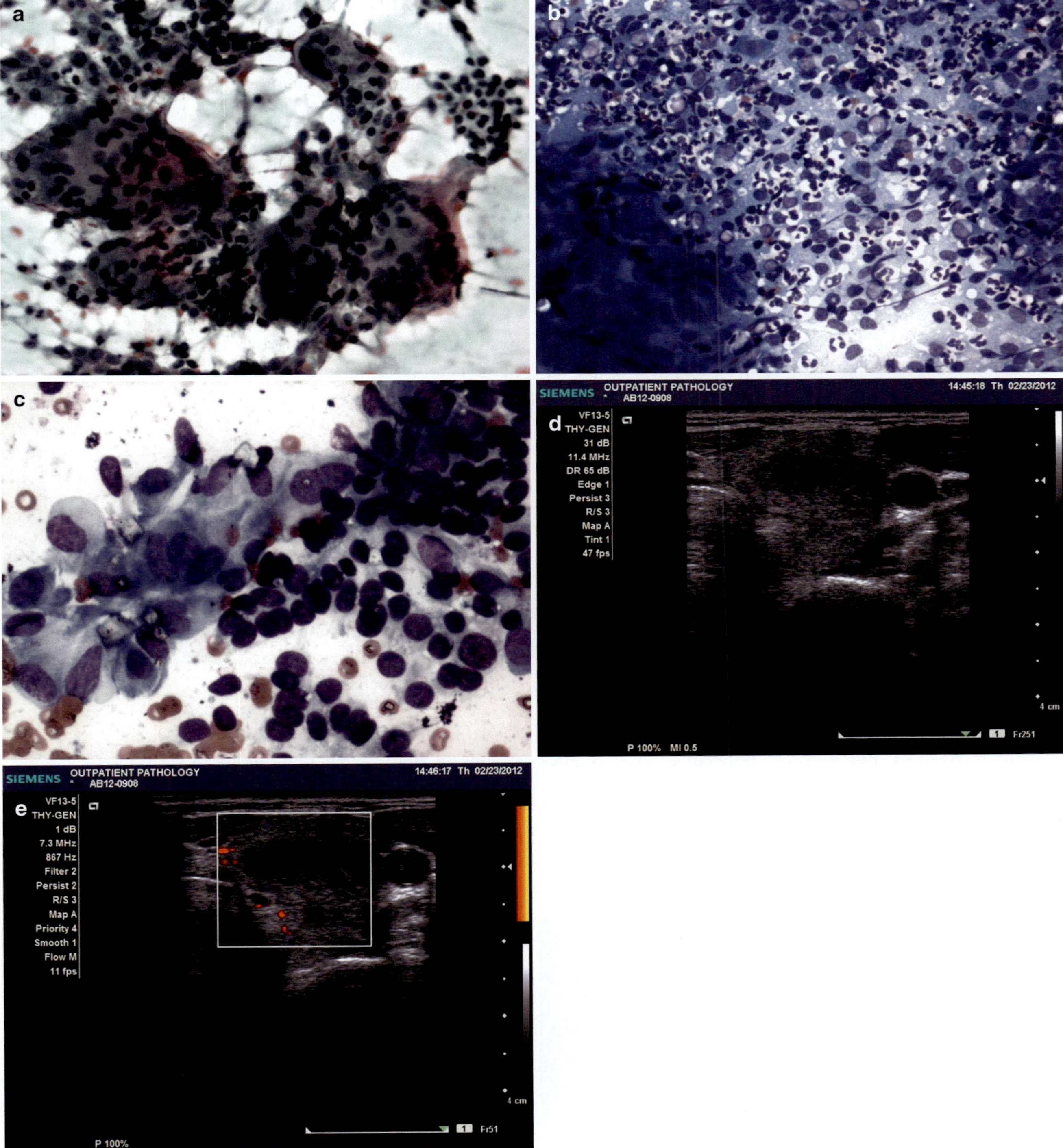

Fig. 3.35 Subacute thyroiditis. Multinucleated giant cells with numerous nuclei (**a**), granulomas (**b**, **c** left lower side), acute inflammatory cells (**b**), and benign follicular cells (**c**) are present. Ultrasound shows poorly defined heterogeneous and irregular areas of hypoechogenicity (**d**) with lack of vascular blood flow by Doppler examination (**e**). (**a**, Papanicolaou stain, low power; **b**, **c** MGG stain, high power)

Acute Suppurative Thyroiditis

Acute suppurative thyroiditis is uncommon. The etiology is bacterial, usually due to staphylococci and streptococci, or fungal secondary to hematogenous or lymphatic dissemination (sepsis in an immunocompromised individual or malnourished infant), contiguous spread from adjacent sites (infections of the upper aerodigestive tract), or superinfection of congenital anomalies such as thyroglossal-duct cyst or pyriform sinus fistula.

Most patients have an underlying thyroid disorder. In the presence of acute suppurative unilateral thyroiditis or abscess in the thyroid or surrounding tissue, a persistent pyriform sinus-thyroid fistula resulting from a fourth branchial cleft anomaly or a persistent embryonal thymopharyngeal duct from the third pouch, usually left-sided should be excluded and surgically treated to avoid recurrent infections. Treatment includes antibiotics and abscess drainage.

Clinical Findings Patients complain of anterior lower neck swelling and pain developing over a period of days to weeks, accompanied by fever, dysphagia, dysphonia, hoarseness, and palpable cervical lymphadenopathy. Thyroid function tests are normal, although there may be transient hyper- or hypothyroidism; autoantibodies are negative.

Histopathology There is acute inflammation and tissue necrosis with eventual abscess formation.

FNA Findings Smears show a purulent smear pattern with necrosis and blood. Organisms may be seen particularly in immunosuppressed patients. Occasional reactive follicular cells may be seen; however, they are not a requirement for specimen adequacy. Samples for bacterial cultures should be obtained.

US Features

- The thyroid gland is diffusely hypoechoic and edematous with intermixed hyperechoic trabeculae and mildly increased vascularity.
- A thyroid abscess may develop in the course of the disease and shows a complex echotexture, irregular borders, and posterior acoustic enhancement in the cystic areas.

Chronic Fibrous (Riedel's) or Ligneous Thyroiditis

This rare entity has an unknown etiology and represents a primary inflammatory dense fibrotic process replacing the thyroid tissue. It is believed to be a manifestation of IgG4 related disease in the thyroid and rarely, it may be part of a multisystemic fibrosclerotic syndrome.

Clinical Findings This process affects predominantly adult or elderly female patients. The fibrosis extends to the tissues surrounding the thyroid, compressing adjacent structures and causing hoarseness and stridor. Shortness of breath and dysphagia develop if the fibrosis extends into the mediastinum. The thyroid gland is enlarged and has a stony consistency. Tenderness or cervical lymphadenopathy is absent. Most patients are euthyroid, but 30% have hypothyroidism. Cases of hypoparathyroidism have been described due to fibrosis. Similar signs and symptoms are seen in anaplastic thyroid carcinoma, lymphoma, and sarcoma.

Histopathology There are areas of complete obliteration of the thyroid parenchyma next to areas with preserved architecture. Microscopically, there is extensive fibrosis that extends to the surrounding perithyroidal tissue planes. Chronic inflammation is patchy. Oncocytes, granulomas, and multinucleated cells are lacking.

FNA Findings Smears are pauci- or acellular, showing rare strands of fibro-collagenous tissue. Rare lymphocytes and bland-appearing spindle cells may be seen. Colloid and follicular cells are usually absent (Fig. 3.36a, b). Open surgical biopsy is often needed for definitive diagnosis and exclusion of malignancy.

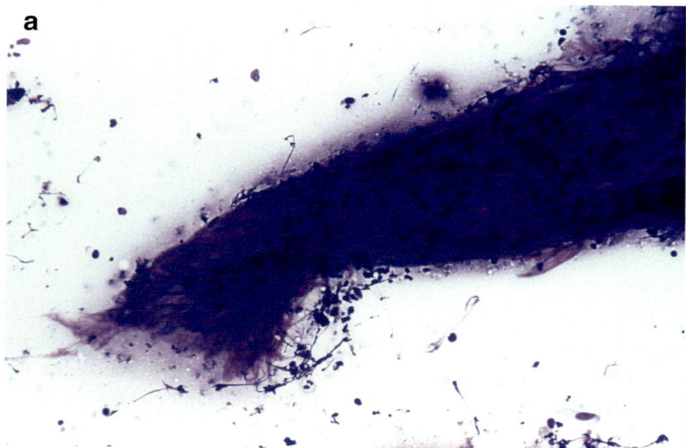
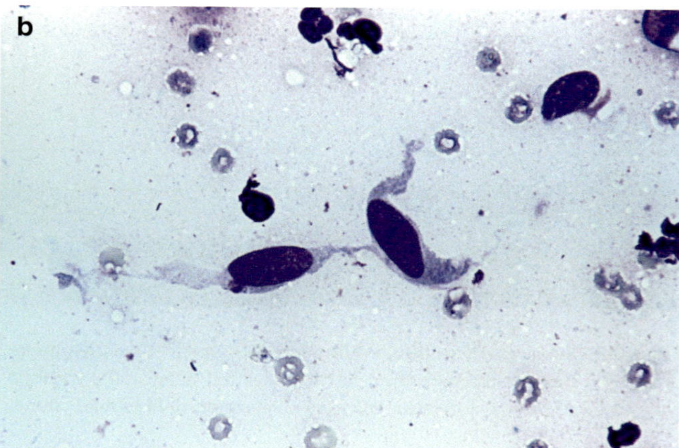

Fig. 3.36 Reidel's thyroiditis (from the American Society of Cytology slide seminar, 2005). Paucicellular smears showing a fibro-collagenous tissue fragment with damaged inflammatory cells (**a**), and rare bland stromal cells (**b**). (**a**, **b**, DiffQuik stain, low and high power)

US Features

- The gland may be enlarged or poorly defined and has a diffuse, homogeneous hypoechogenecity.

FNA Diagnosis of Atypia of Undetermined Significance (AUS)

This 2023 TBSRTC recommended category is reserved for cases of mild atypia, both cellular and architectural, where the atypia is insufficient to classify the nodule as follicular neoplasm, oncocytic follicular neoplasm (when oncocytic cells predominate), or suspicious for malignancy.

AUS is classified depending on the presence of epithelial cells with nuclear atypia or other types of atypia as described and exemplified below. AUS with nuclear atypia has a higher risk of malignancy (20–30%) than other types of atypia. Atypical lymphoid cells and psammoma bodies without atypical follicular cells are rare cases of AUS. AUS cases are followed clinically when a benign diagnosis is obtained on a repeat FNA. AUS interpretation on a repeat FNA must be followed by thyroid molecular testing if available.

Surgery following FNA diagnosis is rare; however, it may be considered when thyroid molecular testing suggests a significative lesion with a high risk of malignancy or malignancy. Approximately, 10–30% of AUS nodules are reported as AUS on a repeat FNA. Nodules with negative thyroid molecular tests have a 3–5% risk of malignancy. Of note, AUS with architectural atypia are more likely to have negative thyroid molecular tests than AUS with nuclear atypia. Thyroid molecular tests are difficult to interpret in AUS with oncocytic predominance due to the complexity of molecular events (near haploid state, mitochondrial DNA mutations).

AUS with Nuclear Atypia

Smears show most cohesive sheets benign follicular cells; rare cells exhibit nuclear atypia with enlargement, pale chromatin, and contour irregularities that raise concern for PTC; intranuclear cytoplasmic invaginations are absent. These findings may be seen in Hashimoto thyroiditis. Extensive nuclear atypia with no or rare intranuclear cytoplasmic invaginations may be seen in NIFTP (Fig. 3.37a, b).

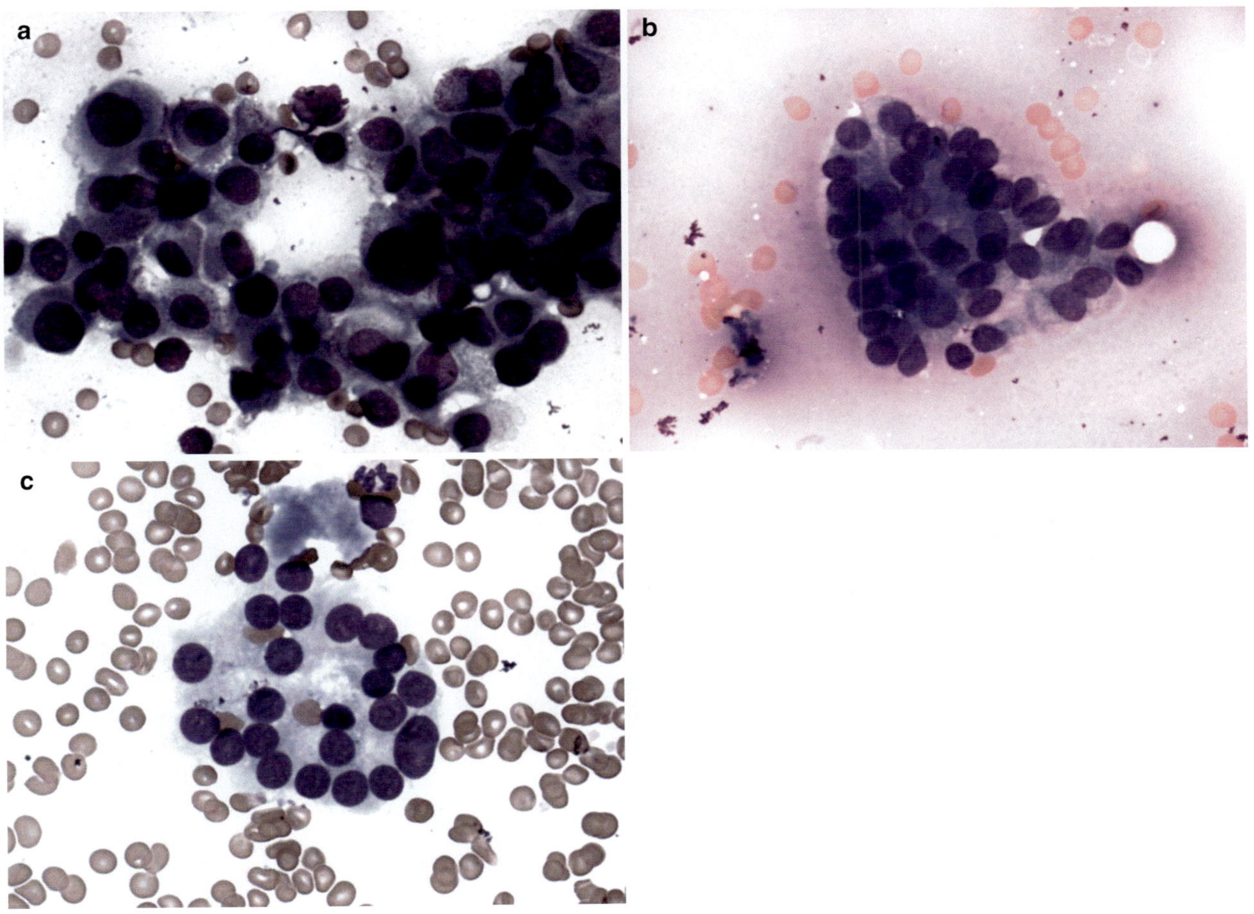

Fig. 3.37 AUS. Nuclear atypia and nuclear overlapping are seen in the first two cases, including anisonucleosis (**a**) and pale chromatin with nuclear groves (**b**). The third case shows poorly formed microfollicles and slight nuclear atypia (**c**). The histopathology diagnoses were follicular adenoma, papillary thyroid carcinoma, and NIFTP, respectively. (**a**, **b**, **c**, MGG stain, high magnification)

Atypical Cyst Lining Epithelial and/or Mesenchymal Cells

Most are diagnosed as benign; however, if nuclear grooves, prominent nucleoli, and rare intranuclear cytoplasmic invaginations are identified, diagnose these findings as AUS. These cells are similar to those seen in PTC (Fig. 3.38a–d).

"Histiocytoid" Cells

These cells are large and can be present single or in small aggregates and raise concern for PTC. Large round nuclei and septate vacuoles are seen. The background shows cystic change with numerous macrophages and few epithelial cells. In contrast to histiocytes, "histiocytoid" cells are positive for epithelial markers and negative for CD68 and CD163. "Histiocytoid" cells are also seen in cystic subtype of PTC (Fig. 3.39a–c).

Architectural Atypia

This category is considered in the following instances. (1) Smears show scant colloid and scant cellularity with well- or poorly formed microfollicles or crowded three-dimensional groups; differential diagnosis includes a poorly sampled parathyroid neoplasm. (2) Smears with adequate cellularity and a predominance of a microfollicular pattern (50–70%) compared to the macrofollicular pattern (cell sheets); of note, when the microfollicular component is >70% the smears should be called follicular neoplasm. (3) Prominent microfollicular pattern without nuclear atypia, usually present in one smear and a cellular pattern of a TFND (colloid, macrophages, and follicular epithelial cell sheets) present in the other smears; consider a parathyroid neoplasm in the presence of microfollicles, complex aggregates, and bare nuclei (Fig. 3.40a–d).

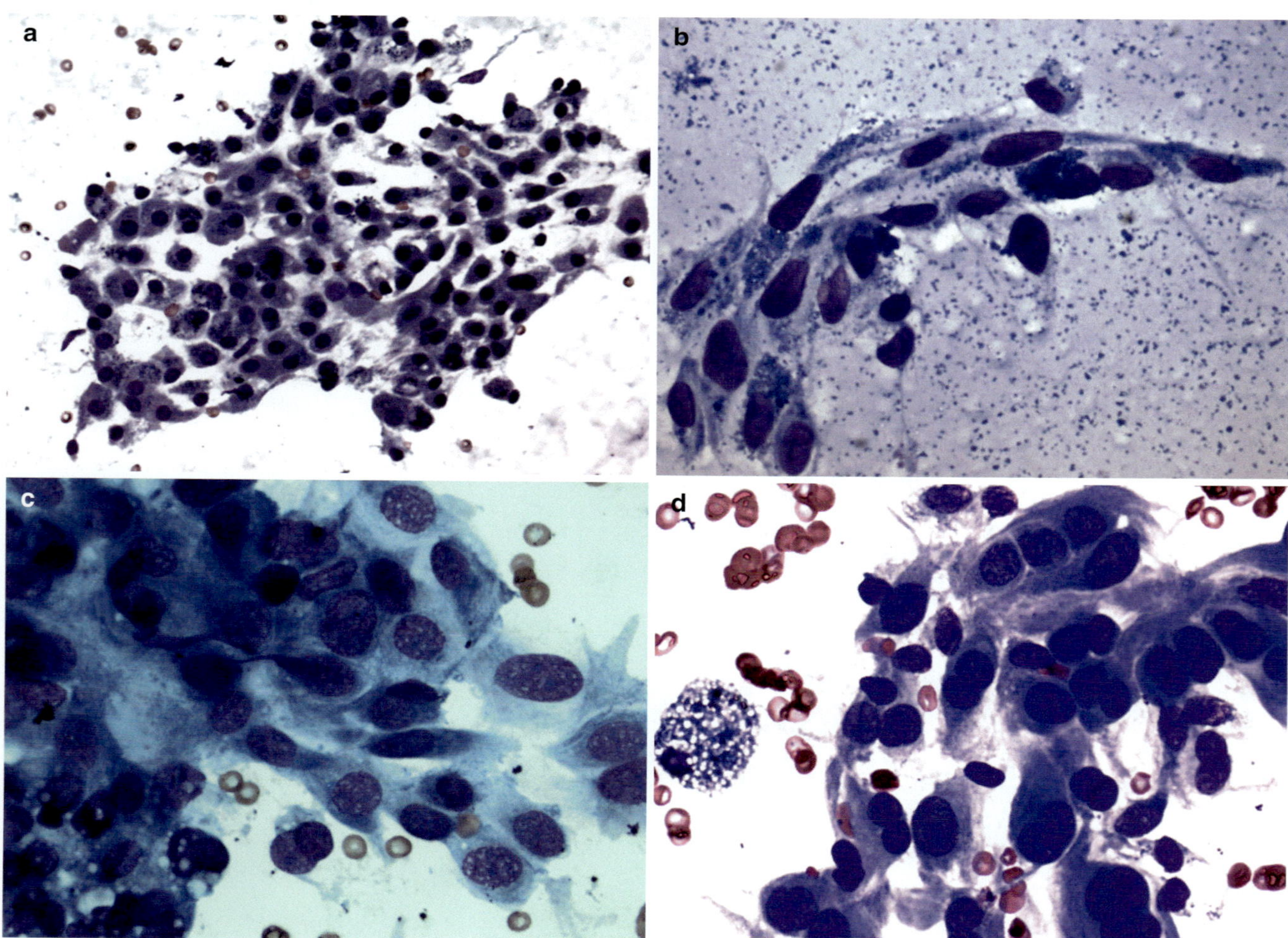

Fig. 3.38 AUS, atypical cyst lining cells. Metaplastic cells with slight anisonucleosis and binucleation but no other features for papillary thyroid carcinoma are present in these four cases. (**a**, MGG stain, medium power; **b**, **c**, **d**, MGG stain high power)

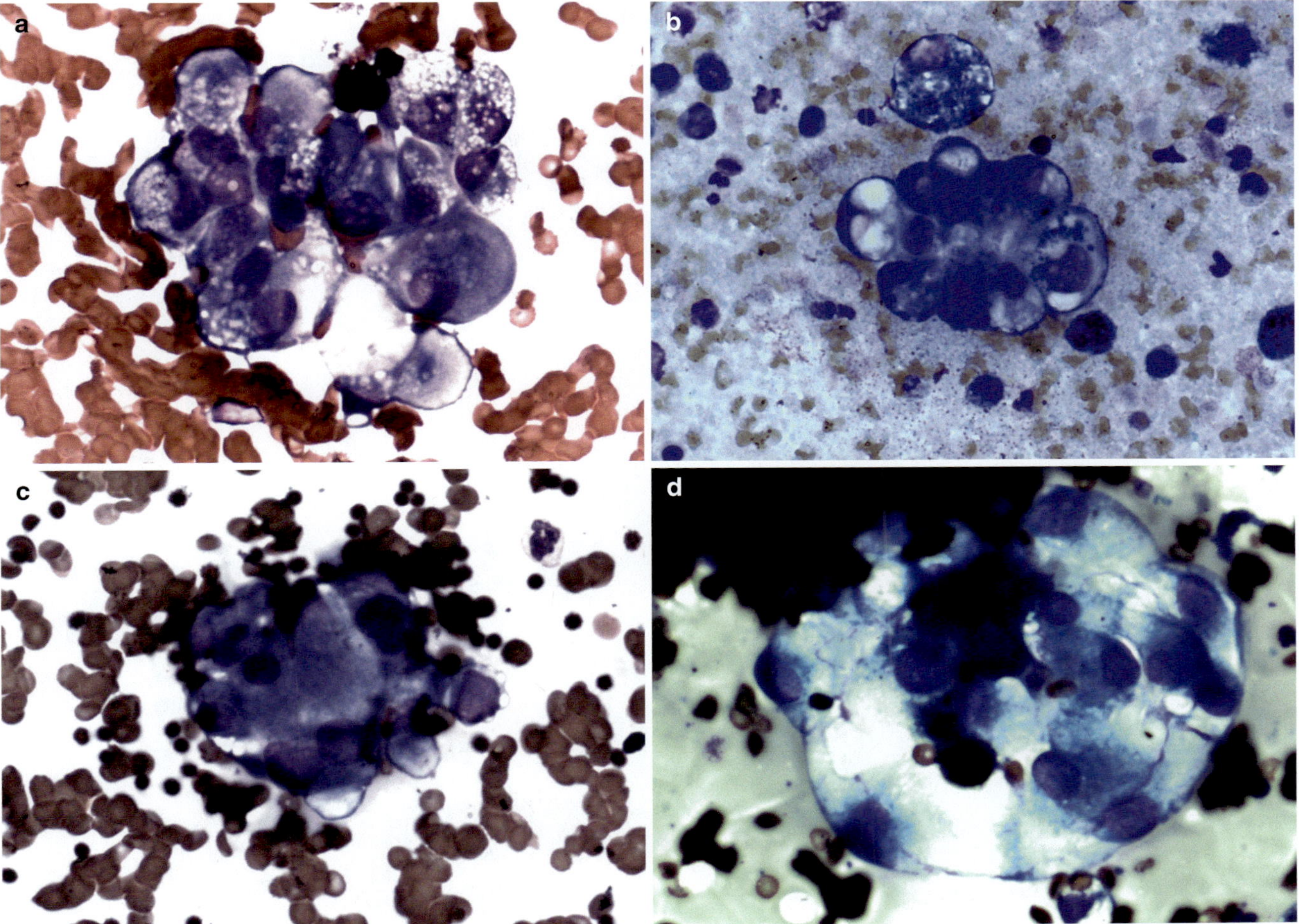

Fig. 3.39 AUS, "histiocytoid" cells. Small aggregates of cells showing prominent cytoplasmic vacuolization are present in a background of cystic change. Histopathology diagnoses in these four cases were papillary thyroid carcinoma with cystic change. (**a–d**, MGG stain, high power)

Oncocyte Atypia

This category is considered in the following instances: (1) Smears of scant cellularity showing oncocytes (exclusively or almost exclusively) and scant colloid; the rationale is not to miss a poorly sampled oncocytic follicular neoplasm. (2) Smears of adequate cellularity showing >70% oncocytes, colloid, and no lymphoid cells; repeat FNA and correlate with clinical findings to exclude Hashimoto's thyroiditis or TFND. (3) Smears from multiple nodules showing features of oncocytic follicular neoplasm, minimal colloid, and no lymphoid cells; AUS is a preferable diagnosis since Hashimoto's thyroiditis or TFND are the most probable causes; correlation with clinical findings is needed (Fig. 3.41a–d).

Atypia, Not Otherwise Specified

This category of nuclear atypia includes anisocytosis, nuclear enlargement, anisonucleosis, prominent nucleoli but does not raise concern for PTC. Clinical correlation to exclude treatment with pharmaceutical drugs such as amiodarone, carbimazole, and radioactive iodine. Finding of Psammoma bodies with no other feature for PTC should be included in the category of atypia NOS; inspissated colloid with radial cracking may be seen in both regular and liquid-based smears and mimic Psammoma bodies (Fig. 3.42a–c).

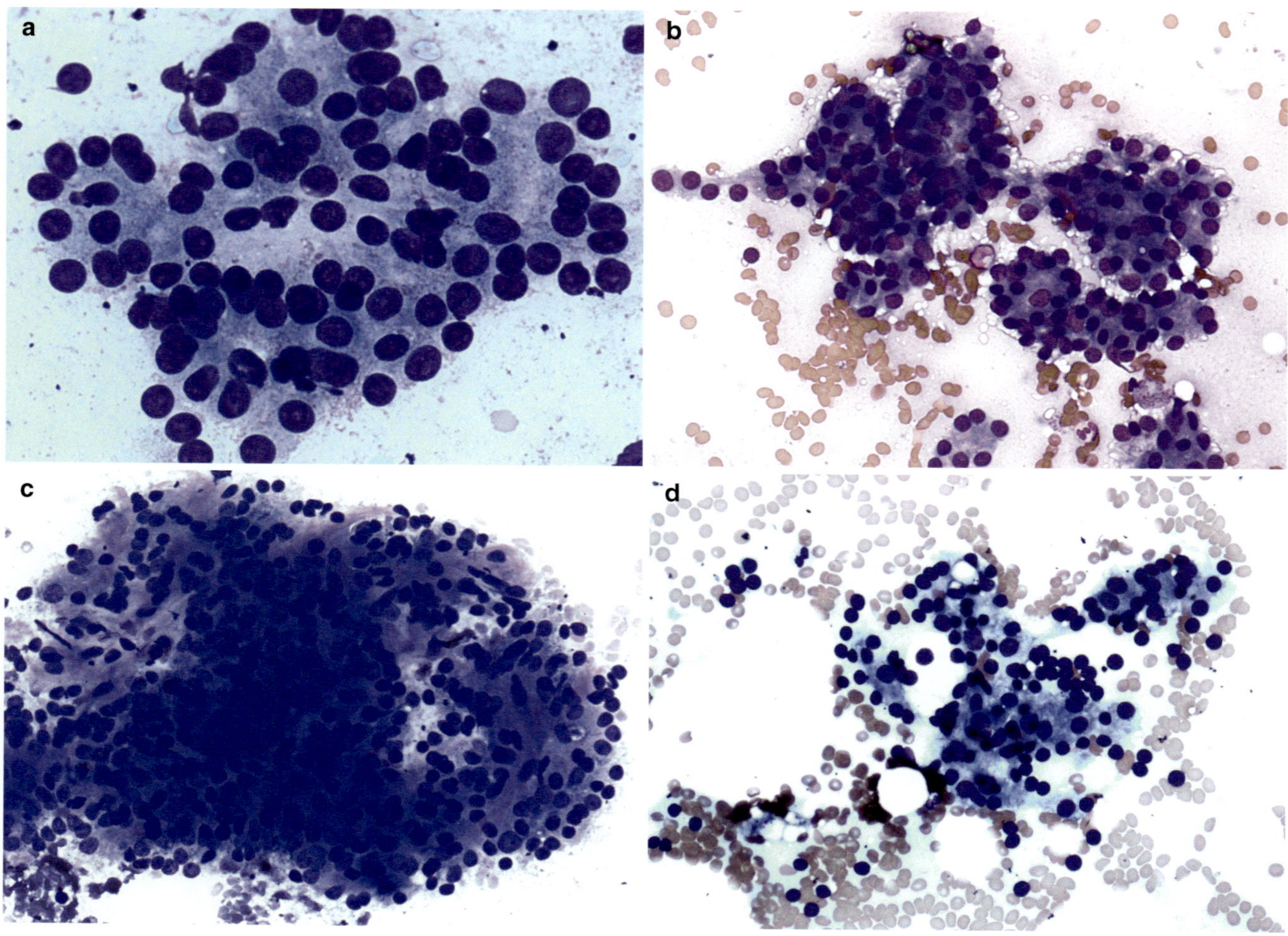

Fig. 3.40 AUS, architectural atypia. Aggregates of poorly formed microfollicles in a background of thin colloid (cells sheets were present in other areas) (**a**). Aggregates of microfollicles composed of cells with hyperplastic change are present in a background of thin colloid (**b**). Aggregates of microfollicles with slight anisonucleosis and oncocytic change (**c**). Poorly formed microfollicles and bare nuclei are present in this sparsely cellular smear (**d**). The histopathologic diagnoses were thyroid follicular nodular disease (benign thyroid nodule) (**a**), follicular adenoma (**b**, **c**), and parathyroid adenoma (**d**). (**a**, MGG stain, high power; **b**, **c**, **d**, MGG stain, medium power)

Atypical Lymphoid Cells

This category of monomorphous lymphoid cells in a rapid growing nodule needs clinical correlation and harvest material for flow cytometry to detect light chain monoclonality.

Extra-nodal marginal zone lymphoma is considered in the presence of a mildly polymorphous lymphoid cell population (Fig. 3.43a, b).

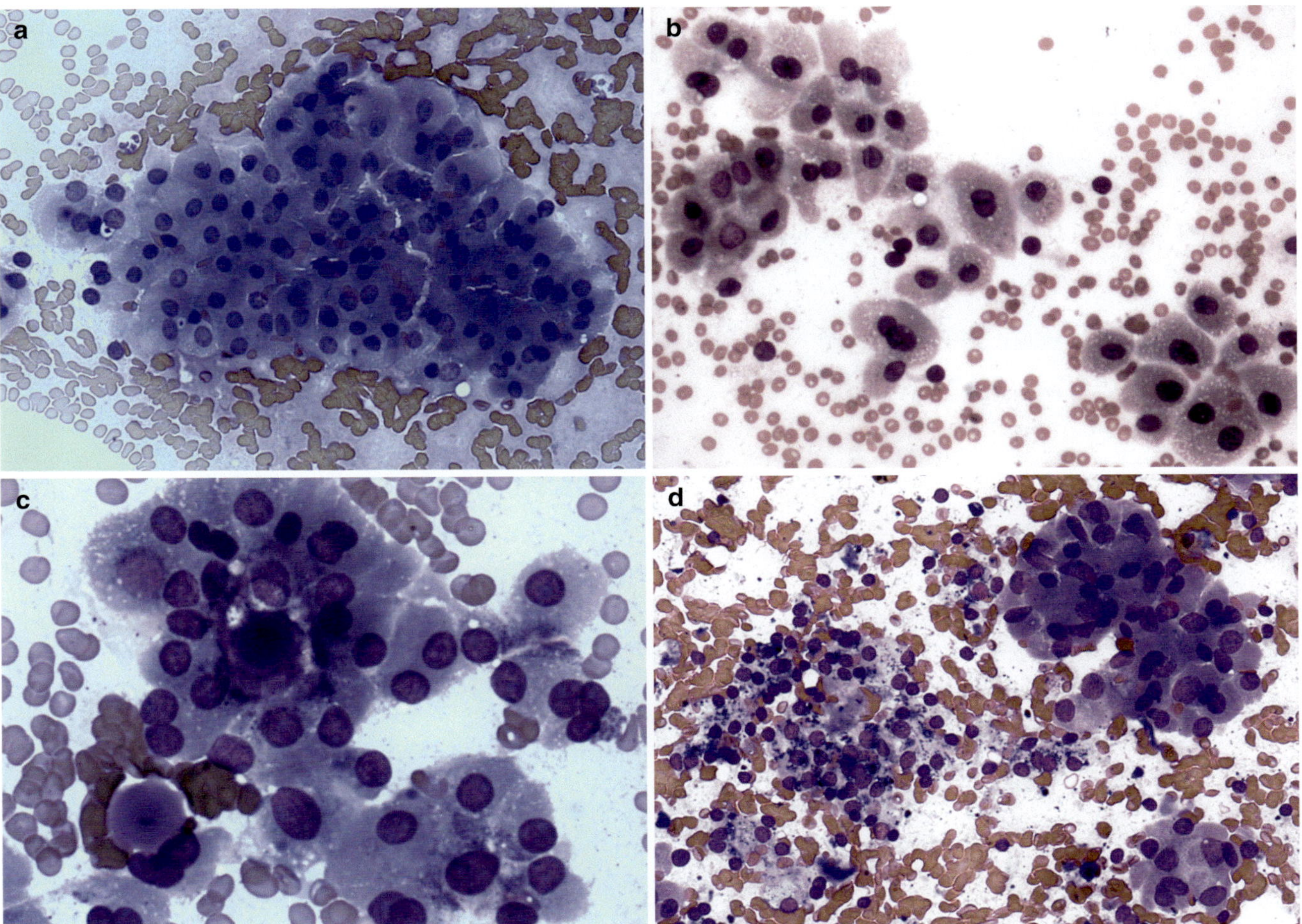

Fig. 3.41 Oncocyte atypia. Numerous sheets of bland appearing oncocytic cells and scant thin colloid (**a**); histopathologic diagnosis was thyroid follicular nodular disease (benign thyroid nodule) with oncocytic differentiation. Oncocytic cells and absent colloid were present in this sparsely cellular smear (**b**); histopathology diagnosis was oncocytic thyroid adenoma. Oncocytic cells with cytologic atypia and absent col- loid (**c**); histopathologic diagnosis was oncocytic thyroid adenoma. Atypical oncocytic cells, colloid, benign follicular cells, and few lymphoid cells (**d**); histopathologic diagnosis was Hashimoto's thyroiditis. (**a**, **d**, MGG stain, medium power; **b**, Papanicolaou stain, medium power; **c**, MGG stain, high power)

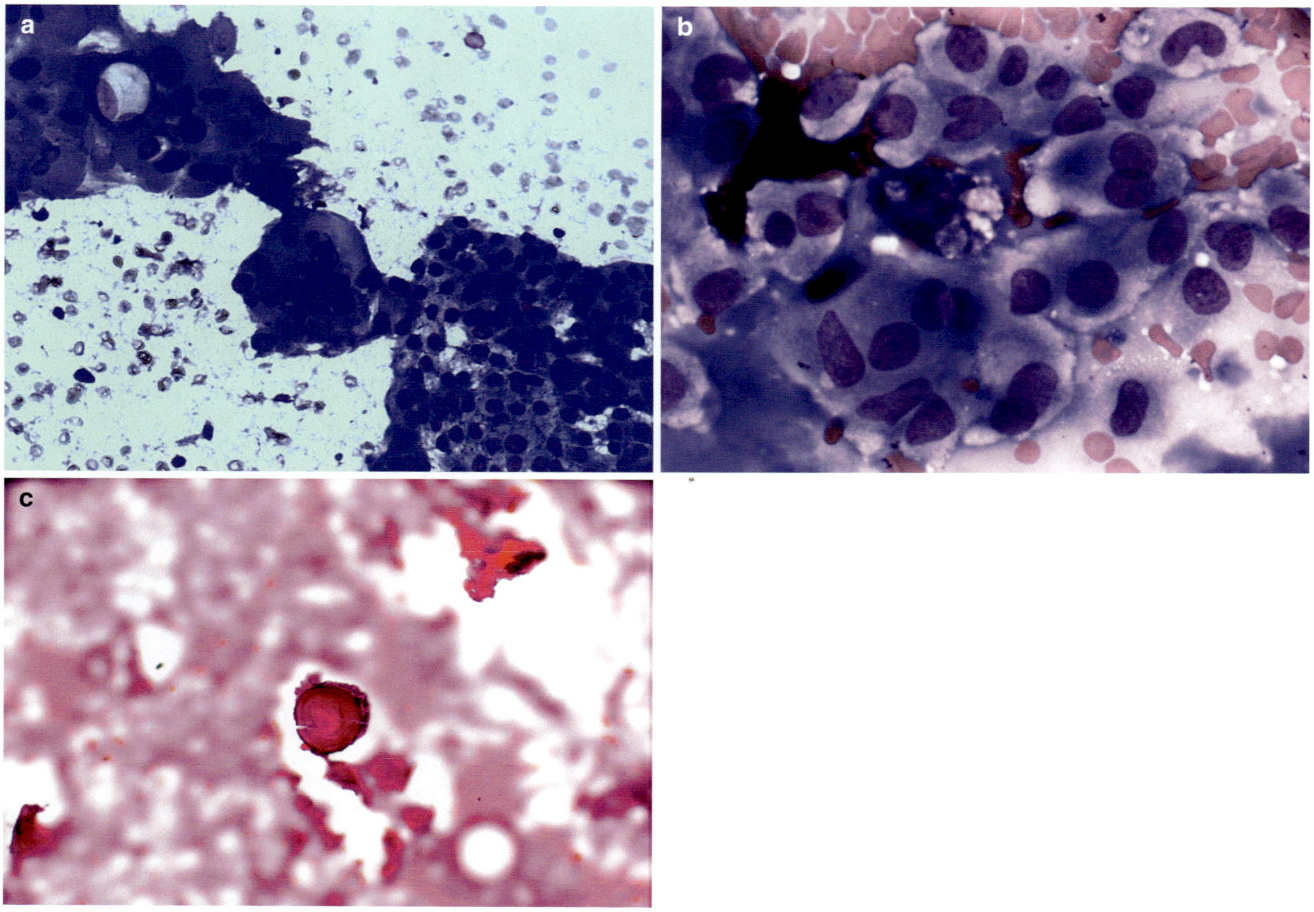

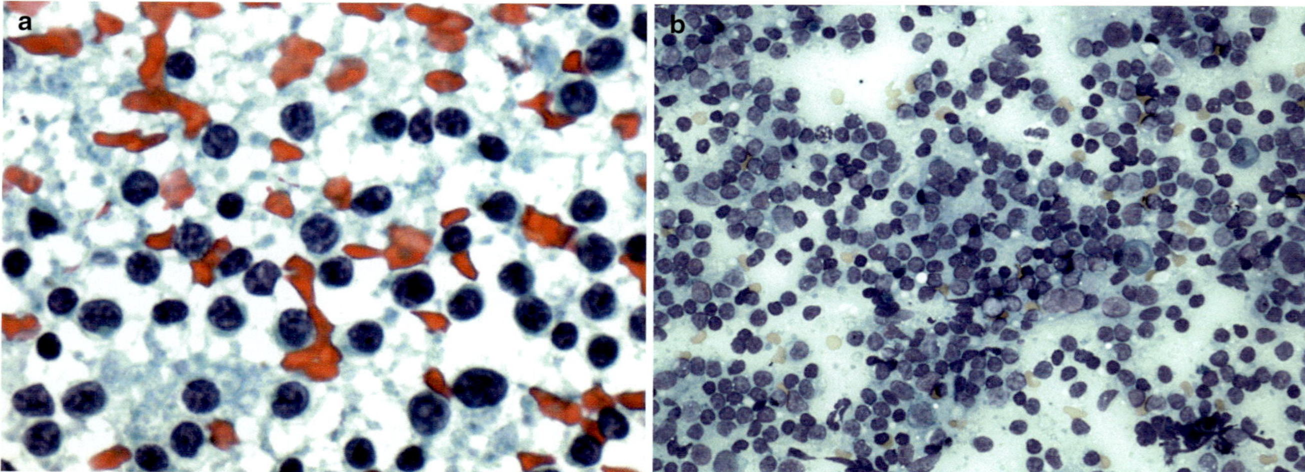

Fig. 3.42 Atypia, not otherwise specified. Atypical cells in a patient with untreated Graves' disease (**a**). Atypical cells present in the smears of a patient with history of amiodarone treated heard disease (**b**). Psammoma body with cracking (**c**); other smears showed papillary thyroid carcinoma. (**a**, MGG stain, medium power; **b**, MGG stain, high power; Papanicolaou stain, high magnification)

Fig. 3.43 Atypical lymphoid cells of small size (**a**) and medium size with slight anisocytosis and anisonucleosis (**b**). Flow cytometry shoed extra nodal marginal zone lymphoma in both cases. (**a**, **b**, MGG stain, medium power)

FNA Diagnosis of Follicular Neoplasm

The FNA diagnosis of "follicular neoplasm" reflects the lack of ability of cytology to distinguish accurately among a hyperplastic nodule in thyroid follicular nodular disease, follicular adenoma, and follicular carcinoma due to overlapping cytologic features. The infiltrating follicular subtype of PTC, NIFTP, and the invasive encapsulated follicular variant of PTC may be considered in this group when inconspicuous nuclear features of PTC are identified. Parathyroid adenoma shows cytologic features similar to those of a follicular neoplasm and is often misinterpreted as such; this issue will be discussed under parathyroid adenoma/carcinoma. Of note, ~30% of follicular-patterned lesions are benign hyperplastic nodules that are included in the thyroid follicular nodular disease category (2022 WHO classification of thyroid tumors).

Follicular Adenoma and Carcinoma

Follicular thyroid adenoma (FTA) is the most common thyroid neoplasm. Follicular thyroid carcinoma (FTC) is rare, although it is more common in iodine-deficient geographic areas.

Thyroid surgery is necessary for differentiation between adenoma and carcinoma. Thus, the diagnosis is made histopathologically only.

Clinical Findings Most patients are euthyroid and have a solitary "cold" nodule on thyroid scan. Few adenomas are "hot" and may cause hyperthyroidism ("Plummer adenoma"). FTAs are usually sporadic and occur predominantly in women in the fifth to sixth decade of life or older. Iodine deficiency, radiation exposure, and familial tumor syndromes (Carney, MEN, McCune-Albright, familial thyroid nodular disease) are other causes. Adenomas have a variable size (1–10 cm).

FTCs often measure >5.5 cm, and they occur predominantly in women with a peak age of 40–60 years; however, it may occur in children and adolescents as well. Metastases are hematogenous rather than lymphatic. Thus, regional lymph node metastases are unusual (<5%). Distant visceral metastases include lung, bone, kidney, etc. The prognosis is slightly worse than that of PTC, with a 75–95% 10-year survival.

Histopathology FTA is surrounded by a thin capsule that is grossly and histologically complete, lacking capsular, vascular, or thyroid invasion. The pattern may be microfollicular, normofollicular, macrofollicular, trabecular, solid, and/or papillary. Cells are usually monomorphic, cuboidal to low columnar, but occasionally there is cellular pleomor-

phism with large bizarre hyperchromatic nuclei; however, other features of malignancy are absent. Nuclear features of PTC are absent. Mitoses are rare or absent. Cystic degeneration, spindle cells, and adipose and cartilaginous metaplasia may be seen particularly in large-sized adenomas. Clear cell changes (cytoplasmic glycogen, lipid, mucin) are more common in PTCs than in adenomas. In contrast, signet ring cells (contain cytoplasmic TG) are more common in adenomas. Adenomas can also show black pigment (minocycline related).

FTC can be subclassified as minimally invasive (capsular invasion only), encapsulated angioinvasive, and widely invasive (thyroid and extrathyroidal soft tissue). It lacks nuclear features of PTC. FTCs measuring less than 2 cm have not been associated with metastatic disease. Widely invasive carcinomas with necrosis and/or mitoses have a worse prognosis.

Immuno-Profile Normal follicular tissue, FTA, and FTC have similar profiles including positivity for TG, TTF-1, PAX8, CD56, low-molecular-weight keratin, EMA, laminin, and type IV collagen. PPARG is rare in adenoma.

Molecular Profile These follicular cell thyroid neoplasms with follicular pattern show a *RAS*-like molecular profile. *RAS* point mutations and *PAX8::PPARG* rearrangements are seen in both FTAs and FTCs. Widely invasive FTCs have higher frequency of allelic loss than minimally invasive FTCs. Of importance, no molecular test can differentiate between FTA and FTC (Diagrams 3.1, 3.2 and 3.3).

- *RAS* mutations (*NRAS*, *HRAS*, and *KRAS*) is related to follicular architecture in thyroid tumors and is typically detected in 20–40% of conventional-type FTAs, 40–50% of conventional-type FTCs, and 10–20% of the invasive encapsulated follicular variant PTC and not in conventional PTC. A lower incidence has been seen in oncocytic tumors.
- *RAS* mutations in FTCs have been correlated with an unfavorable prognosis, poor overall patient survival, and may be correlated with tumor dedifferentiation as they are prevalent in ATC. The *NRAS* codon 61 mutation in follicular carcinomas is positively associated with distant metastases.
- *PAX8::PPARγ* rearrangements occur in ~40% of conventional FTCs, with lower prevalence in oncocytic carcinomas (OTCs). They have also been found in FTAs (2–13%), hyperplastic thyroid nodules, the infiltrative follicular subtype of PTC (38%), and in ATC and PDTCs (7%). Tumors tend to occur at a young age, be of small size, and have vascular invasion.

MAPK SIGNALING PATHWAY

Growth Factors (GFs) bind to
Receptor Tyrosine Kinases (RTKs) such as RET and NTRK

↓

Receptor dimerization & autophosphorilation in the
intracellular domain
(MAPK signaling pathway is activated)

↓

RAS activation

↓

RAS binds, recruits and activates *BRAF*

↓

BRAF activates MAPK/ERK kinase (MEK)

↓

MEK activates the **e**xtracellular signal-**r**egulated **k**inase (ERK)

↓

ERK translocates into the nucleus

↓

ERK regulates

↙   ↓   ↘

Cell differentiation   Cell proliferation   Cell survival

Diagram 3.1 MAPK signaling pathway

RAS in Follicular Carcinoma (40-50%)

Somatic mutation

↓

Amino-acid substitutions of *RAS* gene

↓

NRAS, HRAS, KRAS

↓

Constitutive activation of the Raf-MEK-MAPK and PI3K/AKT
signaling pathways

↓

Dysregulation of specific genes

↓

Abnormal thyroid cell proliferation and differentiation
May correlate with unfavorable prognosis

Diagram 3.2 *RAS* in follicular carcinoma (40–50%)

PAX8::PPARG in Follicular Carcinoma (30-40%)

t(2;3) (q13;p25) rearrangement

↓

In-frame fusion of the promoter and DNA-binding domains of *PAX8*
And

the nuclear receptor domains of *PPARG1*

↓

PAX8::PPARG1 fusion protein

↓

Overexpression of PPARγ1 or
Deregulation of PAX8 pathway

↓

Thyroid carcinoma formation
(solid/trabecular growth pattern, and
higher vascular invasion, often galectin-3 and/or
HBME-1-positive)

Diagram 3.3 *PAX8::PPARG* in follicular carcinoma (30–40%)

- "Hot" FTAs typically have *TSHR* (50–80%) and *GNAS1* (5%) activating mutations.
- The PI3K/PTEN/AKT pathway is rarely activated in FTAs; however, this pathway is activated in FTC associated with Cowden, Carney complex type I, and Werner syndromes.
- Loss of heterozygosity on 7q and 3p loci is frequently encountered in FTCs.

FNA Findings (Follicular adenoma, Fig. 3.44a–d. Follicular carcinoma, Fig. 3.44e–g) Smears are cellular and show microfollicular and trabecular patterns, cell crowding, as well as single cells. A microfollicle is characterized by less than 15 crowded and overlapped cells. Cells may be slightly or markedly enlarged with scant / moderate cytoplasm, a round nucleus, slightly coarse chromatin, and an inconspicuous nucleolus. Rare, atypical cells may be seen. There is nuclear overlapping and molding, but nuclear features for PTC or oncocytic change are either absent or very rare. Colloid is scant or absent; however, dense colloid may be seen in the lumen of the microfollicle. Occasional cell sheets usually comprising less than 25% of smear cellularity and small cell and nuclear size may be seen and indicate a macrofollicular component. Macrophages indicating cystic change may be present in large tumors. True papillae and psammoma bodies are absent; squamous metaplasia is rare. However, in the presence of a microfollicular pattern and focal subtle nuclear features of PTC (irregular nuclear contours, grooves, rare intranuclear cytoplasmic invaginations), consider NIFTP, or IEFV- PTC.

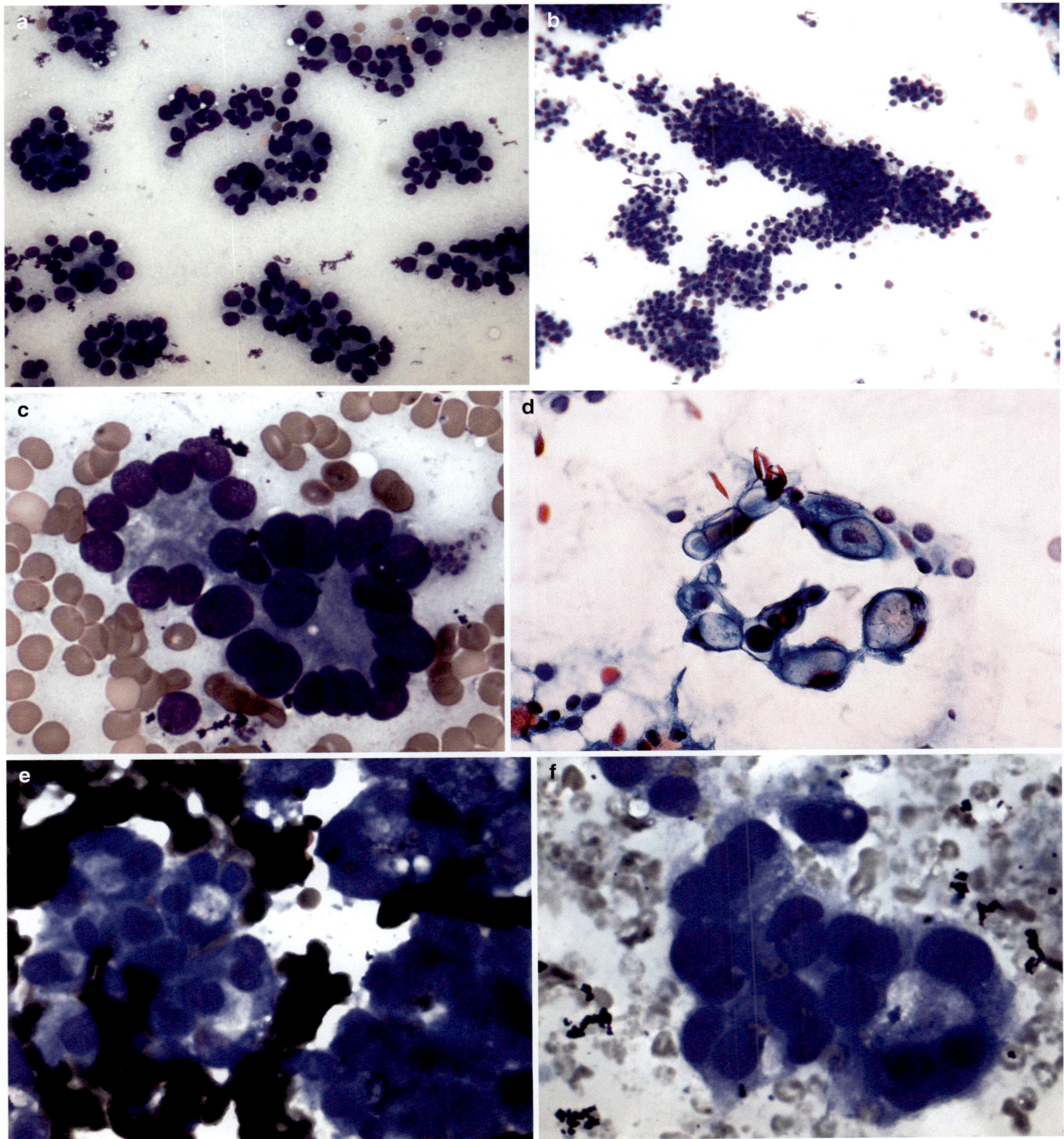

Fig. 3.44 Follicular thyroid adenoma (**a**–**d**). High cellularity and a trabecular arrangement (**a, b**). Microfollicles showing cells with high nuclear to cytoplasmic ratio, large nuclei and molding (**c**). Signet-ring cells (cytoplasmic thyroglobulin) are seen in a different case (**d**). Follicular thyroid carcinoma (**e**–**g**). Cells with oxyphilic change are seen in a microfollicular pattern (**e, f**). Vascular invasion is seen in the resection specimen (**g**). Follicular thyroid adenoma, ultrasound features (**h**–**k**). These two cases show single hypoechoic nodules (1.6 and 5.5 cm in maximum diameter), slightly heterogeneous echotexture, well-defined margins, no halo, and type IV vascular blood flow on Doppler examination. (**a**–**c**, **e** and **f**, MGG stain, high power; **d**, Papanicolaou stain, high power; **g**, Hematoxylin/Eosin stain, low power)

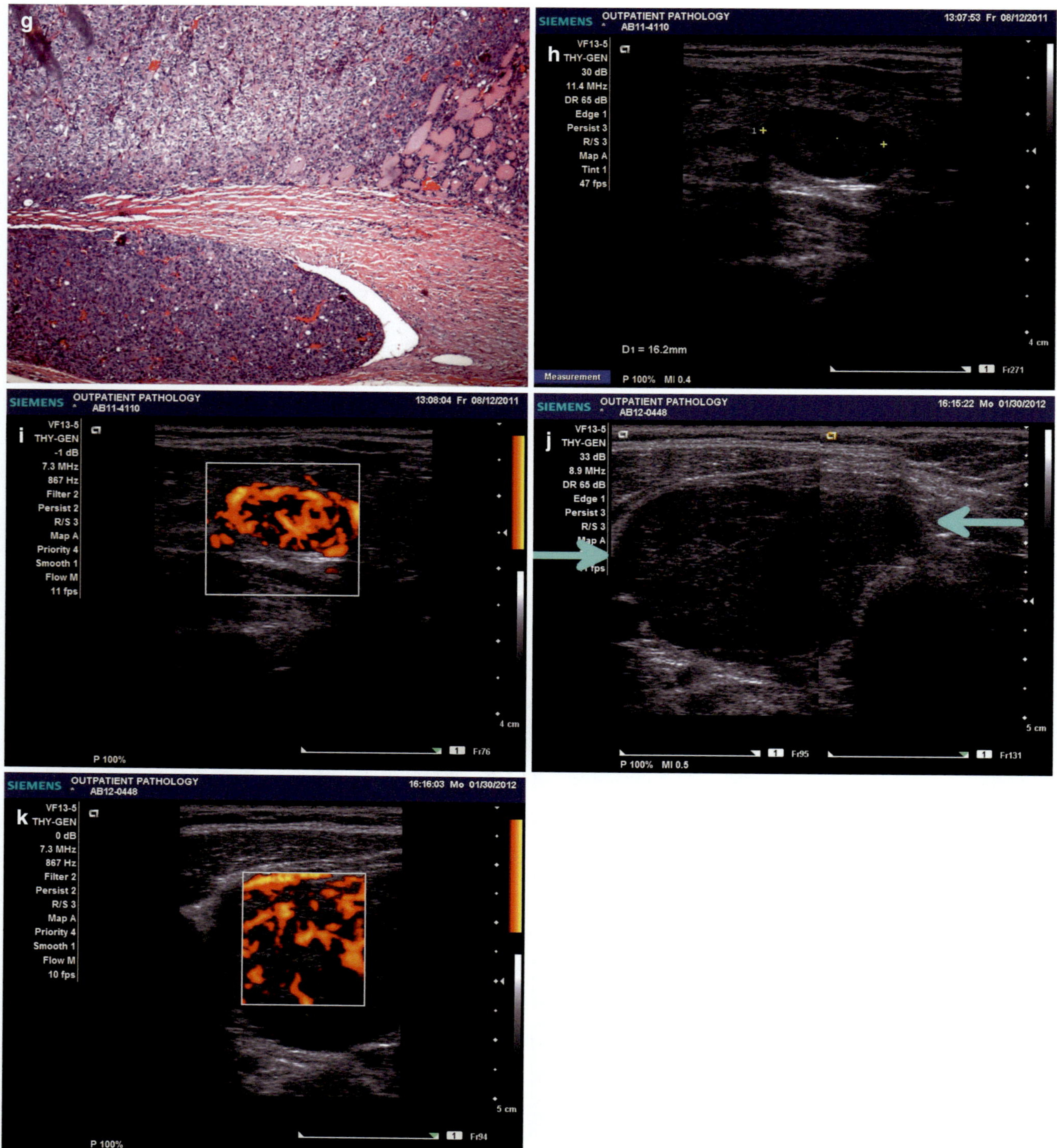

Fig. 3.44 (continued)

US Features (Fig. 3.44h–k)

- US features cannot separate FTA from FTC.
- Nodules are commonly solitary or dominant, hypoechoic, and homogeneous or slightly heterogenous, and solid.
- Oval or round shape, regular and well-defined margins, hypoechoic halo 1–3 mm thick, and an intact capsule are US features suggestive of FTA.
- Inhomogeneous internal texture, an irregular ill-defined margin, and an absent or discontinuous thick and irregular halo suggest FTC. However, these findings are not sensitive or specific, because FTCs may be hyper- or isoechoic and may have a halo.
- Cystic change is absent or minimal and calcifications are rare in FTAs.
- Vascularity is usually present and peripheral in FTAs; however, no vascularity is seen in a few FTAs. Intranodular vascularity is more common in FTCs than in FTAs. A lack of blood flow by Doppler examination in follicular neoplasms makes malignancy unlikely.
- Widely invasive tumors often show a heterogeneous mulberry-like echotexture and ring calcifications.
- Regional lymph node is rare, and they may exhibit a hyperechoic echotexture (Fig. 3.44, Video 3.13).

Oncocytic Follicular Neoplasm

Approximately, 20% of follicular neoplasms are oncocytic; they may be benign or malignant. Oncocytic thyroid adenomas (OTAs) are cured by excision. Oncocytic thyroid carcinomas (OTCs) are highly aggressive.

Clinical Findings Most patients have single or multiple nodules. OTCs are larger than OTAs, tend to occur in an older age group, and are more common in men than in women. Lesions >4 cm are often (80%) malignant. The prognosis seems to be worse than conventional FTC, with a greater risk of distant metastasis (30%), 20–40% mortality at 5 years, and a 40% 10-year survival rate. Lungs and bone are common sites for metastasis. Treatment of OTA is lobectomy. OTC treatment includes thyroidectomy or radiation; the tumor is resistant to radioactive iodine compared to conventional FTC.

Histopathology Oncocytic follicular neoplasms have >75% oncocytic cells containing dysfunctional mitochondria. Oncocytes are of large size, have ample deeply eosinophilic and granular cytoplasm, large nuclei, and prominent nucleoli. Nuclear cytoplasmic invaginations and nuclear groves are rare. Similar to non-oncocytic follicular neoplasms, the distinction between a benign and a malignant oncocytic neoplasm is histologic, following the same histologic criteria (capsular and/or vascular invasion). The architectural pattern may be follicular, trabecular, solid, or papillary. The follicular pattern is commonly seen in adenomas and the solid/trabecular pattern in carcinomas. Carcinomas have a thick capsule. Cellular pleomorphism and prominent nucleoli are common in both. Massive infarction may be present particularly after FNA.

Immuno-Profile No ancillary technique distinguishes between OTA and OTC. Oncocytes show reactivity with TG, mitochondrial antigens, glucose transport 4 (GLUT-4), TTF1, keratin in particular CK7 and CK14, CEA, S-100 protein, and HMB-45.

Molecular Profile Clonal events are absent in 42% of follicular oncocytic neoplasms. No specific chromosomal abnormality has been described. In contrast to PTC with oncocytic features that is diploid, both OTAs and OTCs are aneuploid, including chromosomal gains and losses. *RAS*-like molecular alterations also occur in these tumors, although less frequently than in non-oncocytic follicular tumors. *PAX8::PPARG* rearrangements are virtually never seen in OTC; in contrast, this abnormality is seen in 25% to 50% of FTCs. Mutations or deletions of the mitochondrial and nuclear DNA may be the responsible for the mitochondrial dysfunction and for the increased numbers of mitochondria characteristic of these cells; however, they don't distinguish benign from malignant oncocytic thyroid neoplasms. These tumors show specific genetic alterations including mitochondrial DNA mutations and increased copy number alterations (35% of cases) and identify those patients whose thyroid nodules should undergo surgical resection. *PTEN* and *P53* mutations are present in oncocytic neoplasms, particularly in OTCs (approximately 30%).

FNA Findings (Fig. 3.45a–e) The smears are cellular and composed exclusively or almost exclusively of loosely cohesive oncocytic cells of variable cell, nuclear, and nucleolar size. Syncytial aggregates and crowded groups with or without transgressing capillaries may be seen. Large and small "atypical" oncocytic cells have been described. Small oncocytes have high nuclear to cytoplasm ratio. Large oncocytes may show anisonucleosis (2× variability in nuclear size). Binucleation is common. Cells from OTC are smaller, more monomorphic, and have a high nuclear to cytoplasm ratio than those from OTA. Nuclear atypia is unreliable for the diagnosis of an oncocytic neoplasm, because marked nuclear atypia can be seen in metaplastic non-neoplastic oncocytes of TFND and Hashimoto's thyroiditis. The background lacks colloid, lymphocytes, and plasma cells. PTC (Warthin-like, tall cell, and oncocytic subtypes), MTC, and parathyroid tumors should also be considered in the differential diagnosis. Oncocytic neoplasms lack nuclear features of PTC. MTC

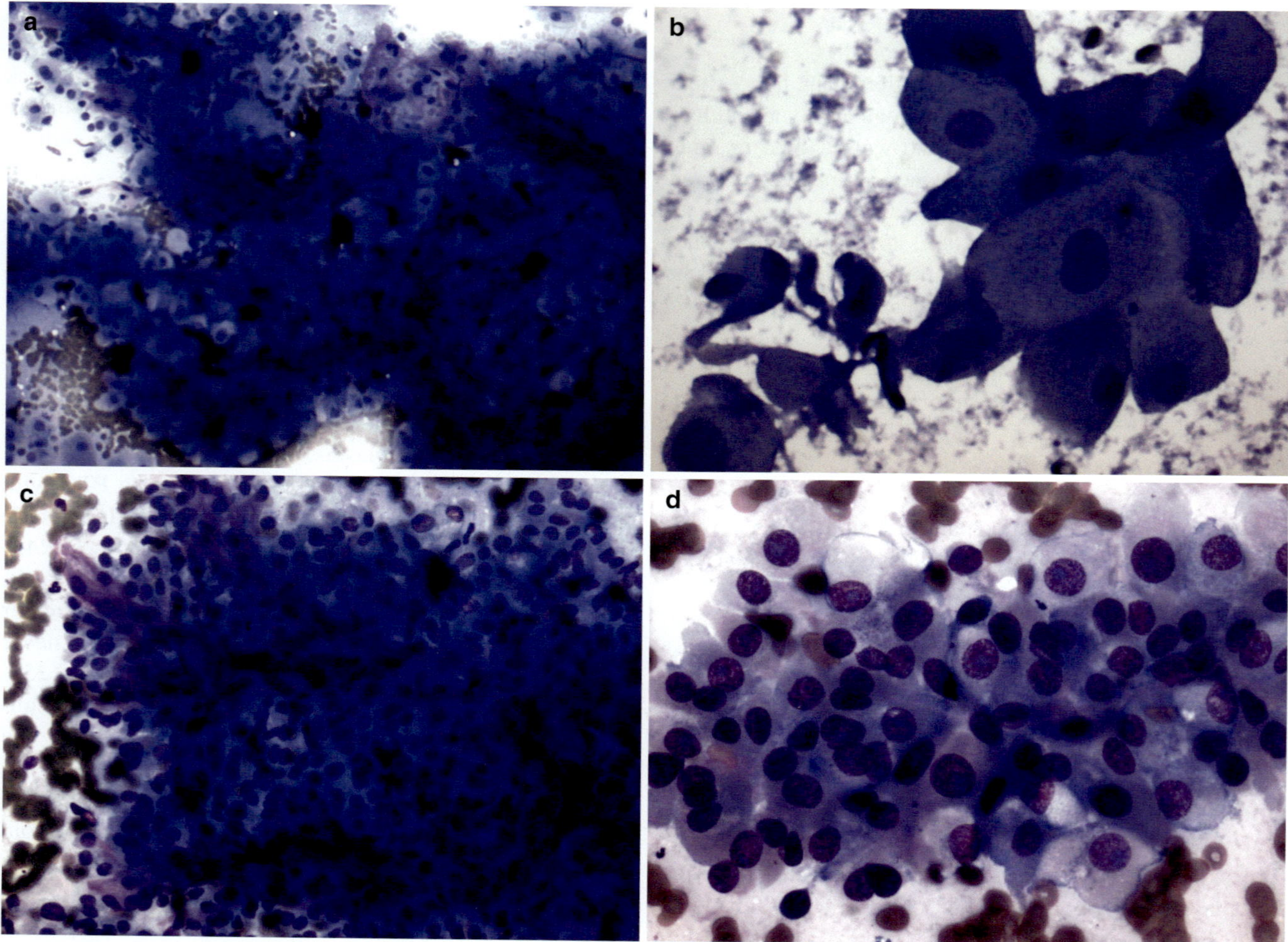

Fig. 3.45 Oncocytic thyroid adenoma (**a**, **b**). Smear shows high cellularity with crowded fragments of large cells and fine capillaries (**a**); cells show anisocytosis, round nuclei with prominent nucleoli and granular eosinophilic cytoplasm (**b**). Oncocytic thyroid carcinoma (**c–e**). Complex aggregate of monomorphic cells supported by a fine capillary network (**c**); bland appearing oncocytic cells are smaller than those of the prior case, monomorphic, and lack cytologic features of malignancy (**d**, **e**). Ultrasound features including Doppler exam of a case of oncocytic thyroid adenoma (**f**, **g**). (**a**, **c** and **d**, MGG stain, high power; **b** and **e**, Papanicolaou stain, high power)

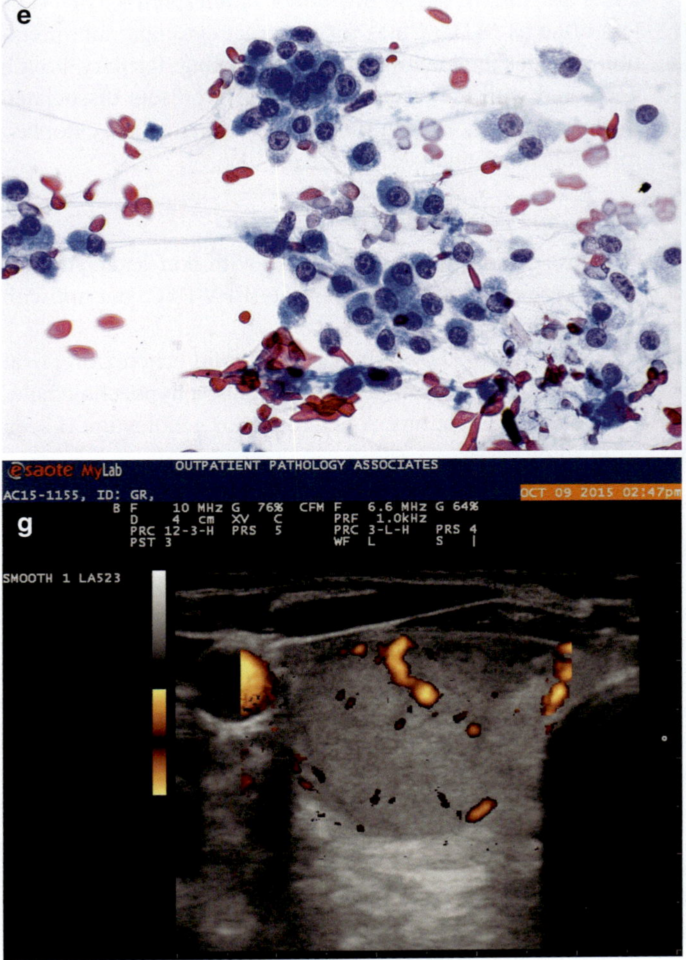

Fig. 3.45 (continued)

cells often lack nucleolus, and parathyroid tumors show a "salt-and-pepper" chromatin. Immunochemical stains are also helpful.

US Features (Fig. 3.45f, g)

- The US criteria are unreliable for differentiation among non-oncocytic follicular neoplasm, OTA, and OTC.

- Nodules have mixed hyper- and hypoechoic echogenicity, are often solid and ill-defined with incomplete halo, and lack punctate echogenic foci.
- Non-specific type-intranodular vascularity as seen in follicular neoplasms may be present.

FNA Diagnosiss of Low-Risk Neoplasms

Hyalinizing Trabecular Tumor

The 2022 WHO classification of thyroid tumors includes hyalinizing trabecular tumor (HTT) in the "low-risk neoplasm" category. HTT is a follicular cell-derived neoplasm with nuclear features of PTC.

Clinical Findings Patients are usually euthyroid and asymptomatic. HTT represents <1% of thyroid neoplasms, is more common in women in the fourth decade of life and is usually found incidentally. Chronic lymphocytic thyroiditis is present in 30% of cases. The clinical course is benign and complete excision is curative; total thyroidectomy or radioactive iodine treatment are not required.

Histopathology This encapsulated tumor has a characteristic trabecular arrangement of follicular cells surrounded by a prominent hyalinized collagenized stroma (type IV collagen). Cells show a cytoplasmic paranuclear yellow inclusion body (intermediate filaments) with a refractile appearance. Capsular or vascular invasion is absent. Stromal calcifications are common. The tumor shows psammoma bodies and shares morphologic features (nuclear inclusions, nuclear membrane irregularities, and groves) with PTC.

Immuno-Profile The tumor is consistently positive for TG, PAX8, TTF-1, and cytokeratin. Immunoreactivity for S-100 protein and neuroendocrine markers may be rarely seen. Cytoplasmic rather than nuclear MIB-1 stain (done at room temperature) is a distinctive feature and clue for the diagnosis. GLIS immunostain is positive; however, it is rarely available in all laboratories. Calcitonin and CEA are negative.

Molecular Profile HTT has a characteristic genetic profile that includes GLIS fusion/translocation (PAX8::*GLIS3*) in most cases and less commonly *PAX8::GLIS1*. These abnormalities have not been found in any other thyroid tumor. Rare cases of HTT share *RET/PTC* translocations as seen in PTC, but no *RAS* or *BRAF* mutations have been found. Of note, *RET/PTC* has also been seen in Hashimoto's thyroiditis, OTA, and TFND (hyperplastic nodules).

FNA Findings The smears are variably cellular and show single dispersed cells and complex cell aggregates embedded in a dense "amyloid-like" metachromatic material. The cells are large, round or spindle, with usually ill-defined cytoplasmic wispy/filamentous borders, dense cytoplasm, and numerous intranuclear cytoplasmic invaginations and nuclear grooves (Fig. 3.46a–d). Psammoma bodies and cytoplasmic paranuclear yellow inclusions (light green on Papanicolaou stain) may be present. True papillae with capillaries are absent. Often, this tumor is interpreted as PTC or less often as MTC. Clues for a correct cytologic interpretation includes the identification of branching fibrillary stroma decorated with tumor cells that are also present dissociated in the smear background, numerous intranuclear cytoplasmic inclusions, and lack of true papillae.

US Features (Fig. 3.46e, f)
- These tumors share US features with non-oncocytic follicular neoplasms, including the IEFV-PTC, but not with those of PTC.
- Tumors often show a hypoechoic solid echotexture, oval to round shape, well-defined margins, a hypoechoic halo, and no calcifications. A heterogenous echotexture is seen in some cases.

Noninvasive Follicular Tumor with Papillary-Like Nuclear Features (NIFTP) (Fig. 3.47a, b)

The term NIFTP (previously called "noninvasive follicular variant of PTC") was proposed in 2016 and the 2017 WHO classification of thyroid tumors endorsed it as NIFTP. The 2022 WHO classification of thyroid tumors includes NIFTP in the low-risk neoplasm category. It is a well-demarcated/encapsulated tumor with a follicular pattern, has an indolent clinical behavior, and should not be considered malignant.

Histopathology Histologic examination requires a meticulous evaluation of the capsule to rule out capsular and/or vascular invasion. Differential diagnosis includes IEFV-PTC, which is a malignant minimally invasive, encapsulated angioinvasive, or widely invasive tumor.

Molecular Profile It is not specific and overlaps with *RAS*-like tumors. *RET* fusions and *BRAF* V600E mutations are characteristic of PTC and absent in NIFTP.

- *RAS* mutations are seen in up to 60% of cases.
- *PAX8::PPARG* rearrangements are seen in up to 30% of cases.
- *THADA* gene fusions are seen in up to 30% of cases.
- *BRAF*-K601E, *EIF1AX*, *EZH1*, *DICER1*, *PTEN*, or *TSHR* mutations are seen in <10% of cases.

FNA Findings Distinction between the NIFTP and IEFV-PTC cannot be made by cytology. Furthermore, US features and molecular alterations overlap between the two entities. Cytologic distinction of NIFTP and IEFV-PTC from conventional PTC, requires the identification of true papilla, and/or prominent nuclear changes of PTC, and/or psammoma bodies to favor PTC. Cytologic interpretation of surgically proven NIFTP include AUS (50–75%), non-oncocytic follicular neo-

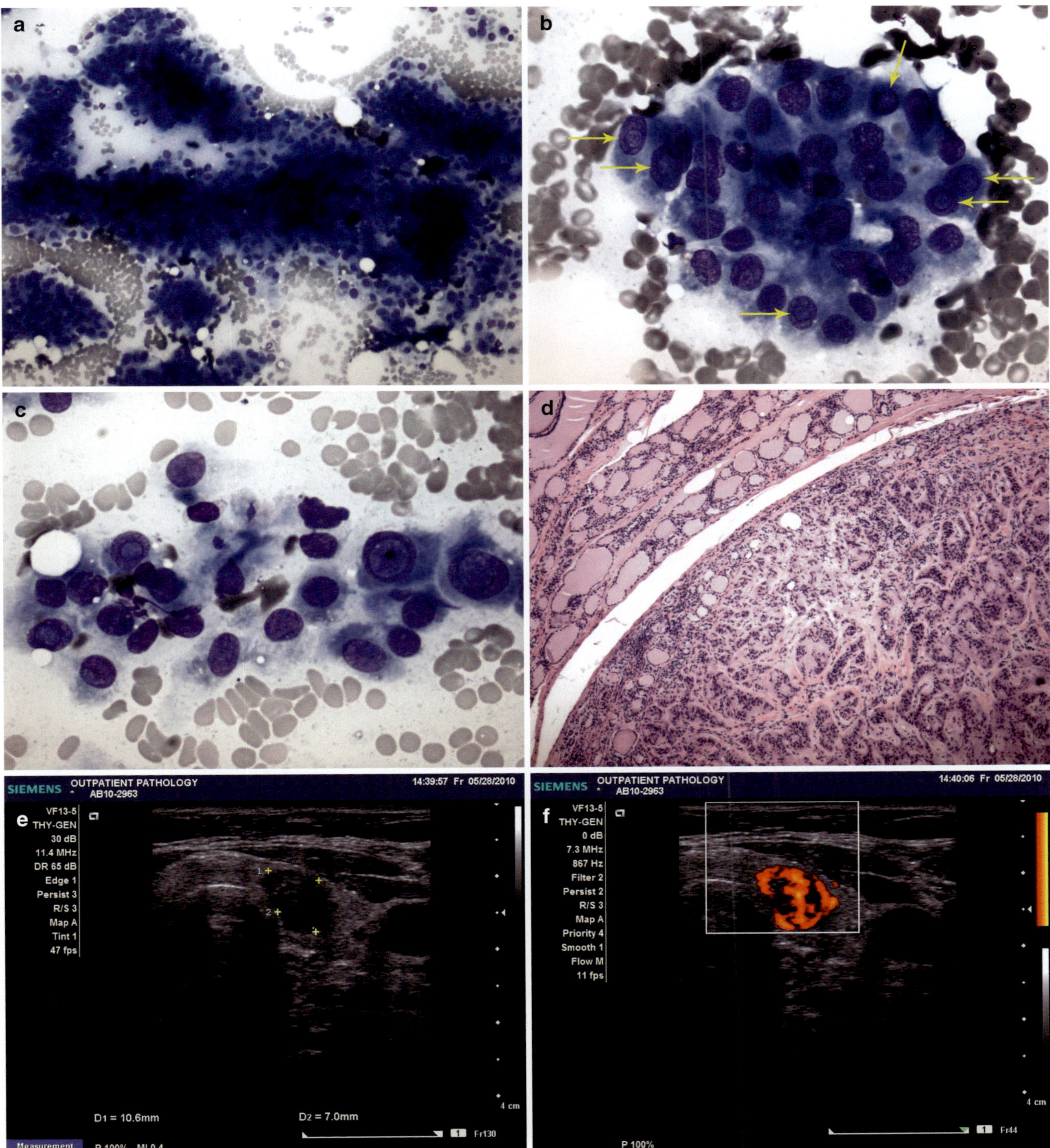

Fig. 3.46 Hyalinizing trabecular tumor. Smear is cellular (**a**) showing complex aggregates of large cells surrounded by an "amyloid-like" stroma (**b**). Cells have ill-defined wispy cytoplasmic borders, nuclear grooves, and numerous intranuclear cytoplasmic invaginations (**b, c**). Tissue section shows a circumscribed tumor with a trabecular architecture supported by a dense hyalinized stroma (**d**). Ultrasound features include an oval well-circumscribed homogeneous hypoechoic nodule with type 4 vascular pattern by Doppler examination (**e, f**). (**a–c**, MGG stain, high power; **d**, Hematoxylin/Eosin, low power)

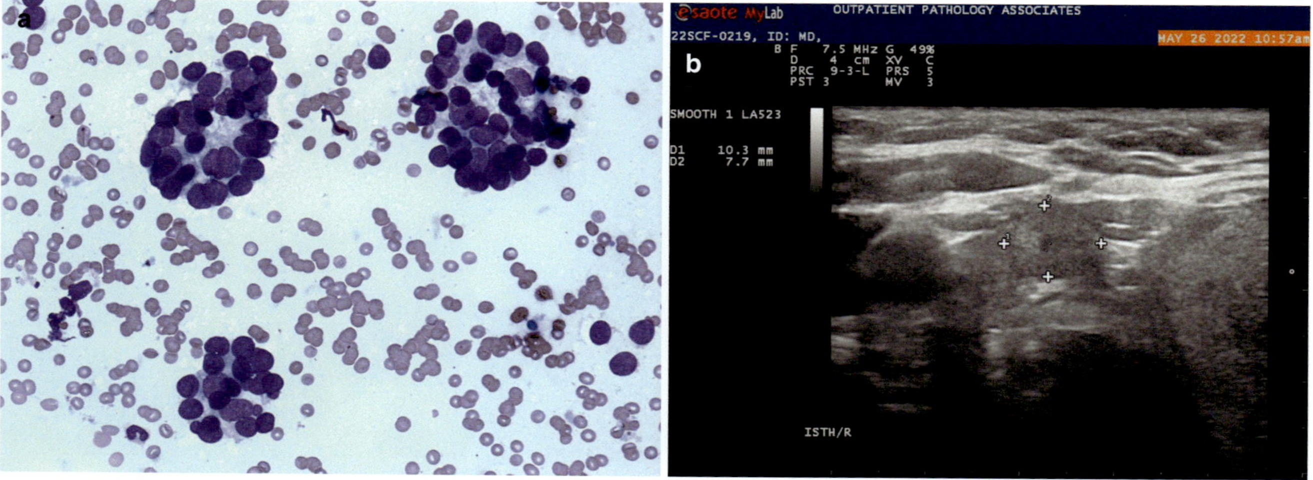

Fig. 3.47 Noninvasive follicular tumor with papillary-like nuclear features. Scattered microfollicles and absence of colloid are present; nuclei are enlarged with pale chromatin and rare intranuclear cytoplasmic invaginations (**a**). US shows a slightly heterogeneous and hypoechoic isthmus nodule (**b**). (**a**, MGG stain, medium power)

plasm (25–30%), and suspicious or malignant in a minority of cases. The 2023 TBSRTC recommends including cases with cytologic features suggestive of NIFTP in the AUS category followed by a comment raising this possibility.

Ultrasound Features Most US features are not specific and include wider that tall shape, well-circumscribed solid echotexture, iso- or hypoechogenicity, and no punctate echogenic foci. Similar features are seen in non-oncocytic follicular adenomas, IEFV-PTC, and minimally invasive FTC. In contrast, findings of deep hypoechogenicity, blurred/microlobulated borders, taller than wide shape, and punctate echogenic foci are features against NIFTP and IEFV-PTC.

FNA Diagnosis of Malignant Thyroid Neoplasms

The American Cancer Society statistics for 2024 estimates that 44,020 (M = 12,500 and F = 31,520) new cases of thyroid cancer will be diagnosed, and 2170 (M = 990 and F = 1180) will die of thyroid malignancy in the USA.

In adults and children, most thyroid malignancies are PTCs (75%–80%) followed by follicular (10%–15%), medullary (1%–2%), and anaplastic (<5%) carcinomas.

The 2022 WHO classification of follicular cell-derived thyroid neoplasms subdivides the malignant neoplasms into:

- Well-differentiated thyroid carcinoma (WDTC).
  - Papillary thyroid carcinoma (PTC).
  - Follicular thyroid carcinoma (FTC).
  - Oncocytic thyroid carcinoma (OTC).
  - Invasive encapsulated follicular variant (IEFV)-PTC.

- Differentiated high-grade thyroid carcinoma (DHGTC).
- Poorly differentiated thyroid carcinoma (PDTC).
- Anaplastic follicular cell-derived carcinoma (ATC).

The histopathology of DHGTC includes thyroid carcinomas with papillary, follicular or solid growth with invasive features, any nuclear cytology, and mitoses (≥5/10HPF) and/or necrosis.

The histopathology of PDTC includes thyroid carcinomas with invasive features, no papillary or follicular component and instead insular, trabecular, and solid histologic tumor architecture, convoluted nuclei with no nuclear features of PTC, and mitoses (≥3/10 HPF) and/or necrosis.

Medullary thyroid carcinoma (MTC) represents <5% of thyroid malignancies.

Thyroid lymphoma, sarcoma, and metastases are rare.

Papillary Thyroid Carcinoma

Papillary thyroid carcinoma (PTC), a *BRAF*-driven neoplasm is the most common type of thyroid malignancy in children and adults, affecting more women than men and predominating in the fifth decade of life. There has been almost a threefold increment in the incidence of PTC in the last 3 decades, mostly due to an increase in detection and not in the true occurrence. Risk factors for PTC include external radiation to the neck during childhood, exposure to ionizing radiation, and genetic susceptibility.

The long-term prognosis is very good, particularly in children and adolescents (close to 100%). The 30-year survival rate is 99% and 95% at 20 years and 30 years after surgery, respectively. Based on its biologic behavior, PTC is treated with total or near-total thyroidectomy with lymph node dissection, depending on the extent of intra- and extrathyroidal and metastatic disease, followed by [131]I. Adverse prognostic factors include male sex, older patients, large tumor size, extracapsular extension or vascular invasion, distant metastases, tall cell, columnar cell, and diffuse sclerosing subtypes at histology, and high postoperative TG levels. Cervical lymph node metastasis does not seem to affect the prognosis. Death secondary to PTC is rare.

DNA ploidy, circulating tumor cells detected by RT-PCR assay for TG RNA, or detection of *BRAF*-V600E mutation are also considered adverse prognostic factors.

Clinical Findings Patients are usually asymptomatic and euthyroid. Lymph node involvement is common particularly in young patients and may be the first manifestation of the disease. Hematogenous metastases are less common. *BRAF* mutations have been associated with lymph node and lung metastases. Extrathyroidal extension is seen in 25% of patients at the time of surgery.

Histopathology The tumor shows a papillary architecture with fibrovascular cores lined with columnar, cuboidal, and at times hobnail epithelium. A follicular component is commonly seen. The cytologic findings include ground-glass nuclei (absent in frozen sections and FNA material), intranuclear cytoplasmic invaginations (present in frozen sections and FNA material), nuclear groves, and nuclear microfilaments seen in rare cases as intranuclear clearing. Psammoma bodies are seen in 50% of cases and, when present, are almost always indicative of PTC; however, they can be seen in MTC. A clear cell change may occur as a result of glycogen accumulation. Chronic inflammation is seen in 25% of cases. The two cardinal features that characterize the classic (conventional) PTC include papillary aggregates supported by fibrovascular cores and cells with nuclear features of PTC.

Immuno-Profile PTC shows positivity for CK/CK19/ TTF-1, TG, HBME-1, PAX8. CK20 is negative. These markers are rarely used because the diagnosis is made by morphology in most cases. However, the most specific and useful markers for determination of the cell lineage are TG and TTF-1. Because the oncocytic cells of Hashimoto's thyroiditis share their immunoprofile with PTC, HBME-1 and CK19 are most useful for differentiating between the two. Ki67 index is low (<1–5%).

Molecular Profile The *BRAF*-like molecular alterations are the most common in PTC. The mitogen-activated protein kinase (MAPK) pathway, physiologically activated by growth factors binding to receptor tyrosine kinases in the cytoplasmic membrane, propagates signals to the nucleus and regulates cell proliferation, differentiation, and survival (Diagram 3.1).

- In PTC, activation of this pathway is secondary to point mutations of *BRAF* genes, or results from *RET/PTC* and *TRK* rearrangements involving the *RET* and *NTRK1* genes, respectively (Diagrams 3.4 and 3.5). RET/PTC is the major molecular marker for PTC and at least 15 types of *RET/PTC* chimeric oncogene have been identified in PTC. All of these mutations and rearrangements are present in 70% of PTCs and were initially thought to be mutually exclusive; however, a simultaneous occurrence of these genetic abnormalities has been shown in some PTCs.

- Activating mutations of the *BRAF* oncogene are highly specific for PTC and related tumor types, are seen in 40–70% of PTCs with the presence of valine in residue 600 of protein (V600E) in most cases and correlate directly with the tumor papillary architecture. Most PTCs carrying the *BRAF* V600E mutation are classic, tall-cell, oncocytic, and Warthin-like subtypes, and sub-

Diagram 3.4 *BRAF* in papillary carcinoma (50%)

BRAF in Papillary Carcinoma (50%)

Oncogenic Point Mutation

↓

BRAF V600E
(Substitution of thymine with adenine = production Glu instead of Val)

↓

Activation and prolonged stimulation of MAPK signaling pathway

↓

Benign Follicular Cell ⟶ Malignant Follicular Cell

95% *BRAF*+PTCs show V600E

Associated with aggressive tumor behavior
& less optimal therapy response including T1
tumors (< 2 cm)

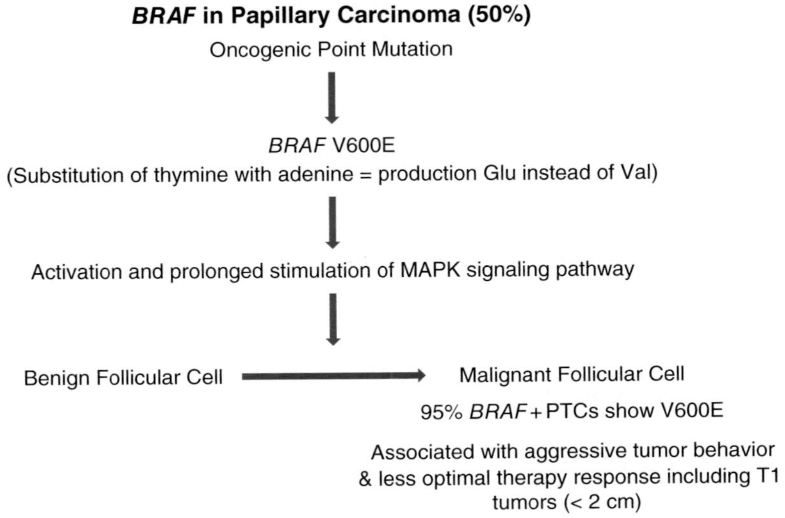

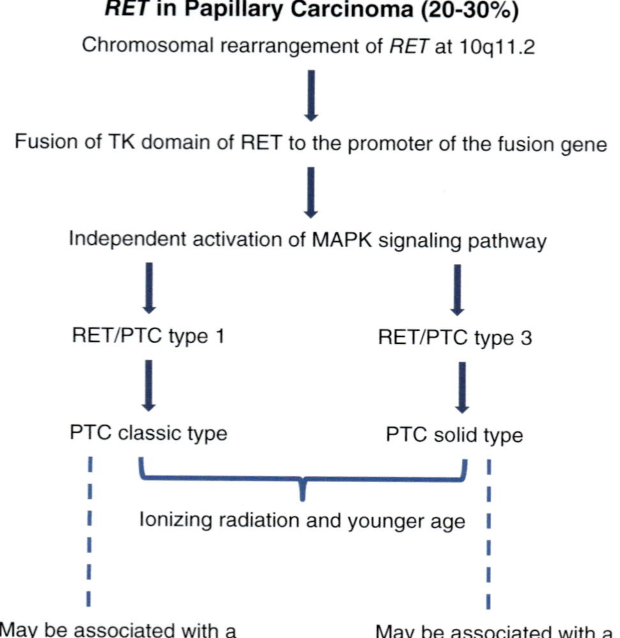

Diagram 3.5 *RET* in papillary carcinoma (20–30%)

capsular sclerosing microcarcinomas. Of note, *BRAF* and *NRAS* gene mutations have been identified in 24% and 8% of diffuse large B-cell thyroid lymphomas, respectively.

- *BRAF* V600E mutation is an early event in thyroid carcinogenesis and has been associated with male gender, older age at diagnosis, classic nuclear features of PTC, infiltrative growth, stromal fibrosis, psammoma bodies, extrathyroidal extension, lymph node metastasis, a higher risk of persistent disease, and more aggressive tumors that are refractory to radioiodine therapy. These prognostic implications are of particular importance in PTCs ≤2 cm, including microcarcinomas. Thus, detection of *BRAF* V600E mutation preoperatively may play a role in a more aggressive surgical approach, post-surgical therapy, and closer follow-up.
- *BRAF* V600E mutations are uncommon in PTC occurring in children and in relation to radiation exposure and have not been found in TFND or FTC. They can be reliably detected by molecular techniques in paraffin-embedded tissue and cell block from FNA samples.
- Gene rearrangements occur in 20–40% of PTCs, mostly involving *RET*, a transmembrane tyrosine kinase receptor. Clonal *RET/PTC rearrangement* is a strong indicator of PTC and has a variable incidence, being detected in 10–20% of adult sporadic PTC, 50–80% of tumors from patients with a history of therapeutic or environmental radiation exposure (detected in 87% of post Chernobyl-related PTC), and 40–70% of PTC in children and young

adults. Of note, activating *point* mutations of the same *RET* oncogene are detected in MTC.

- Fusions involving *PPARG, NTRK1, NTRK3, ALK, LTK, MET, RET, FGFR2 or THADA* are detected in 15% of PTCs; among them, *RET* fusion is the most common, seen in 6%. These alterations are included in the so-called *BRAF*-like molecular group.
- *RET, NTRK1, NTRK3, ALK, BRAF,* and *MET* fusions are the most common genetic alterations (56% of 93 cases) found in classical and follicular subtypes of pediatric PTCs; their presence is associated with an aggressive behavior.
- *NTRK1* is a gene that encodes a transmembrane tyrosine kinase receptor that binds the nerve growth factor. Rearrangement of this gene is identified in 5% of PTCs, and the clinicopathological features are similar to those of PTCs associated with *RET/PTC* rearrangement. However, it is uncommon in PTC related to radiation exposure.
- VEGF, binding to two receptor tyrosine kinases (VEGFR1 and VEGFR2), also triggers MAPK signaling, and the intensity of expression correlates with a poor prognosis and *BRAF* mutation status.
- *TERT* promoter mutation is present in <1% of cases and is associated with aggressive behavior as in DHGTC.

FNA Findings (Fig. 3.48a–e) PTCs of all conventional and subtypes share the same cytomorphologic criteria. Smears are usually cellular and show monolayered sheets, complex tridimensional aggregates (without fibrovascular cores), and single cells. Corrugated or "onionskin" cell sheets and papillary clusters with fibrovascular cores may occasionally be seen. Cellular overlapping, crowding, and molding are important diagnostic features. Cells are enlarged and show dense cytoplasm with well-defined cytoplasmic borders. Squamous metaplasia and focal oncocytic change may also be seen. Enlarged oval or irregularly shaped nuclei with longitudinal linear groves, powdery clear chromatin, and small, eccentrically placed nucleoli and intranuclear cytoplasmic invaginations, are characteristic diagnostic nuclear findings. The background may show stringy, ropy, "bubble-gum"-like colloid and variable numbers of macrophages and lymphocytes. Psammoma bodies and multinucleated giant cell may also been seen.

None of the mentioned features is specific of PTC, and the FNA diagnosis is based on a conjunction of cytologic, architectural, and background features. Intranuclear cytoplasmic invaginations, although crucial for the diagnosis of PTC, are not specific; they are also seen in MTC, DHGTC, PDTC, ATC, and rarely in TFND and chronic thyroiditis. Similarly, psammoma bodies can be seen in MTC, TFND, and chronic thyroiditis.

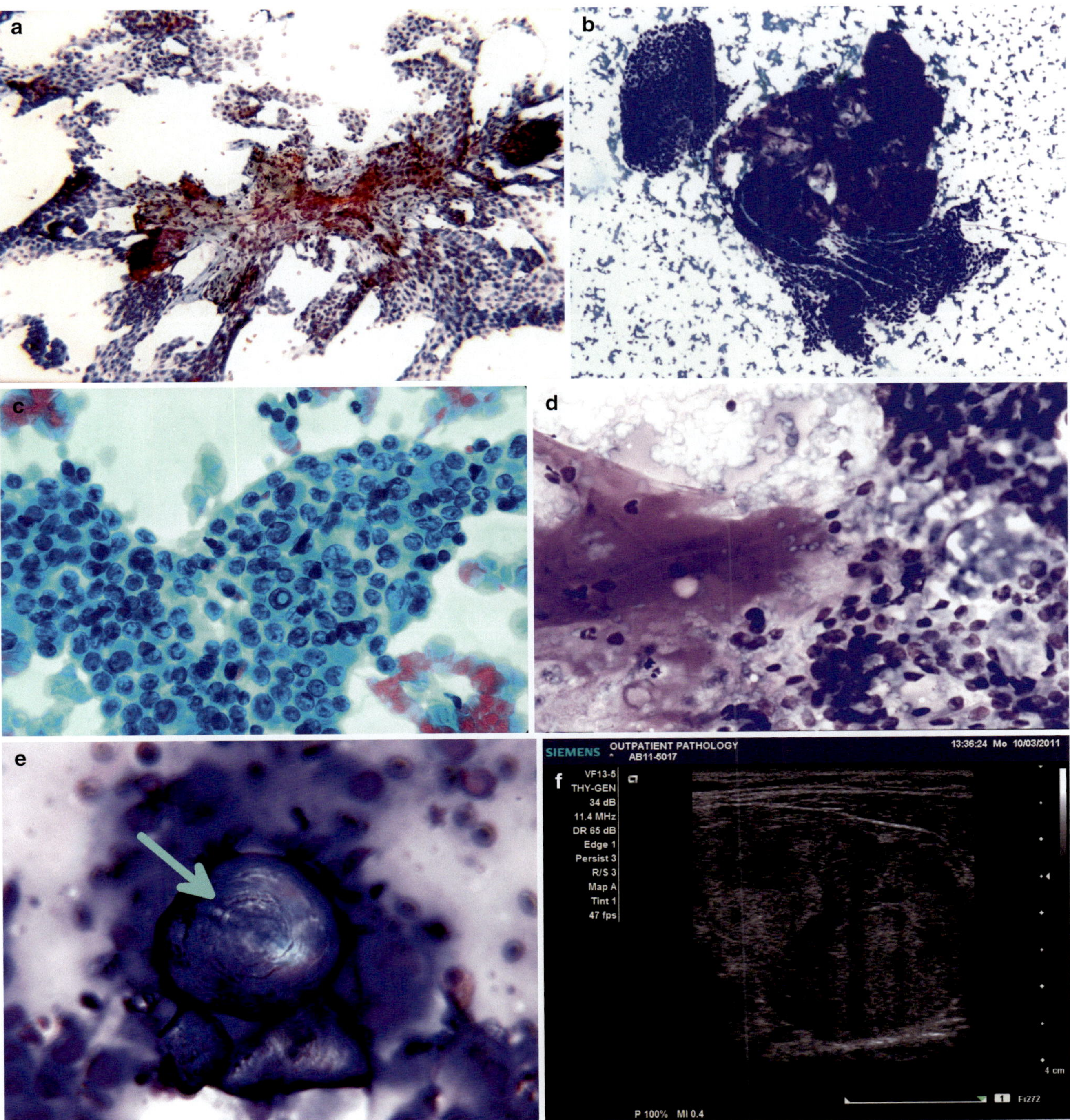

Fig. 3.48 Papillary thyroid carcinoma. FNA cytology of papillary thyroid carcinoma showing papillary fronds (**a**), corrugated sheets of neoplastic cells (**b**), cohesive cell sheets with nuclear grooves and intranuclear cytoplasmic invaginations (**c**), stringing chewing gum-type colloid (**d**), and psammoma bodies (**e**). Ultrasound features of papillary carcinoma (**f–k**) include nodule(s) of variable size, usually solid echotexture with incomplete halo, hypoecho-genicity, irregular lobulated margins, micro-, macro-, or eggshell calcifications, and variable blood flow on Doppler examination. Hyperechogenicity may be seen in rare cases accompanied with chaotic grade 3 vascularity on Doppler examination (**l**, **m**). (**a**, Papanicolaou stain, low power; **b**, DiffQuik stain, low power; **c** and **e**, Papanicolaou stain, medium power; **d**, DiffQuik stain, medium power)

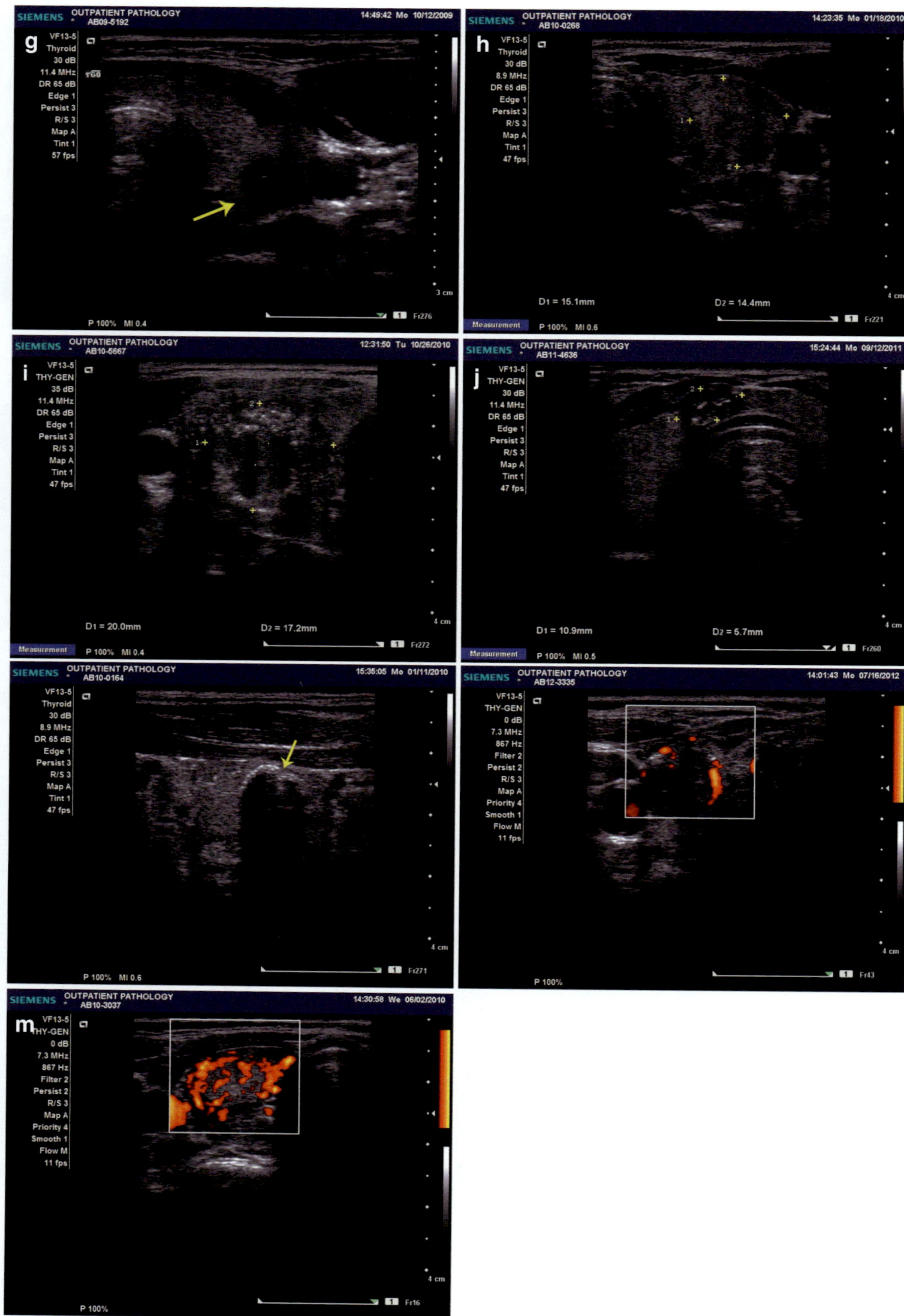

Fig. 3.48 (continued)

In general, the cytoplasmic features including intranuclear cytoplasmic invaginations are best seen in Romanowsky-stained smears; in contrast, nuclear features are best appreciated with Papanicolaou and hematoxylin and eosin stains.

Some of the classical PTC features (cell sheets, smear background, intranuclear cytoplasmic invaginations, pale nuclei, nuclear crowding/overlapping, papillary fragments) seen in conventional preparations may not be observed in FNA specimens processed by liquid-based preparations making the interpretation difficult.

Of note, the cytopathologist must be aware of the cytomorphologic spectrum of PTC, but it is not required to specify the subtype of PTC in the FNA report. Specific architectural, cytoplasmic, nuclear, and background features characterize specific subtypes and will be addressed under the specific subtype.

US Features (Fig. 3.48f–m)

- A halo is seen in 15–30% of cases, frequently incomplete, and represents encapsulation.
- Irregular margins and hypoechogenicity occur in 75–90% of cases.
- Most have a solid composition (70%); however, 20–30% are variably cystic and even purely cystic in rare instances.
- Microcalcifications are seen in 25–45%.
- Coarse and eggshell calcifications are less common; however, an interrupted, displaced, or fractures eggshell calcification is an alarming US finding strongly suspicious for PTC (Fig. 3.48 Video 3.14).
- Multifocality occurs in 10–20% of cases. Associated microcarcinomas are more common.
- Increased vascularity is almost always seen but is not specific. Probably low vascularity has a good negative predictive value for a given nodule.
- In summary, PTCs may be solid and hypoechoic, with microcalcifications, blurred, irregular and lobulated margins, lack of a complete halo, and high intranodular blood flow on power Doppler.
- Invasion of adjacent thyroid and/or extrathyroidal tissue may be present (Fig. 3.48 Video 3.15).
- Lymph node metastasis may be seen with calcifications or cystic degeneration.

Subtypes of PTC

The PTC subtypes considered in the 2022 WHO classification of thyroid neoplasms include infiltrative follicular (includes the macrofollicular), diffuse sclerosing, tall cell, columnar cell, hobnail, solid, Warthin-like, and oncocytic. All share similar nuclear features, and the prognosis may be different when compared with the conventional PTC. However, the initial surgical approach is usually similar.

The microPTC (≤1 cm) generally shows an indolent behavior and the 2022 WHO classification of thyroid tumors suggests the classification be based on the histopathologic subtype rather than tumor size.

The cribriform-morular tumor is no longer a PTC subtype and has been placed in the "thyroid tumors of uncertain histogenesis."

Infiltrative Follicular Subtype

The follicular subtype represents approximately 30% of PTCs in some series. The prognosis is similar to that of the classical/conventional PTC.

Histopathology This subtype shows an entirely or almost entirely microfollicular pattern with nuclear features diagnostic of PTC. The follicular pattern may be microfollicular, normofollicular, or macrofollicular. An abortive papilla, psammoma bodies, and dense colloid support the diagnosis. Associated minor histologic patterns of this subtype include solid and macrofollicular ones, both with nuclear features of classical PTC and well-differentiated features.

Molecular Profile Molecular features are similar to those present in classic/conventional PTC in particular *BRAF-V600E* mutation. *RET/PTC* rearrangement can be seen.

FNA Findings (Fig. 3.49a–c) The smear pattern is that of a microfollicular neoplasm with cells showing nuclear features of PTC. Occasional sheets of cells of normal size are also seen. Dense colloid may be seen in the background and in the follicular lumens. Of note, when nuclear findings are inconspicuous, including intranuclear cytoplasmic invaginations and nuclear grooves, the differential diagnosis includes NIFTP and IEFV-PTC. Correlation with US and molecular findings is necessary in these cases. Therefore, unless diagnostic nuclear features are seen, the USG-FNA diagnosis is usually "follicular neoplasm," with a note addressing the various entities included in the differential diagnosis.

US Features (Fig. 3.49d–e)

- The follicular subtype of PTC often has a benign US appearance, i.e., ovoid to round, iso- to hyperechoic, with a halo.
- Hypoechogenicity is seen in 50% of cases.
- Solid and regular or irregular, well-defined margins.
- A minority (5%) are taller than wide.
- Microcalcifications are rare.

Macrofollicular Subtype

Histologically, more than 50% of the follicles are arranged as macrofollicles.

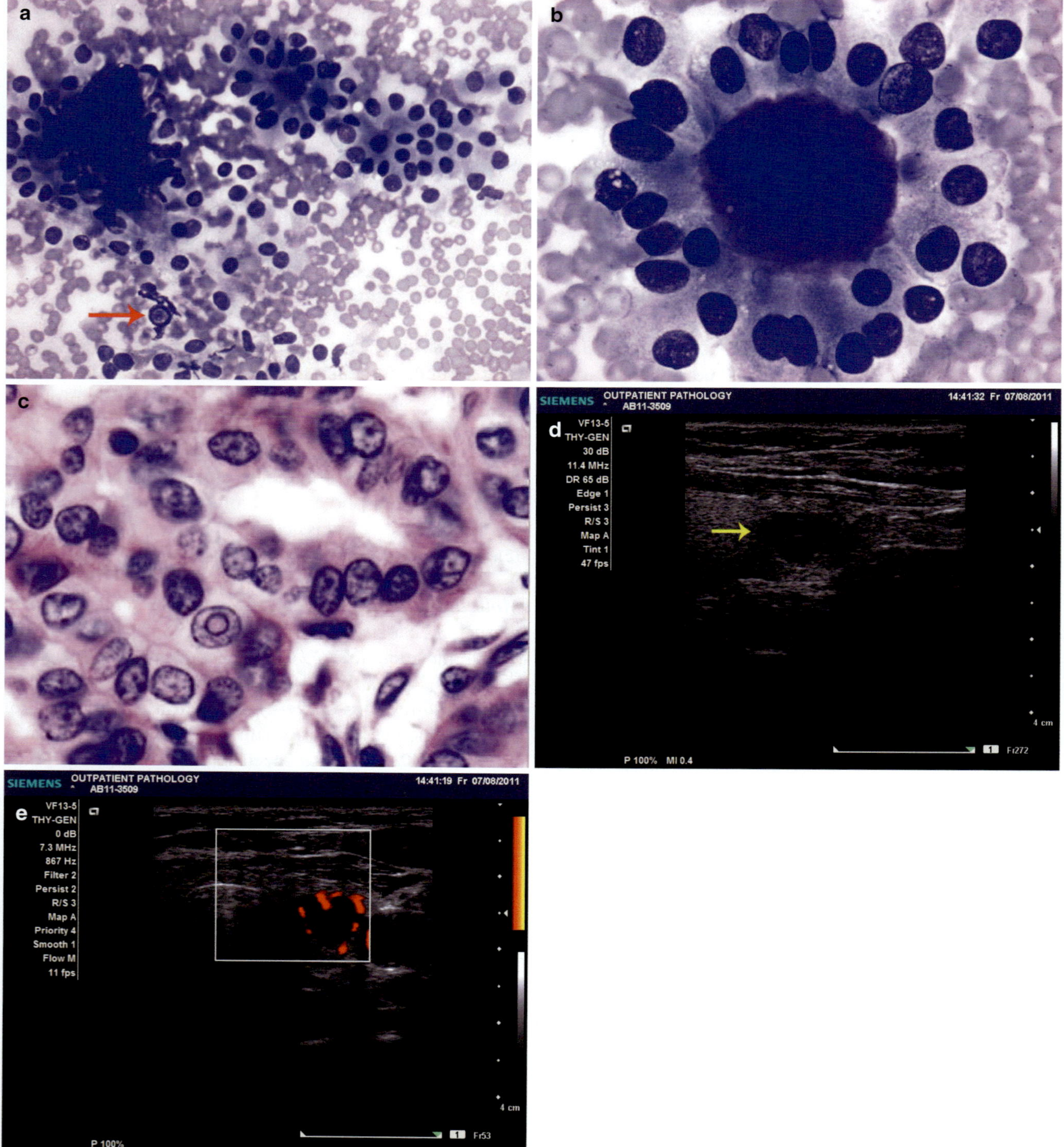

Fig. 3.49 Papillary thyroid carcinoma, follicular subtype. FNA smear shows high cellularity (**a**) with microfollicles containing central dense colloid (**b**) and rare intranuclear cytoplasmic invaginations (**a**, arrow) recapitulating tissue section findings (**c**). Ultrasound features are not specific and include a hypoechoic solid nodule with irregular margins, focal fuzzy edges, and type 2 blood flow by Doppler examination (**e**, **f**). (**a**, **b** DiffQuik stain, high power; **c**, hematoxylin eosin stain, high power. Courtesy Dr. Javier Saenz de Santamaria, Badajoz, Spain)

FNA Findings (Fig. 3.50a–d) The smears are cellular and show sheets of cells of variable size and thin colloid, which, at low power resemble, the findings of a nodule of TFND. The nuclear diagnostic features of PTC must be evaluated at high microscopic power.

Diffuse Sclerosing Subtype

This subtype is uncommon (3% of all PTCs), occurs commonly in pediatric and young female population and in patients with history of radiation. Cervical lymph node and lung metastases are more common than in the classic/conventional PTC, conferring a less favorable prognosis.

Clinical Findings A hard thyroid gland is identified and mimics Riedel thyroiditis. Symptoms of local compression may be present. Regional lymphadenopathy may be identified.

Histopathology There is diffuse involvement of one or both thyroid lobes, extensive solid foci, squamous metaplasia, dense fibrosis, a marked lymphocytic infiltrate, numerous psammoma bodies, and vascular permeation. Extrathyroidal invasion is common.

Immunoprofile Tumor cells show positivity for TG, TTF1, and CK19. Napsin A may be positive and PAX8 may be negative.

Molecular Profile *RET/PTC* rearrangement has been identified in 60% of cases (resulting in the activation of RAS/RAF/MAPK pathway). *NCOA4::RET* is seen in cases after radiation. *BRAF* mutations are seen in up to 20% of cases (50% in Korea) and *ALK* translocations in 13%.

FNA Findings (Fig. 3.51a, b) Smears may be modestly cellular and show numerous psammoma bodies along with

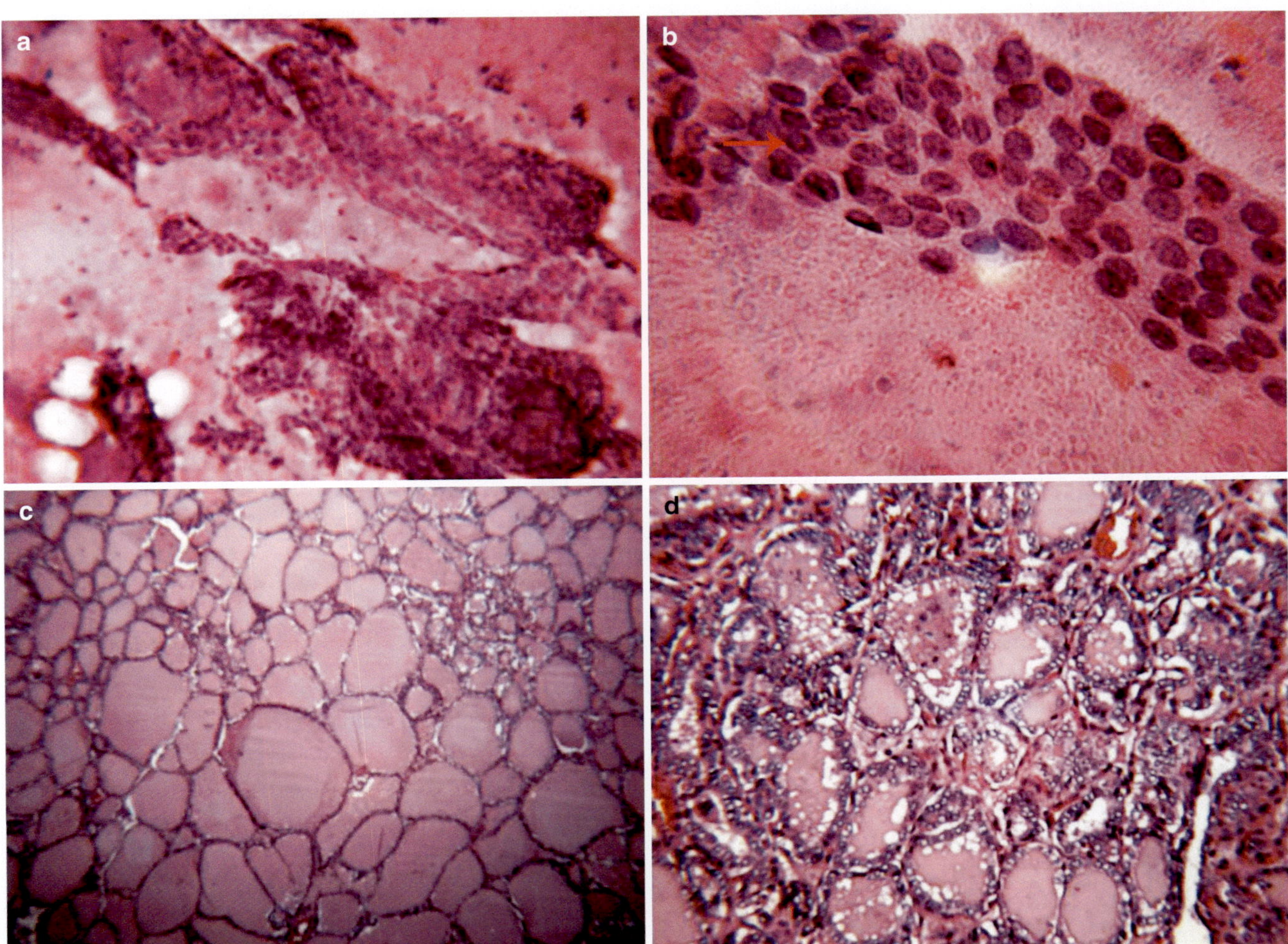

Fig. 3.50 Papillary thyroid carcinoma, macrofollicular subtype. FNA smear shows large cell sheets and colloid, findings that at low magnification resemble those of benign thyroid nodule. Nuclear hypochromasia, grooves, and rare intranuclear cytoplasmic invaginations (**b**, red arrow) are seen at high magnification (**a**, **b**). Similarly, the histologic examination requires careful search for nuclear features of papillary carcinoma (**c**, **d**). (**a–d**, hematoxylin eosin stain, low and medium power)

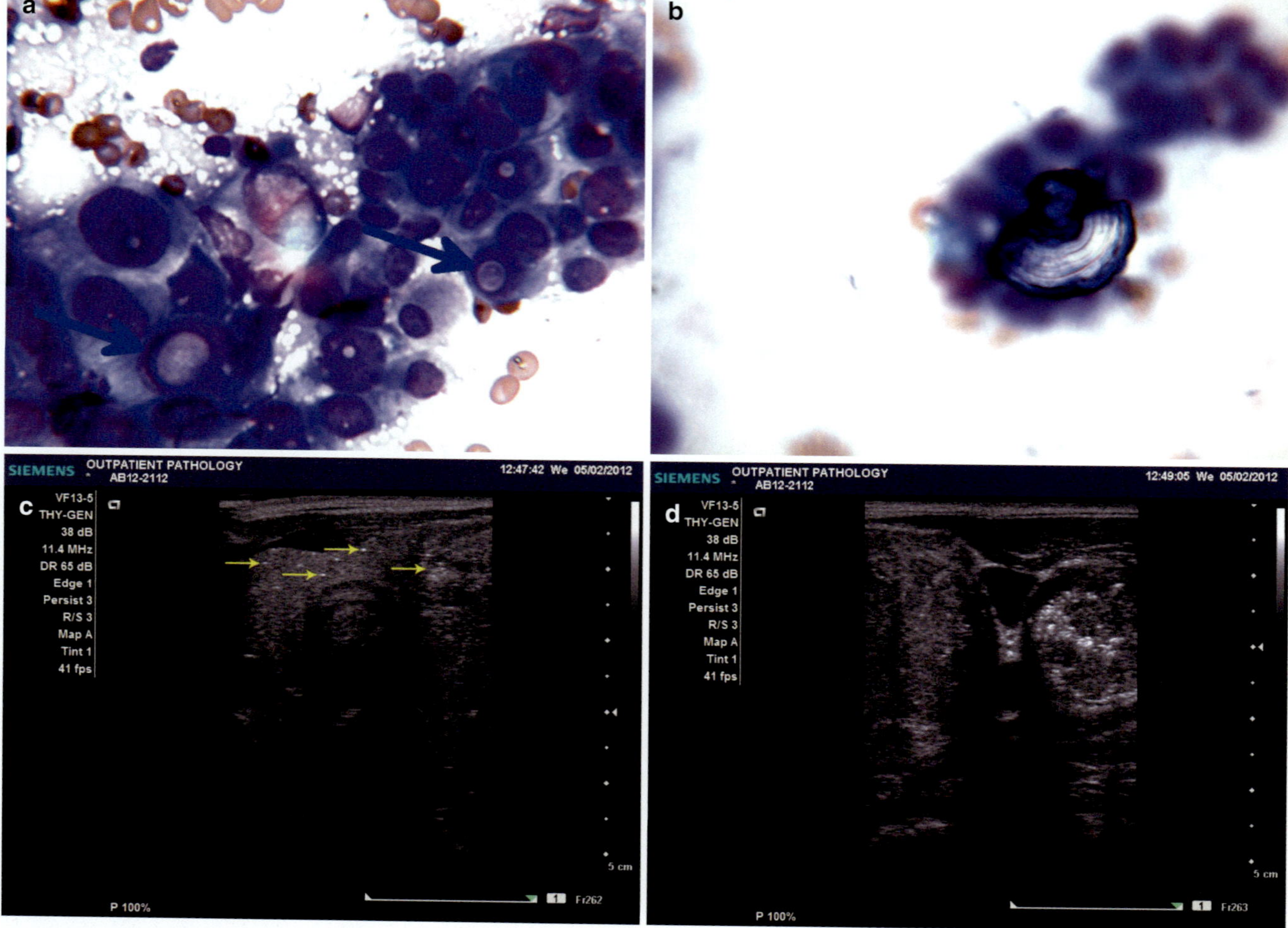

Fig. 3.51 Papillary thyroid carcinoma, diffuse sclerosing subtype. FNA smears show cytologic features of papillary carcinoma including complex cellular aggregates and intranuclear cytoplasmic invaginations (**a**, blue arrows), and numerous psammoma bodies (**b**). Ultrasound shows numerous diffuse microcalcifications scat-tered in the thyroid parenchyma (**c**, arrows), a large left thyroid lobe iso- to hyperechoic mass (**d**, left side of frame), and lymph node metastasis (**d**, right side of frame) both with numerous diffuse microcalcifications ("snowstorm" pattern). (**a**, **b**, MGG stain, high power view)

cytologic features of PTC, including sheets of follicular cells with pleomorphic nuclear enlargement, irregular nuclear membranes, grooves, and intranuclear cytoplasmic invaginations commonly present in a background of chronic thyroiditis. In contrast to conventional PTC, this subtype has fewer nuclear inclusions and nuclear grooves, and the chromatin is darker than in conventional PTC. Three-dimensional ball-like clusters are also present. Squamous metaplastic cells may be seen.

US Features (Fig. 3.51c, d)

- Large, heterogenous solid tumors with irregular margins often involving one entire thyroid lobe diffusely; the involvement may be bilateral.
- There is hyper- or hypoechogenicity.
- Scattered microcalcifications are present ("snowstorm" pattern), most commonly diffuse and rarely focal.
- Metastatic cervical lymph nodes are almost always present.

Cystic Subtype

This PTC subtype occurs in 5% of PTCs, and the associated lymph node metastases are often cystic.

Histopathology The amount of cystic change varies, and most retain a papillary architecture.

FNA Findings (Fig. 3.52a, b) Smears show a background of abundant thin, watery fluid, numerous macrophages with variable cytoplasmic hemosiderin, and tumor cells often with vacuolated cytoplasm ("histiocytoid" cells).

The epithelial component may be inconspicuous, but usually shows sufficient diagnostic criteria with convincing nuclear features for diagnosis. Cells may be arranged in small aggregates, papillae, and small follicles. Cyst lining epithelium and metaplastic cells may be present. This subtype should be kept in mind in cases showing a dominant or entirely cystic and/or hemorrhagic smear pattern.

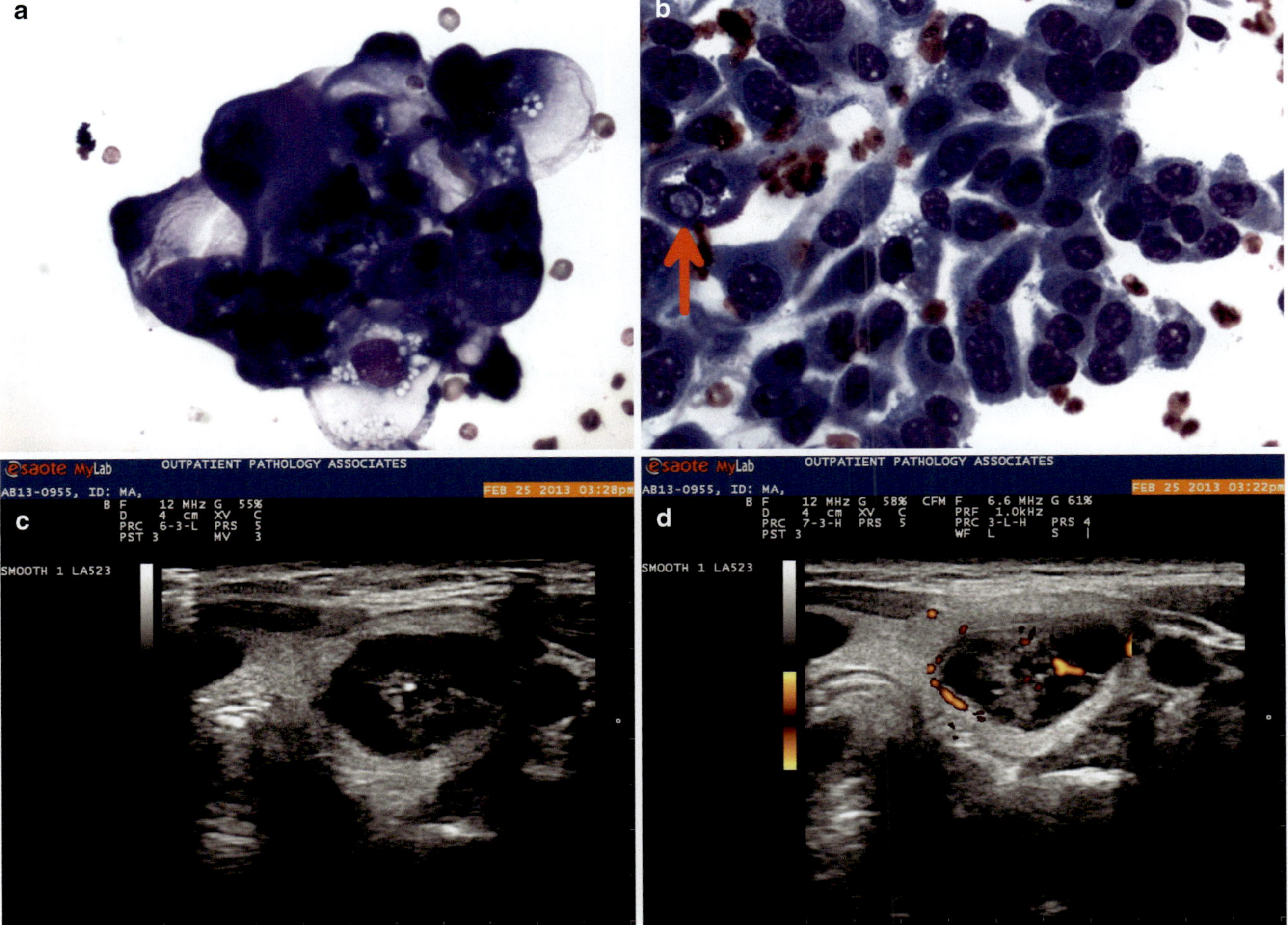

Fig. 3.52 Papillary thyroid carcinoma, cystic subtype. FNA smear shows aggregates of large cells with ballooned cytoplasm containing large vacuoles ("histiocytoid" cells) in a background of watery fluid (**a**). Occasional intranuclear cytoplasmic invaginations are seen in the meta-plastic cells (**b**, red arrow). Ultrasound shows a predominantly cystic complex nodule with a bright dot corresponding to the 27-gauge needle tip in the solid component (**a**); blood flow by Doppler examination is evident in the solid portion (**d**). (**a**, **b**, MGG stain, high power)

US Features (Fig. 3.52c, d)

- Cystic tumors are often taller than wide and have spiculated margins.
- A solid hypervascular nodule is almost always seen in the cyst wall.
- A "comet tail" sign can be observed, particularly in cystic metastases to lymph nodes.
- Microcalcifications may be seen in the solid component.

Oncocytic Subtype (Fig. 3.53a–f)

The growth pattern may be papillary or follicular. In this subtype, the cells are polygonal and have abundant granular eosinophilic cytoplasm and nuclear features of PTC.

When the oncocytic subtype of PTC shows heavy lymphocytic infiltrate in the papilla, the tumor is named **Warthin-like subtype** of PTC and has *BRAF* mutations and *RET/PTC* rearrangements. The prognosis is similar to that of the classic PTC.

FNA Findings Smears are variably cellular and show a predominance of oncocytic cells arranged in papillae, sheets, or as isolated cells with nuclear changes of PTC. The background shows rare or no lymphocytes.

When a papillary architecture is prominent and lymphoid cells are numerous, a **Warthin-like subtype** must be considered. When lymphocytes are absent, the differential diagnosis includes oncocytic neoplasms. Thus, this subtype should be searched for when the smear pattern shows a predominance of oncocytic cells. However, if a lymphoplasmacytic infiltrate is present, the **Warthin-like subtype** may be overlooked, and the tumor diagnosed as Hashimoto's thyroiditis. Of note, nucleoli are more prominent in Hashimoto's thyroiditis than in any of the oncocytic-rich subtypes.

Tall-Cell Subtype

This tumor tends to occur in elderly people, particularly men. The course is aggressive and often presents as a bulky

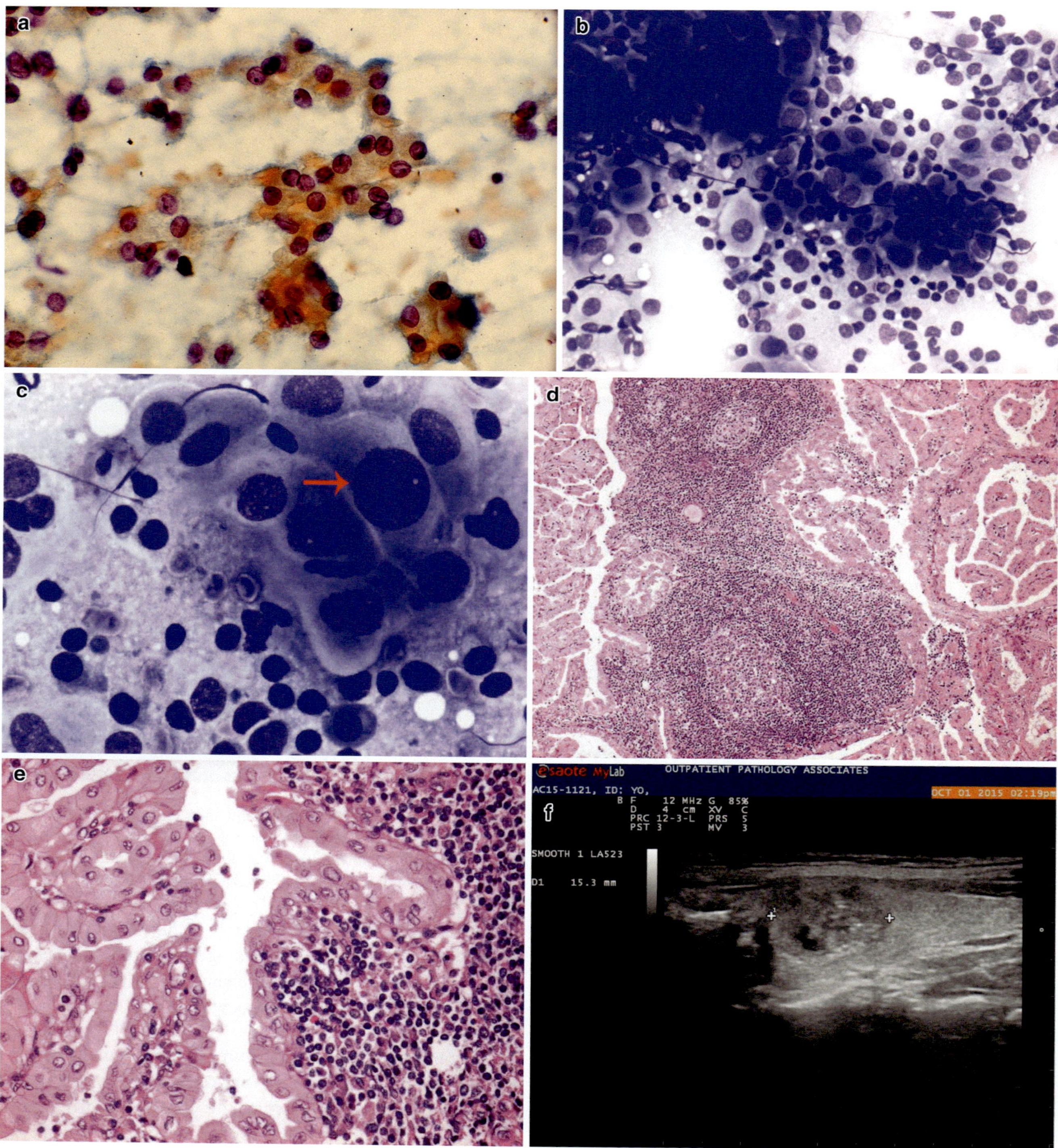

Fig. 3.53 The smears of the papillary thyroid carcinoma, oncocytic subtype, show small sheets and circumferential aggregates of cells with eosinophilic cytoplasm, nuclear features of papillary carcinoma, and lack of lymphoid cells (**a**). The smears of the papillary thyroid carcinoma, Warthin's subtype, show aggregates of large cells exhibiting eosinophilic granular cytoplasm and nuclear features of papillary carcinoma in a background of numerous lymphocytes and plasma cells (**b**, **c**). Histologic sections confirm the diagnosis (**d**, **e**). US shows a hypoechoic nodule with heterogeneous echotexture and lobulated margin (**f**). (**a**, Papanicolaou stain, medium power; **b**, DiffQuik stain, medium power; **c**, DiffQuik stain, high power; **d**, **e**, hematoxylin eosin stain, low and medium power. Courtesy Dr. Javier Saenz de Santamaria, Badajoz, Spain)

tumor with extrathyroidal extension and often lymph node metastasis. It accounts for ~10% of all thyroid PTC cases and it is refractory to radioactive iodine therapy.

Immunoprofile PTC shows positivity for CK/CK19/ TTF-1, TG, HBME-1, and PAX8.

Histopathology The growth pattern is papillary and at least 30% of the tumor shows "tall" cells (at least three times taller than wide). The cytoplasm is eosinophilic, and the nuclear features are those of PTC. Of note, the percentage of tall cells must be calculated and addressed in the final report, since it conveys an aggressive behavior particularly if it is >10%.

Molecular profile The tumor expresses a *BRAF* V600E mutation in 90% of cases and has been associated with *RET/PTC3* translocation. *RAS* mutations have not been identified. *TERT* promoter mutations are seen in 30% of cases and are associated with a worse outcome. It has the highest DNA copy number alterations of all PTC subtypes.

FNA Findings Smears show papillary fragments with no nuclear pseudostratification and tall tumor cells (at least three times taller than wide) showing cytoplasmic eosinophilia and nuclear features of PTC, including multivacuolated/septated ("soap bubble like") intranuclear cytoplasmic invaginations. Cells are elongated and cylindrical with and eccentrically place nuclei that results in a "tadpole" or "tail-like" shape. In contrast to classic/conventional PTC, the nuclei are less powdery, the nucleolus is more prominent, and mitoses may be identified.

US Features

- Microlobulated markedly hypoechoic nodules with microcalcifications.
- Extrathyroidal extension.

Columnar Cell Subtype

The columnar cell subtype of PTC is an aggressive and rare neoplasm (<5% of all PTCs). The tumors are large and invasive and occur more common in elderly men.

Histopathology The architecture is papillary and shows prominent nuclear pseudostratification, which is reminiscent of that of the endometrium. The nuclei are oval and hyperchromatic with supra- or subnuclear cytoplasmic vacuoles.

Immunoprofile CDX2 is positive in 50% of cases. TTF1, TG, and PAX8 are also positive.

Molecular Profile *BRAF*-V600E mutations occur in 40% of cases. Secondary oncogenic mutations (*TERT* or

TP53) and multiple chromosomal gains and losses occur in most cases and correlate with an aggressive tumor behavior.

FNA Findings (Fig. 3.54a–c) Cells are arranged in aggregates, sheets, and papillae and show clear cytoplasm and nuclear pseudostratification. The nuclear features of PTC, such as nuclear grooves and intranuclear cytoplasmic invaginations, are focal and less prominent, the nuclei are hyperchromatic, and colloid and cystic changes are typically absent. Mitoses can be found. These features may be a factor in not making an accurate diagnosis.

Solid Subtype (Fig. 3.55a–d)

The solid subtype of PTC is rare in adults (2% of adult PTCs) and is common in children without or with history of radiation (>30% of children following Chernobyl accident). These tumors have a worse prognosis compared with that of classic/conventional PTCs.

Histopathology The solid and/or trabecular and/insular pattern predominates (>50% of the tumor) and lacks a papillary or a follicular pattern. The tumor cells have nuclear features of PTC. Necrosis is absent.

Molecular Profile The prevalence of *BRAF* mutations is low; in contrast *RET* or *NTRK1/3* fusions are more prevalent in this tumor. *RET/PTC3* rearrangement is seen in tumors following Chernobyl accident.

FNA Findings Smears are cellular and lack colloid. Tumor cells are cohesive forming syncytial 3-dimensional and trabecular fragments, and non-cohesive as single cells. Cells show typical nuclear features of PTC. True papillae with fibrovascular cores are absent. The presence of Necrosis and mitoses are absent in this tumor and are important to distinguish it from DHGTC or PDTC (have necrosis and/or mitoses).

Hobnail Subtype

The hobnail subtype is rare (<1% of all PTCs). This aggressive PTC subtype is composed of papillary and micropapillary formations decorated with cells showing apical nuclei with loss of cell polarity and cohesiveness.

The *BRAF*-V600E mutation is seen in 80% of cases. *TP53* mutations (55%), *TERT* promoter mutations (45%), and *PIK3CA* mutations (28%) are also common. No *RAS* mutations have been identified.

Cytologically, there is overlapping with tall cell, columnar cell, and diffuse sclerosing subtypes. Furthermore, histologic diagnosis can be made only in the presence of clinical findings of an aggressive tumor.

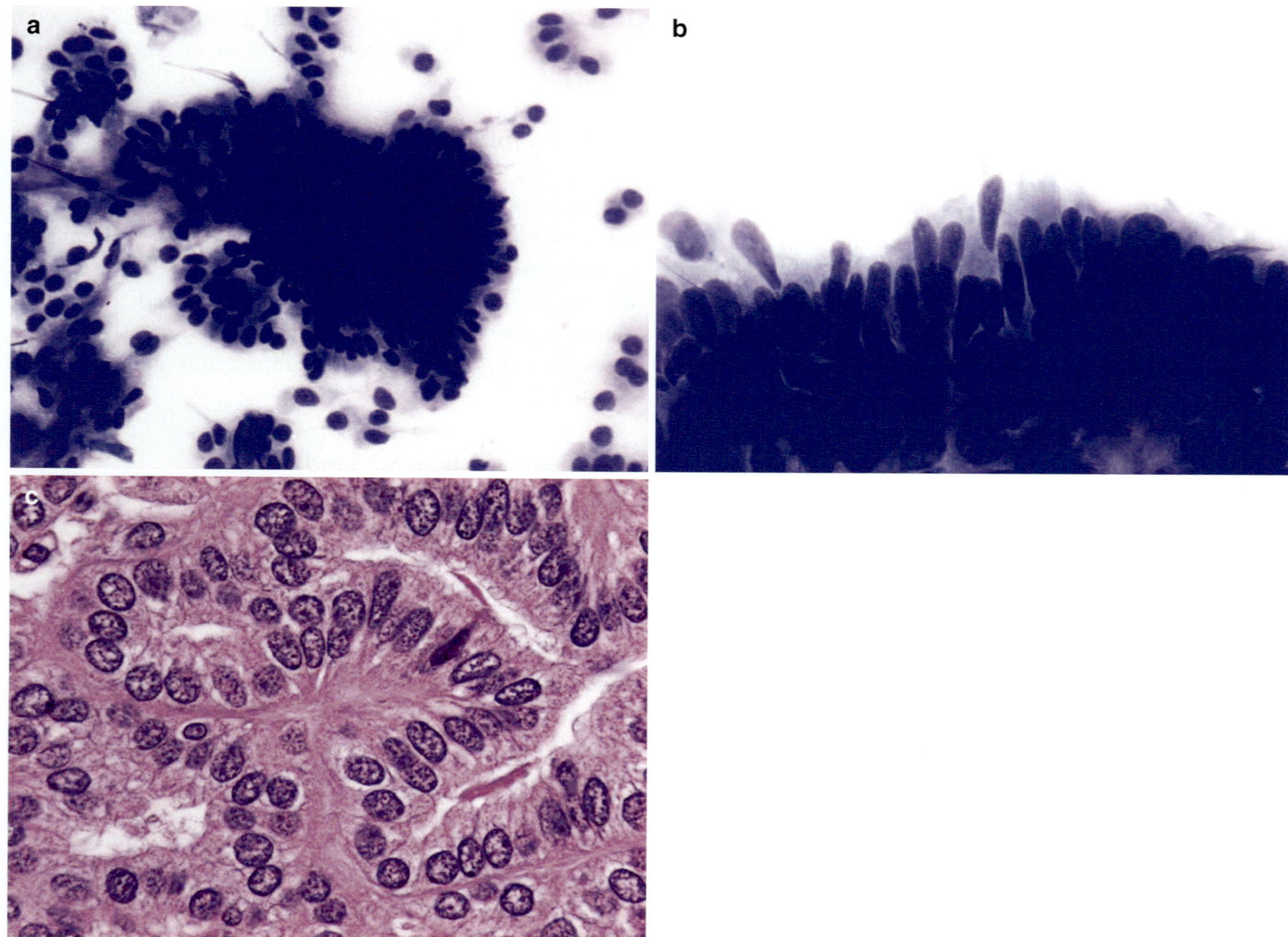

Fig. 3.54 Papillary thyroid carcinoma, columnar cell subtype. Smears show complex cellular aggregates and pseudopapillary structures composed of elongated cells with slight clear cytoplasm and pseudostratification reminiscent of that of the endometrium (**a**, **b**). This cell pattern correlates with the tumor tissue sections (**c**). (**a**, **b**, DiffQuik stain medium and high power; **c**, hematoxylin eosin stain, medium power. Courtesy Dr. Javier Saenz de Santamaria, Badajoz, Spain)

Thyroid Cancer Recurrences

These usually occur in the thyroid bed. Lymph node metastasis can also occur, often in neck compartments III, IV, and VI. USG-FNA is required for exclusion of a non-neoplastic process such as a fibrous nodule, a suture-related foreign-body-type granulomatous reaction, reactive lymph node, regenerated thyroid tissue (common in Hashimoto's thyroiditis), parathyroid neoplasm (usually adenoma), etc. (Fig. 3.56a–f, Videos 3.16 and 3.17).

US Features
- Nodules of recurrent thyroid cancer in the thyroid bed are often hypoechoic, irregular, and variably vascular. Hyperechogenicity may correlate with fibrosis.

Lymph Node Metastsasis in PTC

Lymph node metastases of PTC are present in 50% of cases at diagnosis and may be the first manifestation of the carcinoma in up to 20%. Ninety percent are micrometastases to neck lymph nodes and do not influence disease-free survival. Close to 90% of lymph node metastases involve the level VI compartment, regardless of involvement of other compartments. Pure solitary lymph node cystic metastases are seen particularly in patients under the age of 35 years.

Surgical management is altered in the presence of neck US-visible metastases, and patients undergo central or lateral neck dissection and total or near-total thyroidectomy for improved survival. Lymph node detection by other imaging

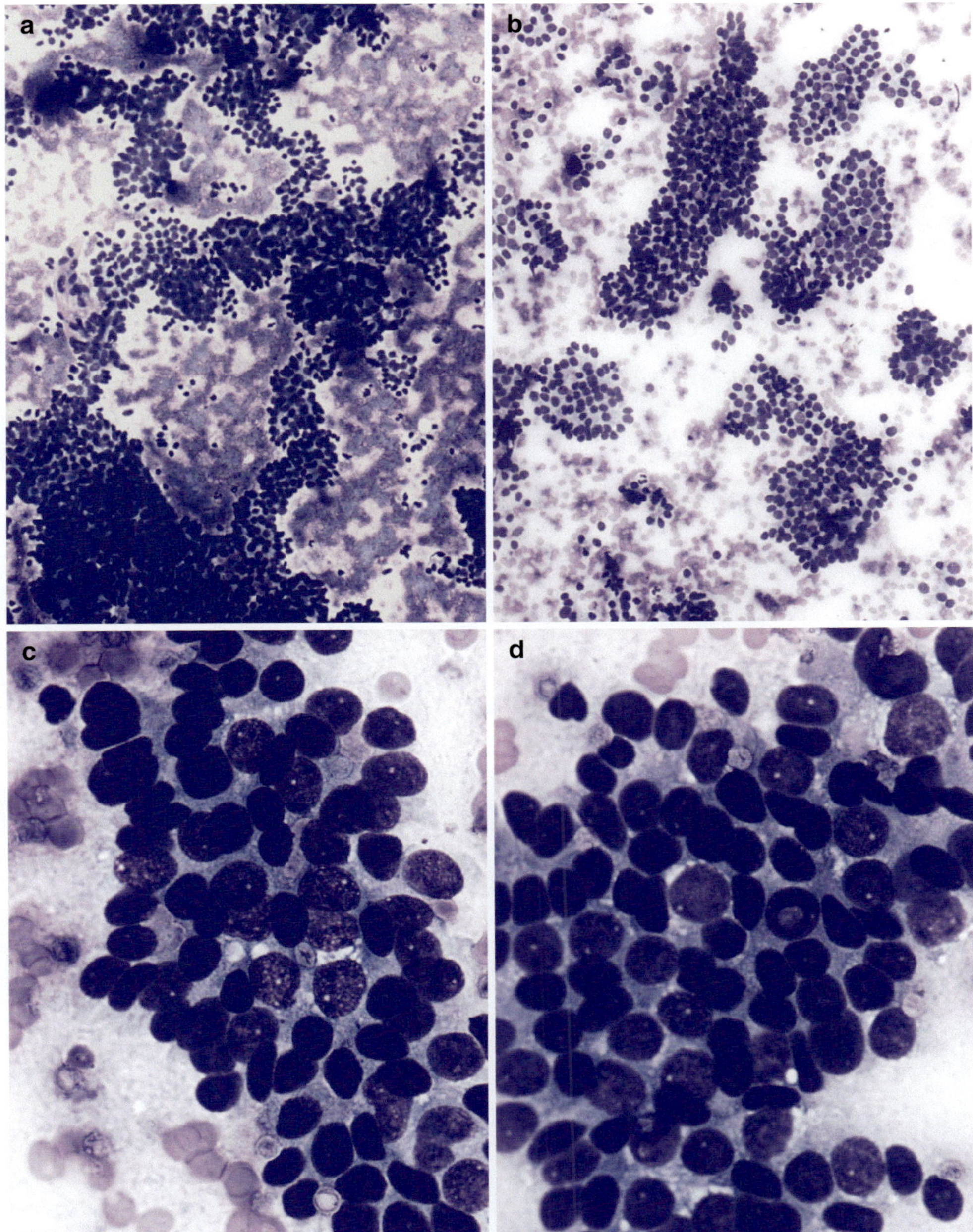

Fig. 3.55 Papillary thyroid carcinoma, solid subtype. Cellular smear with anastomosing groups and sheets of tumor cells showing cytologic atypia including nuclear overlapping, slight anisonucleosis, and intranuclear cytoplasmic invaginations. No papillary fragments are seen. Scant dense colloid was present other areas of the smears. (**a, b**, DiffQuik stain, low power; **c, d**, DiffQuik stain, high power)

modalities (CT, MRI, PET) is not recommended by ATA guidelines. US has limited resolution in evaluation of the level VI compartment, particularly posterior tracheal and tracheoesophageal groove lymph nodes.

USG-FNA of lymph nodes should include cytology and needle rinses for TG level measurements in all cases of differentiated thyroid cancer. Suspicious lymph nodes less than 5–8 mm in the greatest diameter may be followed by US; if the node grows or threatens vital structures, USG-FNA should be performed.

FNA Findings (Fig. 3.57a, d, f, g) Because lymph node metastases may show variable degrees of cystic degeneration, the FNA shows characteristic features of PTC, hemorrhagic necrotic fluid, and variable numbers of macrophages. Pure solitary lymph node cystic metastases show only macrophages, and they must be considered in the differential diagnosis of congenital neck cysts, particularly when there is no US-visible primary thyroid malignancy. High TG levels in the aspirated fluid help in the diagnosis. Cystic metastatic squamous cell carcinoma, although uncommon in young patients, should also be included in the differential diagno-

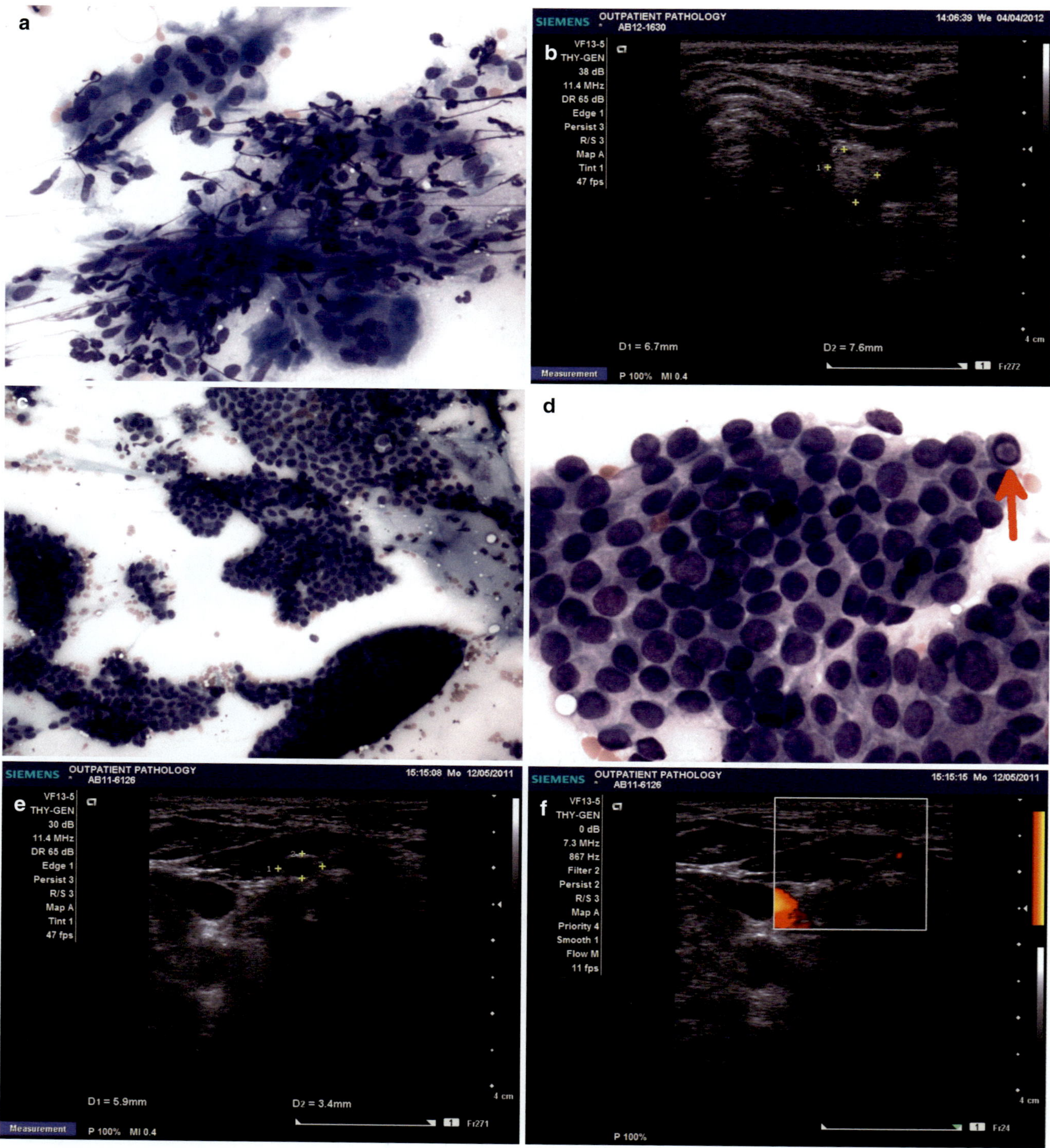

Fig. 3.56 Thyroid bed nodules. Granulation tissue and foreign body type giant cell reaction is noted in this benign nodule (**a**); the patient had thyroidectomy for PTC 15 years before and the US evaluation showed a slightly hyperechoic nodule (**b**). Recurrent PTC was the diagnosis in the smears obtained from this 0.6 cm hypoechoic, round, well circumscribed, and bulging nodule (**c–e**). Doppler examination showed no vascular blood flow (**f**). (**a**, **c**, **d** MGG stain, medium and high power)

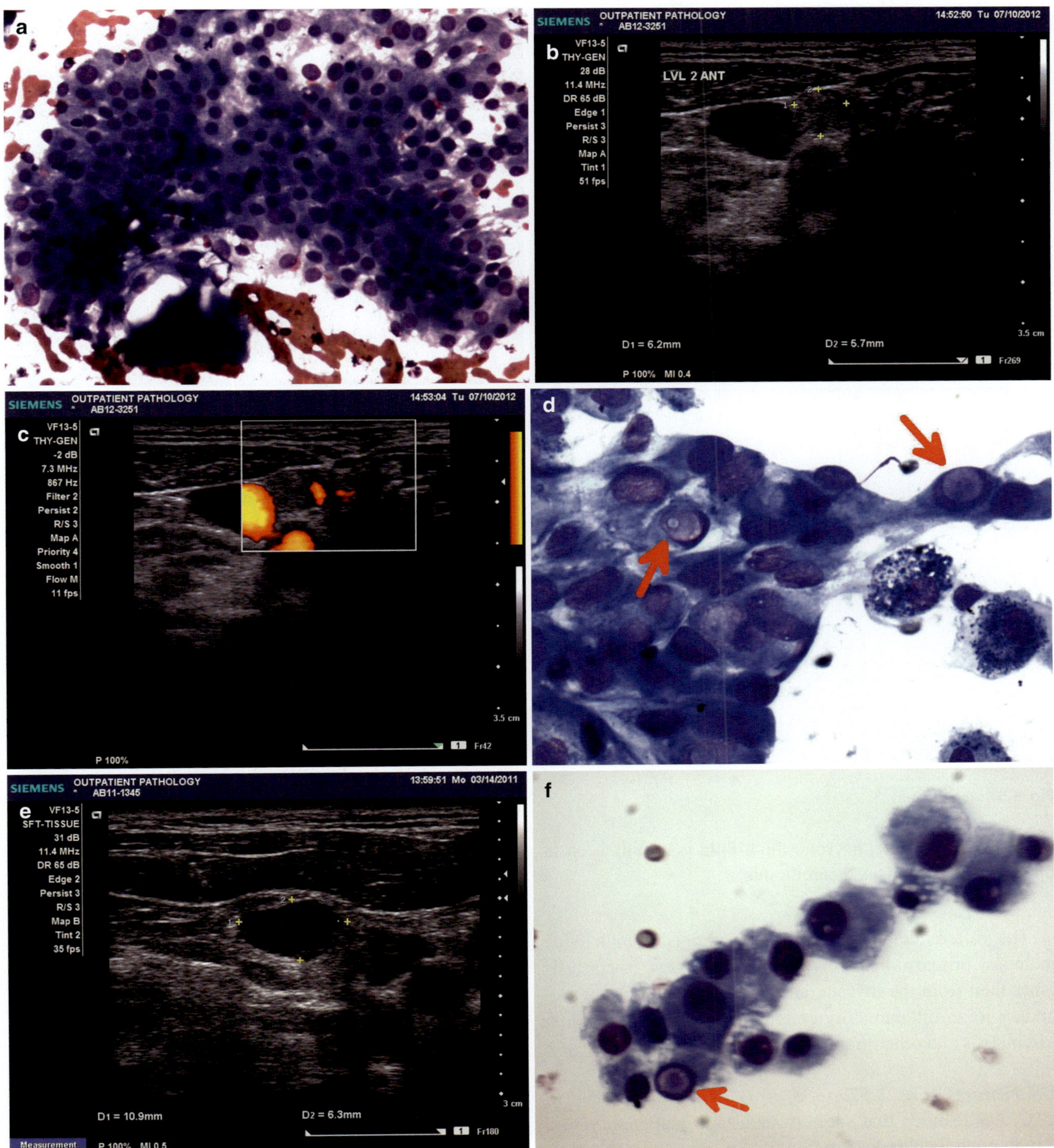

Fig. 3.57 Differentiated thyroid cancer metastatic to neck lymph nodes. A complex aggregate of bland-appearing epithelial cells with oxyphilic change (**a**) were seen in the smears obtained from a 0.6 cm right level II heterogeneous and slightly hyperechoic lymph node with focal peripheral vascularity (**b, c**) 22 years after having total thyroidectomy for thyroid carcinoma. An aggregate of metaplastic-appearing cells with intranuclear cytoplasmic invaginations and macrophages (**d**) were obtained from a 1.1 cm hypoechoic cystic cervical lymph node with irregular and fuzzy margins (**e**, radio 3 to 6) in a patient with history of PTC. Large cells with vacuolated cytoplasm, intranuclear cytoplasmic invaginations (**f**) and psammoma bodies (**g**) were obtained from a patient with history of PTC. The US of the neck showed a level IV 1.8 cm heterogeneous mass with lobulated and fuzzy margins and slight central blood flow by Doppler examination (**h, i**). (**a, d, f** MGG stain, high power; **g**, Papanicolaou stain, medium power)

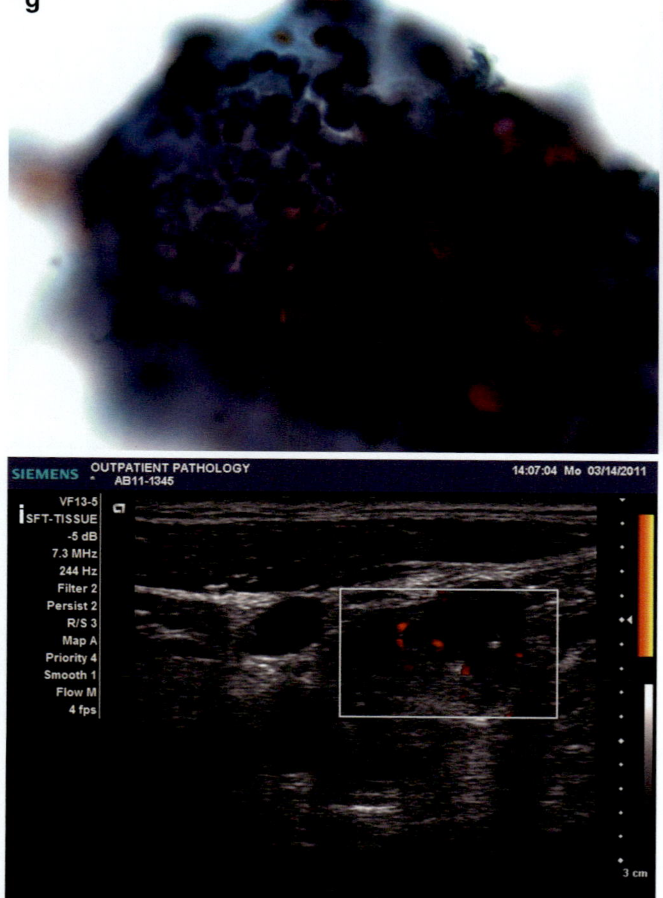

Fig. 3.57 (continued)

sis; less hemorrhagic, necrotic thick fluid is usually seen in metastatic squamous cell carcinoma.

The differential diagnosis of an enlarged lymph node includes primary hematolymphoid processes, metastasis other than from the thyroid, and lymphoid hyperplasia secondary to an inflammatory or infectious process, including sarcoidosis and other granulomatous processes.

US Features (Fig. 3.57b, c, e, h, i) While not limited to PTC, US features that suggest metastatic malignancy to a lymph node include loss of fatty hilum, rounded rather than oval shape, marked hypoechogenicity, cystic change, microcalcifications, and increased vascularity. Nodal metastasis may show the following US characteristics:

- They are located in the middle and lower jugular chains (compartments III and IV) and ipsilateral in 70–85%. Pre- and paratracheal nodes (compartment VI) are also common but less often found at US.

- They have absent echogenic hilar line. A hilar line may be seen in reactive lymph nodes; however, is not seen by US in reactive nodes less than 5 mm in diameter.
- They have a round (antero-posterior/transverse ratio > 0.5 in the transverse view) appearance instead of flattened or oval shape (<0.5 ratio).
- They have well-defined margins.
- They may have a chaotic vascularity.
- They are hypoechoic and occasionally have a marked hypoechogenicity.
- They have microcalcifications in 50% and mainly seen in solid metastases. Dense macrocalcifications or entirely calcified lymph nodes may be seen post ^{131}I therapy.
- Variable cystic degeneration is seen in 20–50%. Pure solitary cystic metastasis, although rare, is seen particularly in young patients.
- Features such as size and well-defined borders are less important than the other mentioned US features.

Invasive Encapsulated Follicular Variant (IEFV) PTC

The 2022 WHO classification of thyroid neoplasms classifies IEFV-PTC as low-risk malignant neoplasm rather than an overt malignancy. This tumor has a good prognosis, and the treatment is conservative (lobectomy) similar to that of NIFTP.

Histopathology IEFV-PTC is an encapsulated tumor with capsular or vascular invasion, follicular growth pattern (micro-, normo-, or macrofollicular), no papillae formation, and subtle nuclear features of PTC.

Immunoprofile IEFV-PTC shows positivity for TTF1, PAX8, and TG. HBME-1, galectin 3, and CK19 are also positive.

Molecular Profile This tumor shares *RAS*-like molecular profile like FTA and FTC.

FNA Findings IEFV-PTC cannot be reliably distinguished from NIFTP on cytology as capsule invasion cannot be evaluated on FNA specimens. Cytologically, the identification of a follicular-patterned aspirate with subtle nuclear changes of PTC (nuclear enlargement, nuclear contour irregularity, and nuclear clearing) should be best classified as follicular neoplasm (IEFV-PTC versus NIFTP) rather than malignant or suspicious for malignancy. However, a follicular subtype of PTC should be suspected in the presence of a microfollicular pattern and distinct nuclear features of PTC. Clinical correlation with US and molecular studies is mandatory (Fig. 3.58a, b).

US Features US features are non-specific and include solid echotexture, smooth margins, wider than tall shape on a transverse view, and a variably present hypoechoic rim (Fig. 3.58c, d).

Medullary Thyroid Carcinoma

Medullary thyroid carcinoma (MTC) arises from the neuro-endocrine calcitonin-secreting parafollicular or "C" cells found in the middle to upper third of the lateral thyroid lobes, accounts for approximately 1–2% of thyroid carcinomas, and can be sporadic (75%) or heritable (25%). The heritable form may be a part of multiple endocrine neoplasia [MEN 2A (pheochromocytoma and hyperparathyroidism), MEN 2B (pheochromocytoma, mucosal neuromas, gastrointestinal ganglioneuromatosis, and marfanoid habitus)], or be isolated, with no other tumors (familial MTC syndrome). MTC is likely to be present when the serum calcitonin level is >10 pg/mL. Ultrastructurally, "C" cells contain neurosecretory dense-core granules.

Clinical Findings Patients with sporadic MTC are in the fifth decade of life or older, and they almost always have a solitary tumor. The heritable form is autosomal dominant with virtually complete penetrance and is more aggressive than the sporadic form, affects young patients usually in the first three decades of life, and is often multifocal and bilateral.

MTC is an aggressive tumor that spreads through hematogenous and lymphatic channels. Most patients have regional cervical and mediastinal lymph node and/or distant organ metastases (bone, liver, and lung) at diagnosis. Total thyroidectomy and radical neck dissection is an effective treatment only before metastatic dissemination. Tyrosine kinase inhibitors with vandetanib (targets *RET, EGFR, VEGFR*) and carbozantinib (targets *RET, c-MET, VEGFR2*) can be used for patients with advanced disease. The tumor does not respond to chemotherapy, radioactive iodine, or radiotherapy. Poor prognostic factors include old age and an advanced tumor stage at diagnosis. The 5-year survival rate is 75%.

Genetic testing for *RET* proto-oncogene mutations should be performed in patients with parafollicular C cell hyperplasia or sporadic MTC. Thyroid US screening should also be performed in patients with *RET* proto-oncogene mutations and no clinical evidence of thyroid disease.

Histopathology MTC is usually, but not always invasive and may present as firm encapsulated masses. The heritable form may be multifocal. The classic tumor shows a solid proliferation of round to polygonal cells with granular cytoplasm, vascular stroma, hyalinized collagen, and amyloid. The architectural pattern may be trabecular, carcinoid-like, paraganglioma-like, neuroblastoma-like, angiosarcoma-like, papillary, pseudopapillary, or glandular. The cytomorphology is also highly variable ranging from small to large pleomorphic cells. Calcifications may be present, and true psammoma bodies may be identified. The histologic heterogeneity is challenging for the diagnosis; however, it does not influence the prognosis. The 2022 WHO classification of thyroid neoplasms recommends grading of MTC (low- and high-grade) based on Ki-67 proliferation index, mitotic count, and tumor necrosis.

High-grade MTC (comprises 10–20% of cases) must show at least one of mitotic count ≥5/10 high-power fields, tumor necrosis, and Ki67 proliferation index >5%. Low grade MTC lacks elevated mitotic count, high Ki67, and tumor necrosis.

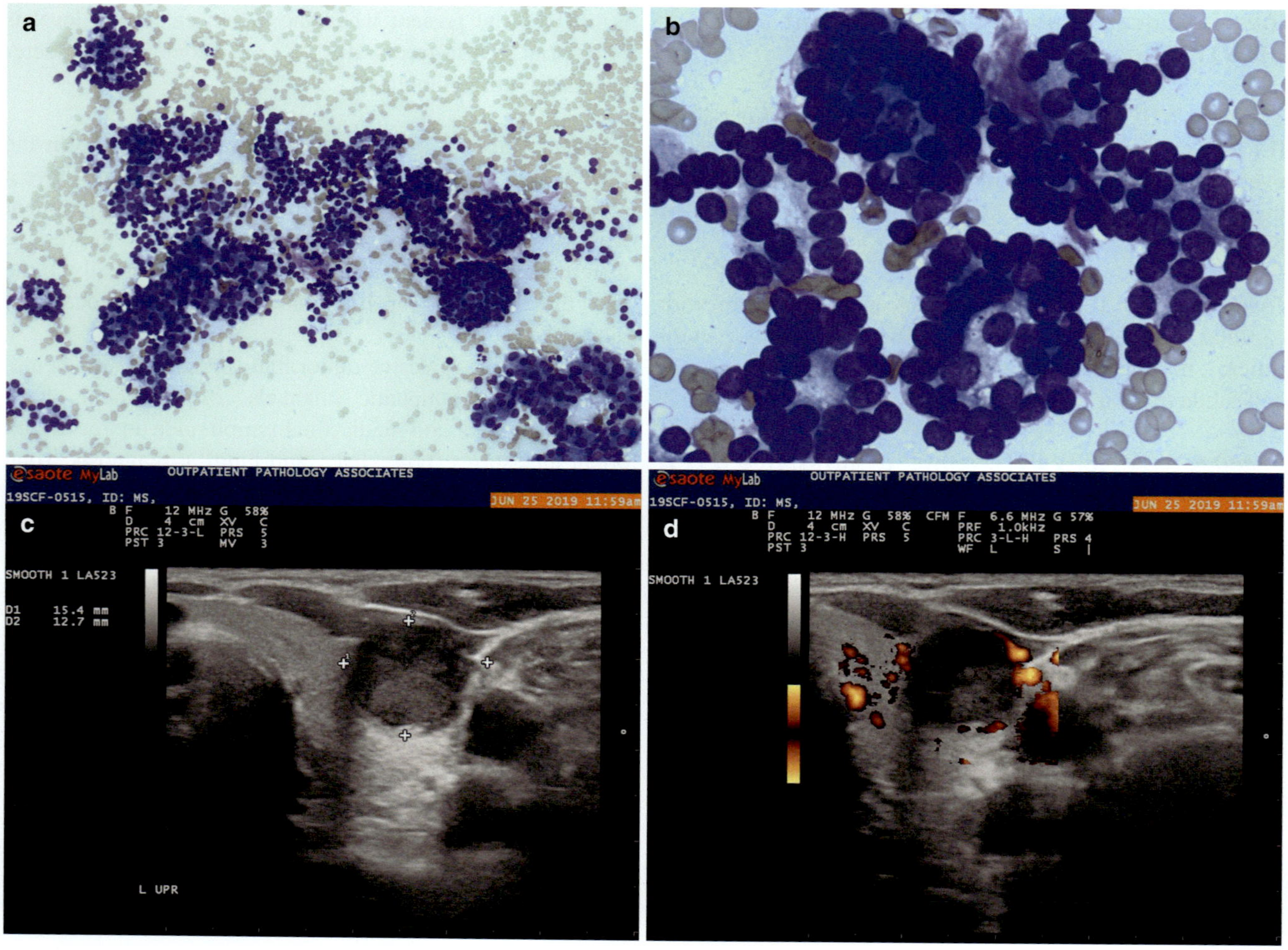

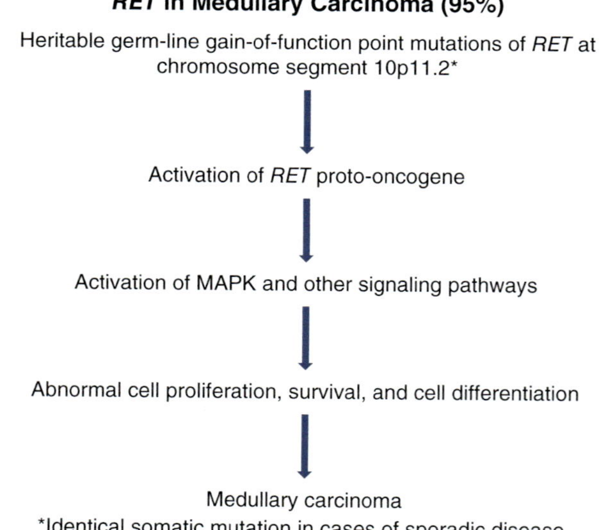

Fig. 3.58 Invasive encapsulated follicular variant-papillary thyroid carcinoma (IEFV-PTC). USG-FNA of this follicular-patterned neoplasm was diagnosed "follicular neoplasm, NIFTP versus IEFV-PTC versus PTC follicular subtype. The smears showed micro follicles with nuclear overlapping, no colloid, and mild cytologic atypia (**a**, **b**). US showed a 15.4 × 12.7 mm heterogeneous hypoechoic nodule with mild peripheral vascular flow (**c**, **d**). Histopathology showed capsular invasion. Molecular test showed a *RAS*-like profile negative *BRAF*-like profile

Immuno-Profile Tumor cells are positive for keratin, CEA, TTF-1, neuroendocrine markers (chromogranin, synaptophysin), and calcitonin, and negative for TG. Cells also express PAX8 (variable with polyclonal but negative with monoclonal PAX8), BCL2, and MYC. Congo-red stain for amyloid is positive. Oncocytic cells that may resemble MTC cells, stain positively for TG, and negatively for calcitonin and chromogranin.

Molecular Profile Somatic and germline *RET* mutations are seen in sporadic and heritable MTC respectively. Activation of the *RET* proto-oncogene by point mutations located on chromosome segment 10p11.2 is seen in 95% of heritable and 50% of sporadic forms of MTC (Diagram 3.6). It is known that clinical behavior varies according to the germline and somatic *RET* mutations. The tree forms of MEN2 (A, B, and familial) have specific activating point mutations in the *RET* proto-oncogene. MEN2A often carry *RET* mutations in codon 634 encoding cyste-

RET in Medullary Carcinoma (95%)

Heritable germ-line gain-of-function point mutations of *RET* at chromosome segment 10p11.2*

↓

Activation of *RET* proto-oncogene

↓

Activation of MAPK and other signaling pathways

↓

Abnormal cell proliferation, survival, and cell differentiation

↓

Medullary carcinoma
*Identical somatic mutation in cases of sporadic disease.

Diagram 3.6 *RET* in medullary carcinoma (95%)

ine, have high risk of lymph node metastasis, and often affect patients by age 20 years. Most MEN2B patients have *RET* mutation in exon 16 that is found as a germline mutation and correlates with an aggressive disease. Familial forms carry mainly *RET* mutations in codons 609, 611, and 618 as well as in the intracellular exons 13 and 15. Of note, screening of at-risk family members for MTC should be done by testing for germline mutations in the *RET* proto-oncogene. This screening may also detect MEN-2 in 5% of sporadic MTC cases, and these patients may benefit from prophylactic total thyroidectomy. Of note, *PROM1* gene has been found to be significantly overexpressed in aggressive MTC associated with *RET* M918T mutation that confers resistance to therapy; thus, decrease in *PROM1* expression opens a venue for targeted therapy at this level.

FNA Findings (Fig. 3.59a–g) Smears are moderately to highly cellular, showing cell aggregates and numerous single cells with ill-defined cytoplasmic borders and mild to moderate pleomorphism. Cells may be spindle, cuboidal, plasmacytoid, oncocytic, squamoid, clear, small, giant multinucleated, pleomorphic, pigmented, or melanin-producing. Binucleation is common; multinucleation is less often identified. Neuroendocrine features are present and include plasmacytoid cells, red cytoplasmic granules seen with Romanowsky stains, "salt and pepper" chromatin, inconspicuous nucleoli, binucleation, and ill-defined cytoplasmic borders. Intranuclear cytoplasmic invaginations are present in 50% of cases. Cytoplasmic vacuoles and psammoma bodies may be present, although rarely. Again, the architecture and cytomorphology are highly variable and is a challenge for the diagnosis. Necrosis and mitoses may be identified; however, grading is not currently recommended on cytology specimens. Amyloid is present in most cases as dense amorphous "puffy cloud"-appearing matter in the background.

Calcitonin levels in needle rinses provide a valuable information; a very high level, usually >80 pg/mL, is diagnostic of MTC.

The differential diagnosis includes oncocytic neoplasms, oncocytic PTC, HTT, PDTC, ATC, parathyroid neoplasms, paraganglioma, and metastases including melanoma, among others. Cytomorphology including nuclear and nucleolar features, calcitonin levels in needle rinses and serum, and judicious uses of immunohistochemistry are helpful. Of note, calcitonin immunostain is positive in MTC and negative in the above-mentioned neoplasms. Likewise, neuroendocrine markers are positive in MTC, parathyroid, and paraganglioma and negative in the others. Calcitonin immunostain and Congo red stain for amyloid can be made in cytology smears and cell block.

US Features (Fig. 3.59h–k) A solid hypoechoic mass with dense and coarse echogenic calcific foci is present in 80–90% of cases, representing amyloid with associated calcifications, and these may have a posterior acoustic shadowing.

- Involvement is localized in the mid- to upper third of the lobe in the early sporadic form and diffuse and/or bilateral in the familial type.
- Disorganized and chaotic hypervascularity may be present.
- Cervical and mediastinal lymph node metastases are hypoechoic, with echogenic foci similar to those of the primary tumor. Cystic change is rare.

Differentiated High-Grade Thyroid Carcinoma

Differentiated high-grade thyroid carcinoma (DHGTC) is associated with aggressive clinicopathological features and poor clinical outcomes. The aggressive clinical behavior is intermediate between that of differentiated thyroid carcinomas (PTC, FTC, OTC) and ATCs. They do not respond to radioactive iodine therapy.

Clinical Findings Compared to differentiated thyroid cancers, patients with DHGTC are older with tumors of larger tumor size, extrathyroidal extension, distant metastasis, and high tumor staging (Fig. 3.60a).

Histopathology Tumors retain their architectural and/or cytologic features of PTC, FTC, OTC that are present in 65%, 25%, and 12% of cases, respectively. DHGTC requires the presence of ≥ 5 mitoses/10 high power fields and/or necrosis. In contrast, PDTCs lack architectural features of differentiated thyroid carcinomas, solid, trabecular and insular features are most prevalent, and require the presence of ≥ 3 mitoses/10 high power fields.

Molecular Profile DHGTCs are associated with high-risk molecular alterations (68% of cases). *TERT* mutations and *TP53* gene mutations (aggressive tumor markers) are present in 40% of cases. *RAS*-like or *BRAF*-like molecular alterations (90% of cases) indicate the preceding tumor was FTC or PTC respectively.

FNA Findings Marked cytologic atypia, anisocytosis, anisonucleosis, necrosis, and/or mitosis are present in 25% of cases. The specific diagnosis of DHGTC may be challenging by FNA cytology, however, diagnosis of malignancy including PTC and PDTC can be made. The identification of necrosis and/or mitoses, malignant cells with significant nuclear pleomorphism, and a microfollicular pattern and/or nuclear

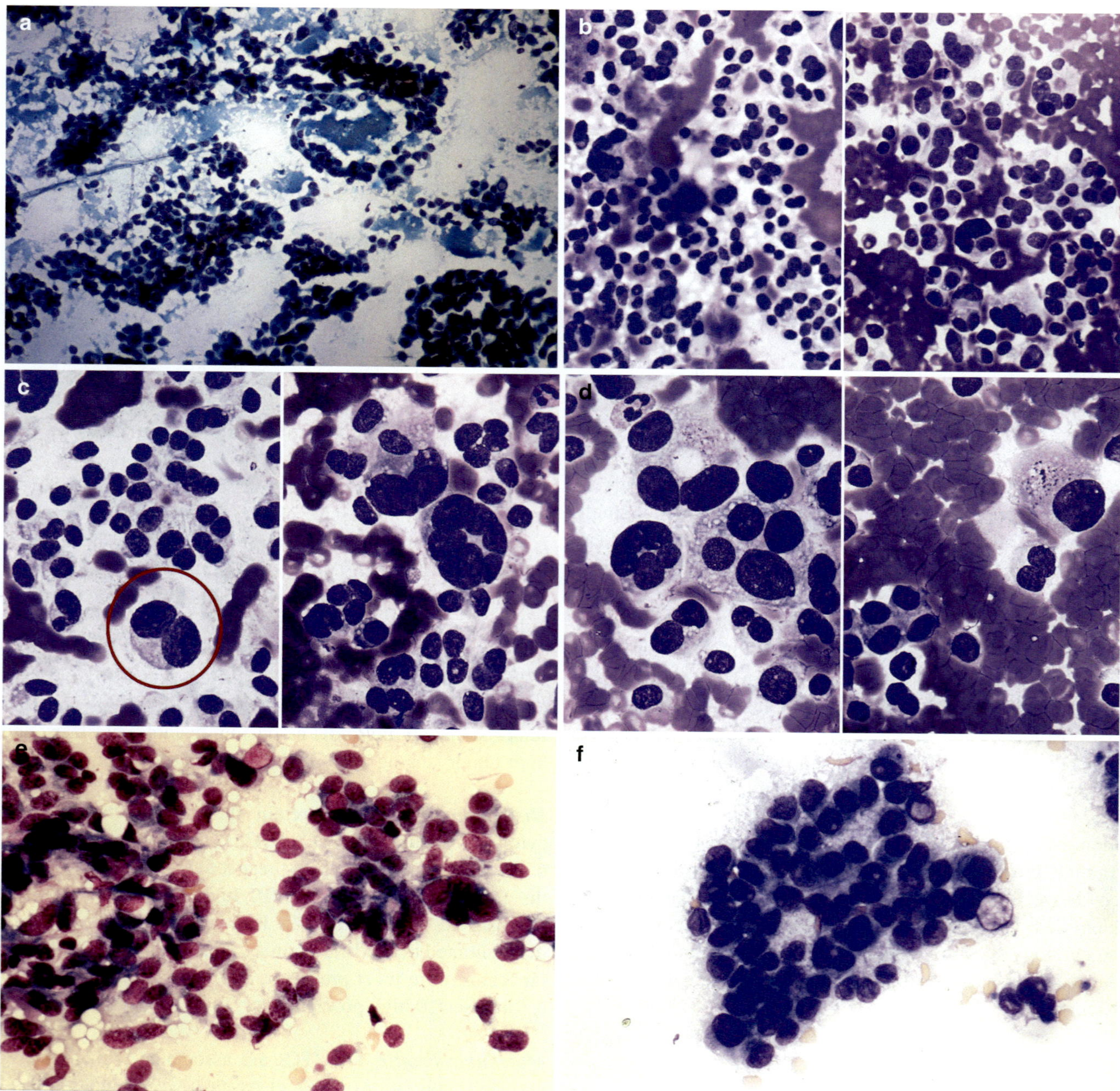

Fig. 3.59 Medullary thyroid carcinoma. The smears show characteristic features including high cellularity (**a**, **b**), cellular pleomorphism with aggregated and dissociated cuboidal, multinucleated, spindle, and plamacytoid cells exhibiting hyperchromasia, lack of nucleoli, and granular ("salt and pepper") chromatin (**c**–**e**). Variable numbers of intranuclear cytoplasmic invaginations (**f**) may be present resembling PTC. The finding of fine cytoplasmic metachromatic granules supports the diagnosis (**d**). The smear background shows amyloid in variable amounts and textures (**a**, **g**), which may be identified by Congo-red stain in cytology preparations and evaluated under polarized light (**g**).The US often shows a large hypoechoic mass with irregular borders, ill-defined margins, variable calcific foci, and high vascularity. One case shows a large ill-defined slightly hyperechogenic mass (**h**), and the other a 2.2 cm oval mass invading the surrounding thyroid parenchyma (**i**, left upper and right lower borders), microcalcifications (arrows), and correlate with vascular pattern by Doppler examination (**j**). US exam from a different case of medullary thyroid carcinoma shows a hypoechoic taller than wide mass with numerous microcalcifications (**k**). (**a**, **e** Papanicolaou stain, low and high power; **b**–**d**, **f**, **g** DiffQuik stain, high power; **g**, Congo-red stain, high power) (**b**–**d**, **g** Courtesy Dr. Javier Saenz de Santamaria, Badajoz, Spain)

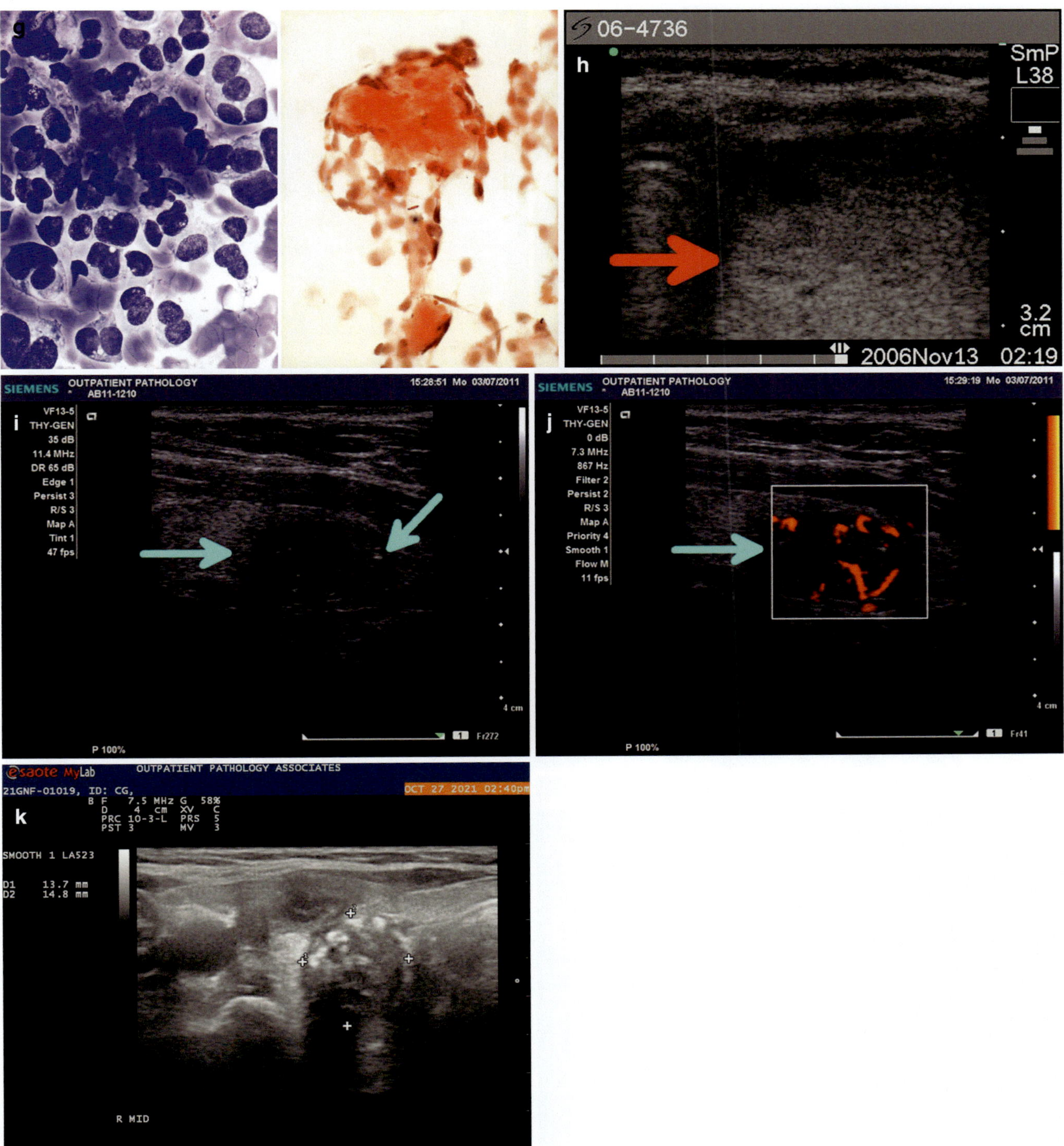

Fig. 3.59 (continued)

features of PTC are useful findings to consider the diagnosis of DHGTC (Fig. 3.60b-d).

US Features Findings are not specific; however high TIRADS (4 or 5) is present in most cases (Fig. 3.60e, f).

Poorly Differentiated Thyroid Carcinoma

Poorly differentiated carcinoma (PDTC) is a rare thyroid malignancy (5%) that falls between differentiated thyroid carcinomas (PTC, FTC, and OTC) and ATC. The clinical

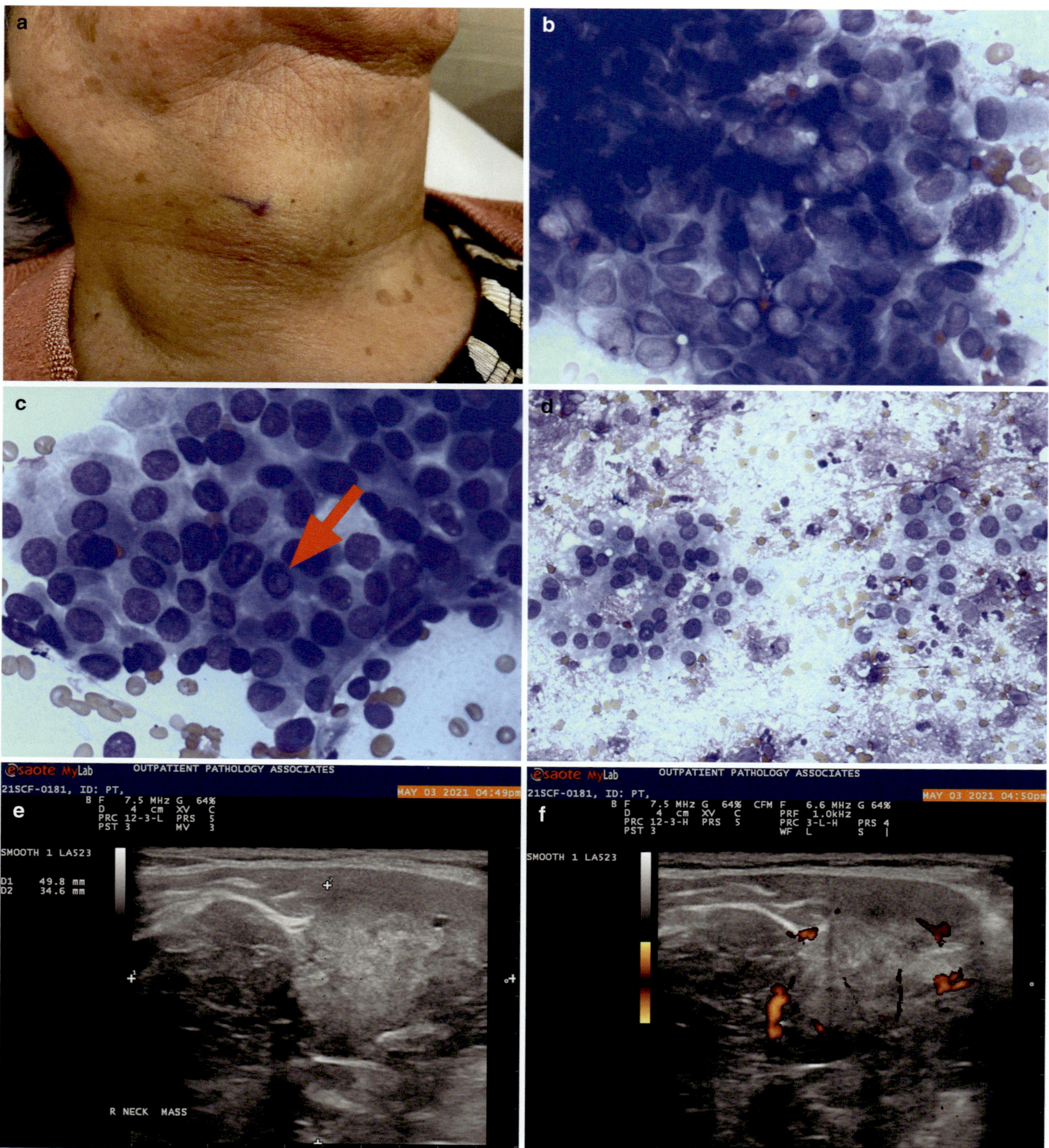

Fig. 3.60 Differentiated high-grade thyroid carcinoma. Large right thyroid mass extending to the adjacent right neck (**a**). Smears show aggregates of malignant cells with marked cytologic atypia and features suggestive of papillary thyroid carcinoma (**b**). Intranuclear cytoplasmic invaginations (**c**, arrow) and an atypical mitosis (right mid edge of frame) surrounded by cells of conventional papillary thyroid carcinoma are also seen. Focal necrosis is present (**d**). Ultrasound exam shows a large heterogenous tumor mass with areas hyper-, iso-, and hypoecho-genicity, lobulated ill-defined margins, and focal vascular blood flow by Doppler exam (**e, f**)

behavior is aggressive and also falls between differentiated thyroid carcinoma and ATC. The mean 5-year survival rate is 50%. The definitive diagnosis is made histologically. In contrast to differentiated thyroid carcinomas (PTC, FTC, OTC), PDTC is treated with a more aggressive surgical approach, often postoperative ^{131}I, and in some cases adjuvant therapy (external-beam radiotherapy and chemotherapy) for advanced and/or distant metastatic disease. Molecular target therapy may improve the prognosis of patients with advanced PDTC.

Clinical Findings PDTC occurs in patients older than those with the differentiated thyroid carcinomas and often presents at an advanced stage, recurs locally, and metastasizes to the cervical lymph nodes and distant organs particularly, lung and bones (Fig. 3.61a).

Histopathology Tumor cells are small and uniform and form a characteristic nesting growth pattern surrounded by a delicate rim of stroma (insular type). Solid (may contain microfollicles) and trabecular patterns are also present (non-insular type). Features of PTC are absent; however, mitoses ≥3/10 high power fields and/or tumor necrosis are/or convoluted nuclei are present. Occasionally, differentiated thyroid cancers may show focal poorly differentiated features but necrosis, mitoses, and convoluted nuclei must be absent.

Immuno-Profile The tumor shows positivity for TG and TTF-1. Ki-67 is positive in up to 30% of cases. Calcitonin and CEA are negative. Often there is focal weak positivity with neuroendocrine markers.

Molecular Profile Molecular alterations include those seen in differentiated thyroid carcinomas *(BRAF-* like and *RAS-*like mutations) and those of poorly differentiated carcinomas *(TP53* mutation in 40% and *CTNNB1* mutation in 30%, with expression of p53 and β-catenin by immunohistochemistry, respectively). *RAS-*like mutations are seen in 20–50% of cases and *PAX8::PPARG* translocation in 7%. *TERT, CTNNB1, AKT1,* and *P53* molecular abnormalities are present in up to 50%.

FNA Findings (Fig. 3.61b–h) The smears show high cellularity, a nesting (insular) and trabecular pattern, and often necrosis. The smear pattern is usually homogeneous; however, some cases show cell pleomorphism. Tumor cells lack features of PTC and have scant cytoplasm, a high nuclear-to-cytoplasm ratio, small round or convoluted nuclei, and hyperchromasia. The nuclei may show a "salt and pepper" chromatin, inconspicuous nucleolus, and mild atypia. The architecture, marked crowding, dissociated cells, and a high nuclear-to-cytoplasmic ratio are

helpful for the diagnosis. A microfollicular, papillary, or oncocytic cell pattern may be seen when there is a differentiated thyroid carcinoma component. Tumor necrosis and/or mitoses are common. However, the FNA diagnosis in most cases is either carcinoma including PTC (25%) or follicular neoplasm (45%), and the specific diagnosis is made in 30%.

The differential diagnosis includes MTC, ATC, parathyroid carcinoma, and metastases, particularly melanoma and hematolymphoid malignancies. FTC may show necrosis and rare mitoses; however, in contrast to PDTC nuclear and architectural features are present. Judicious use of immunohistochemistry and serum calcitonin levels is helpful. Of importance, TTF1 is positive in both PDTC and MTC. ATC shows marked cellular pleomorphism and TG and TTF1 are usually negative.

US Features (Fig. 3.61i–k)
- Tumors are usually large and show US features of extrathyroidal extension.
- The shape is irregular, lobulated, and has irregular indistinct borders.
- Heterogenous echotexture and hypoechogenicity with areas of cystic necrosis is noted.
- A peripheral halo is absent.
- There is variable and chaotic vascularity; the viable areas are vascular.
- Cervical lymphadenopathy is common.

Anaplastic Thyroid Carcinoma

Clinical Findings Anaplastic thyroid carcinoma (ATC) is a rare (1–2% of thyroid carcinomas) and highly aggressive malignancy with a poor prognosis that affects middle-aged to elderly patients who may or may not have a history of differentiated thyroid carcinoma (PTC, FTC, OTC). The average survival rate is 9 months; patients usually die of compression of the aerodigestive tract. Patients usually are euthyroid and have compressive and obstructive symptoms in the upper airways and esophagus. They may have recurrent laryngeal nerve palsy and neck pain resulting from local tumor invasion. The clinical and imaging differential diagnosis for this rapidly enlarging thyroid mass is non-Hodgkin lymphoma.

Poor prognostic factors include *TERT* promoter mutations, concomitant *BRAF, RAS,* and *TERT* promoter mutations, *EIF1AX* mutation, and chromosome 13q loss and 20q gains.

Treatment includes surgery (if the tumor is resectable), and/or radiotherapy and/or chemotherapy to shrink the tumor and allow resectability. Radioactive iodine therapy is ineffective in ATC. Targeted therapy depends on the molecular

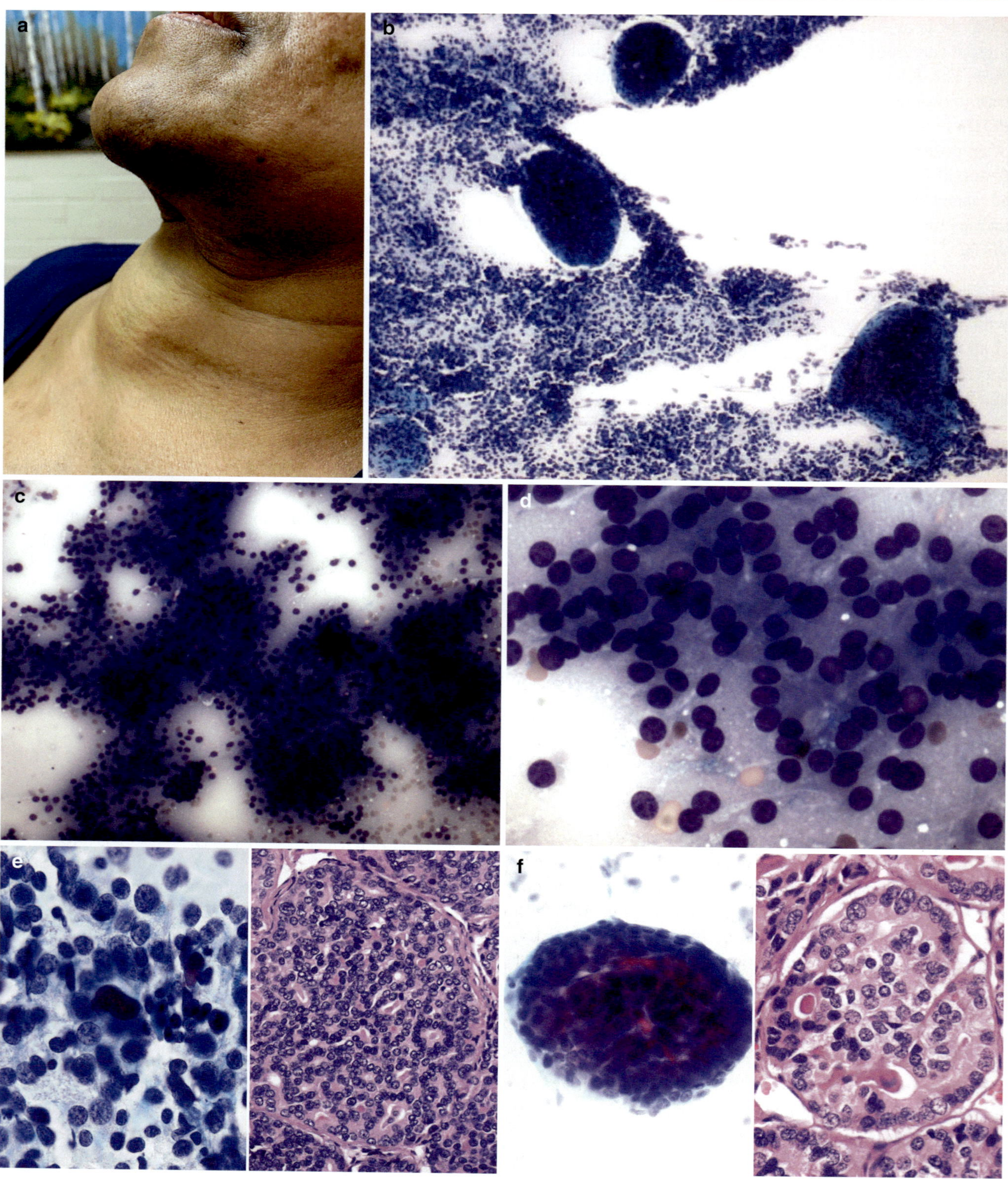

Fig. 3.61 Poorly differentiated thyroid carcinoma. Large bulging thyroid mas with nodular appearance (**a**). Insular (**b**, **f**) and trabecular/microfollicular (**c–e**, **g**) patterns are seen in these tumors. Occasional cellular pleomorphism (**f**) is present. Immunostains for thyroglobulin and TTF1 are positive (**h**). Cytology and histology findings of this case of insular carcinoma show unequivocal correlation (**e**, **f**). Ultrasound exam shows a large odd-shaped, heterogeneous, and hypoechoic mass with irregular, angulated, and microlobulated margins invading the surrounding thyroid parenchyma and skeletal muscles (**i–k**). (**b**, **g**, DiffQuik stain, low and high power; **c**, **d** MGG stain, medium and high power; **e**, **f** DiffQuik and hematoxylin eosin, high power; **h**, immunoperoxidase stain) (**b**, **e–h** Courtesy Dr. Javier Saenz de Santamaria, Badajoz, Spain)

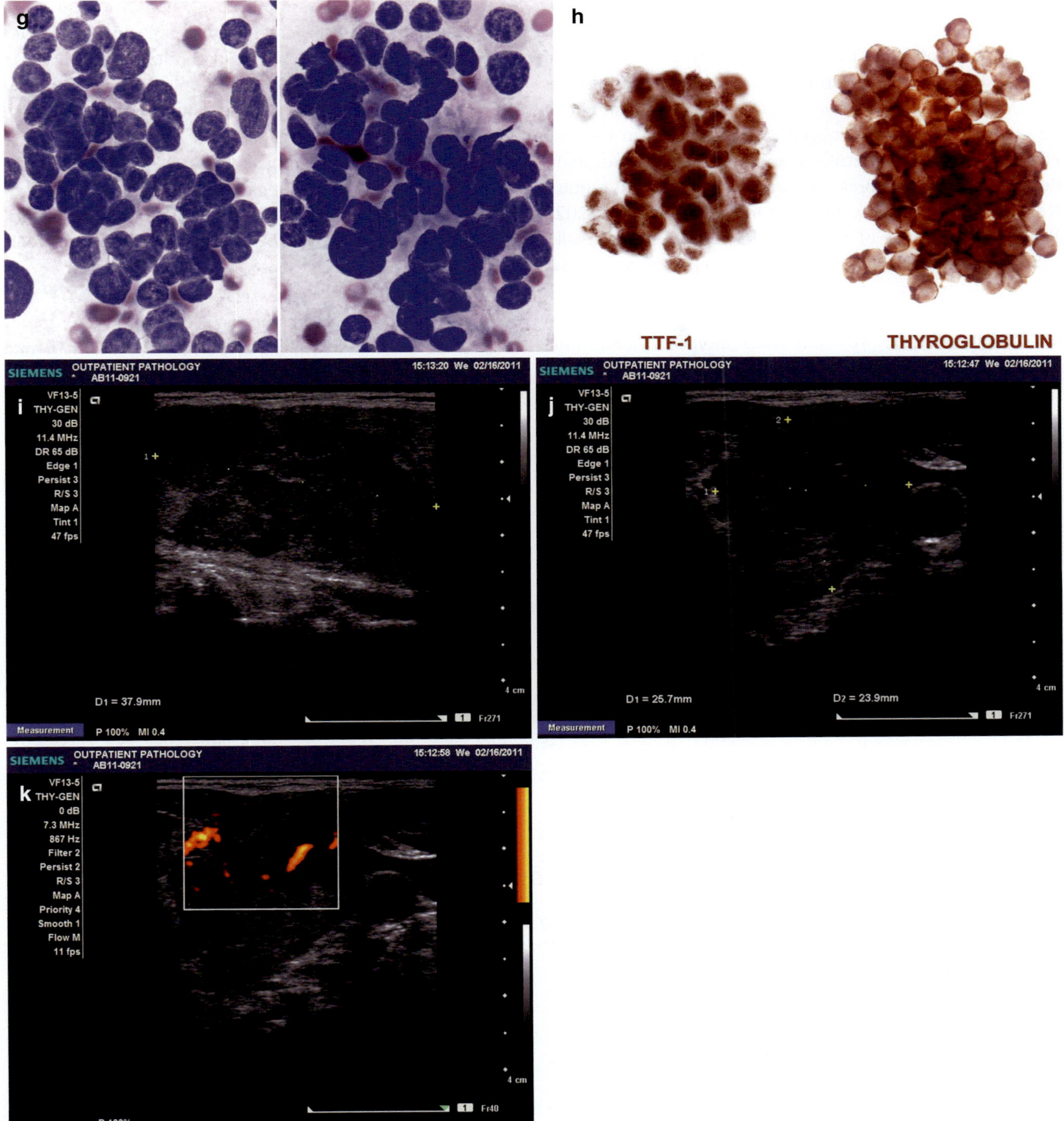

Fig. 3.61 (continued)

Histopathology Microscopically, ATC) is composed of mitotically active undifferentiated cells with a loss or focal follicular cell differentiation and atypical mitoses. Coexistent PTC, FTC, OTC, or PDTC may be identified. There is a variety of features including squamous cells, alterations present and includes dabrafenib, trametenib, crizotinib, ceritinib, alectinib, pralsetinib, selpercatinib, larotectrinib, and entrectinib. Therapy with checkpoint inhibitors such as pembrolizumab is also available.

foci of keratinization, epithelioid cells, spindle cells, small cells, giant cells, osteoclast-like multinucleated giant cells, foci of neutrophilic infiltrate, bone, cartilage, and skeletal muscle differentiation, variable fibrosis and hyalinization, hemorrhage, and tumor necrosis. A clear cell change may be seen as a result of glycogen accumulation. Various histologic tumor cell patterns (squamous, angiomatoid, rhabdoid, lymphoepithelioma-like, and paucillular that mimics Riedel thyroiditis) may be identified. However, the 2022 WHO classification of thyroid tumors does not consider subtypes based on the predominant pattern. Primary squamous cell carcinoma that was listed separate in the 2017 WHO classification is now considered a histologic pattern of ATC based on the prevalent *BRAF* molecular alterations present in most tumors. Of note, squamous cell differentiation can be seen in other thyroid tumors (PTC, FTC, PDTC, MTC, DHGTC), mucoepidermoid thyroid carcinoma, and intrathyroidal thymic carcinoma and may mimic ATC; however, except for MTC that may have necrosis and cell pleomorphism, the other tumors lack these features. Metastasis from squamous cell carcinoma is also a possibility to be considered in the differential diagnosis.

Immuno-Profile Positivity for keratin (50–70% of cases), PAX8 polyclonal antibody (varies with histologic pattern, up to 100% in squamous, 60% in sarcomatoid), and p53 is seen. Ki67 labeling index is >50%. Vimentin is also positive), particularly in the spindle cells; stromal positivity for laminin and focal positivity for CEA and EMA are seen in the squamous type. TG and TTF-1 are usually negative; however, they are positive in coexisting differentiated thyroid carcinoma and PDTC.

Molecular Profile Genetic profiles demonstrate a stepwise progression of burden and frequency of molecular alterations present from differentiated thyroid carcinoma to PDTC to ATC. The molecular alterations present in ATC are similar to those seen in PDTC but occur with greater frequency. Molecular abnormalities include *BRAF*-like, *RAS*-like, *TERT* promoter, and *TP53* mutations seen in up to 80% of cases. *TP53* mutations coding for p53 are seen in 50%–80% of cases. Alterations in cell cycle genes (*CDKA2A*, *CDKA2B*, *CCNE1*) are also present. *RET/PTC* and *PAX::PPARG* rearrangements are usually absent.

Mutations of MMR genes (*MLH1*, *PMS2*, *MSH2*, and *MSH6*), DNA mismatch repair genes (*MSH*, *MLH1*), tumor suppressor genes (*TP53*, *NF2*, *NF1*, *RB1*, *MEN1*), and *P13K/AKT* pathway genes (*PIK3CA*, *PTEN*, *AKT1*, *AKT2*) are also variably present. *PIK3CA* and *PTEN* mutations that are observed in a minority of cases frequently coexist with *RAS* and *BRAF* V600E mutations, suggesting an origin from and/or coexistence with differentiated thyroid carcinoma.

RET and *NTRK* gene fusions, *ALK* mutations, and *ALK* fusions are also present. Mutation in the gene *CTNNB1* coding for β-catenin is found in 66% of cases.

The PI3K/PTEN/AKT pathway is altered (Diagram 3.7). Epithelial-mesenchymal transition [loss of E-cadherin (CDH1) expression due to activation of E-cadherin repressors] is accepted as a key mechanism in the development and progression of ATC.

Of note, all ATCs, including squamous cell carcinoma should be tested for the presence of *BRAF*-V600E mutations. The detection of *RET* fusions, *BRAF*-V600E mutations, and

Diagram 3.7 Synergistic signaling pathways

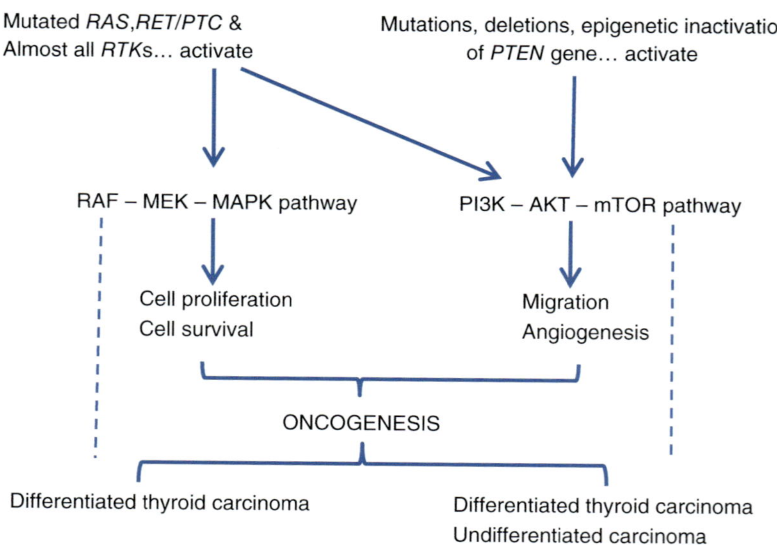

NTRK1/3 and *ALK* fusions are important for the potential use of targeted therapy.

FNA Findings (Fig. 3.62a–e) The USGFNA sampling should avoid necrotic areas. Smears show high cellularity and highly pleomorphic malignant cells with nuclear enlargement, irregular nuclear membranes, clumped chromatin, macronucleoli, necrosis with variable numbers of acute inflammatory cells, and atypical mitoses. Cells may have squamous features, be multinucleated (osteoclast type and bizarre), and have a spindle appearance. The background shows variable necrosis and scattered neutrophils.

The differential diagnosis includes metastases to the thyroid, particularly from lung, melanoma, and sarcomatoid renal cell carcinoma. MTC may be considered in cases with absent necrosis or multinucleated cells, because they are almost always absent in MTC. Again, judicious use of immunostains is helpful. We should emphasize that a diligent search of malignant cells should be conducted in hypocellular specimens so that a misdiagnosis of Riedel thyroiditis is avoided.

US Features (Fig. 3.62f, g)
- Diffuse and usually large mass with heterogenous and hypoechoic echotexture, frequently seen in a background of multinodular goiter (clinical diagnosis).
- Dense coarse amorphous calcification is present in 60%.
- Necrosis is common (80%) and may be extensive.
- Cervical lymphadenopathy is common (80%), usually heterogenous, and shows necrosis.
- US evidence of local invasion of adjacent neck structures including blood vessels is seen.
- Areas of viable tumor are vascular, and areas of necrosis are hypovascular.

Thyroid Lymphoma

Thyroid lymphoma, either primary or secondary, is rare. Secondary involvement is more common, because 20% of disseminated non-Hodgkin lymphomas (NHLs) involve the thyroid. Plasmacytoma, Hodgkin lymphoma, Langerhans cell histiocytosis, Rosai-Dorfman disease, and extramedullary hematopoiesis (Fig. 3.63a, b) can involve the thyroid gland, often presenting as thyroid nodules.

Clinical Findings Patients with primary NHL usually have Hashimoto's thyroiditis; however, only a minority of patients with Hashimoto's develop NHL, usually 20 or 30 years after the diagnosis. Patients are usually women with a median age of 60 years. The clinical presentation is similar to that of ATC, including a rapidly enlarging thyroid mass, dysphagia, and hoarseness. The response to chemotherapy, and/or radiotherapy, and/or immunotherapy with rituximab is favorable, and the prognosis is better than that for patients with ATC. The prognosis is better for extranodal marginal-zone lymphoma than for diffuse large B-cell lymphoma.

Histopathology Almost all thyroid lymphomas are B-cell NHL, mainly of the diffuse large cell type (70%), less commonly of the marginal zone B-cell lymphoma of mucosa associated lymphoid tissue (MALT) type (15%), and only rarely are true follicular lymphomas. Primary thyroid T cell lymphomas are exceedingly rare.

Immuno-Profile A consideration in the evaluation of B-cell lymphomas in a background of chronic lymphocytic thyroiditis is the detection of clonal B-cell populations that have not yet evolved into lymphoma. Thus, careful interpretation of results is advised. Clinical correlation is necessary.

Molecular Profile *BRAF* and *NRAS* gene mutations have been identified in 24% and 8% of diffuse large B-cell thyroid lymphomas, respectively. *HRAS* and *KRAS* mutations or *PAX8::PPARG* have not been detected.

FNA Findings (Fig. 3.63c–e) Smears are cellular and show a monomorphic non-cohesive lymphoid cell population in a background of red blood cells and numerous lymphoglandular bodies. Cells of marginal-zone lymphoma are of medium size (twice the size of small lymphocytes) and have a plasmacytoid appearance. Cells of large-cell lymphoma may have a fragile cytoplasm, and numerous stripped nuclei may be present along with intact cells showing a basophilic cytoplasm and prominent nucleoli. Occasionally, there is a mixed lymphoid cell population.

US Features (Fig. 3.63f–h)
- A diffuse or focal hypoechoic homogeneous mass is often seen. Occasionally, the thyroid is nodular, mimicking TFND (multinodular goiter clinically) or enlarged with no obvious abnormality.
- The focal lymphomatous nodule may be profoundly hypoechoic (pseudocystic) with posterior acoustic enhancement resembling a thyroid cyst.
- In contrast to ATC, calcifications, cystic degeneration, and necrosis are rare.
- Vascularity is variable, from almost absent to marked and chaotic.
- The background thyroid parenchyma often has US features of Hashimoto's thyroiditis.
- Associated lymph nodes may be large, round, homogeneous, and very hypoechoic with posterior acoustic enhancement, and they often lack calcifications or necrosis.

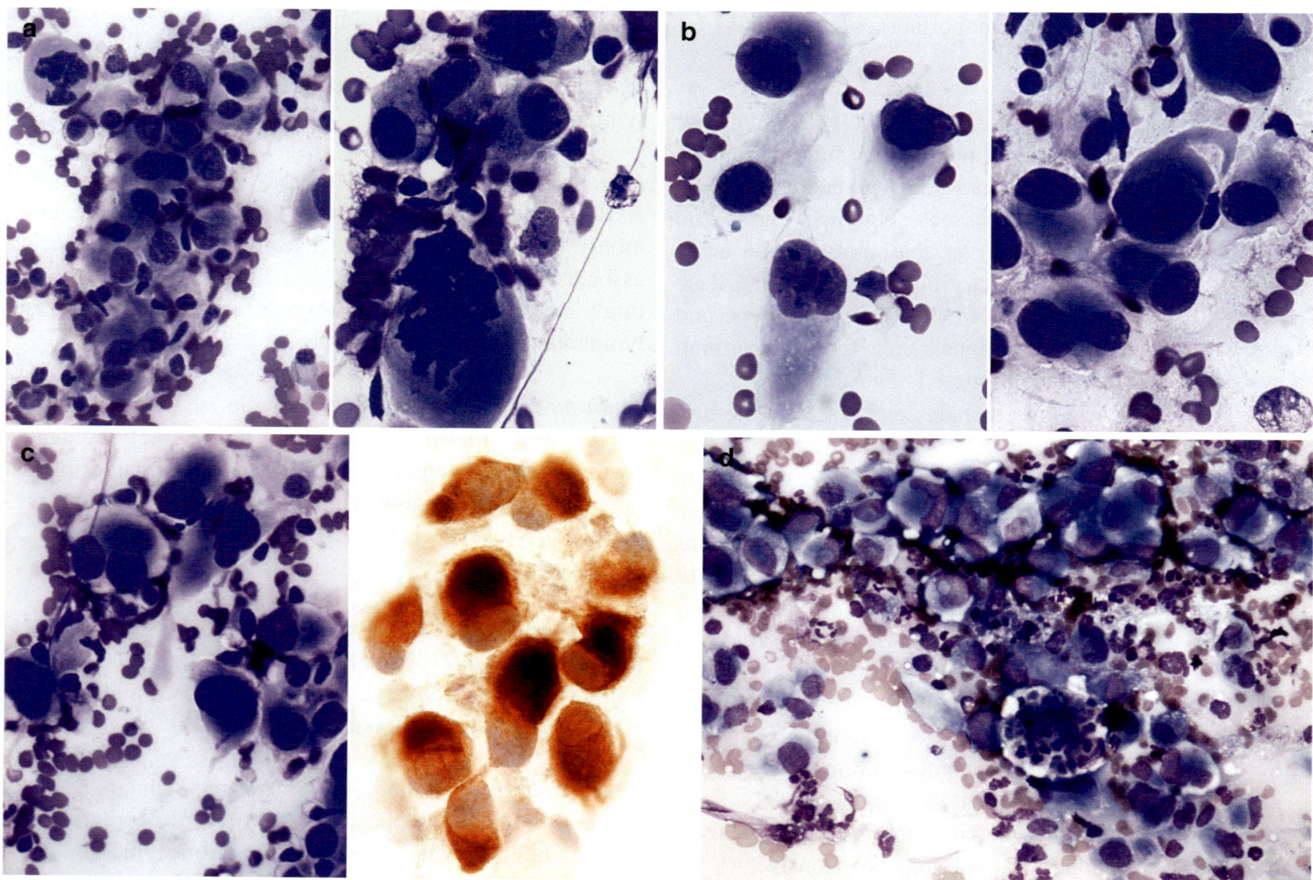

Fig. 3.62 Undifferentiated (anaplastic) carcinoma. Smears show large single and multinucleated pleomorphic cells with atypical mitoses, variable amounts of cytoplasm and a necrotic background with neutrophils both extra- and intracellular (**a**, **b**, **d**, **e**). A rhabdoid phenotype with dense cytoplasmic aggregates of intermediate filaments may be evident and show immunostain positivity for vimentin (**c**). Ultrasound in this particular case shows a large hypoechogenic mass with slight heterogeneous echotexture, slightly irregular, lobulated and fuzzy borders with moderate vascularity by Doppler examination (**f**, **g**). (**a–c** Courtesy Dr. Javier Saenz de Santamaria, Badajoz, Spain)

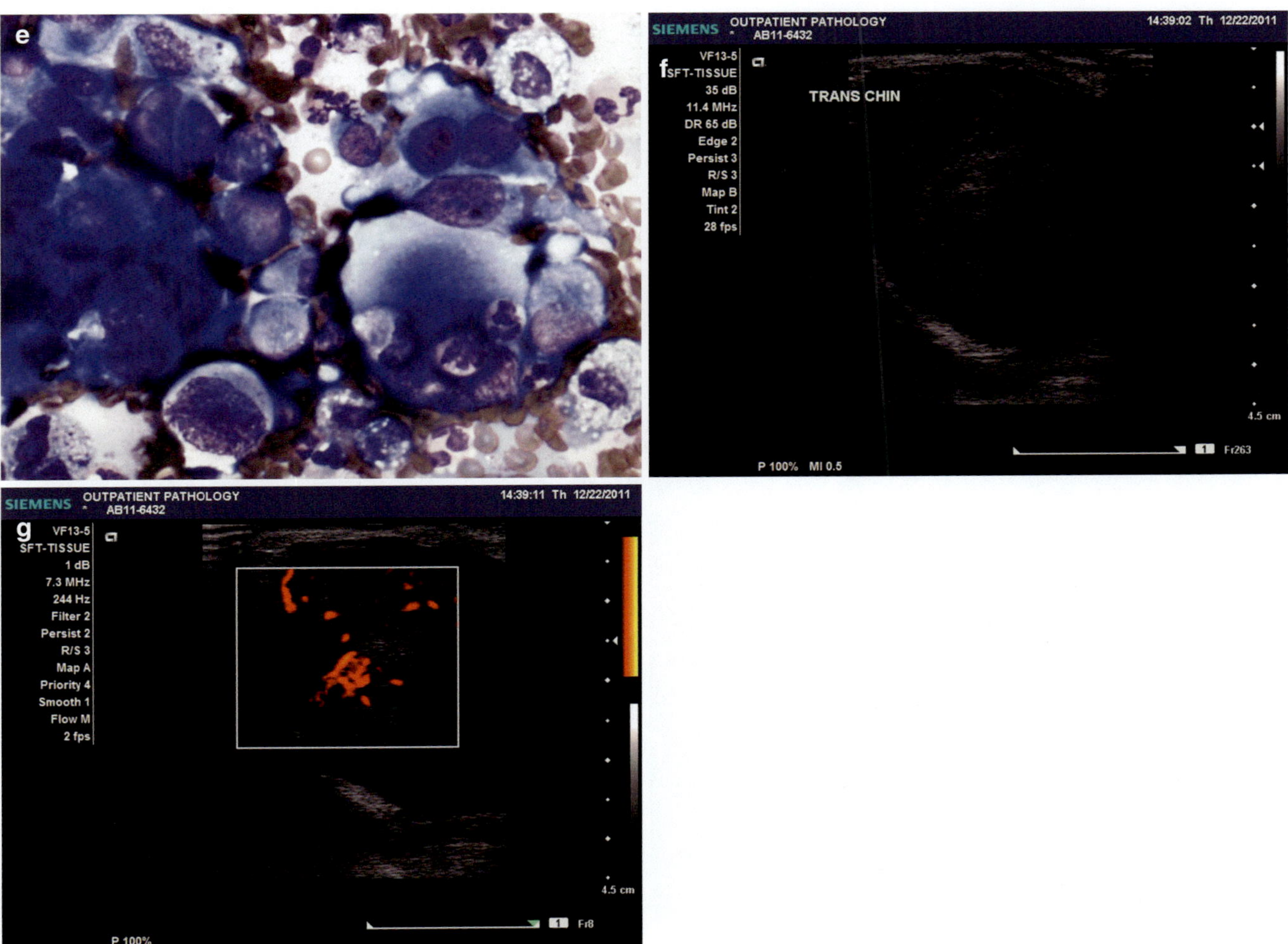

Fig. 3.62 (continued)

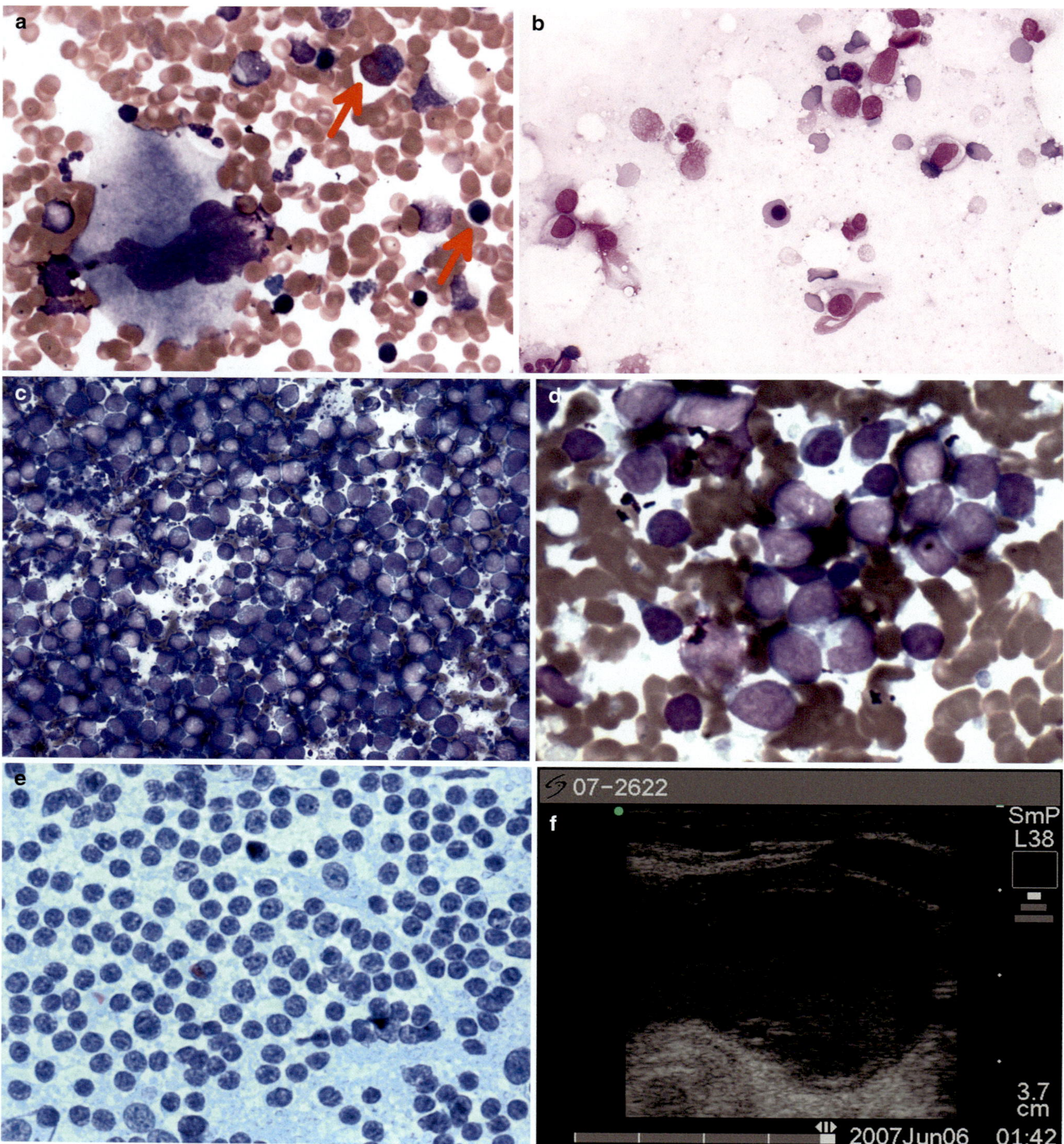

Fig. 3.63 Smears of extramedullary hematopoiesis showing a single megakaryocyte, nucleated red blood cell (**a**, right arrow; **b**, center), myeloblasts (**b**), and one immature eosinophil (**a**, upper arrow). Smear from non-Hodgkin lymphoma show a monotonous population of small cells (**c**) with nuclear clefts (**d**), coarse chromatin, and conspicuous nucleoli (**e**). These two cases of lymphoma show similar US features including large a homogeneous hypoechoic solid mass with posterior acoustic enhancement and minimal vascularity by Doppler examination (**f–h**). (**a–d**, MGG stain high power; **e**, Papanicolaou stain, high power)

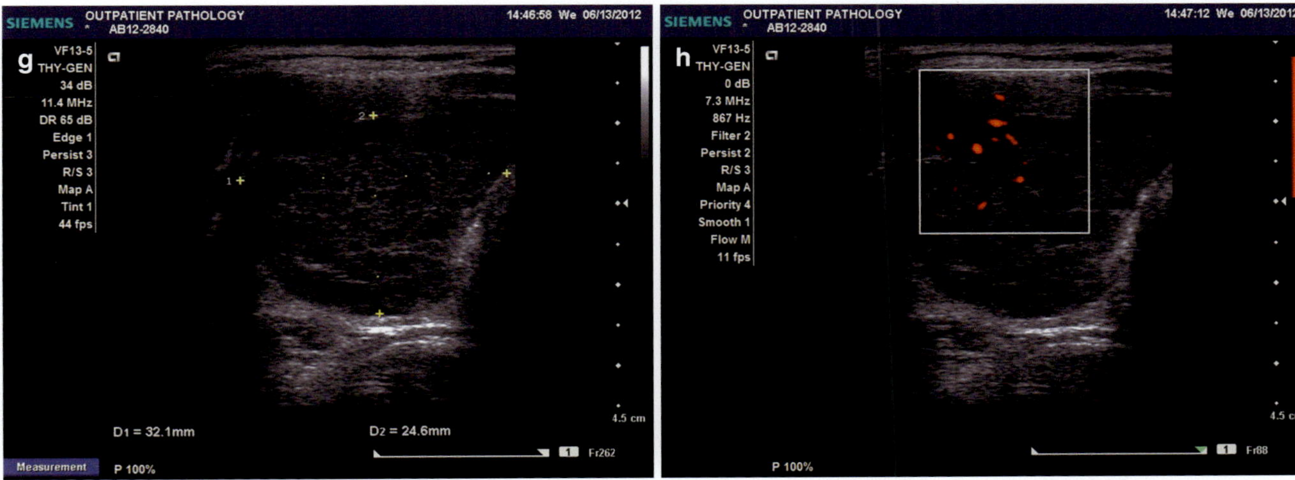

Fig. 3.63 (continued)

FNA Diagnosis of Malignant Thyroid Tumors of Uncertain Histogenesis

Cribriform-Morular Thyroid Carcinoma

This tumor is no longer considered a PTC subtype; The 2022 WHO classification of thyroid tumors includes cribriform-morular thyroid carcinoma (CMTC) in the category of carcinomas of uncertain histogenesis driven by Wnt/beta-catenin pathway activation. The architecture of this tumor shows cribriform and solid morular formations, as the name implies. The diagnosis may lead to early detection of associated familial adenomatous polyposis or Gardner syndrome.

Clinical Findings The inherited form of CMTC carries a germline mutation of the *AFP* gene, almost always occurs in young women, and is associated with familial adenomatous polyposis. A sporadic form occurs in patients with somatic mutations of the APC gene. Regional lymph node metastases are rare. Inherited tumors are often multifocal and/or bilateral than the sporadic tumors. Sporadic CMTC are treated with lobectomy; the familial form may be treated with total thyroidectomy. Targeted therapy with lenvatinib may be considered to treat patients with recurrent disease or distant metastasis.

Histopathology The tumor is well circumscribed or encapsulated. Architectural patterns are follicular, trabecular, solid, or papillary lined with columnar cells with nuclear features of PTC. Squamoid morules may be present in some cases. Capsular invasion, angioinvasion, or extrathyroidal extension can be seen some cases. Tumor necrosis, mitoses, or neuroendocrine differentiation are features seen in aggressive tumors.

Immunoprofile Tumor cells are positive for TTF-1, negative for TG, and weak or negative for PAX8. Nuclear and cytoplasmic positivity with beta-catenin in seen. High expression of estrogen and progesterone receptors is also present.

Molecular Profile Tumor cells of both sporadic and inherited forms have Wnt/beta-catenin pathway that results in nuclear and cytoplasmic positivity for beta-catenin. *BRAF-V600E* mutation is absent. Uncommon molecular alterations include *RET/PTC* rearrangements and *PIK3CA* or *RAS* mutations.

FNA Findings Smears are cellular with elongated cells arranged in papillary aggregates, a cribriform pattern, and morules. Cells are tall and columnar or spindled with nuclear hyperchromasia and exhibit nuclear clearing and nuclear grooves; however, intranuclear cytoplasmic invaginations are less common than in PTC or absent. Squamous morules are present. The aggregates and sheets show round to slit-like empty spaces. The background shows macrophages, but colloid is absent.

Mucoepidermoid Thyroid Carcinoma

Mucoepidermoid thyroid carcinoma (METC) has been described only rarely in the thyroid. The diagnosis is histologic and should be made after exclusion of PTC with a squamous or mucoepidermoid component, or a metastatic deposit. Solid epidermoid and mucin producing cell nest pattern in a background of fibrous tissue is present. Mucin, necrosis, psammoma bodies, and lymphocytes may be identified; however, no eosinophils are seen. Nuclear fea-

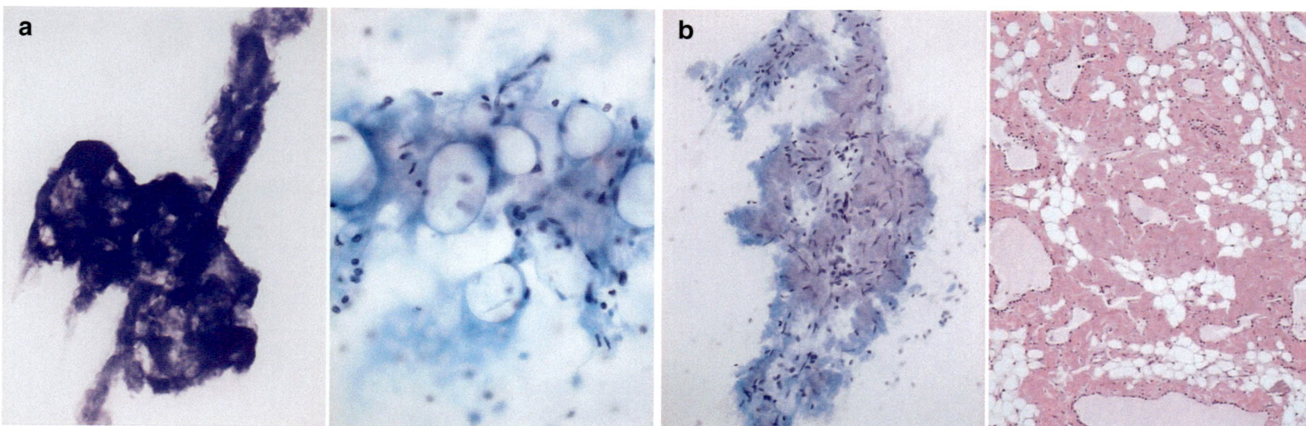

Fig. 3.64 Amyloid goiter. Smear shows ill-defined fragments of amorphous cottony material ("puffy clouds") admixed with benign stromal elements (**a**, **b**), which correlate with the tissue findings (**b**). (**a**, **b** DiffQuik and Papanicolaou stains, high power; **b**, hematoxylin eosin, medium power. Courtesy Dr. Javier Saenz de Santamaria, Badajoz, Spain)

tures of PTC are variably present. The long-term prognosis is good. TG and TTF1 are focally positive.

Sclerosing Mucoepidermoid Thyroid Carcinoma with Eosinophilia

A distinct subtype of METC is the sclerosing type with eosinophilia, which often arises in a background of Hashimoto's thyroiditis with fibrosis. The eosinophils tend to cluster around the moderately pleomorphic squamous cells. Keratin and p63 are positive. TTF-1 may be focal and variable. PAX8 and TG are usually negative. Molecular analysis shows no follicular cell thyroid carcinoma-related abnormalities. Gene fusions present in the salivary gland counterpart are negative in sclerosing METC with eosinophilia. The clinical course appears to be more aggressive than other differentiated thyroid carcinomas (PTC, FTC, OTC).

Other rare tumors of the thyroid gland include teratomas, which usually occur in the first decade of life, neuroblastomas, thymic and parathyroid tumors, and amyloidosis causing the called "amyloid goiter" (Fig. 3.64a, b). Mixed medullary-follicular, mixed medullary-papillary, thyroid paraganglioma, and primary small cell carcinoma are other neuroendocrine tumors described in the thyroid.

Secretory carcinoma of thyroid, primary thymoma of the thyroid, and spindle epithelial tumor with thymus-like differentiation (SETTLE) are also rare thyroid neoplasms.

FNA Diagnosis of Mesenchymal Tumors

Lipoma, hemangioma, leiomyoma, schwannoma, and granular cell tumor have been described in the thyroid. Sarcomas including spindle, epithelioid, and pleomorphic cell types are exceedingly rare and should be considered after exclusion of ATC. Angiosarcoma has also been described in the thyroid, particularly in patients from European Alpine countries (Fig. 3.65a–c).

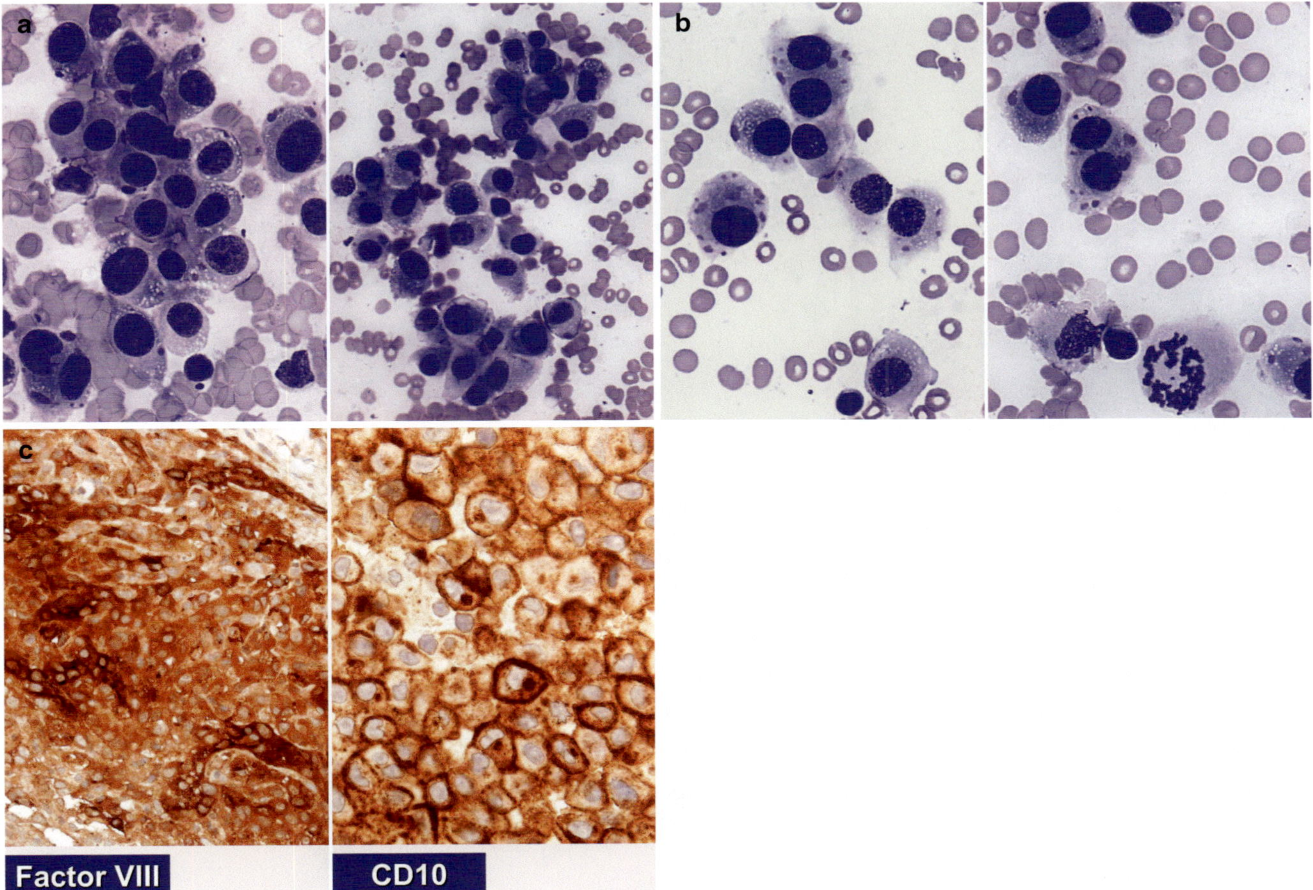

Fig. 3.65 Primary thyroid angiosarcoma. Epithelioid angiosarcoma resembles either primary or metastatic poorly differentiated malignancy. Cells have mild to moderate pleomorphism and may show small cytoplasmic vacuoles (**a**, **b**). Immunocytochemical stains for factor VIII and CD10 are confirmatory (**c**). (**a**, **b**, DiffQuik stain, high power; **c**, immunocytochemistry, high power. Courtesy Dr. Javier Saenz de Santamaria, Badajoz, Spain)

FNA Diagnosis of Metastasis to the Thyroid

Clinically significant metastases to the thyroid gland are not unusual and are seen in approximately 2% of patients who have surgery for suspected thyroid cancer and 10% of patients who die of malignancy other than thyroid. The most common primary sites for thyroid metastases include the kidney (48%), colorectum (10%), lung (8%), breast (8%), and sarcomas (4%). Aggressiveness of the tumor and host susceptibility account for the incidence and time of detection of the metastasis after the primary tumor. Local invasion from primary malignancies of adjacent organs is less common and is seen only in advanced disease.

Clinical Findings Thyroid metastases are commonly solitary (40%); however, they may be multiple or diffuse and are commonly the result of an advanced and disseminated malignancy. Regional lymphadenopathy is common in thyroid metastasis. Forty four percent of metastases to the thyroid

occur in glands with underlying primary thyroid neoplasms and benign thyroid conditions. In general, the clinical suspicion for a metastatic malignancy is high except for renal cell carcinoma. Renal cell carcinoma can present as a thyroid nodule years or decades after the diagnosis of the primary tumor.

FNA Findings Cytologic features are those described in the primary tumors. Briefly, renal cell carcinoma shows aggregates of cells with finely granular, clear, or micro vacuolated cytoplasm, large round to oval nuclei, and often large nucleoli. In melanoma, the smear is cellular with cellular pleomorphism including anaplastic, spindle, and plasmacytoid cells, eccentric nuclei, prominent nucleoli, and occasional intranuclear cytoplasmic invaginations; fine granular cytoplasmic pigment may be present. A uniform population of polygonal cells may be seen in metastatic adenocarcinoma. The smear background often shows necrosis and acute inflammation (Fig. 3.66a–h).

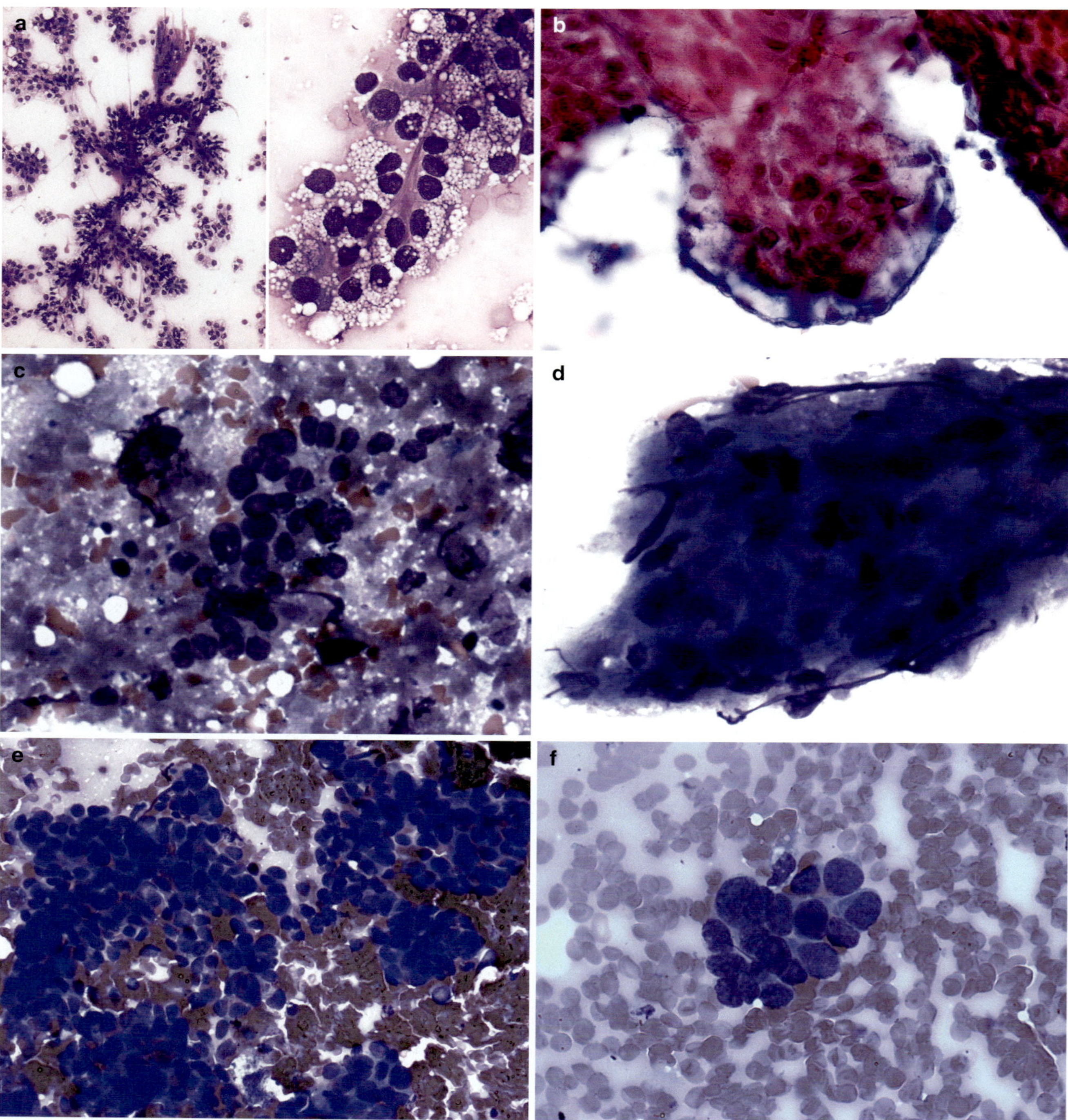

Fig. 3.66 Metastases to the thyroid. Examples of metastatic clear-cell renal-cell carcinoma (**a**), metastatic squamous cell carcinoma of the esophagus (**b**), metastatic squamous cell carcinoma of the base of tongue (**c**, **d**), metastatic adenocarcinoma of the breast (**e**, **f**), and metastatic adenocarcinoma of the lung (**g**, **h**). Ultrasound of the metastatic adenocarcinoma of the lung shows no specific features including a hypoechoic, solid, round, well-circumscribed left thyroid mass with posterior acoustic enhancement mass (**i**, **j**). (**a**, DiffQuik stain, low and high power; **b**, **h**, Papanicolaou stain, high power; **c**, **d**, **f**, MGG stain, high power; **e**, MGG, medium power; **g**, Papanicolaou stain, low power)

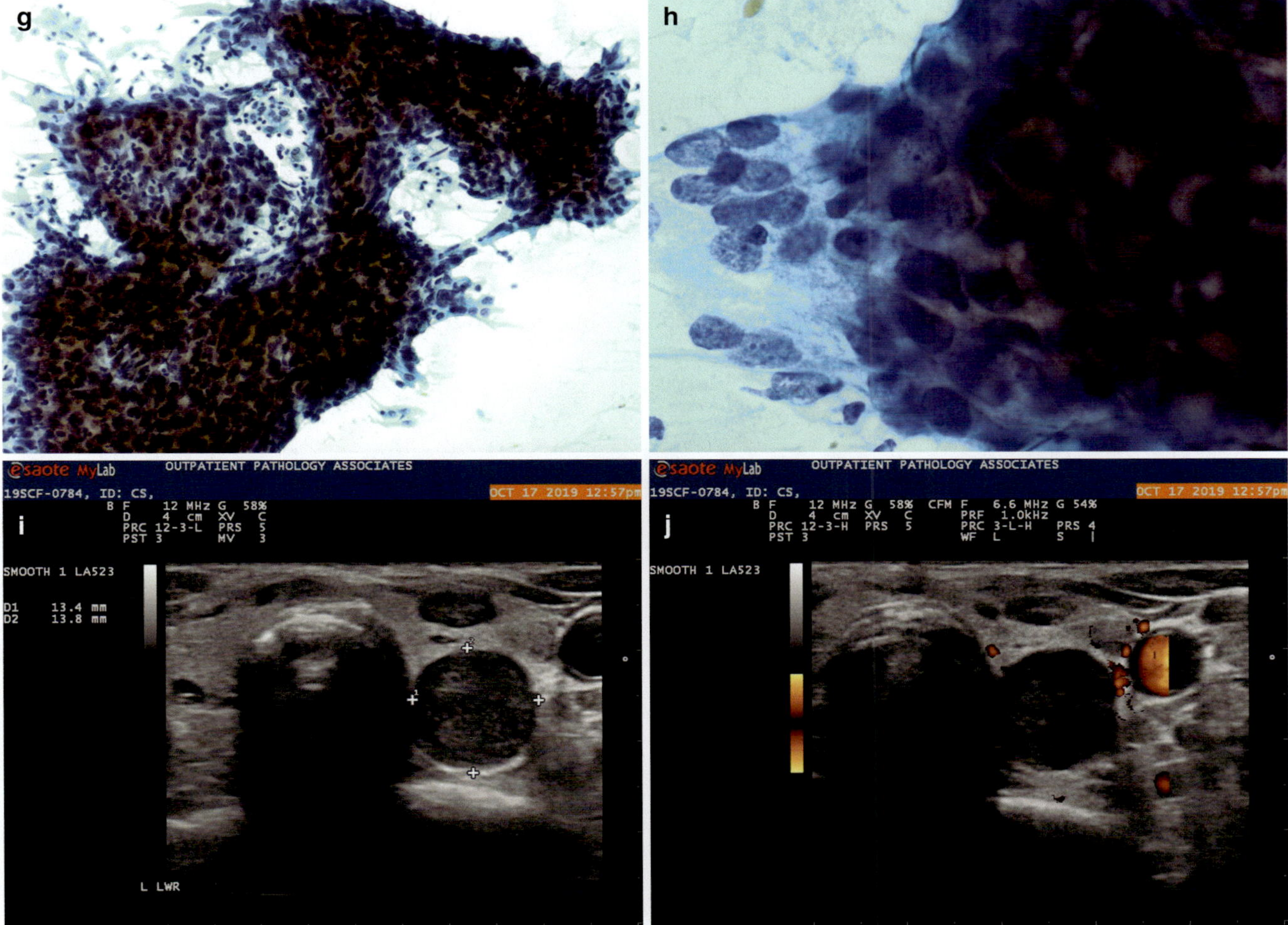

Fig. 3.66 (continued)

The clinical history, cytomorphology, comparison with the primary tumor tissue, and wise use of immunohisto-chemical markers are of paramount importance for the diagnosis. In metastatic carcinoma, it is important to remember that a lung primary shows a TTF-1 inmunoreactivity. The presence of cytoplasmic mucin in the malignancy strongly favors a metastatic deposit; however, mucoepidermoid thyroid carcinoma must be excluded. Small cell carcinoma of lung mimics PDTC; however, TTF-1 immunopositivity is seen in both, but neuroendocrine markers are seen in small cell carcinoma.

US Features (Fig. 3.66i, j)
- Solid, large, and well-defined hypoechoic and homogeneous mass affecting predominantly the lower poles of the thyroid.
- Diffuse involvement is unusual; a heterogeneous echo pattern may be seen.
- Calcifications and necrosis are uncommon.
- A non-specific vascular pattern is seen on Doppler examination.
- Cervical lymph node and systemic involvement is often present.

AUS: FNA Diagnosis and Ancillary Tests

USG-FNA cytology is highly accurate and has a sensitivity and specificity of more than 95% in the diagnosis of benign and malignant thyroid nodules (in our experience evaluating over 81,000 samples). Follicular and oncocytic cell neoplasms remain the most challenging in FNA cytology and constitute the majority of the TBSRTC indeterminate category. In contrast to published statistics that report 15–20% rate for indeterminate diagnoses, our rate is well below 4%.

Cytologic Considerations for Reducing the Indeterminate FNA Diagnosis Rate

1. The presence of lymphoid cells, both single and entangled, along with cell sheets (macrofollicles), which may be oncocytic, strongly suggests chronic thyroiditis including Hashimoto's. The differential diagnosis is broad and correlation with clinical findings including serology and US features is needed (Fig. 3.67a).
2. A two-cell pattern including microfollicles and macrofollicles indicates a mixed micro- and macrofollicular pattern nodule. If macrofollicles (cell sheets) comprise more than 25%, repeat USG-FNA in 6 months. If microfollicles comprise 25–75%, the category is AUS. A predominantly microfollicular pattern (>75%), the category is follicular neoplasm. A predominantly macrofollicular pattern nodule in a pediatric patient may be a *DICER1* mutated nodule, which show minimal or no nuclear atypia and may be a TFND, FTA, or FTC (Fig. 3.67b).
3. Modest cellularity with few microfollicles is not sufficient for a diagnosis of a microfollicular-patterned nodule. Render a descriptive (AUS) diagnosis and repeat

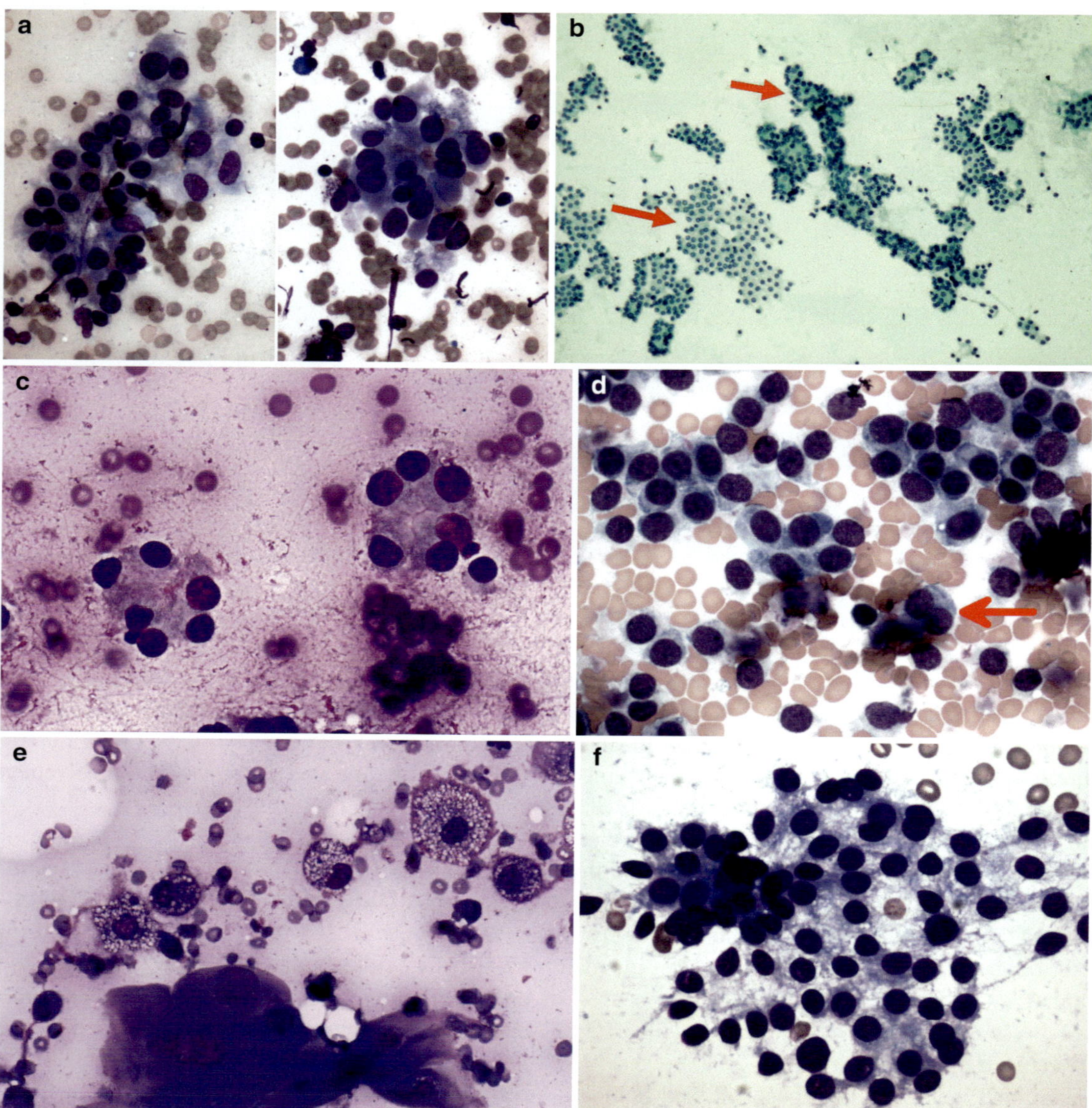

Fig. 3.67 Cytologic clues to avoid erroneous diagnoses. Oncocytiic cells forming microfollicles are often seen in chronic thyroiditis and TFND, and a follicular oncocytic neoplasm or atypia of undetermined significance should be avoided (**a**). The predominance of a macrofollicular pattern in a mixed macrofollicular (**b**, left arrow) microfollicular (**b**, top arrow) pattern-nodule merits repeat FNA under US guidance in 3–6 months. The diagnosis of microfollicular tumor should be avoided in the presence of rare microfollicles (<25%); thus, repeat FNA under US guidance in not less than 3 months (**c**). When cellular findings suspicious for malignancy are seen (medullary carcinoma in this case), correlate the cytology with clinical findings (serum calcitonin levels in this case) (**d**, arrow indicates a distinct type of binucleation). Metaplastic cells and macrophages are findings that may be seen in PTC (**e**) and further sampling under US guidance is required, particularly when there is a solid component. Pseudo-microfollicles may be seen in benign thyroid nodules with atrophic pattern; small nuclear and cell size, fragile cytoplasm, and lack of molding are seen in atrophy and not in true microfollicles (**f**)

Table 3.4 Reflex ancillary tests based on the cytopathology interpretation

USG-FNA diagnosis	Ancillary tests	Remarks
AUS	Molecular studies	Results guide therapy
Follicular neoplasm	Molecular studies	Results guide therapy
Differentiated thyroid carcinoma (PTC, FTC, OTC)	Molecular studies	Results guide therapy
PDTC	Molecular studies	Results guide therapy
ATC	IHC for keratin Molecular studies	IHC preferably done in cell block material *BRAF*-V600E mutation is prevalent in the squamous type Rule out metastases (melanoma, lung, pancreas, breast, kidney, etc.)
Lymphoma	Immunophenotype by flow cytometry	Submit one or two dedicated passes in RPMI medium for flow cytometry studies
MTC	Serum calcitonin, IHC for calcitonin, CEA, TG, synaptophysin, chromogranin	IHC preferably done in cell block material Results guide therapy
Metastasis *from* the thyroid	IHC for PAX8, TG and TTF-1 Needle rinses (in 1 mL of normal saline) for TG and TG antibody level measurement	IHC preferably done in cell block material Results guide therapy Store needle rinses at 4 °F
Metastasis *to* the thyroid	IHC for PAX8, TG, TTF-1. If negative, clinical correlation and proceed with additional IHC tests	IHC preferably done in cell block material TTF-1 is positive in lung tumors
Parathyroid	IHC for PTH, TG, TTF-1, and chromogranin Needle rinses (in 1 mL of normal saline) for PTH level measurement	IHC preferably done in cell block material Store needle rinses in the freezer

AUS atypia of undetermined significance, *FNA* fine needle aspiration, *IHC* mmunohistochemistry, *RPMI* Roswell Park Memorial Institute, *CEA* carcinoembryonic antigen, *TTF-1* thyroid transcription factor, *TG* thyroglobulin, *PTH* parathyroid hormone, *PTC* papillary thyroid carcinoma, *FTC* follicular thyroid carcinoma, *OTC* oncocytic thyroid carcinoma, *PDTC* poorly differentiated thyroid carcinoma, *ATC* anaplastic thyroid carcinoma, *MTC* medullary thyroid carcinoma

USG-FNA in not less than 3 months and harvest a sample for thyroid molecular tests (Fig. 3.67c).

4. Nuclear features short of malignancy are not sufficient for the diagnosis of malignancy. Render a descriptive diagnosis (AUS or suspicious for malignancy) and repeat USG-FNA in not less than 3 months and harvest a sample for thyroid molecular tests (Fig. 3.67d).

5. A cystic background and scattered metaplastic cells and "histiocytoid cells" may be seen in PTC. Render an AUS descriptive diagnosis and repeat USG-FNA in not less than 3 months, with sampling of the solid-phase component and harvest a sample for thyroid molecular tests (Fig. 3.67e).

6. "Pseudomicrofollicles," seen in benign thyroid nodules with atrophy show cell and nuclear sizes similar or slightly bigger than those of red blood cells, lack intact cytoplasm, and lack molding and overlapping in contrast with true microfollicles (Fig. 3.67f).

Currently, ancillary tests including immunohistochemical and molecular markers complement the USG-FNA diagnoses of AUS (TBS category 3), follicular neoplasm (TBS category 4), or suspicion of malignancy (TBS category 5). The value of these tests in the diagnosis of specific thyroid malignancies and indeterminate FNA results varies from institution to institution and depends heavily on the molecular or immunohistochemistry laboratory and the expertise of the cytopathologist, who should use these tests judiciously and in selected cases.

Table 3.4 provides general guidelines to perform additional tests based on cytomorphologic findings to help clarify the TBSRTC diagnosis under consideration.

Overview of Molecular Alterations in Thyroid Tumors

Currently, the cytopathology report based on TBSRTC, the use of ancillary tests including molecular markers and immunohistochemistry, and the histopathology report based on the 2022 WHO classification of thyroid tumors, are the cornerstones for an accurate diagnosis of thyroid neoplasms.

Molecular Markers

The development of thyroid carcinoma is a multistep process that involves gene abnormalities that occur at the DNA level and measurable changes in mRNA or microRNA expression profiles.

In follicular cells, the mitogen-activated protein kinase (MAPK) signaling pathway regulates cell proliferation, differentiation, and survival and is physiologically activated by growth factors binding to receptor tyrosine kinases. The signal is transmitted to the nucleus through proteins and cytoplasmic kinases including RAS, BRAF, MEK, and ERK. Thyroid tumors frequently have genetic alterations leading to the non-regulated spontaneous activation of the MAPK and/or PI3K/AKT/mTOR signaling pathways (Diagram 3.1 and Table 3.5).

A seven-gene panel of mutations and rearrangements frequently seen in approximately 70% of thyroid cancers includes hotspot mutations in *BRAF*, *NRAS*, *HRAS*, and *KRAS*, and fusion genes *RET/PTC1*, *RET/PTC3*, and *PAX::PPARG* is the most commonly tested. *NTRK1–3* gene rearrangements and fusions that are present in 5% of PTCs may be included in the panel as the eight gene.

- *BRAF* is a serine threonine kinase. Mutations are seen in 40% of PTCs and in about 50% of tumors with indeterminate FNA diagnosis. The most common is *BRAF*-V600E activating mutation; other mutation is *BRAF*-K601E. A negative BRAF result in a patient with an indeterminate FNA diagnosis will create more uncertainty, and the clinical management must be based on the cytology diagnosis. If there is a false-positive BRAF result, although unlikely in a patient with an indeterminate FNA diagnosis, the result will be an unnecessary surgery for a neoplasia that in most cases is not life-threatening.

Table 3.5 Common genetic alteration in thyroid tumors

Tumor	Genetic alteration (in various proportions)
Papillary thyroid carcinoma	*BRAF*-V600E-like molecular profile
Follicular carcinoma	*RAS*-like molecular profile
Oncocytic neoplasm	No molecular alterations in 40% of cases Haplodisation-type copy number variants in 35% of cases Mitochondrial DNA alterations
Medullary carcinoma	*RET* point mutations *PROM1* gene overexpression
Differentiated high-grade thyroid carcinoma Poorly differentiated carcinoma	*BRAF*-V600E-like molecular profile *RAS*-like molecular profile *CTNNB1* (β-catenin) mutations *TERT* promoter *TP53* mutations Cell cycle genes Chromatin remodeling genes DNA mismatch genes
Anaplastic carcinoma	*CTNNB1* (β-catenin) mutations *TERT* promoter, *TP53* mutations, cell cycle genes, chromatin remodeling genes, DNA mismatch genes *BRAF*-V600E-like molecular profile *RAS*-like molecular profile

- *NRAS*, *HRAS*, and *KRAS* are oncogenes mutated in several tumors. Mutations of these genes have been reported in 45% of FTCs and 30% of FTAs. They have been reported in invasive and noninvasive follicular-patterned tumors including NIFTP and IEFV-PTC.
- The fusion genes *RET/PTC1* and *RET/PPTC3* are seen in PTCs (10% of cases). The specificity of *RET/PTC* has been questioned because of the identification of *RET/PTC* in non-neoplastic follicular cells, Hashimoto's thyroiditis, oncocytic tumors, and other benign lesions.
- *PAX8::PPARG* fusions are seen primarily in FTCs (40% of cases). This fusion may be seen in FTA and infiltrative follicular subtype of PTC (38%).
- *NTRK1* and *NTRK3* gene rearrangements are seen in 5% of PTCs and may be higher in pediatric cases of PTC.
- *ETV6-NTRK3* is the most common rearrangement seen in radiation-associated PTC; however, its prevalence in PTC in adults is 1%.
- *PAX8::GLIS3* and *PAX8::GLIS1* fusions are seen in HTT and permit the differentiation from PTC.

Additional genes that have been implicated in thyroid cancer include *EIF1AX*, *TERT*, *TP53*, *PIK3CA*, *AKT1*, *TSHR*, *GNAS*, *RET*, *ALK*, *PTEN*, *CTNNB1*, and *THADA*.

- *EIF1AX* is not specific for thyroid cancer as have been identified in benign tumors.
- *TERT* promoter mutations are found in association with aggressive tumors. They have not been found in MTC or benign tumors.
- *TP53*, *PIK3CA*, and *AKT1* genes are associated with aggressive behavior and tumor progression. They may be present in association with molecular alterations listed in the seven/eight gene panel.
- *TSHR* and *GNAS* are genes that predict tumors with a benign behavior. They have been found (rarely) in FTCs.
- *RET* proto-oncogene germline or somatic mutations, are seen in MTC heritable or sporadic forms respectively. *RAS* somatic mutations are also seen in MTC.
- *ALK* fusions have been found in PTC (2%), PDTC (9%), ATC (4%), and MTC (2%).
- *PTEN* somatic mutations are extremely rare and have found associated with primarily benign thyroid nodules including FTA, OTA, NIFTP, and rarely with PTC of follicular subtype and PDTC.
- *CTNNB1* (β-catenin gene) mutations, commonly found in desmoid-type fibromatosis has been identified in PTC with prominent myofibroblastic stromal component.
- *THADA* fusions have been reported in 1% of PTCs.
- Mitochondrial DNA mutations and recurrent chromosome-level copy number molecular alterations are characteristic of oncocytic tumors. Additional alterations (*TERT* pro-

moter, *TP53*, etc.) may be found in oncocytic tumors with aggressive behavior.

- MicroRNAs are short noncoding RNAs that regulate gene expression. Some microRNAs are up- or down-regulated in different types of thyroid tumors. The microRNA expression profile is used as a diagnostic tool to stratify the risk of malignancy of tumors with AUS or follicular neoplasm cytology diagnosis.

Molecular Classification of Thyroid Neoplasms

Thyroid neoplasms are classified as two molecular groups (*BRAF*-V600E-like and *RAS*-like) or three molecular groups (*BRAF*-V600E-like, *RAS*-like, and non-*BRAF*-V600E-like/non-*RAS*-like). PTC is representative of the *BRAF*-V600E-like group.

The molecular profile of the *BRAF*-V600E-like group includes *BRAF*-V600E mutations and *ALK*, *BRAF*, *RET*, *NTRK1/3*, and *MET* gene fusions.

The *RAS*-like group molecular profile includes *NRAS*, *KRAS*, *HRAS*, *EIF1AX*, *EZH1*, *DICER1*, and *PTEN* mutations, *BRAF*-K601E, and *PPARG* and *THADA* gene fusions.

When the three molecular group classification is applied *PAX8::PPARG* gene fusion and mutations of *EIF1AX*, *EZH1*, *IDH1*, *SOS1*, *SPOP*, *DICER1*, and *PTEN* genes are classified as non-*BRAF-V600E*-like/non-*RAS*-like.

Additional genetic changes occur in DHGTC, PDTC, and ATC that include *TERT* promoter, *TP53*, cell cycle genes, chromatin remodeling genes, and mismatch genes.

Molecular alterations present in thyroid tumors permit the stratification into low (single *RAS* mutation or *RAS*-like alterations), intermediate (*BRAF*-V600E mutation, other *BRAF*-like, and copy number alterations), and high (*TERT*, *TP53*, *AKT1*, and/or *PIK3CA*) molecular risk groups.

Molecular markers are currently not recommended for routine use in diagnosis of thyroid tumors; however, they have been incorporated in the management guidelines of thyroid tumors. The American Thyroid Association guidelines recommendation is that *BRAF*, *RAS*, *RET/PTC*, and *PAX8::PPARγ* gene alterations complements FNA cytomorphology and clinical findings including US for patients with indeterminate FNA cytology (AUS, FN) to provide the risk of malignancy and help guide management. In addition, molecular testing of thyroid FNA specimens can provide predictive and prognostic markers for patients with diagnosed thyroid cancer.

Cytology material is particularly suitable for molecular analysis of thyroid nodules. The rate of PTC in *BRAF*-positive nodules tested by FNA is 99.8%, showing that this test is highly accurate in the diagnosis. However, in our experience, PTC is also confidently diagnosed by FNA cytology in more than 99% of cases; thus, in an experienced cytology laboratory, molecular testing that looks for *BRAF*

mutation or *RET/PTC* rearrangement analysis may be unnecessary for the diagnosis of PTC. Similarly, the clinical history, FNA cytology, and serum calcitonin levels will allow one to diagnose almost all medullary carcinomas, and *RET* proto-oncogene analysis may not be necessary.

Besides the established thyroid cancer biomarkers, *BRAF*, *RET/PTC*, *RAS*, and *PAX8::PPARγ* that represent well-understood mutations with regard to activating pathways of growth, recently, up-regulated genes (*MRC2*, *HMGA2*, *SFN*) with a potential effect on neoplastic growth have been described as useful discriminators for thyroid cancer in indeterminate FNA diagnosis. Also, it has been suggested that microRNA analysis could be a useful adjunct in the management algorithm of patients with thyroid nodules, based on 100% sensitivity and 86% specificity (96% specificity when oncococytic lesions were excluded) at differentiating malignant from benign and indeterminate thyroid lesions diagnosed by FNA cytology.

It is important to stress that (1) thyroid molecular tests are expensive, performed in only in few molecular laboratories, not easily accessible, and not standardized yet; (2) a molecular seven-gene panel that includes *BRAF*-V600E, and *RAS* point mutations and *RET/PTC* and *PAX8::PPARγ* rearrangements will be able to identify a group of patients (70%) with almost 100% probability of malignancy; however, 30% of thyroid cancers have no detectable molecular markers, a fact that is difficult to ignore clinically; and (3) thyroid molecular markers have high specificity for malignant lesions, but do not have a good negative predictive value for cytology-indeterminate lesions. It has been shown that 7.6%–16.2% of patients with indeterminate cytology diagnosis (well above the 3.9% in our laboratory) and negative molecular testing had thyroid carcinoma on surgical excision. Thus, it is still necessary to find out what is the appropriate clinical management when a patient with an undetermined FNA diagnosis has molecular-panel-negative results.

The efficacy of these studies must be assessed carefully, considering the laboratory standards and clinical scenario, including imaging studies. The so-called reflex BRAF testing is clinically beneficial for the patient and for the healthcare system when the cytology diagnosis is indeterminate or suspicious for PTC in less than the acceptable 5% rate, otherwise health care becomes molecular test-dependent and unnecessarily expensive. We must emphasize that the operator needs training to obtain a diagnostic specimen and/or the cytopathologist needs to reassess the diagnostic criteria to lower the rate of undetermined FNA diagnoses.

Therapeutic Implications of Molecular Markers

1. *Surgical therapy*. Conventional therapy for most patients with differentiated thyroid cancer (PTC, FTC, OTC) includes surgery, radioactive iodine, and TSH-suppressive

thyroid hormone therapy. When metastatic disease occurs, radioactive iodine can be curative. However, for those patients with differentiated thyroid cancer whose disease progresses despite conventional therapy, molecular alterations may guide the selection of systemic therapy directed to tumor molecular profile.

2. *Targeted therapy.* A minority of patients with differentiated thyroid carcinoma develop a more aggressive, metastatic, recurrent, and life-threatening disease. Targeted therapies for thyroid cancer with kinase inhibitors based on molecular and cellular pathogenetic pathways can be of use in patients who are not surgical candidates, patients with metastatic thyroid carcinoma unresponsive to traditional therapy, or preoperatively to convert an unresectable tumor into a resectable one. Patients with ATC or progressive metastatic MTC also benefit from neoadjuvant biologically targeted therapy. The hypothesis is that the targeting of these kinases could block tumor growth and ultimately induce cell death.

   Drugs that target cell proliferation, angiogenesis, apoptosis, immunosuppression, metabolomic reprograming, and epigenetic changes have been tested.

Therapy by categories includes the following:

1. *Tyrosine kinase inhibitors.* These agents can target a single kinase (such as BRAF) or multiple kinases in the MAPK signaling pathway, which is activated in most PTCs. Inhibitors of RET, RAS, RAF, and MEK kinases target different points in the same pathway.
   (a) RAF inhibitors: induce growth arrest and apoptosis.
   (b) Vemurafenib: *BRAF*-V600E inhibitor reduces the phosphorylation of ERK, increases cell cycle arrest, inhibits tumor growth and metastasis on specifically mutant *BRAF* V600E, with no effect on wild type *BRAF* or other RAF kinases.
   (c) Dabrafenib: targets *BRAF*-V600E mutation and is used for *BRAF*-V600E-mutated ATC, DTC, and PDTC.
   (d) Selumetinib: MEK inhibitor that reduces the phosphorylation of ERK, increases cell cycle arrest, inhibits tumor growth and metastasis, and seems to target *BRAF* V600E.
   (e) Trametinib: MEK inhibitor. Combined with dabrafenib benefit patients with metastatic ATC with *BRAF*-V600E mutation.
   (f) Selumetinib and trametinib target *RAS* mutation and are used for redifferentiation of RAS-mutated PTC, FTC, or PDTC.

2. *Anti-angiogenic thyrosine kinase inhibitors.*
   (a) Sorafenib: multikinase inhibitor that targets *VGFR1–3, RET, FLT3, BRAF,* and *BRAF*-V600E. It is approved for patients with advanced, iodine-refractory thyroid cancer. The anti-RET activity makes this agent a potential use for MTC. Side effects are serious.
   (b) Lenvatinib: multikinase inhibitor that targets *VGFR1–3, FGFR, PDGFR, RET,* and *KIT*. It is approved for the treatment of advanced, progressive differentiated iodine-refractory thyroid cancer. Side effects are serious.

3. *PI3K/Akt pathway targets.* This pathway plays a role in thyroid carcinogenesis, cell differentiation, invasion, and metastasis. The main three players of this pathway are PI3K, Akt, and mTOR. Activating mutations of the *PI3K* gene (*PI3KCA*) and inactivating mutations of the tumor suppressor gene *PTEN* have been identified in FTC and ATC.
   (a) Everolimus targets *mTOR* mutation, represses tumor growth and cancer progression, and is used for DTC, MTC, and ATC. Response to this treatment may be modest.

4. *Other targeted therapy for specific molecular alterations.*
   (a) Selpercatinib and pralsetinib targets *RET* fusion and *RET* mutation and are used for RET-fused thyroid carcinoma and MTC.
   (b) Larotrectinib, reprotectinib, and entrectinib target *NTRK* fusion and are used for thyroid carcinoma with *NTRK* fusion. The last two are used for *NTRK* or *ALK* or *ROS* fusion thyroid carcinoma.
   (c) Crizotinib, repotrectinib, and entrectinib target *ALK* fusion and are used for *ALK* fusion thyroid carcinoma.
   (d) Reprotectinib and entrectinib target *ROS*1 fusion and are used for *NTRK* or *ALK* or *ROS* fusion thyroid carcinoma.

5. *Immunotherapy.* The expression of immunosuppressive markers (CTLA-4 and PD-L1) is high in several solid tumors including *BRAF*-mutated thyroid tumors compared with wild-type tumors and are associated with poor prognosis. Of note, high PD-L1 expression inhibits T cell activation in the tumor microenvironment and the tumor escapes the immune response.
   (a) Pembrolizumab: is an anti PD-L1 antibody and is a good therapy for advanced thyroid cancer.
   (b) A combination therapy of *BRAF*-V600E inhibitor and anti-PD1/PD-L1 antibody is promising for metastatic cancer.

6. *Modulators of apoptosis.* Apoptosis is targeted by *PPARγ* activators, including ruxolitinib and bortezomib.
   (a) Ruxolitinib is a janus-activated kinase inhibitor (JAK) that inhibits JAK1 and JAK2 protein kinases. It induces apoptosis and pyroptosis in ATC, a tumor that has significantly upregulated the JAK1/2-STAT3 signaling pathway.

(b) Bortezomib. It sensitizes thyroid cancer to a *BRAF* inhibitor and can be used in combination with vemurafenib, a *BRAF*-V600E inhibitor for aggressive thyroid cancer.

Earlier studies claimed that *BRAF* and *RAS* mutations and *RET/PTC* rearrangements were mutually exclusive in PTC, but recent studies have shown the coexistence of *RET/PTC*, *BRAF* V600E, *RAS*, and phosphatase and tensin homolog (*PTEN*) rearrangements in some PTCs. *RAS* and *RET/PTC* are genetic alterations that can activate the MAPK cascade. Thus, it may be more effective to provide therapeutic agents with a broader inhibitory profile (kinases and growth factor receptors) than using single targeted therapy agents.

The success of the above-mentioned biological targeted therapies has not been dramatic and varying on the agent and dosage, side effects such as hypertension, heart conduction system abnormalities, photosensitivity, mucositis, nausea, vomiting, diarrhea, fatigue, a high incidence of cutaneous squamous cell carcinoma have been reported. Targeting angiogenesis by blocking of VEGF tyrosine kinase receptors is very promising for the management of differentiated thyroid carcinoma and MTC because of the synergistic effect on angiogenesis and on MAPK signaling pathways (Diagram 3.7). However, we are still waiting for the development of a selective agent to a specific target within the neoplastic cell that prevents the development and maintenance of the malignant phenotype with high therapeutic efficacy and without side effects.

Handling of Cytologic Specimens for Molecular Marker Studies

The following summarizes the steps involved in the procurement, handling, and submission of material for molecular testing from thyroid nodules obtained by USG-FNA.

Because paired samples for cytology and molecular tests are obtained during the same procedure, this should be performed not sooner than 3 months after prior FNA to avoid finding reactive cytologic changes that may interfere with the cytology interpretation and correlation with the molecular test results.

1. Perform the USG-FNA of the thyroid nodule with 25- or 27-gauge needles, as described before.
2. Prepare the smears for cytologic interpretation in the conventional manner, as described before.
3. Rinse the FNA needles with the solution provided by the molecular-test manufacturer.
4. Perform two passes exclusively for the molecular test. Rinse the needle in the solution as in step 3.
5. If the molecular test is performed by an outside laboratory, submit the vial for molecular tests following the instructions of the manufacturer.

6. Stain the rest of the cytology smears by using standard staining techniques, preferably Romanowsky and Papanicolaou stains.
7. The cytopathologist should perform the cytologic interpretation without knowing the molecular test results to avoid bias.

Minimally Invasive Procedures Guided By US

Percutaneous ethanol injection is used to destroy thyroid nodules by chemical ablation (sclerosing effects of alcohol by cell dehydration and protein denaturation). It may be curative for thyroid cysts that recur after initial drainage, particularly if it is unilocular and simple. Recurrences are common in large, multilocular, and predominantly cystic complex nodules, and surgery is often the final therapy.

Percutaneous laser and radiofrequency ablation are used to destroy thyroid nodules (symptomatic cold nodules and cysts, autonomous functioning nodules, recurrent thyroid cancer) using hyperthermia. They have been proposed for decreasing the volume and improving local symptoms in patients who decline surgery or are at surgical risk. The ablation is done with local anesthesia, and the results are promising.

Further Reading

AACE/ACE-AME. Clinical practice guidelines for the diagnosis and management of thyroid nodules. Endocr Pract. 2016;22(Suppl 1):1–59.

Abele JS. The case for pathologist ultrasound-guided fine-needle aspiration biopsy. Cancer. 2008;114(6):463–8.

Abele JS. Putting aspiration back into thyroid fine-needle biopsy-the re-emerging role of vacuum assistance. Cancer Cytopathol. 2012;120(6):366–72.

Abele JS, Levine RA. Diagnostic criteria and risk-adapted approach to indeterminate thyroid cytodiagnosis. Cancer Cytopathol. 2010;118(6):415–22.

Agarwal S. Anaplastic thyroid carcinoma. PathologyOutlines.com website. 2024. https://www.pathologyoutlines.com/topic/thyroid-Undiff.html. Accessed 28 Jun 2024.

Ahuja AT. The thyroid and parathyroids. In: Ahuja A, Evans R, editors. Practical head and neck ultrasound. London: Greenwich Medical Media; 2000. p. 35–64.

Aiken AH. Imaging of thyroid cancer. Semin Ultrasound CT MR. 2012;33(2):138–49.

Alexander EK, Marqusee E, et al. Thyroid nodule shape and prediction of malignancy. Thyroid. 2004;14(11):953–8.

Alexander EK, Kennedy GC, et al. Preoperative diagnosis of benign thyroid nodules with indeterminate cytology. N Engl J Med. 2012;367(8):705–15.

Ali SZ, VanderLaan PA. The Bethesda system for reporting thyroid cytopathology definitions, criteria, and explanatory notes. 3rd ed. Cham: Springer Nature; 2023.

American Thyroid Association Guidelines Taskforce on Thyroid, N., C. Differentiated Thyroid, et al. Revised American Thyroid

Association management guidelines for patients with thyroid nodules and differentiated thyroid cancer. Thyroid. 2009;19(11):1167–214.

Baloch ZW, Asa SL, et al. Overview of the 2022 WHO classification of thyroid neoplasms. Endocr Pathol. 2022;33(1):27–63.

Bardales RH, Suhrland MJ, et al. Cytologic findings in thyroglossal duct carcinoma. Am J Clin Pathol. 1996;106(5):615–9.

Baskin HJ, Duick DS, et al. Thyroid ultrasound and ultrasound-guided FNA. New York: Springer; 2013.

Bishop JA, Owens CL, et al. Thyroid bed fine-needle aspiration: experience at a large tertiary care center. Am J Clin Pathol. 2010;134(2):335–9.

Boos LA, Dettmer M, et al. Diagnostic and prognostic implications of the PAX8-PPARgamma translocation in thyroid carcinomas—a TMA-based study of 226 cases. Histopathology. 2013;63:234.

Brose MS. In search of a real "targeted" therapy for thyroid cancer. Clin Cancer Res. 2012;18(7):1827–9.

Buehler D, Hardin H, et al. Expression of epithelial-mesenchymal transition regulators SNAI2 and TWIST1 in thyroid carcinomas. Mod Pathol. 2013;26(1):54–61.

Bychkov A, Jun CK. What's new in thyroid pathology 2024. Updates from the new WHO classification and Bethesda system. J Pathol Transl Med. 2024;58:98.

Chan JKC. Tumors of the thyroid and parathyroid glands. In: Fletcher CDM, editor. Diagnostic histopathology of tumors, vol. 2. Philadelphia: Churchill Livingstone Elsevier; 2007. p. 997–1079.

Chui MH, Cassol CA, et al. Follicular epithelial dysplasia of the thyroid: morphological and immunohistochemical characterization of a putative preneoplastic lesion to papillary thyroid carcinoma in chronic lymphocytic thyroiditis. Virchows Arch. 2013;462(5):557–63.

Chung AY, Tran TB, et al. Metastases to the thyroid: a review of the literature from the last decade. Thyroid. 2012;22(3):258–68.

Cibas ES, Ali SZ. The Bethesda system for reporting thyroid cytopathology. Thyroid. 2009;19(11):1159–65.

Clark DP, Faquin WC. Thyroid cytopathology. New York: Springer; 2010.

Cozens N. Thyroid and parathyroid. In: Allan PL, Baxter GM, Weston MJ, editors. Clinical ultrasound, vol. 2. London: Elsevier; 2011. p. 867–89.

Dellis RA, Lloyd RV, et al. Tumors of the thyroid and parathyroid. In: Pathology and genetics tumours of endocrine organs. Lyon: IARC Press; 2004. p. 49–133.

Duick DS, Levine RA, Lupo MA. Thyroid and parathyroid ultrasound and ultrasound-guided FNA. 4th ed. Cham: Springer Nature; 2018.

Filie AC, Asa SL, et al. Utilization of ancillary studies in thyroid fine needle aspirates: a synopsis of the National Cancer Institute thyroid fine needle aspiration state of the science conference. Diagn Cytopathol. 2008;36(6):438–41.

Finkelstein A, Levy GH, et al. Papillary thyroid carcinomas with and without BRAF V600E mutations are morphologically distinct. Histopathology. 2012;60(7):1052–9.

Frates MC, Benson CB, et al. Management of thyroid nodules detected at US: Society of Radiologists in ultrasound consensus conference statement. Radiology. 2005;237(3):794–800.

Geisinger KR, Stanley MW, et al. Thyroid gland fine needle aspiration. In: Modern cytopathology. Philadelphia: Churchill Livingstone; 2004. p. 731–80.

Gharib H, Papini E, et al. American Association of Clinical Endocrinologists, Associazione Medici Endocrinologi, and EuropeanThyroid association medical guidelines for clinical practice for the diagnosis and management of thyroid nodules. Endocr Pract. 2010;16(Suppl 1):1–43.

Guo Y, Zhu L, Duan Y, et al. Ruxolitinib induces apoptosis and pyroptosis of anaplastic thyroid cancer via the transcriptional inhibition of DRP1-mediated mitochondrial fission. Cell Death Dis. 2024;15:125.

Hassell LA, Gillies EM, et al. Cytologic and molecular diagnosis of thyroid cancers: is it time for routine reflex testing? Cancer Cytopathol. 2012;120(1):7–17.

Haugen BR, Alexander EK, et al. American Thyroid Association management guidelines for adult patients with thyroid nodules and differentiated thyroid cancer: the American Thyroid Association guidelines task force on thyroid nodules and differentiated thyroid cancer. Thyroid. 2016;26(1):1–133.

Juhlin CC, Mete O, et al. The 2022 WHO classification of thyroid tumors: novel concepts in nomenclature and grading. Endocr Relat Cancer. 2022;30:2.

Juliano AF, Cunnane MB. Benign conditions of the thyroid gland. Semin Ultrasound CT MR. 2012;33(2):130–7.

Jun CK, Bychkow A, Kakudo K. Update from the 2022 World Health Organization classification of thyroid tumors: a standardized diagnostic approach. Endocrinol Metab. 2022;37:703–18.

Kim EK, Park CS, et al. New sonographic criteria for recommending fine-needle aspiration biopsy of nonpalpable solid nodules of the thyroid. AJR Am J Roentgenol. 2002;178(3):687–91.

Kim TY, Kim WB, et al. Metastasis to the thyroid diagnosed by fine-needle aspiration biopsy. Clin Endocrinol (Oxf). 2005;62(2):236–41.

Laha D, Nilubol N, Boufraqech M. New therapies for advanced thyroid cancer. Front Endocrinol. 2020;11:82.

Lee YYP, Wong KT, et al. Ultrasound investigations in head and neck cancer patients. In: Bernier J, editor. Head and neck cancer: multimodality management. New York: Springer; 2011. p. 221–33.

Ljung BM. Thyroid fine-needle aspiration: smears versus liquid-based preparations. Cancer. 2008;114(3):144–8.

Maliszewska A, Leandro-Garcia LJ, et al. Differential gene expression of medullary thyroid carcinoma reveals specific markers associated with genetic conditions. Am J Pathol. 2013;182(2):350–62.

Moysich KB, McCarthy P, et al. 25 years after Chernobyl: lessons for Japan? Lancet Oncol. 2011;12(5):416–8.

Nikiforov YE. Thyroid carcinoma: molecular pathways and therapeutic targets. Mod Pathol. 2008;21(Suppl 2):S37–43.

Nikiforov YE. Molecular diagnostics of thyroid tumors. Arch Pathol Lab Med. 2011;135(5):569–77.

Nikiforov YE, Ohori NP, et al. Impact of mutational testing on the diagnosis and management of patients with cytologically indeterminate thyroid nodules: a prospective analysis of 1056 FNA samples. J Clin Endocrinol Metab. 2011;96(11):3390–7.

Pekova B, Sikorova V, et al. RET, NTRK, ALK, BRAF, and MET fusions in a large cohort of pediatric papillary thyroid carcinomas. Thyroid. 2020;30(12):1771–80.

Roh MH, Jo VY, et al. The predictive value of the fine-needle aspiration diagnosis "suspicious for a follicular neoplasm, hurthle cell type" in patients with Hashimoto thyroiditis. Am J Clin Pathol. 2011;135(1):139–45.

Rosai J, Tallini G. Thyroid gland. In: Rosai and Ackerman's surgical pathology. Edinburgh: Mosby Elsevier; 2011. p. 487–564.

Ruggeri RM, Campenni A, et al. What is new on thyroid cancer biomarkers. Biomark Insights. 2008;3:237–52.

Sharma A, Gabriel H, et al. Subcentimeter thyroid nodules: utility of sonographic characterization and ultrasound-guided needle biopsy. AJR Am J Roentgenol. 2011;197(6):W1123–8.

Sherman SI. Targeted therapies for thyroid tumors. Mod Pathol. 2011;24(Suppl 2):S44–52.

Snozek CL, Chambers EP, et al. Serum thyroglobulin, high-resolution ultrasound, and lymph node thyroglobulin in diagnosis of differentiated thyroid carcinoma nodal metastases. J Clin Endocrinol Metab. 2007;92(11):4278–81.

Stelow EB, Woon C, et al. Interobserver variability with the interpretation of thyroid FNA specimens showing predominantly Hurthle cells. Am J Clin Pathol. 2006;126(4):580–3.

Tessler F, Middleton W, Grant E, et al. ACR thyroid imaging, reporting and data system (TI-RADS): white paper of the ACR TI-RADS Committee. J Am Coll Radiol. 2017;14(5):587–95.

Torous VF, Jitpasutham T, et al. Cytologic features of differentiated high-grade thyroid carcinoma: a multi-institutional study of 40 cases. Cancer Cytopathol. 2024;132:525. https://doi.org/10.1002/cncy.22874.

Tsumagari K, Abd Elmageed ZY, et al. Bortezomib sensitizes thyroid cancer to BRAF inhibitor *in vitro* and *in vivo*. Endocr Relat Cancer. 2018;25(1):99–109.

Virk RK, Van Dyke AL, et al. BRAF(V600E) mutation in papillary thyroid microcarcinoma: a genotype-phenotype correlation. Mod Pathol. 2013;26(1):62–70.

WHO Classification of Thymors. Editorial Board. Endocrine and Neuroendocrine Tumors. WHO classification of tumor series. 5th ed. Lyon: International Agency for Research on Cancer; 2022.

Wunderbaldinger P, Harisinghani MG, et al. Cystic lymph node metastases in papillary thyroid carcinoma. AJR Am J Roentgenol. 2002;178(3):693–7.

Zajdela A, de Maublanc MA, et al. Cytologic diagnosis of orbital and periorbital palpable tumors using fine-needle sampling without aspiration. Diagn Cytopathol. 1986;2(1):17–20.

The Parathyroid Gland

Ricardo H. Bardales

Parathyroid glands usually have the size of a grain of rice, measure approximately 5 × 3 × 1 mm, weigh 20–40 mg, and are surrounded by a fibrofatty tissue capsule. The location of the superior parathyroid glands is in the posterior mid to upper thirds of the thyroid lobes, usually at the level of the thyroid isthmus. The location of the lower parathyroid glands, usually caudal to the inferior aspect of the thyroid lobes, is more variable than that of the upper glands, and they may even be in ectopic locations such as in the mediastinum, around the carotid sheath, in the carotid bifurcation, and in the aorto-pulmonary window. Supernumerary glands may be seen in 5% to 15% of individuals. Rarely, the parathyroid glands may be intrathyroidal, usually within the upper pole.

Embryologically, the lower and upper parathyroid glands develop from the third and fourth branchial clefts, respectively. The lower parathyroid glands share their embryologic origin with the thymus, all migrating caudally, leaving the parathyroid glands in the dorsal extra-capsular aspect of the lower thyroid poles. The upper parathyroid glands descend with the thyroid gland and locate in the dorsomedial extra-capsular aspect of the upper thyroid poles.

Histologically, the parathyroid glands are composed of one basic cell type, the chief cell which may have morphologic variations (oncocytic, clear, transitional), reflecting different physiologic states of activity. Chief cells have a central nucleus and pale granular cytoplasm, which has secretory granules (parathyroid hormone or PTH) and variable amounts of glycogen. Increased secretory granules, prominent Golgi apparatus, and less glycogen are seen in response to hypocalcemia, reflecting increased PTH production. Oncocytic cells have a deep eosinophilic cytoplasm that is rich in mitochondria, but they have fewer secretory granules.

Water-clear cells have clear cytoplasm and are more commonly seen in hyperplastic glands than in normal glands. Transitional cells may also be present. In addition, parathyroid glands contain variable amounts of stromal fat that increases with the age of the individual; however, functional parenchymal elements remain constant. Cytoplasmic immunoreactivity with antibodies to PTH, CK19, and neuron-specific enolase is seen in all cell types.

Of note, the neuroendocrine differentiation of parathyroid tissue is limited and, except for chromogranin A and synaptophysin-positive reactions that are seen in most cases (synaptophysin is less frequent and variable), CD56 immunostaining is negative. Positive CD56 immunostaining helps in the differential diagnosis; as it is seen in follicular thyroid neoplasms, primary and metastatic neuroendocrine tumors, NK lymphoma, and plasma cell myeloma among others.

Hyperparathyroidism

Primary hyperparathyroidism is the most common cause of hypercalcemia, occurring in 1/500–1/1000 of the population; most patients are asymptomatic. Most cases of primary hyperparathyroidism are caused by parathyroid neoplasms.

Currently, based on a better understanding of the pathogenesis of parathyroid disease, the 2022 WHO classification of parathyroid tumors brings new concepts: (1) redefines parathyroid hyperplasia as "multiglandular parathyroid disease" or "multiple glandular parathyroid adenomas" due to the identification of multiple clonal neoplastic proliferations in the affected glands; (2) the term "parathyroid hyperplasia" is reserved to define secondary and tertiary hyperparathyroidism (commonly the result of chronic renal failure); (3) the concept of parafibromin deficiency (parafibromin is a protein encoded by the *CDC73* gene and has multiple suppressive functions) is broadened to "parafibromin-deficient parathyroid neoplasm" and is applied to a parathyroid neoplasm that shows negative parafibromin immunostaining; (4)

Supplementary Information The online version contains supplementary material available at https://doi.org/10.1007/978-3-031-73702-2_4.

R. H. Bardales (✉)
Precision Pathology, Outpatient Pathology Associates, Sacramento, CA, USA

the term "atypical parathyroid adenoma" is replaced by the term "atypical parathyroid tumor" to reflect a parathyroid neoplasm of uncertain malignant potential in the presence of worrisome clinical and laboratory findings along with atypical histologic and immunohistochemical findings. Therefore, there is a need for a thorough and complete pathologic examination of the surgically excised specimen and the appropriate use of immunohistochemistry including parafibromin, paramount to distinguish between benign and malignant parathyroid tumors. Loss of parafibromin favors carcinoma over a benign tumor, confers a worse prognosis in confirmed parathyroid carcinoma, and predicts a high risk of recurrence in atypical parathyroid tumor. In summary, the 2022 WHO classification of parathyroid tumors includes: parathyroid adenoma, multiglandular parathyroid disease also called multiple glandular parathyroid adenomas, atypical parathyroid tumor, and parathyroid carcinoma.

Most abnormal parathyroid glands are enlarged and cellular. A single parathyroid adenoma is the cause of primary hyperparathyroidism in 80–85% of cases; whereas multiple glandular parathyroid adenomas account for 15%. Parathyroid carcinoma is a rare cause (0.1–5%) of primary hyperparathyroidism.

All patients with hyperparathyroidism should undergo US so that the adenomatous/hyperplastic gland(s) are located, and coexisting thyroid nodules are identified, because the incidence of coexisting thyroid cancer is 2–6%. Thus, US of parathyroid glands is conducted as a part of the hyperparathyroidism workup; however, parathyroid gland enlargement may be identified incidentally at the time of thyroid or head and neck US evaluation for some other indication.

Parathyroid Adenoma

Parathyroid adenomas are more frequent in women than in men and occur at any age, including childhood, but are particularly common in the fourth decade of life. Patients with a small parathyroid adenoma (<1 cm, 40–100 mg) may have normal or low serum calcium levels and no clinical findings of hyperparathyroidism. Hypercalcemia and clinically evident disease are usually present in the presence of adenomas larger than 1 cm. Giant parathyroid adenomas (several centimeters) rarely occur.

Most parathyroid adenomas are single, and 75% involve one of the inferior glands. Multiple glandular parathyroid adenomas are examples of parathyroid involvement in hyperparathyroidism jaw-tumor (HPT-JT) syndrome and MEN syndromes (MEN1 more than MEN2A and MEN2B, MEN4, MEN5) and more frequently affecting the superior parathyroid glands than the inferior ones.

Histologically, adenomas are well circumscribed and have a thin capsule. They are usually solid; however, they may have calcifications and cystic and hemorrhagic degeneration. Stromal fat is usually absent in adenomas but can be abundant in lipoadenomas (>50% of the tumor). Adjacent subcapsular normal or atrophic tissue is present in >50% of cases. Solid adenomas are cellular and are usually composed of chief cells; but a common finding is a combination of the other cell morphologic variants. Cellular elements are arranged to form small follicles that, when large can be mistaken for thyroid tissue, particularly in intraoperative consultations. Chief cells show a scant cytoplasm, small round nuclei, smooth nuclear contours, powdery chromatin, and an absent or inconspicuous nucleolus. Mild anisocytosis and slight hyperchromasia may be present, as may be a fine network of capillaries. A trabecular architecture and cell sheets, cell groups, mitoses, necrosis, cellular atypia, enlarged nucleoli are absent. Multiple glandular parathyroid adenomas can contain nodular aggregates of chief cells and other cell variants and often lack the rim of normal or atrophic parathyroid tissue. Band fibrosis is absent in adenoma, but may be seen in secondary and tertiary hyperparathyroidism, adenomas of large size, and a sequela of prior ethanol ablation of the tumor. Focal areas of fibrosis and bleeding can be seen as a result of prior FNA. Lymphoid cells and sometimes plasma cells may be present. "Colloid-like" material simulating thyroid tissue may be seen in large follicles (Figs. 4.1 and 4.2).

Oncocytic parathyroid adenoma is composed of >75% oncocytic cells (mitochondria-rich) and is commonly larger than in chief-cell parathyroid adenoma, and in a nonfunctioning adenoma. Clear-cell parathyroid adenomas are composed entirely of clear cells that exhibit distended and vacuolated glycogen-rich cytoplasm with well-defined cytoplasmic membranes, and they have hyperchromatic peripherally placed nuclei. The term "cystic parathyroid adenoma" may be used when cystic change is present in >50% of the tumor; associated areas of fibrosis or calcification may be present and should not be interpreted as signs of an atypical parathyroid tumor or a carcinoma.

Immunostains for PTH, chromogranin A, synaptophysin (most cases), GATA3, APC, CAM5.2, CK7, CK8, CK18, and CK19 will be positive. Thyroid follicular markers such as thyroglobulin, TTF1, PAX8, and galectin 3 are negative (Figs. 4.1 and 4.2). PGP9.5 is negative and Ki67 is <1%. Parafibromin immunohistochemistry shows a strong nuclear reaction, except for rare parathyroid adenomas arising in patients with pathogenic germline *CDC73* variants. Of note, a small subset of cystic parathyroid adenomas may harbor somatic mutations of the *CDC73* gene. The histologic diagnosis of "parafibromin-deficient parathyroid neoplasm" should be made in these cases, and a further genetic evaluation should be performed as the appropriate clinical setting indicates.

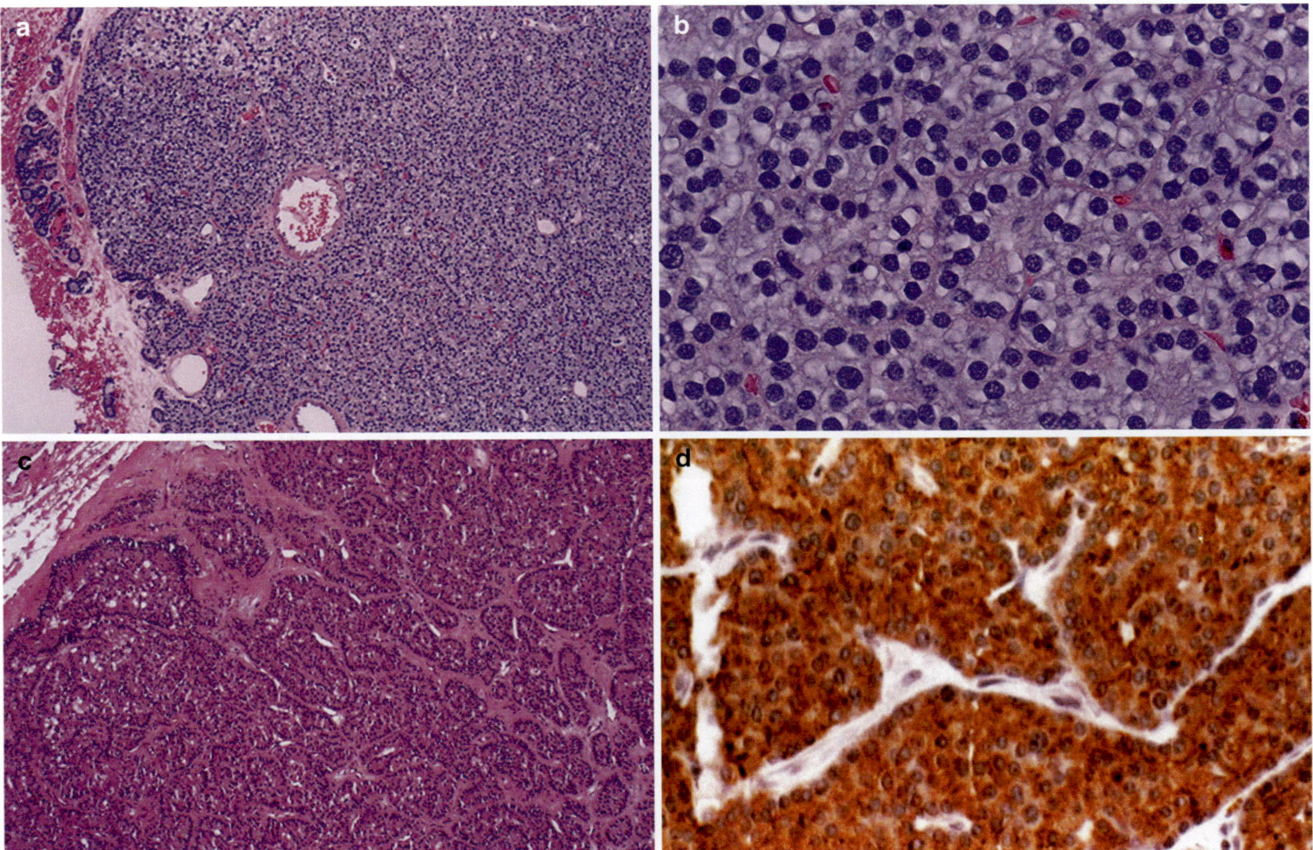

Fig. 4.1 Histologically, this adenoma shows a thin capsule, a remnant of normal parathyroid tissue at the periphery (**a**), and a follicular architecture composed of small- to medium-sized cells without atypia (**b**). This resected parathyroid shows fibrous bands and a trabecular architecture suggestive of an atypical parathyroid tumor (**c**). Immunostain for paratohormone is positive (**d**). (**a-c**, H&E stain, low and medium magnification; **d**, immunoperoxidase stain, medium magnification)

Molecular-genetic abnormalities of single parathyroid adenomas are diverse and variable and are not conclusively different from those found in multiple parathyroid adenomas. Clonality studies suggest that these abnormalities are related to the "nodular architecture" seen in both entities. Furthermore, alterations in the overexpression of Cyclin D1 and chromosome 11q13 regions are seen in both. A gene expression classifier (Veracyte and Interpace) platform is helpful for distinguishing a parathyroid tumor from a thyroid follicular nodule.

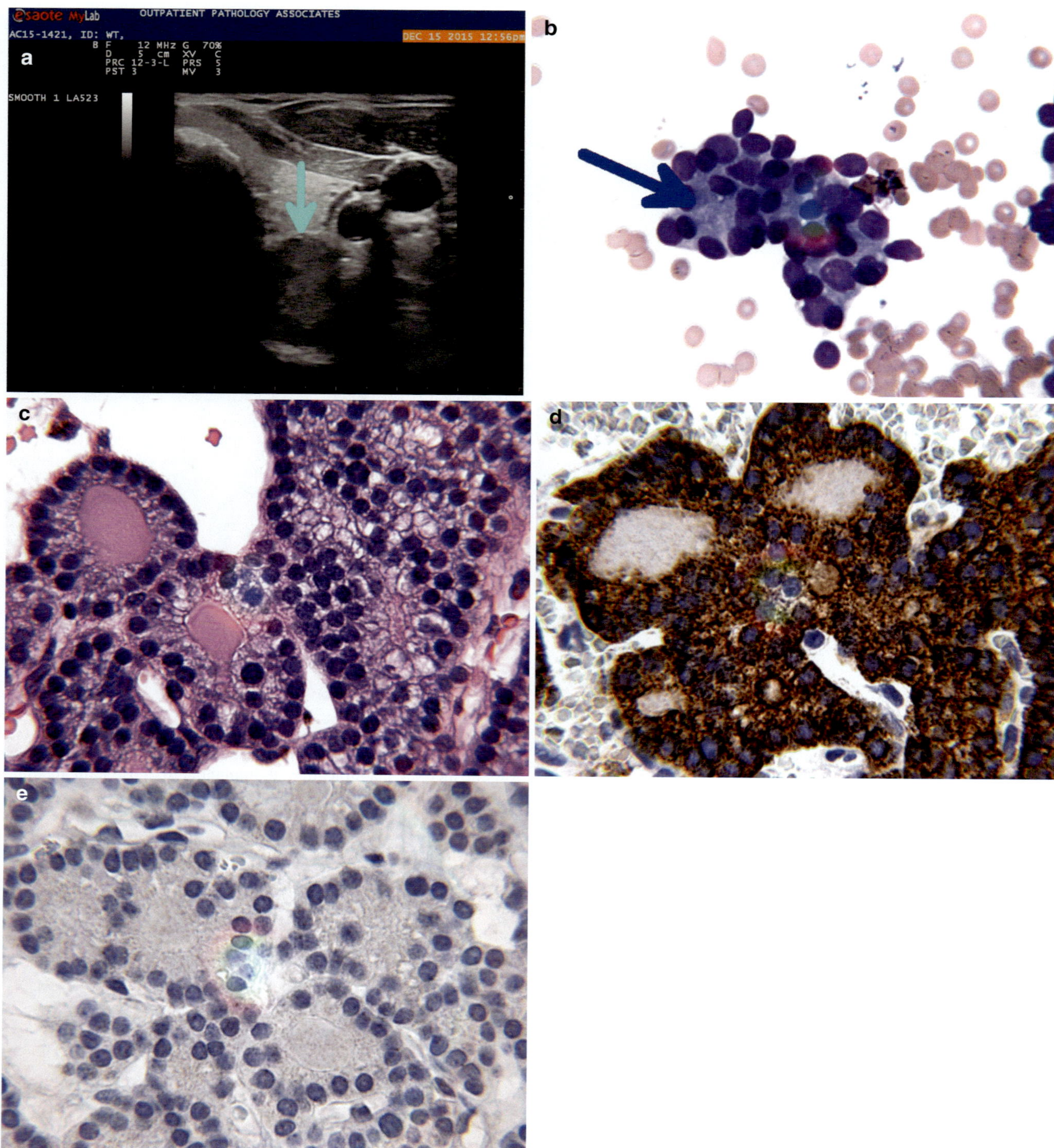

Fig. 4.2 Ultrasound of this left lower parathyroid adenoma shows a well-circumscribed hypoechoic tumor (**a**, arrow), microfollicles (**b**), central "colloid-like" within the follicles (**c**, parathyroidectomy), positive immunostain for chromogranin (**d**), and negative immunostain for TTF-1 (**e**). The histopathology of this parathyroid adenoma resembles that of a microfollicular thyroid nodule. (**b**, MGG stain, high magnification; **c**, H&E stain, medium magnification; **d, e,** immunoperoxidase stains, medium power)

Atypical Parathyroid Tumor

This is a parathyroid neoplasm of uncertain malignant potential that is composed predominantly of chief cells and that shows clinical, pathologic, and immunohistochemical features suggestive, but not conclusive for parathyroid carcinoma. The histopathology evaluation requires submission of the entire surgically excised specimen.

The following are strong considerations for the diagnosis of atypical parathyroid tumor:

– Clinical findings suspicious for malignancy: palpable neck mass, parathyroid gland >3 cm, hypercalcemia >12 mg/dL, serum PTH >3× over the upper normal limit, adhesions found intraoperatively.
– Aberrant immunophenotype: Ki67 > 5%, expression of PGP9.5, galectin 3, hTERT, or aberrant p53, loss of APC, p27, Bcl2, MDM2, RB, or E-cadherin, and loss of parafibromin.
– Atypical histopathologic findings: band-like fibrosis in the absence of a prior FNA or ethanol injection, tumor within, but not through the capsule, trabecular or sheet-like architecture, cellular atypia, enlarged nucleoli, necrosis, mitosis >5 per 50 high power fields, atypical mitoses. These findings should prompt the search for conclusive histologic evidence of carcinoma. If invasion into surrounding tissues, metastases, angioinvasion, or perineural (or intraneural) invasion is not identified, the diagnosis of "parafibromin-deficient parathyroid neoplasm (adenoma vs. atypical parathyroid tumor vs. carcinoma)" is made and further genetic evaluation is conducted to rule out *CDC73*-related potentially hereditary disease even in the absence of a suggestive personal history. In general, atypical parathyroid tumors display a genetic profile that resembles parathyroid carcinoma more closely than parathyroid adenoma.

Most atypical parathyroid tumors do not recur after surgery and behave like adenomas; however, tumor recurrence or metastasis has been reported. Therefore, clinical and biochemical follow-up is recommended.

Parathyroid Carcinoma

Parathyroid carcinoma is rare and may be seen as a component of MEN 1. A hereditary predisposition for parathyroid carcinoma is seen in approximately 15% of patients with the HPT-JT syndrome (parathyroid cysts, parathyroid carcinomas, fibro-osseous lesions of the jaw), an autosomal dominant disorder that affects adolescents and young adults. Parathyroid carcinoma is suspected in patients who have a firm, palpable neck mass, symptoms related to local invasion of adjacent neck structures, nodal metastasis, very high calcium (>14 mg/dL), and intact PTH serum levels >3× the upper limit of normal. Rarely, parathyroid carcinoma may be non-functional. The survival at 5 years is 85%; at 10 years, it ranges from 49% to 77%. Regional lymph node metastases are found in 25% of cases and distant metastases in <3%.

Histologically, parathyroid carcinoma requires one of the following: (1) capsular, vascular, lymphatic, or perineural (or intraneural) invasion; (2) local invasion into adjacent tissue; or (3) documented metastatic disease. Tumors show conspicuous dense, fibrous tissue bands as well as cuboidal and/or spindle cells arranged in a trabecular pattern, and they commonly exhibit a high mitotic count (>5 mitoses per 50 high power fields) that correlates with the K67 labeling index (>5%). Carcinomas composed of chief cells are more common than are oncocytic-cell carcinomas.

The following responses to immunohistochemical stains help in the diagnosis of parathyroid carcinoma: loss of the nuclear and/or nucleolar parafibromin stain (which is a protein that is formed as the result of germline-inactivating mutations of the tumor suppressor gene *HRPT2*, also known as *CDC73* which is responsible for the HPT-JT syndrome); loss of APC, p27, Bcl2, MDM2, RB, or E-cadherin; and expression of PGP9.5, galectin 3, hTERT, or aberrant p53. Of note, germline *CDC73* inactivation is found in up to 30% of patients with sporadic parathyroid carcinoma.

Chief-Cell Hyperplasia

Chief-cell hyperplasia can be secondary to renal failure or malabsorption. The parathyroid glands are enlarged in the classic condition; however, at times one gland may be grossly enlarged, with all glands being histologically hyperplastic. Parathyroid calcification is more common in hyperplasia than in adenoma or carcinoma. The diagnosis of chief-cell hyperplasia cannot be made histologically without the aid of clinical and laboratory information. Although it is difficult to evaluate, the compressed rim of normal parathyroid tissue seen in adenoma helps in making the distinction from hyperplasia.

Water-Clear-Cell Hyperplasia

Water-clear-cell hyperplasia is rarely associated with hyperparathyroidism and is not associated with MEN syndrome. It affects predominantly the superior parathyroid glands, which may be large, weighing 100 g or more. Cells arranged in a solid or pseudo-glandular pattern have well-defined cytoplasmic membranes, peripheral nuclei of variable sizes, and membrane-bound cytoplasmic vacuoles which are probably related to the Golgi apparatus.

Ultrasound (US) Examination and USG-FNA of Solid Parathyroid Tumors

In this chapter, I include my personal experience in the evaluation of 38 parathyroid gland tumors (36 solid and 2 cysts) identified in 36 patients with the use of USG-FNA with US correlation over a period of 13 years. The pertinent literature is revised.

Normal parathyroid glands usually are not seen by US, and parathyroid gland enlargement <5 mm may be undetectable by US.

US is used in the evaluation of parathyroid glands to look for parathyroid hyperplasia or adenoma in patients who have borderline or elevated calcium levels with or without symptoms of hyperparathyroidism.

The patient must lie supine with the neck hyperextended. High-frequency US transducers in the range of 11.5–14 MHz are commonly used; however, transducers with low-frequency in the range of 7.5–10 MHz are recommended for evaluation of deep-neck structures and inferior parathyroid glands, particularly in patients who have a voluminous neck.

The US search for an enlarged parathyroid gland is conducted first in the extrathyroidal mid-posterior aspect of thyroid lobes and the regions caudal to the thyroid gland poles. It may be difficult to visualize enlarged glands located in the tracheoesophageal groove or superior mediastinum by US. The positive predictive value of US in parathyroid adenomas is 97.5%, and that of 99Tc MIBI or Sestamibi scan is 83.7%. Thus, the US evaluation has greater sensitivity than does the Sestamibi scan; it is less expensive and includes no ionizing radiation. In addition, the examination is rapid and allows for simultaneous thyroid evaluation. However, US is unable to detect small parathyroid tumors, particularly if they are located in the upper mediastinum, and has limitations regarding the distinction of parathyroid tumors from reactive lymph nodes adjacent to the thyroid gland (a location commonly found in chronic thyroiditis), follicular thyroid neoplasms, or thyroid nodules adjacent to the thyroid gland (as may be seen in long-standing chronic thyroiditis) without measurement of PTH levels in needle rinses (PTH has more sensitivity than does cytology). Of importance, the PTH is thermo-sensitive, and the collected sample must be stored at or below 0 °F (−18 °C), while it waits to be processed.

The experience of the sonographer is the most important factor in the detection and localization of an enlarged parathyroid gland (>100 mg). CT and MRI are useful for detecting mediastinal and retro-tracheal parathyroid glands.

US Features of Parathyroid Solid Tumors (Fig. 4.3)

- Parathyroid adenomas and carcinomas may share similar US features.
- The fibrofatty capsule of the parathyroid tumor, which separates the tumor from the thyroid tissue, appears as a thin echogenic "separation" line between the two and is seen in 88% of cases in my experience. This line is usually not US-visible in an intrathyroidal parathyroid tumor.
- The tumor is homogeneous, hypoechoic relative to the thyroid gland, and of variable size and shape; it molds to the surrounding structures. It can be nearly anechoic (pseudo-cystic) or isoechoic to hyperechoic in some cases.
- Tumors have a well-defined echogenic line that separates them from the thyroid gland. The surface is flattened because it lies against the fascial planes. These tumors are oval, round undulating, or display an odd variable shape if they about the surrounding thyroid gland, or when they are located adjacent to and lower than the thyroid pole.
- In parathyroid hyperplasia, the lesions are more spherical in shape than they are in adenoma.
- Calcifications are uncommon in adenomas, but they are more commonly seen in parathyroid carcinoma and hyperplasia.
- Intrathyroidal adenomas are rare (1–2% of cases) and are hypoechoic with a sharp edge/border and prominent vascularity, similar to a "hot" thyroid nodule. The echogenic line is usually inconspicuous or absent.
- Hypervascularity is common, with a predominant arterial pattern. Visualization of the feeding polar inferior thyroid artery in the vascular pedicle is a helpful feature (Video 4.1). The vascular pedicle is caudal in the inferior glands and cranial in the superior glands. "Vascular arc" is another pattern of blood flow that can be seen in some parathyroid tumors.
- Avascular tumors (10%) are usually less than 1 cm in diameter, cystic, and deep-seated.
- Large tumors may be partially or entirely cystic; multiple cysts are more common than a single cyst.
- Parathyroid carcinoma is suspected in the presence of a mass with irregular borders, invasion of adjacent structures, immobility on swallowing, and/or abnormal regional lymph nodes. Lymph node metastasis is seen in 25% of cases of parathyroid carcinoma.
- The parathyroid tumor must be distinguished from the *longus colli* muscle, esophagus, blood vessels, small lymph nodes without US-visible fatty hilum, and thyroid nodules (Fig. 4.4).

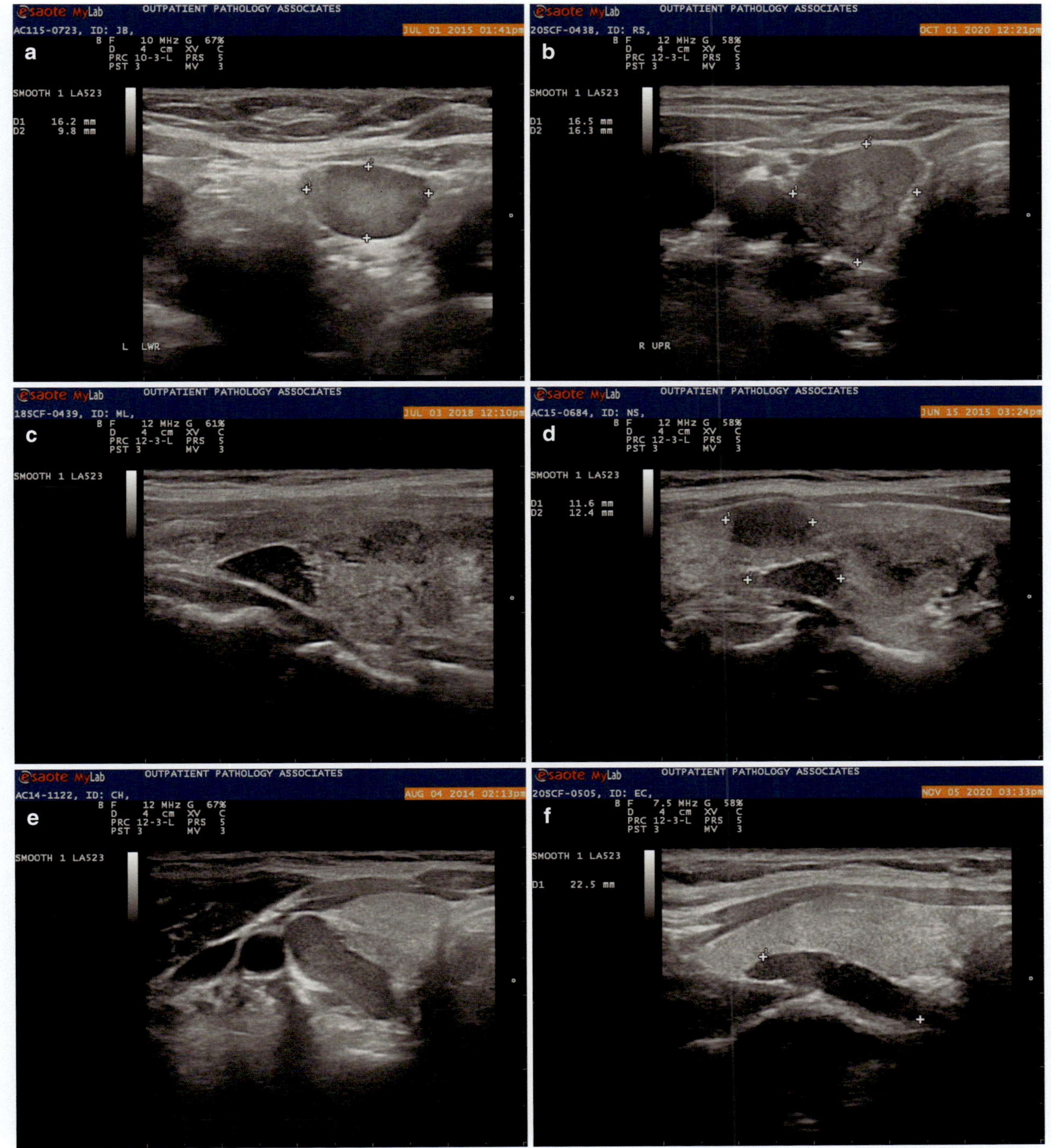

Fig. 4.3 Ultrasound features of a parathyroid adenoma. Solid, hypoechoic, and echogenic rim (**a**, left lower, transverse view). Solid, isoechoic, and echogenic line (**b**, right upper, transverse view). Solid, deeply hypoechoic, echogenic rim, and "triangular shape" (**c**, mid-upper posterior, longitudinal view). Solid, deeply hypoechoic, echogenic rim, "triangular shape," and adjacent hypoechoic thyroid nodule (**d**, mid-posterior, longitudinal view). Solid, hypoechoic, echogenic rim, and "fat worm shape." Note that the upper surface of the adenoma is concave and is being pushed inferiorly by the surrounding thyroid lobe (**e**, right lower, transverse view). Solid, deeply hypoechoic, echogenic rim, and "fat worm shape" (**f**, right lower posterior, longitudinal view). Solid, hypoechoic, echogenic rim, and "mouse shape" (**g**, mid-posterior, longi-tudinal view). Solid, taller than wide, isoechoic with hypoechoic halo, and echogenic rim. Note the hypoechoic vascular pedicle that connects the adenoma with the artery and corresponds to the feeding vessel (**h, i**, right lower, transverse view). Solid, isoechoic, echogenic rim, and cha-otic vascularity by Doppler examination (**j, k**, right lower, longitudinal view). Intrathyroid parathyroid adenoma: solid, iso- to hypoechoic, no echogenic rim, and peripheral vascularity by Doppler examination (**l, m**, right mid lower, transverse view). Cystic parathyroid adenoma: solid isoechoic component is seen in the lower portion, and needle tip in the anechoic upper portion (**n**, right lower, transverse view); needle tip is seen in the mass post-fluid drainage (**o**, right lower, transverse view). (**a–o**, US, high frequency, transverse view)

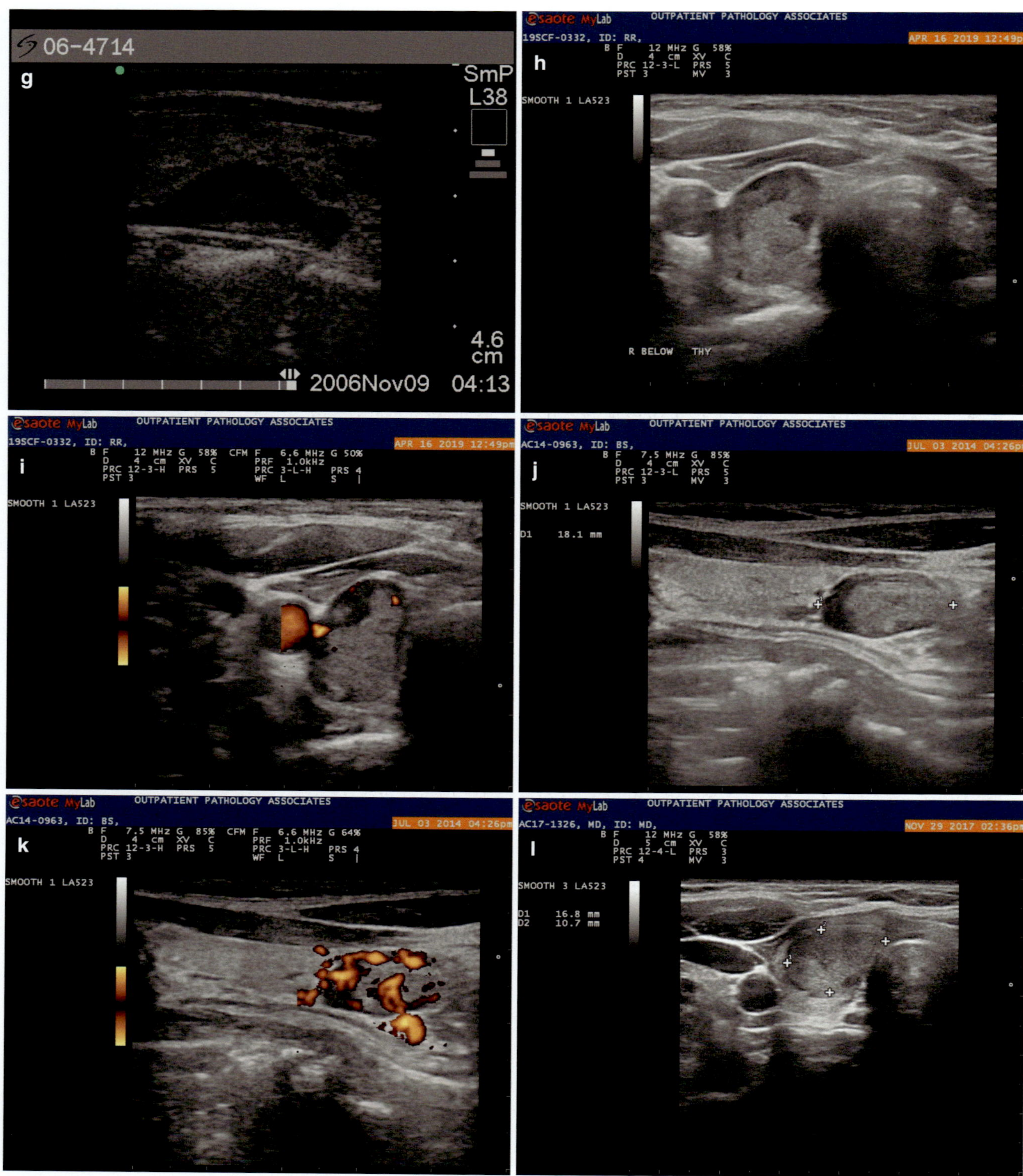

Fig. 4.3 (continued)

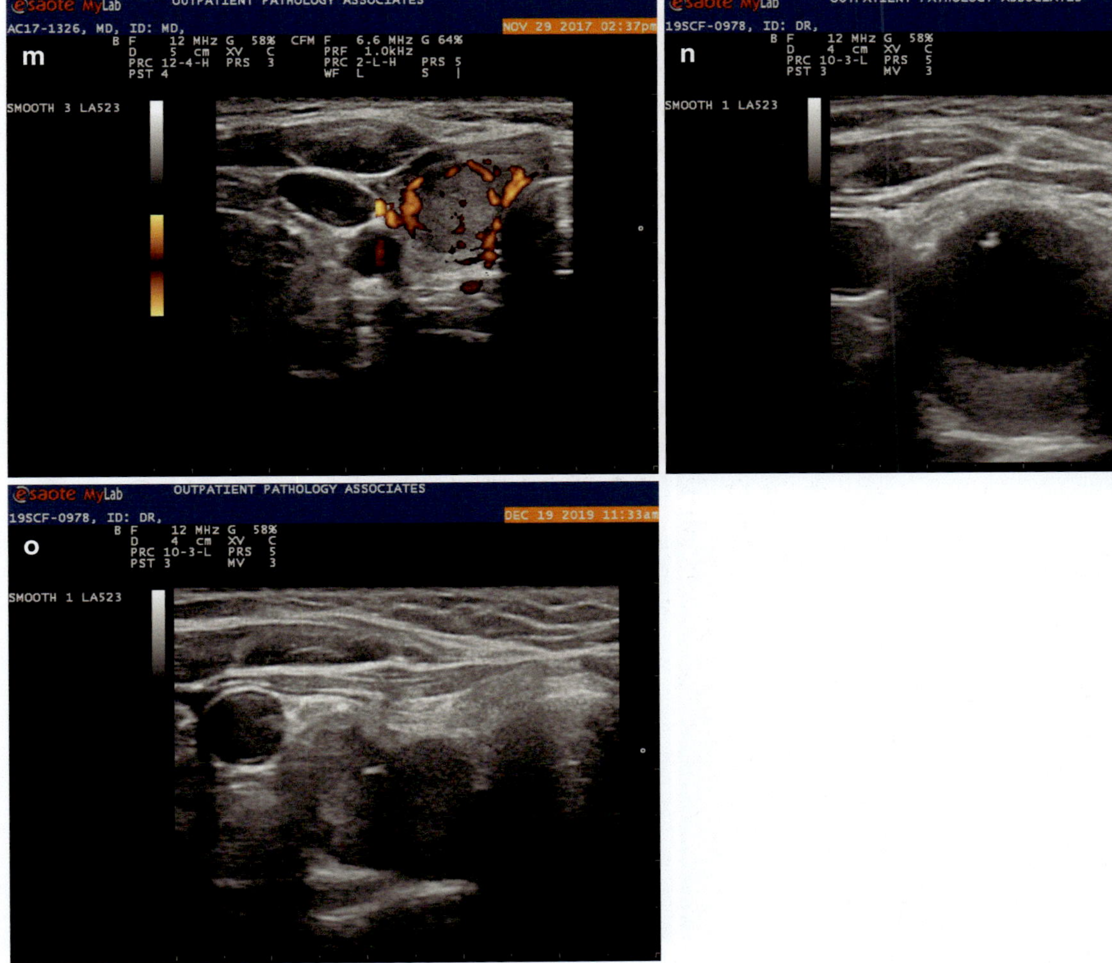

Fig. 4.3 (continued)

- Pressing the US probe firmly against the thyroid and asking the patient to swallow are maneuvers that may help to distinguish a parathyroid tumor from a thyroid nodule. The parathyroid tumor will move separately from the thyroid gland with a nodule.

Ultrasound-Guided FNA of Parathyroid Solid Tumors (Videos 4.2, 4.3, and 4.4)

Not all parathyroid tumors need USG-FNA; however, USG-FNA is helpful when there are multiple tumors, or when the tumor is in an intrathyroidal or atypical neck location, particularly after a negative Sestamibi scan or failed surgery, or prior to ethanol ablation. USG-FNA can also play a role in localizing the tumor in recurrent disease, and it can be used for obtaining material for cytology and for measurement of PTH levels in needle rinses.

Sampling should be done by capillarity (Zajdela technique) with the use of a 27-gauge needle. One or two quick thrusts per second in 1 or 2 s are sufficient for obtaining diagnostic material. Samples are bloody, and the operator will see how rapidly blood appears in the hub of the needle. Thus, the sampling needle must be withdrawn, and the material must be immediately smeared onto a glass slide to avoid clotting.

Relative contraindications for USG-FNA may include morbid obesity, respiratory movement problems, partial or complete obscuring by vessels, and patients who are receiving anticoagulation treatment.

FNA Findings in Parathyroid Solid Tumors (Fig. 4.5)

Parathyroid solid tumors and cysts may be mistaken clinically to be thyroid nodules. Furthermore, the cytologic findings of parathyroid tumors are very similar to those of thyroid follicular tumors, and without clinical and US correlation, differentiating between the two is difficult.

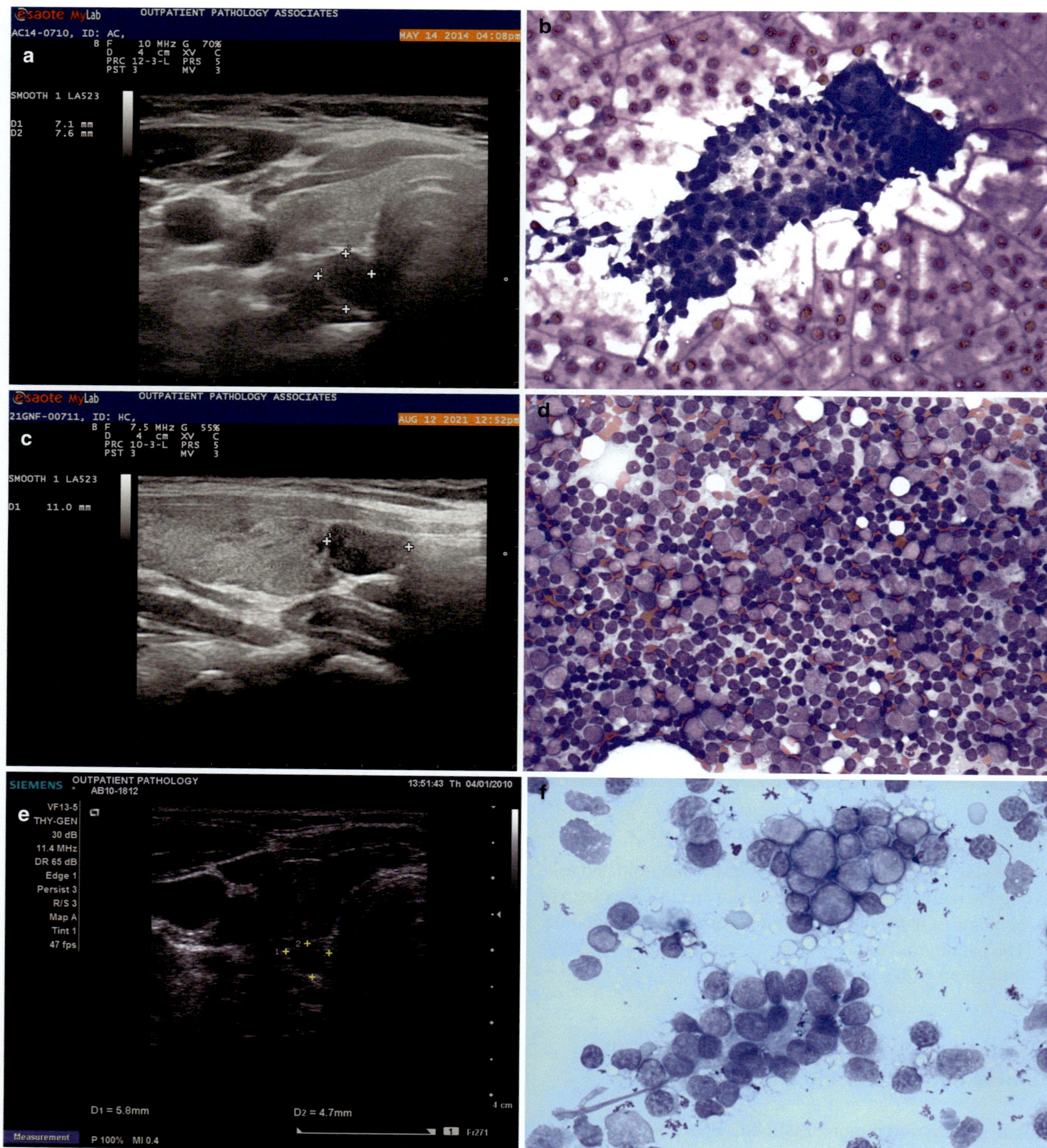

Fig. 4.4 US mimics a parathyroid tumor. Ultrasound images show extrathyroidal small, solid, hypoechoic, round- to oval-shaped masses below the lower poles, each exhibiting an echogenic rim identical to that seen in parathyroid tumors (**a**, **c**, **e**). Cytology smears show evidence of a benign thyroid nodule (**b**, and Video 4.2), benign reactive lymphoid cell hyperplasia (**d**, and Video 4.3), and benign lymphocytes in a case of chronic thyroiditis with a detached thyroid nodule (**f**, and Video 4.4). PTH levels in needle rinses in all cases were negative. (**a**, **c**, **e**, US, high frequency, transverse view; **b**, MGG stain, medium magnification; **d**, **f**, MGG stain, high magnification)

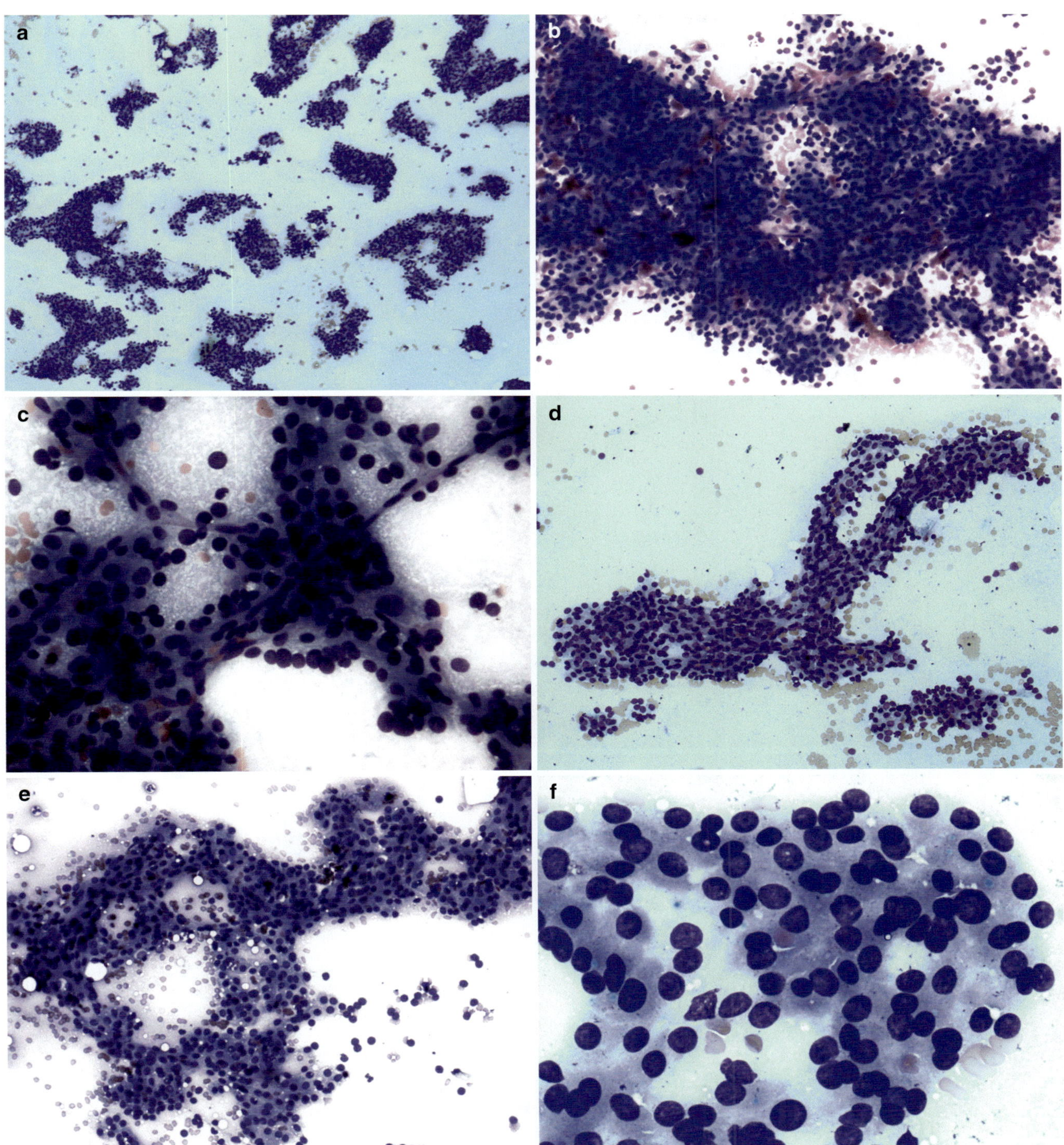

Fig. 4.5 Smears from *parathyroid adenoma* show: hypercellularity with cell aggregates of various shapes and sizes (**a**), cell aggregates supported by a network of fine capillaries (**b**, **c**), coalescing microfollicles forming branching and circumferential aggregates (**d**, **e**), chief cells (monomorphous, cuboidal, with round nuclei, slight anisonucleosis, granular chromatin, and absent nucleoli) forming loose and cohesive microfollicles (**f**, **g**), chief cells with ample and dense cytoplasm forming less conspicuous microfollicles (**h**), oncocytic cells with no distinguishable microfollicular pattern (**i**), numerous stripped nuclei and disrupted microfollicles (**j**), numerous chief cells with a single minute cytoplasmic vacuole (**k**), anisonucleosis and giant nuclei may be seen in some cases (**l**, **m**), variable amounts of colloid (**n**, **o**, **p**), macrophages and lymphocytes (**q**, **r**). Ultrasound and cytology of a parathyroid gland that is visible by US in the thyroid bed of a patient with a history of papillary thyroid carcinoma who was referred to our clinic to rule out recurrent or metastatic papillary carcinoma (**s**, **t**). Smears from a pigmented melanocytic *parathyroid carcinoma* (**u–x**) show features similar to those found in a parathyroid adenoma; granular cytoplasmic pigment and macrophages laden with melanin are also seen in this case. (**a**, MGG stain, low power; **b**, **d**, **e**, **j**, MGG stain, medium magnification; **c**, **f–h**, **k–r**, **t**, MGG, high magnification; **u–x** DiffQuik stain, high magnification; **i**, Papanicolaou stain, high magnification; **s**, US, high frequency, transverse view)

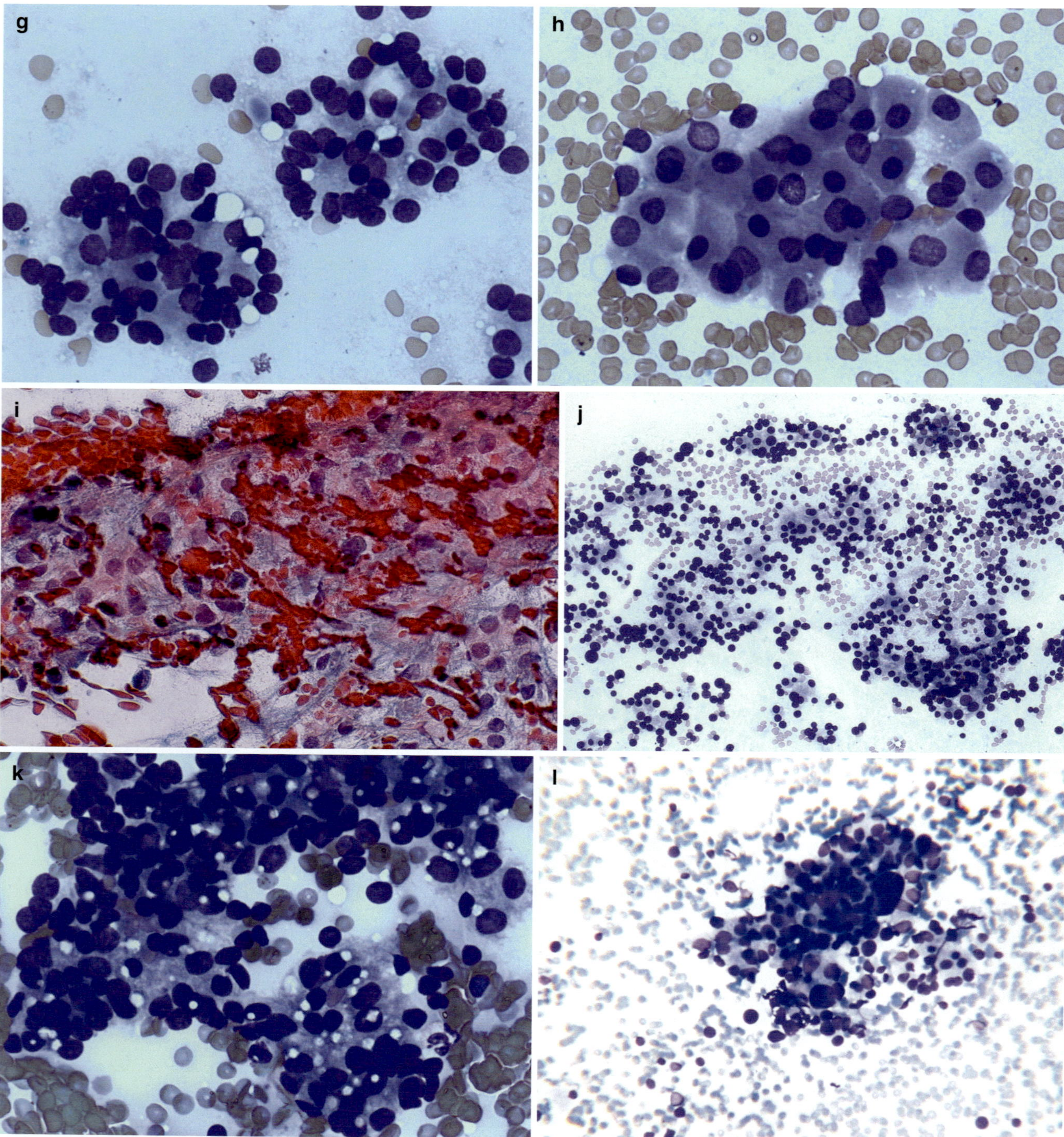

Fig. 4.5 (continued)

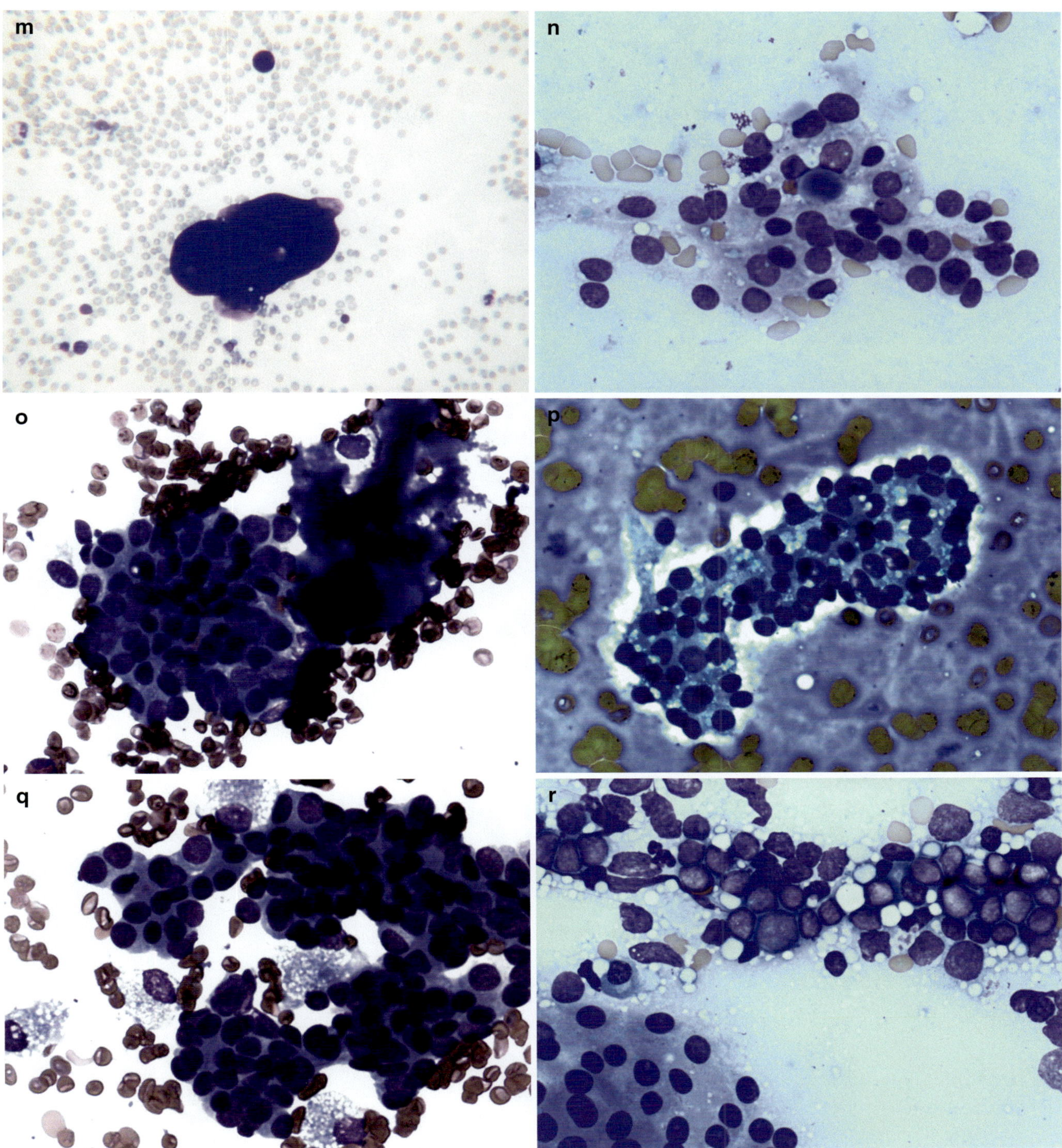

Fig. 4.5 (continued)

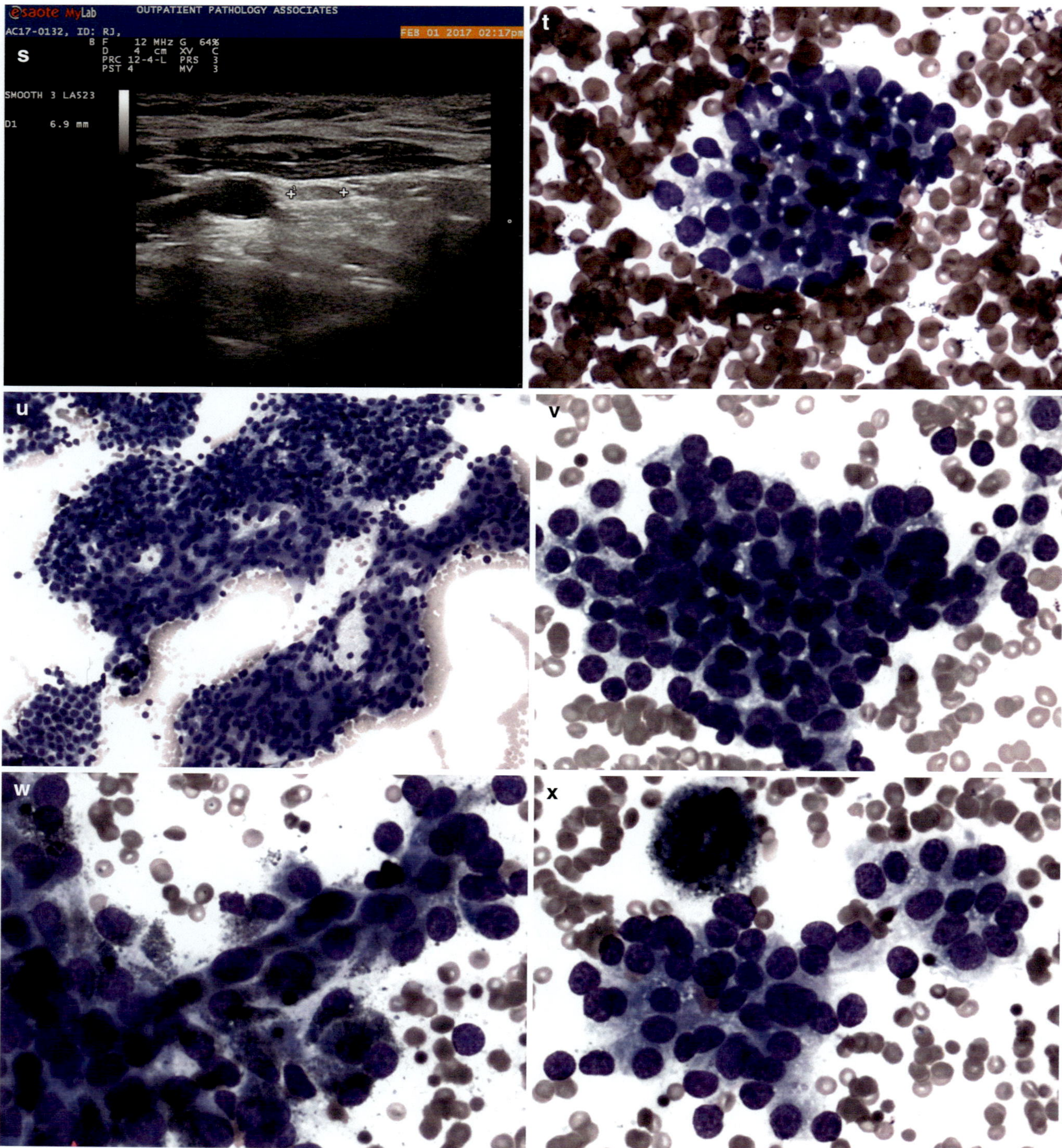

Fig. 4.5 (continued)

Smears are cellular (82% of cases in my experience) and show predominantly isolated and coalescing microfollicles, branching aggregates, papillary structures, and variable numbers of dispersed single cells with cytoplasm. Epithelial cells are cuboidal with eccentric round or oval nuclei, inconspicuous nucleoli, granular coarse chromatin, and either non-oncocytic scant cytoplasm (chief cells) or oncocytic ample cytoplasm, and they may show intranuclear cytoplasmic inclusions. Nuclear size is usually ≤3 times the size of erythrocytes and >3 times in some cases. Mild anisonucleosis is common; however, marked anisonucleosis and anisocytosis may be seen in some cases (Fig. 4.5m). It is my experience that, in the presence of a cellular microfollicular pattern, the finding of cells with a single cytoplasmic micro-vacuole (present in 23% of cases) and numerous bare nuclei (present in 53%) should raise the possibility of a parathyroid neoplasm. Variable amounts of proteinaceous fluid, few lymphoid cells, and macrophages indicating cystic change may be present in the background.

Although parathyroid adenoma is far more frequent than other parathyroid tumors (carcinoma, atypical parathyroid tumor, and tumors of other origins, including carcinomas), cytopathology without ancillary tests cannot distinguish between them. When oncocytic cells predominate, the differential diagnosis includes oncocytic thyroid neoplasms or even metastatic malignancies extending to the thyroid or parathyroid gland. When clear cells predominate, the differential diagnosis includes metastasis from renal-cell clear-cell carcinoma. Thyroglobulin and PTH measurements in needle rinses, and immunostains for PTH, TTF1, and thyroglobulin, are helpful in the differential diagnosis. Metastases to the parathyroid gland are exceedingly rare; one case of metastatic breast carcinoma was reported by Fulciniti F. et al.

Ultrasound (US) Examination and USG-FNA of Parathyroid Cysts

Parathyroid cysts are rare and are more frequent in women than in men. Patients do not have hypercalcemia or hyperparathyroidism and are asymptomatic except for feeling local pressure. The mean diameter is 4 cm.

US Features of Parathyroid Cysts (Fig. 4.6)

- The cysts may be large and may be found within the lower neck region or in the upper mediastinum.
- 2/3 of the cysts originate in the inferior parathyroid glands, and 95% are located below the inferior thyroid border.
- They may "dissect" the tissue planes and compress the adjacent structures, i.e., the trachea, esophagus, or recurrent laryngeal nerve.
- The cysts are well-defined and thin walled.

FNA Findings of Parathyroid Cysts (Fig. 4.7)

The fluid has a characteristic and almost pathognomonic clear, transparent, and water-like appearance, but can be yellow and cloudy, similar to thyroid cyst contents. The drained volume is variable but may be 100 mL or more.

Variable numbers of macrophages may be present.

The cyst wall has parathyroid tissue and is lined with cuboidal epithelium; high PTH levels in needle rinses confirm the diagnosis. Of importance, the PTH is thermosensitive, and the collected sample must be stored at or below 0 °F (−18 °C), while it waits to be processed.

The differential diagnosis includes thymic and thyroid cysts.

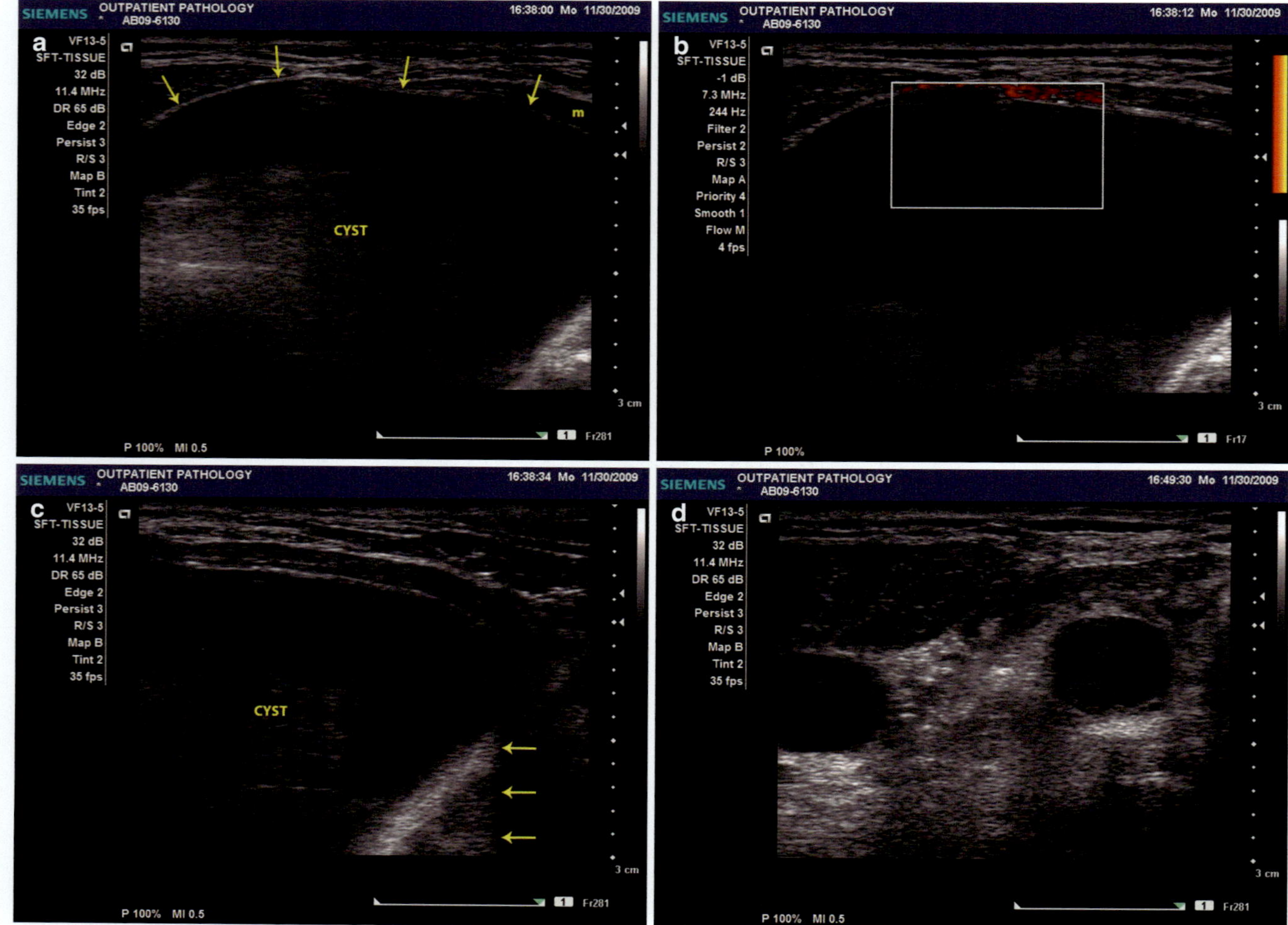

Fig. 4.6 Ultrasound features of two parathyroid cysts. These large anechoic masses are compressing the muscle (**m**) and show a thin, uniform wall (**a**, arrows), no vascular blood flow (**b**), and posterior acoustic enhancement that is seen best in the lateral (**c**, arrows) and posterior (**e**) aspects of the cysts. A bright echogenic rim is more prominent in the smaller cyst (**e**, **f**). The cysts completely collapsed after fluid drainage (**d**, **g**). The needle-tip image is seen bright in the upper portion of the cyst (**g**) and faintly in the tissue corresponding to the collapsed cysts (**d**, **g**) (**a-g**, US, high frequency, transverse view)

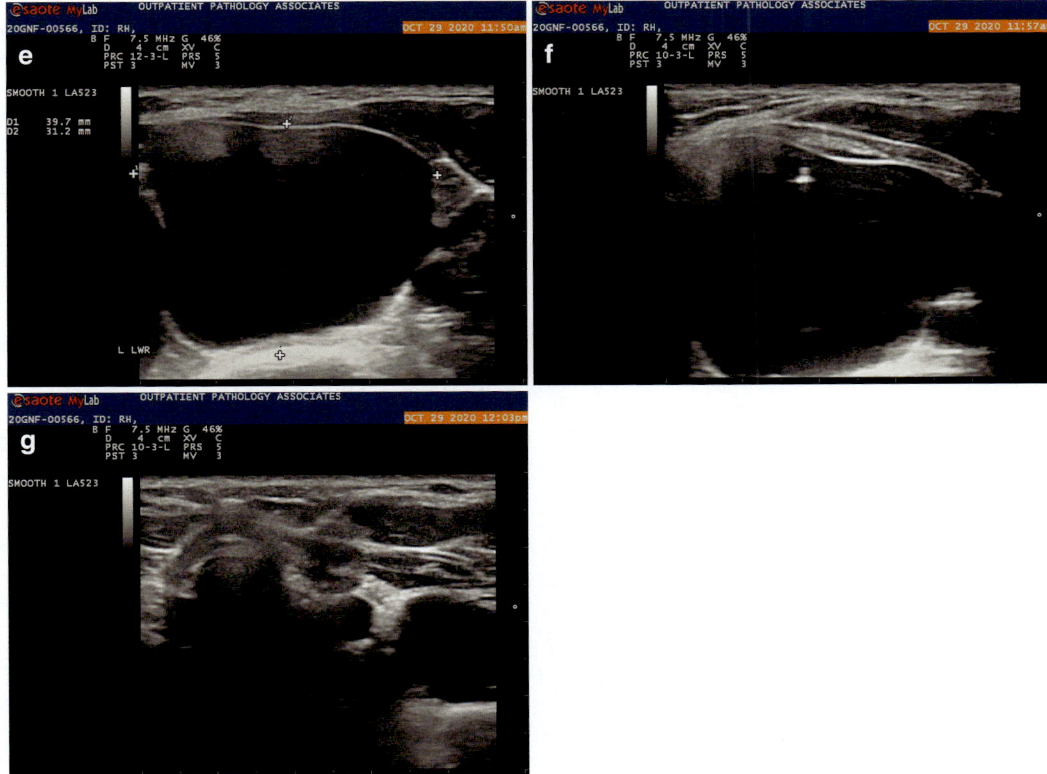

Fig. 4.6 (continued)

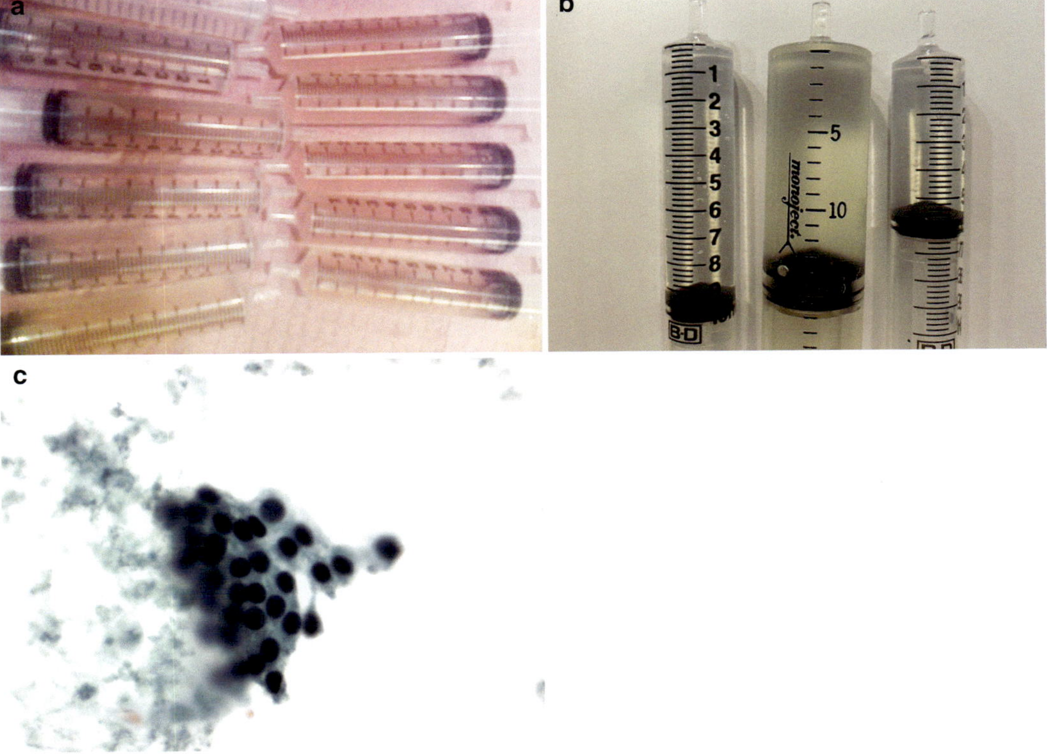

Fig. 4.7 Parathyroid cyst contents. Approximately, 100 cc of clear fluid was drained from the larger cyst (**a**) and 30 cc of water-clear fluid from the smaller cyst (**b**), corresponding to the US images shown in Fig. 4.6. PTH levels in the fluid were high in both cysts and supported the diagnosis. A rare small sheet of cyst-lining cuboidal epithelial cells was identified in the smears from the smaller cyst (**c**) (**c**, MGG stain, high magnification)

Further Reading

Agarwal AM, Bentz JS, et al. Parathyroid fine-needle aspiration cytology in the evaluation of parathyroid adenoma: cytologic findings from 53 patients. Diagn Cytopathol. 2009;37(6):407–10.

Ahuja AT. The thyroid and parathyroids. In: Ahuja A, Evans R, editors. Practical head and neck ultrasound. London: Greenwich Medical Media; 2000. p. 35–64.

Bardales R. The invasive cytopathologist. In: Ultrasound guided fine-needle aspiration of superficial masses. New York: Springer; 2014.

Baskin HJ, Duick DS, et al. Thyroid ultrasound and ultrasound-guided FNA. New York: Springer; 2008.

Cozens N. Thyroid and parathyroid. In: Allan PL, Baxter GM, Weston MJ, editors. Clinical ultrasound, vol. 2. London: Elsevier; 2011. p. 867–89.

Dellis RA, Lloyd RV, et al. Tumors of the thyroid and parathyroid. In: Pathology and genetics tumours of endocrine organs. Lyon: IARC Press; 2004. p. 49–133.

Dimashkieh H, Krishnamurthy S. Ultrasound guided fine needle aspiration biopsy of parathyroid gland and lesions. Cytojournal. 2006;3:6.

Duick DS, Levine RA, et al. Thyroid and parathyroid ultrasound and ultrasound-guided FNA. 4th ed. Cham: Springer; 2018.

El-Naggar AK. Celular and molecular pathology of head and neck tumors. In: Bernier J, editor. Head and neck cancer: multimodality management. New York: Springer; 2011. p. 57–79.

Erickson LA, Mete O, Juhlin CC, Perren A, Gill AJ. Overview of the 2022 WHO classification of parathyroid tumors. Endocr Pathol. 2022;33:64–89.

Fulciniti F, Pezzullo L, et al. Metastatic breast carcinoma to parathyroid adenoma on fine needle cytology sample: report of a case. Diagn Cytopathol. 2011;39(9):681–5.

Ippolito G, Palazzo FF, et al. A single-institution 25-year review of true parathyroid cysts. Langenbecks Arch Surg. 2006;391(1):13–8.

Khati N, Adamson T, et al. Ultrasound of the thyroid and parathyroid glands. Ultrasound Q. 2003;19(4):162–76.

Leonardo E, Bardales R. Practical immunocytochemistry in diagnostic cytology. Cham: Springer Nature; 2020.

Lieu D. Cytopathologist-performed ultrasound-guided fine-needle aspiration of parathyroid lesions. Diagn Cytopathol. 2010;38(5):327–32.

Owens CL, Rekhtman N, et al. Parathyroid hormone assay in fine-needle aspirate is useful in differentiating inadvertently sampled parathyroid tissue from thyroid lesions. Diagn Cytopathol. 2008;36(4):227–31.

Paker I, Yilmazer D, et al. Intrathyroidal oncocytic parathyroid adenoma: a diagnostic pitfall on fine-needle aspiration. Diagn Cytopathol. 2010;38(11):833–6.

Papanicolau-Sengos A, Brumund K, et al. Cytologic findings of a clear cell parathyroid lesion. Diagn Cytopathol. 2011;41:725.

Phillips CD, Shatzkes DR. Imaging of the parathyroid glands. Semin Ultrasound CT MR. 2012;33(2):123–9.

Rosai J. Parathyroid glands. In: Rosai J, editor. Rosai and Ackerman's surgical pathology. Edinburgh: Elsevier Mosby; 2011. p. 565–84.

Tseng FY, Hsiao YL, et al. Ultrasound-guided fine needle aspiration cytology of parathyroid lesions. A review of 72 cases. Acta Cytol. 2002;46(6):1029–36.

Uljanov R, Sinkarevs S, et al. Immunohistochemical profile of parathyroid tumours: a comprehensive review. Int J Mol Sci. 2022;23:6981.

Wei CH, Harari A. Parathyroid carcinoma: update and guidelines for management. Curr Treat Options Oncol. 2012;13(1):11–23.

Ricardo H. Bardales

Normal Salivary Glands

The three pairs of major salivary glands include the parotid, submandibular, and sublingual. The minor salivary glands are numerous and are located in the mouth and oropharynx.

All salivary glands are exocrine and have serous or mucous acini and excretory ducts. Serous acini have basally located nuclei, granular basophilic cytoplasm, and cytoplasmic zymogen PAS+ diastase-resistant granules, and they secrete amylase (Fig. 5.1). Mucous acini have basally located nuclei, clear vacuolated cytoplasm, and cytoplasmic sialomucin vacuoles, and they secrete mucin. The ductal system begins distally in the intercalated ducts, which are lined with cuboidal epithelium. The cells have central nuclei in communication with the larger striated ducts which are lined by mitochondria-rich columnar eosinophilic cells. The more proximal interlobular ducts are lined by pseudostratified columnar epithelium with scattered mucinous cells. Myoepithelial cells surround the secretory acini and the intercalated ducts. The intraglandular ducts drain into the main duct (Stensen's duct) that runs over the masseter muscle and enters the cheek mucosa into the oral cavity at the level of the upper molars.

The parotid gland is a serous gland and contains lymphoid aggregates; lymph nodes may be present and contain ducts or occasionally acini. The submandibular gland is mixed serous and mucous; caps of serous cells may be seen in the mucous acini. The sublingual gland is also mixed, but is predominantly mucous. The minor glands may be predominantly serous or mucous.

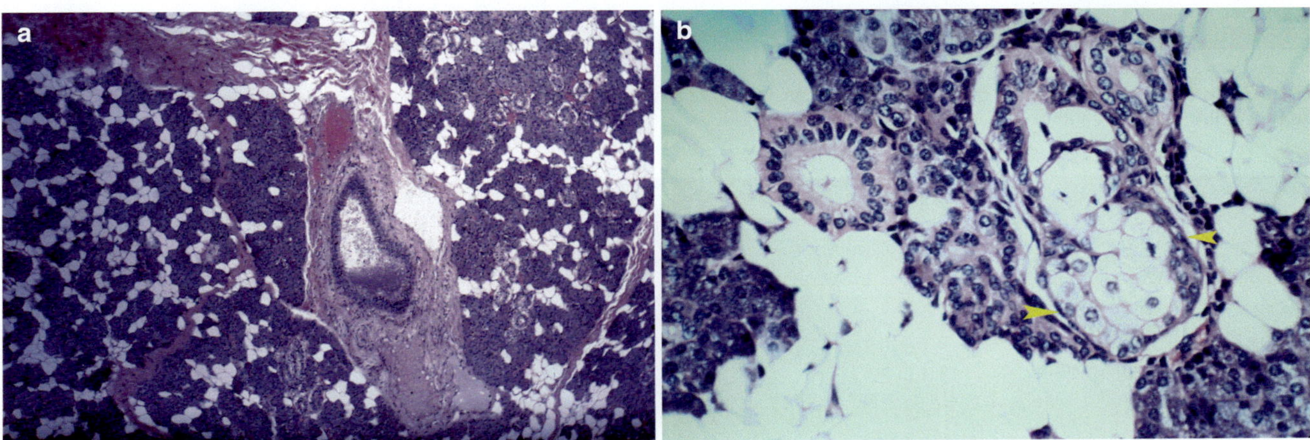

Fig. 5.1 Normal histology of the parotid gland at low (**a**) and high magnification (**b**). Note the presence of adipose tissue and sebaceous glands (**b**, arrowheads). (Hematoxylin and eosin stain)

Supplementary InformationThe online version contains supplementary material available at https://doi.org/10.1007/978-3-031-73702-2_5.

R. H. Bardales (✉)
Precision Pathology, Outpatient Pathology Associates,
Sacramento, CA, USA

Ultrasound Findings

The parotid space extends from the external auditory canal superiorly to the angle of the mandible inferiorly, neighbors the nasopharyngeal area in the medial aspect, and is separated from the carotid space by the posterior belly of the digastric muscle. The space contains the parotid gland, facial nerve, retromandibular vein, external carotid area, and lymph nodes. The normal parotid gland has a homogeneous echotexture and is hyperechoic in comparison to adjacent muscles, more than the submandibular gland (Fig. 5.2). The echogenicity is directly proportional to the intraglandular fatty tissue. The facial nerve cannot be visualized; however, the retromandibular vein, seen as a well-defined hypoechoic tubular structure, is the landmark for the facial nerve.

Intraparotid lymph nodes may be visualized, measure <5 mm, and are usually located in the superficial lobe (Fig. 5.3). An accessory parotid gland may be seen in 20% of patients and is located anterior to the masseter muscle within the cheek (Fig. 5.4). The normal no obstructed Stensen's duct, usually not visible by US can be distended, tortuous, and visible outside the gland secondary to a distal obstruction (Fig. 5.5, Video 5.1).

The submandibular and sublingual spaces lay inferolateral and superomedial, respectively, and are divided by the mylohyoid muscle. The submandibular space (level Ib in terms of the neck lymph node regions) contains the anterior belly of the digastric muscle, the superficial lobe of the submandibular gland, lymph nodes, the facial artery and vein, the inferior part of the XII nerve, and fat.

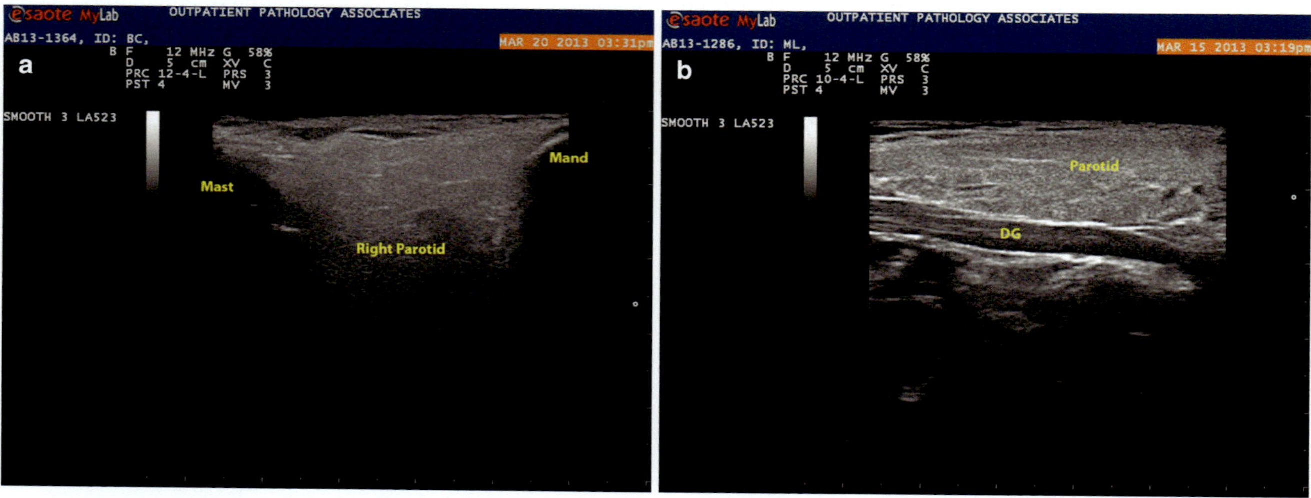

Fig. 5.2 Normal US of the parotid space and parotid gland (**a**, right parotid; **b**, left parotid). *Mand* mandible, *Mast* mastoid process, *DG* posterior belly digastric muscle

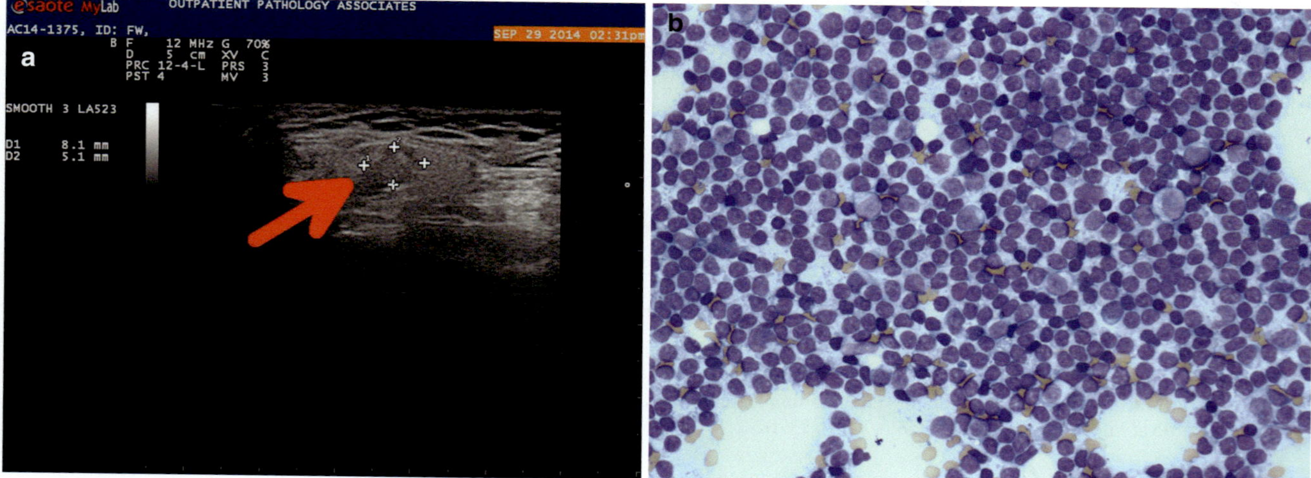

Fig. 5.3 US parotid gland showing an intraparotid lymph node (**a**). US-guided FNA shows reactive lymphoid hyperplasia (**b**) (**b**, MGG stain, medium magnification)

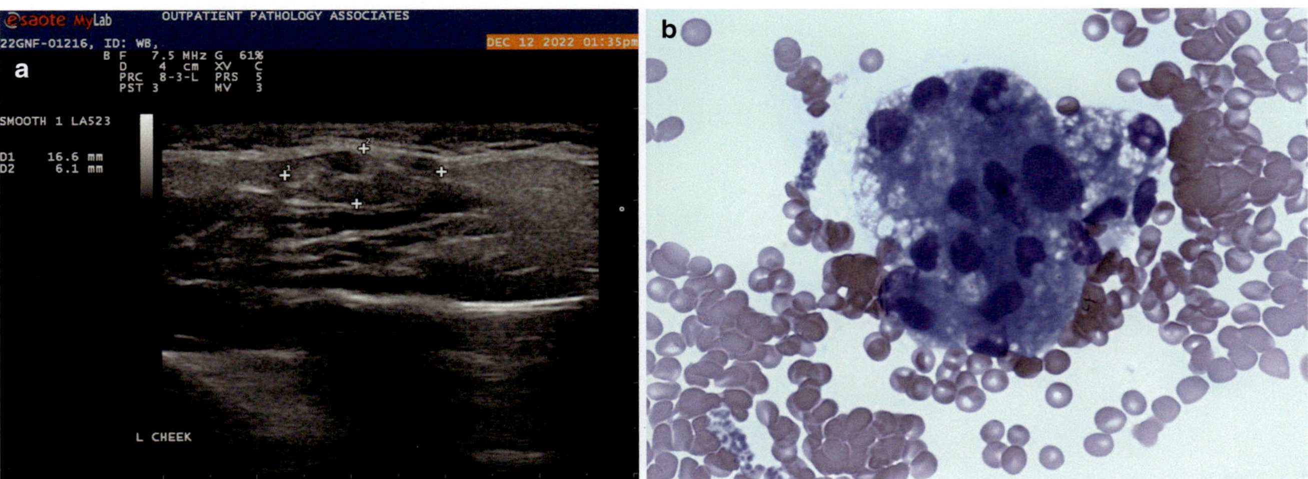

Fig. 5.4 Extra-glandular parotid gland tissue. US of the left cheek region shows an isoechoic, heterogeneous, and ill-defined mass (**a**). US-guided FNA shows benign salivary gland acini (**b**) (**b**, MGG stain, high magnification)

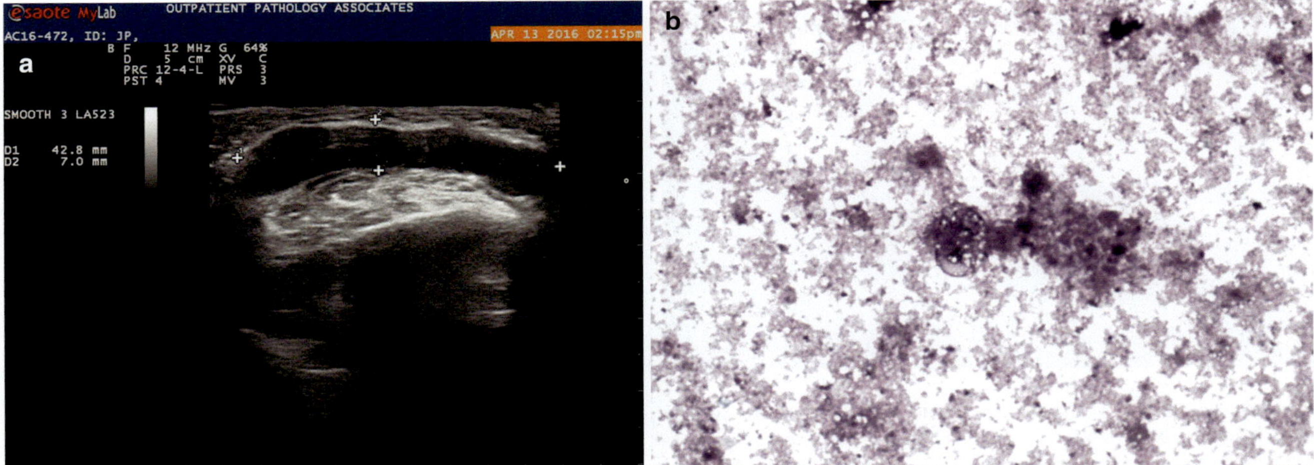

Fig. 5.5 Dilated Stensen's duct. An anechoic dilated duct with smooth and well-circumscribed borders were the US findings of a slightly palpable, serpiginous, and slightly fluctuant mass located medial to the parotid gland extending toward the lateral cheek (**a**). US-guided FNA yielded turbid whitish fluid; smears show scattered degenerated macrophages and a granular background (**b**) (**b**, Papanicolaou stain, high magnification)

Different from the parotid gland, the lymph nodes are around and not within the submandibular gland. The sublingual space contains the anterior hyoglossus muscle, the deep lobe of the submandibular gland, sublingual gland and ducts, submandibular duct, lingual artery and vein, lingual nerve, and cranial nerves IX and XII. The submandibular and sublingual glands are homogeneous and slightly hyperechoic relative to the adjacent musculature (Fig. 5.6). The Wharton's duct is not normally seen, only when dilated (Fig. 5.7a–c).

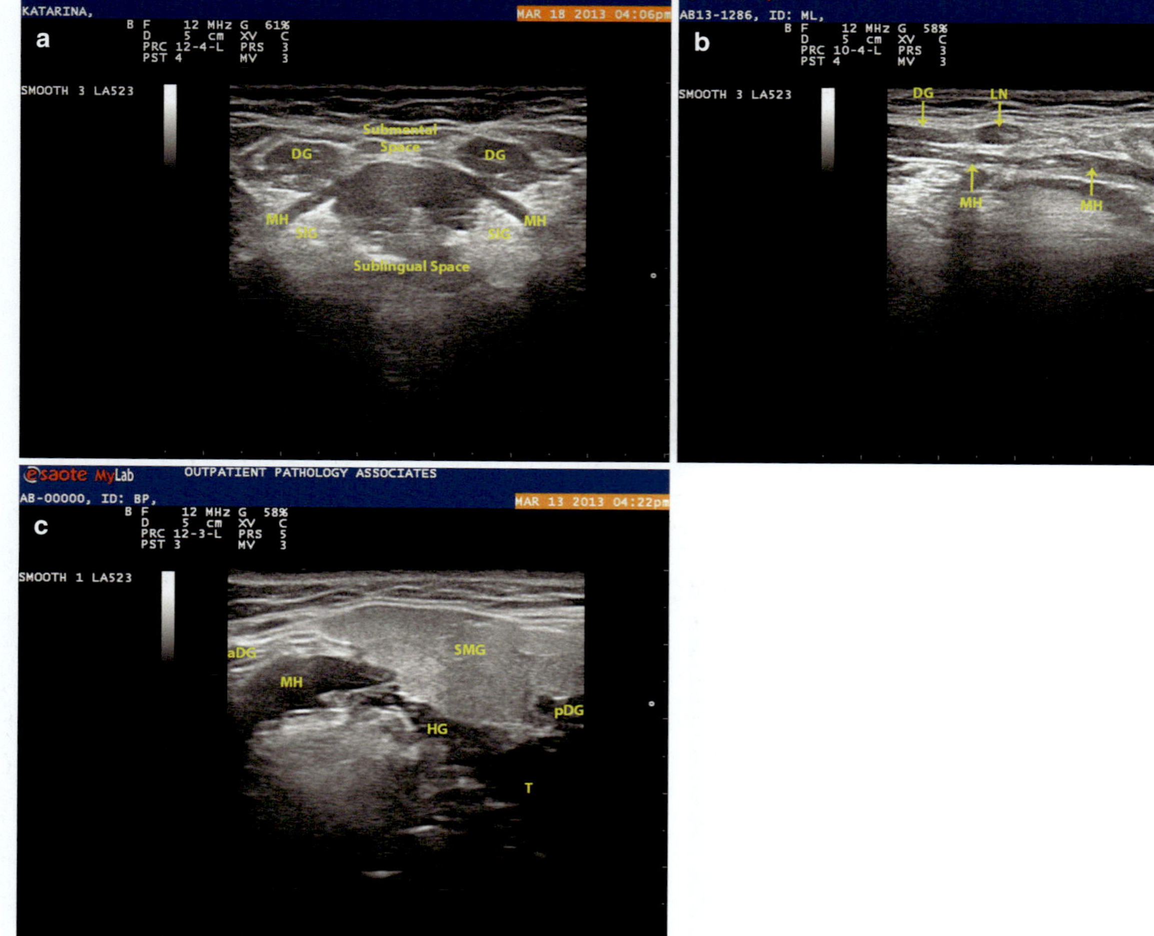

Fig. 5.6 Normal US of the submental and sublingual (a, transverse view; b, longitudinal view), and submandibular (**c**) gland spaces and the submandibular gland. *DG* digastric muscle, *MH* mylohyoid muscle, *SlG* sublingual gland, *LN* lymph node, *SmG* submandibular gland, *DGa* anterior belly digastric muscle, *DGp* posterior belly digastric muscle, *HG* hyoglossus muscle, *T* tonsil

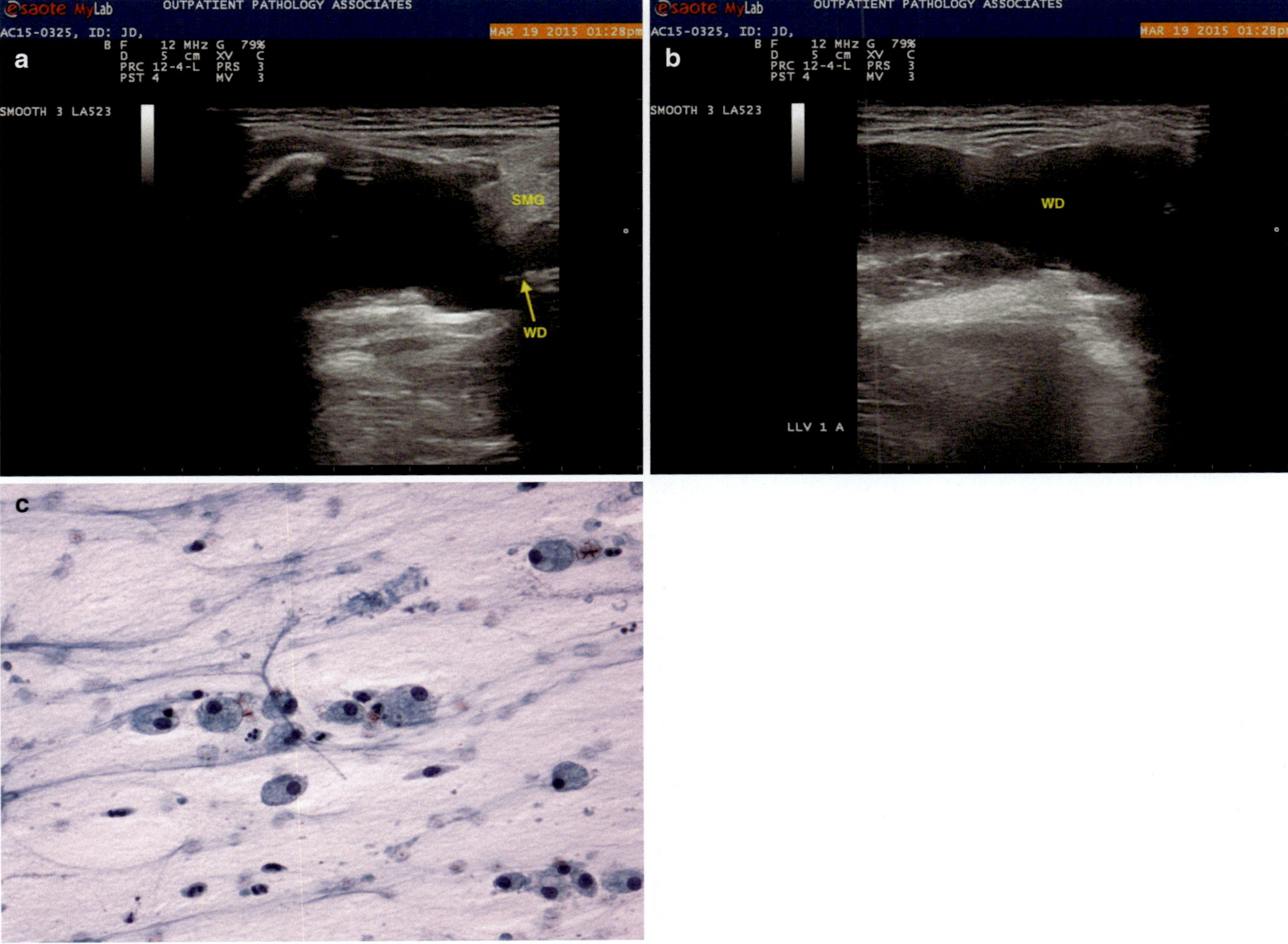

Fig. 5.7 Dilated Wharton's duct. An anechoic dilated duct extending from the left submandibular gland (**a**) toward the submental region (**b**) is seen by US. US-guided FNA smears show a proteinaceous fluid and macrophages (**c**) (**c**, Papanicolaou stain, high magnification). *SMG* submandibular gland, *WD* Wharton's duct

US and Salivary Gland Masses

US imaging alone is usually sufficient for the initial evaluation of most salivary gland masses. It can be easily performed in an outpatient clinic, is cost-effective, and frequently avoids more costly imaging studies. However, US has limitations, it cannot visualize the deep lobe of the parotid gland and the minor salivary glands. Thus, masses arising deep in the parotid gland, oral cavity, tracheobronchial tree, or pharynx cannot be evaluated by US. In cases of salivary gland malignancies, US cannot evaluate bone, perineural, or deep-soft-tissue involvement, or the retropharyngeal lymph nodes. Despite these limitations, US should be part of the initial clinical evaluation of any accessible salivary gland mass, particularly when it develops in the parotid, submandibular, or sublingual areas. Of note, 20% and 80% of masses clinically considered as being in the parotid or submandibular gland, respectively, are extra-glandular and reinforce the use of US. US characterizes a salivary gland mass, distinguishes focal from diffuse disease and solid from cystic masses, evaluates associated lymphadenopathy, and permits needle guidance and accurate sampling by fine-needle aspiration (USG-FNA). USG-FNA is the preferred diagnostic modality for any symptomatic or asymptomatic salivary gland mass.

Salivary glands should be evaluated in at least two perpendicular planes (sagittal and transverse) and the contralateral gland be scanned looking for bilateral masses or systemic processes that affect both glands. When there is a concern for malignancy, the neck lymph nodes should always be assessed in search for a related or unrelated disease.

US Features of Benign and Malignant Salivary Gland Masses

1. *Tumor edge.* Benign tumors and cysts have well-defined, regular, and smooth margins. Malignant tumors have irregular and ill-defined contours (Fig. 5.8).

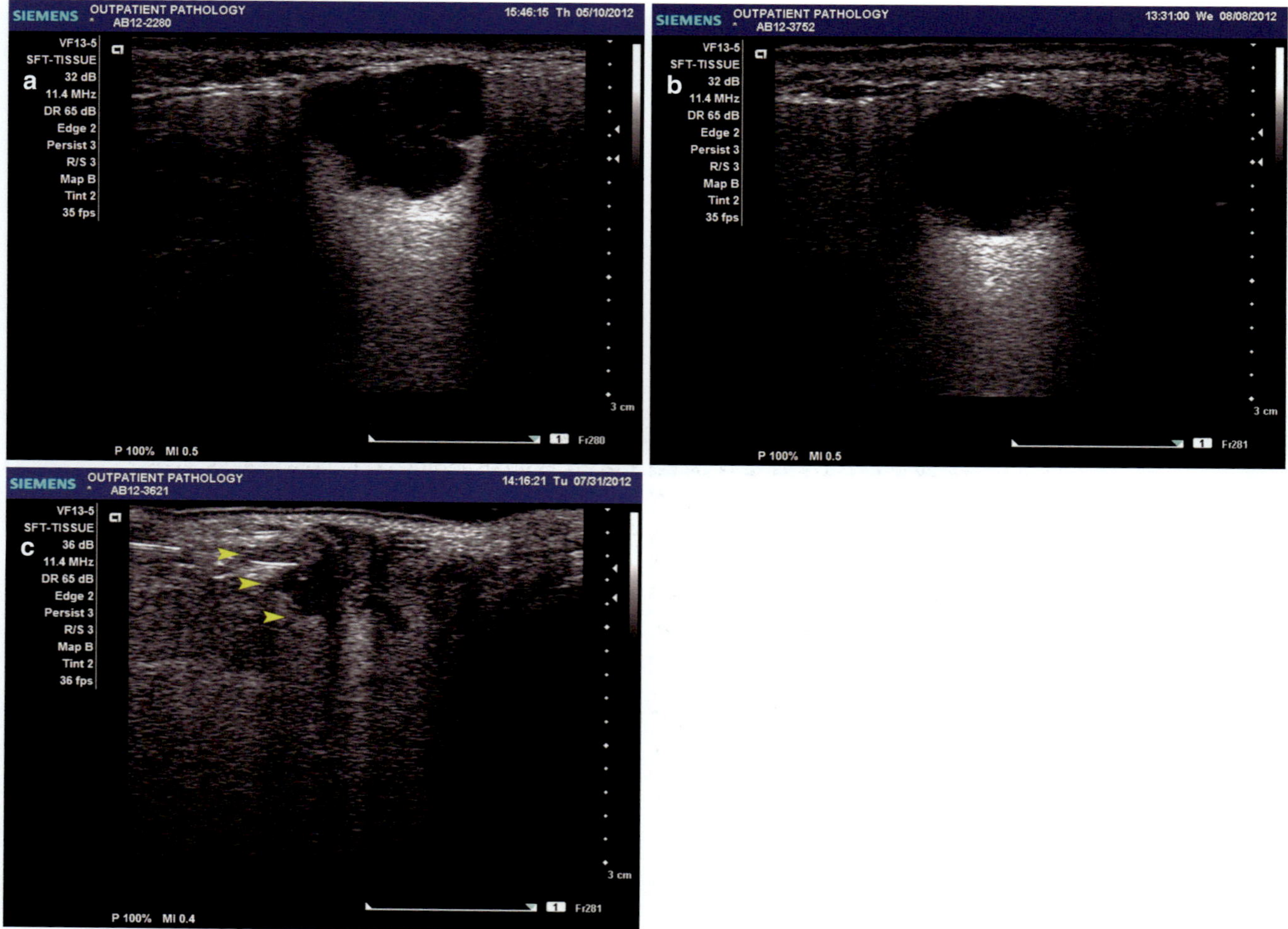

Fig. 5.8 Tumor edge. Smooth, well-defined, and lobulated borders are often seen in benign mixed tumors (**a**). Round and well-defined edges are seen in cystic lesions (**b**). Spiculated infiltrative borders (arrow heads) are seen in malignant tumors (**c**, adenoid cystic carcinoma)

2. *Internal architecture.* Cysts are anechoic and have posterior acoustic enhancement. Benign tumors have a homogeneous echotexture and may have posterior acoustic enhancement, as often seen in pleomorphic adenomas. Malignant tumors have heterogenous internal architecture and may have areas of necrosis and cystic change/hemorrhage in addition to irregular borders. However, benign tumors may have cystic change and complex internal architecture, i.e., Warthin's tumors or large pleomorphic adenomas. Calcification usually indicates a long-standing process and may have posterior acoustic shadowing, as seen in pleomorphic adenoma (Fig. 5.9).
3. *Tumor extent.* Extracapsular invasion into the surrounding tissue, including skeletal muscle, subcutaneous tissue, and skin may be seen, particularly in high-grade or long-standing malignant tumors (Fig. 5.10).
4. *Tumor vascularity.* Vascular blood flow is variable. Malignant tumors may show increased internal vascularity. Pleomorphic adenomas may have peripheral vascularity (Fig. 5.11).
5. *Lymphadenopathy.* An indirect sign of malignancy is the presence of cervical lymph nodes with abnormal US features in the region of lymphatic drainage.

The US distinction between benign and malignant salivary gland masses is not clear, and features overlap. Low-grade malignancies often share similar US features with benign tumors, and chronic inflammation with those of malignant tumors. Despite these limitations, US imaging helps to separate benign from malignant tumors with accuracy.

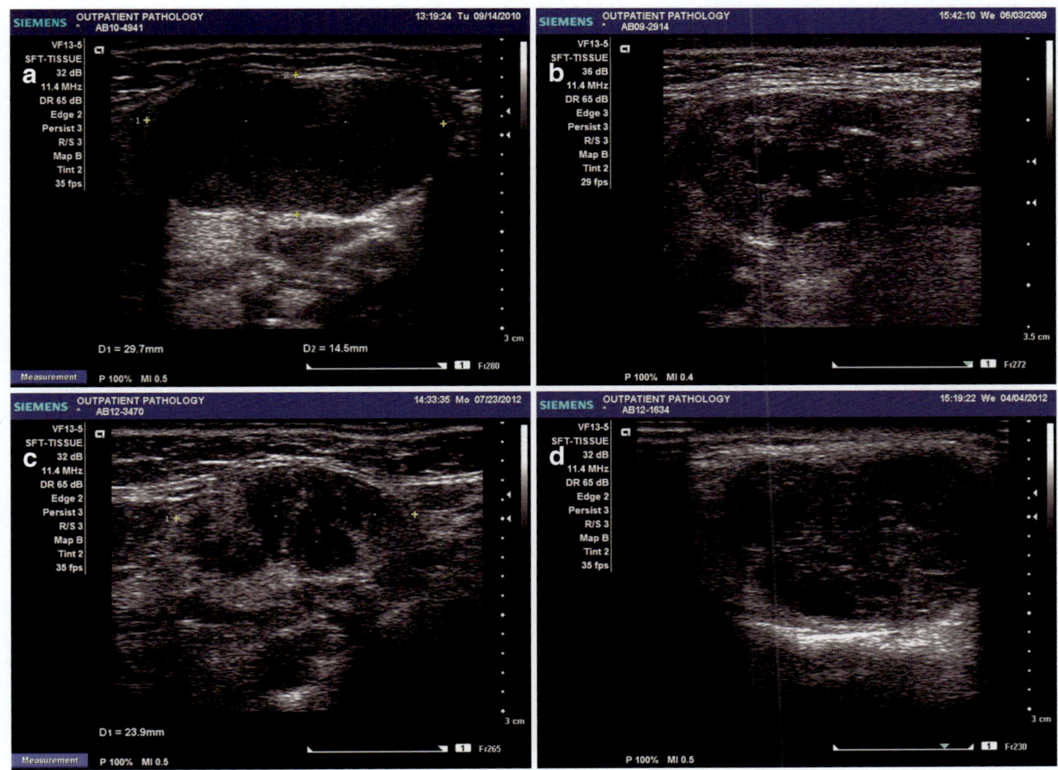

Fig. 5.9 Internal architecture. Homogeneous echo texture is commonly seen in monomorphic and pleomorphic adenomas (**a**, monomorphic adenoma). Heterogeneous echo texture may be seen in malignant tumors (**b**, mucoepidermoid carcinoma), chronic sialadenitis (**c**), and benign tumors (**d**, Warthin's tumor)

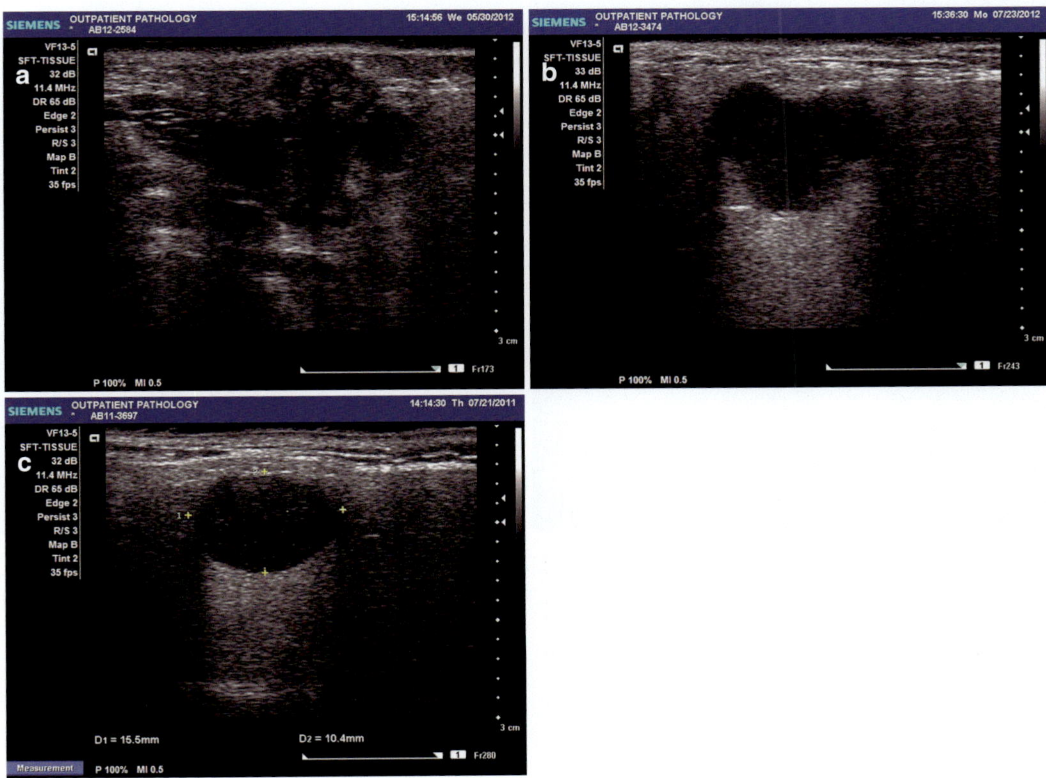

Fig. 5.10 Tumor extent. Malignant tumors show spiculated and fuzzy borders with infiltration into surrounding tissue (**a**, basal cell carcinoma). Smooth and distinct borders are commonly seen in benign conditions (**b**, monomorphic adenoma; **c**, Warthin's tumor)

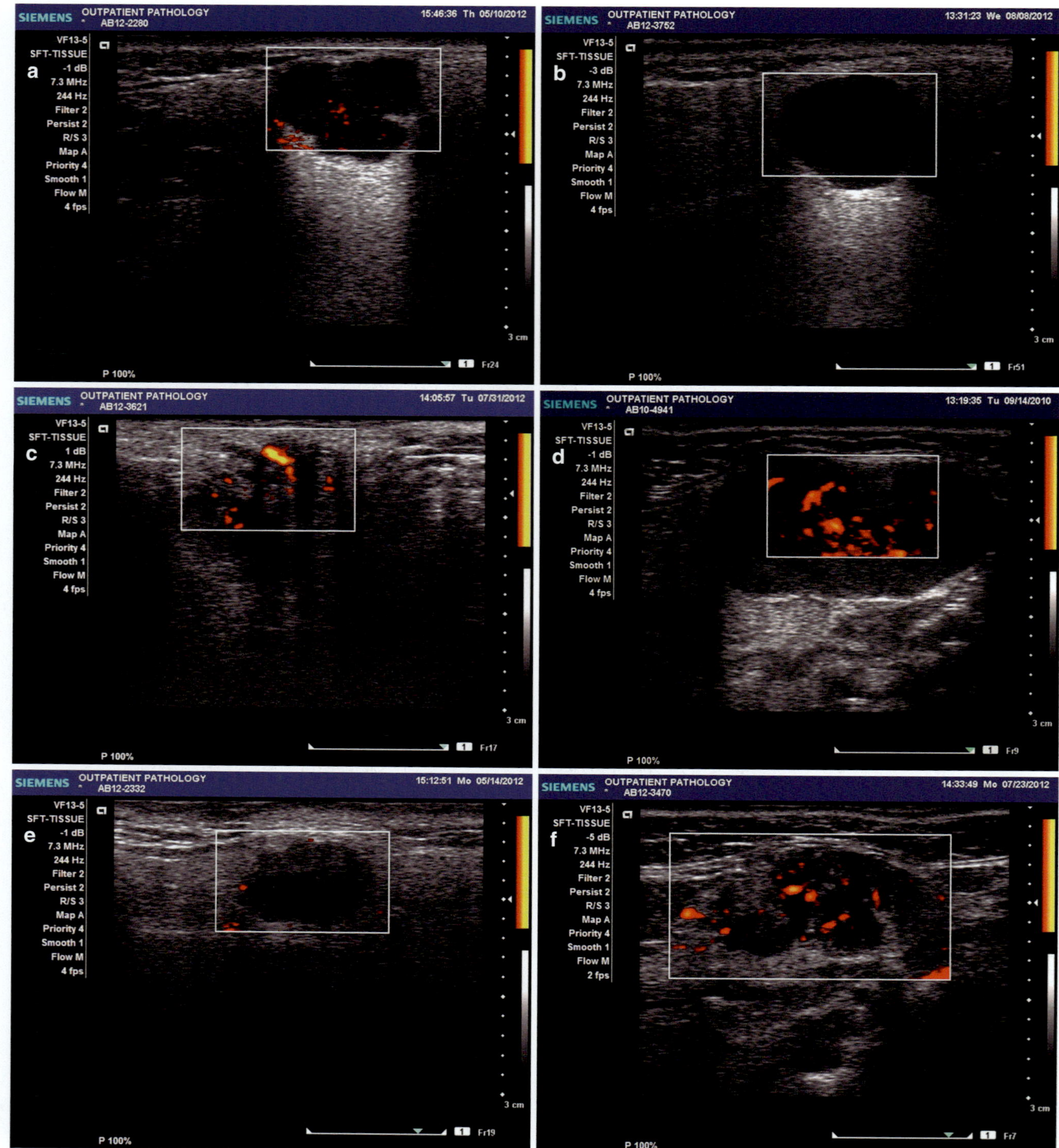

Fig. 5.11 Tumor vascularity. Vascularity is variable and usually high in high-grade tumors. However, Warthin's tumors commonly have high internal vascularity. The tumors shown correspond to those benign and malignant tumors and lesions listed in 5.8a–c (**a**, pleomorphic adenoma; **b**, cyst; **c**, adenoid cystic carcinoma), 5.9a–d (**d**, monomorphic adenoma; **e**, mucoepidermoid carcinoma; **f**, chronic sialadenitis; **g**, Warthin's tumor), and 5.10a–c (**h**, basal cell carcinoma; **i**, monomorphic adenoma; **j**, Warthin's tumor)

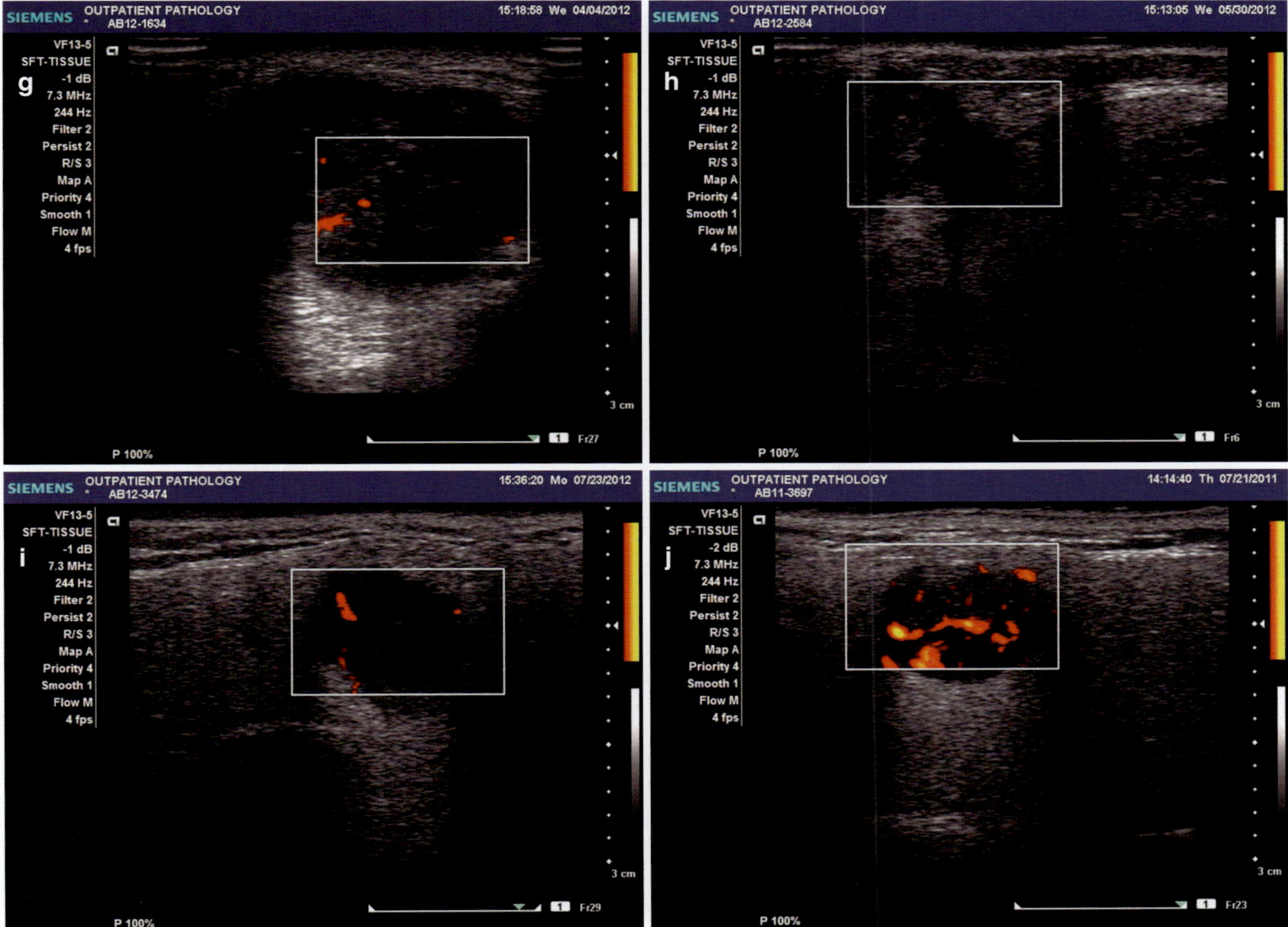

Fig. 5.11   (continued)

Classification of Salivary Gland Pathologies

Many changes in the histopathologic classification of salivary gland pathology have occurred during the last 50 years, essential for patient treatment and prognosis. The fifth edition of the World Health Organization classification from 2022 provides a clear classification with incorporation of new entities and reclassification of existing ones, with an emphasis on the genetic alterations, helpful to provide the landmarks for targeted anti-cancer therapies. Genomic alterations characterized in many salivary gland tumors have been shown to be tumor-type specific and have been included in the definition of mucoepidermoid carcinoma, adenoid cystic carcinoma, secretory carcinoma, polymorphous adenocarcinoma, hyalinizing clear cell carcinoma, mucinous adenocarcinoma, and microsecretory adenocarcinoma. Microsecretory adenocarcinoma and sclerosing microcystic adenocarcinoma as new malignant entities, and keratocystoma, intercalated duct adenoma, and striated duct adenoma as new benign neoplasms are included in this classification. The 39 salivary gland pathologies, divided into four categories: non-neoplastic epithelial lesions, malignant and benign epithelial tumors, and mesenchymal tumors are listed in Table 5.1. Many of these entities can be diagnosed by FNA cytology complemented with the use of cell block immunohistochemistry and material harvested for genetic and molecular studies.

Table 5.1 Salivary Gland Pathologies: 2022 WHO Classification and Main Genetic Findings

	Main genetic alteration and prevalence	IHC
Malignant epithelial tumor		
Adenoid cystic carcinoma	MYB fusion/activation 80% MYBL1 fusion/activation 10% NOTCH mutation ~14%	Myb NICD
Polymorphous adenocarcinoma		
Classic subtype	PRKD1 mutation 73%	
Cribriform subtype	PRKD1 fusion 38% PRKD3 fusion 19%	
Basal cell adenocarcinoma	CYLD mutation 29%	
Intraductal carcinoma		
Intercalated duct subtype	NCOA4-RET fusion 47%	
Apocrine subtype	PIK3CA and HRAS mutations, high	
Sebaceous adenocarcinoma	MSH2 loss 10%	
Mucinous adenocarcinoma	AKT1 E17K mutation 100% TP53 mutation 88%	
Sclerosing microcystic adenocarcinoma		
Microsecretory carcinoma	MEF2C-SS18 fusion >90%	
Salivary gland carcinoma NOS and emerging entities (poorly differentiated and oncocytic carcinoma)		
Epithelial-myoepithelial carcinoma	HRAS mutation 78%	HRAS
Myoepithelial carcinoma	PLAG fusion 38%	
Squamous cell carcinoma		
Salivary duct carcinoma	AR copy gain 35% HER2 amplification 31% TP53 mutation 56% PIK3CA and HRAS mutation 33% PTEN loss 38%	AR Her2
Carcinosarcoma		
Lymphoepithelial carcinoma		
Sialoblastoma		
Secretory carcinoma	ETV6-NTRK3 fusion >90%	Pan-Trk

(continued)

Table 5.1 (continued)

	Main genetic alteration and prevalence	IHC
Mucoepidermoid carcinoma	CRTC1-MAML2 fusion 40–90% CDKN2A deletion 25%	Areg[a]
Acinic cell carcinoma	NR4A3 fusion/activation 86%	NR4A3
Carcinoma ex pleomorphic adenoma	PLAG1 fusion/amplification 73% HMGA2 fusion/amplification 14% TP53 mutation 60%	Plag1
Hyalinizing clear cell carcinoma	EWSR1-ATF1 fusion 93%	
Benign epithelial tumor		
Pleomorphic adenoma	PLAG1 fusion/amplification >50% HMGA2 fusion/amplification ~15%	Plag1 Hmga2
Myoepithelioma	PLAG1 fusion ~40%	
Basal cell adenoma	CTNNB1 mutation 37–80% AXION1 mutation ~36%	b-catenin LEF-1
Warthin's tumor		
Oncocytoma		
Sebaceous adenoma		
Ductal papilloma		
Sialadenoma papilliferum	BRAFV600E mutation 50–100%	
Cystadenoma		
Lymphadenoma		
Canalicular adenoma		
Sclerosing polycystic adenoma		
Keratocystoma		
Intercalated duct adenoma		
Striated duct adenoma		
Other salivary gland entities		
Sialolipoma		
Nodular oncocytic adenosis		
Lymphoepithelial sialadenitis		

WHO World Health Organization, *IHC* immunohistochemistry

Modified from Żurek, M., Fus, Ł., Niemczyk, K. et al. (2023) Salivary gland pathologies: evolution in classification and association with unique genetic alterations. <u>Eur Arch Otorhinolaryngol</u> **280**, 4739–4750. https://doi.org/10.1007/s00405-023-08110-w

[a]Areg (amphiregulin) is an epidermal growth factor receptor and has been shown to be the downstream target of CRTC1-MAML2 fusion

Ultrasound-Guided FNA of Salivary Gland Masses

From the clinical perspective, it is relevant to remember that masses often develop in the parotid, submandibular, sublingual, and minor salivary glands in decreasing order. They may be present in heterotopic salivary gland tissue in various sites of the head and neck, including along Stensen's duct, and most are malignant, with mucoepidermoid carcinoma being the most common. Patient age is relevant because benign mixed tumor and Warthin's tumor occur in adulthood and mucoepidermoid carcinoma is the most common salivary gland tumor in children. Local pain, facial nerve damage, and signs of local tumor invasion often indicate malignancy, but their absence does not exclude such a diagnosis.

Masses affecting the salivary glands may be broadly classified as infectious/inflammatory, non-neoplastic, and neoplastic with a vast resulting number of mass lesions. Superimposed alterations such as degeneration, chronic inflammation, cystic change, or metaplasia of various types add challenges to the already at times difficult pathologic diagnosis.

We agree with Stanley MW et al., that a practical approach to interpreting FNA material based on a pattern diagnosis recognition based on first-impression key findings will result in a narrow differential diagnosis for that particular pattern. We will adopt this approach to discuss common salivary gland masses. Briefly, the salivary gland patterns include (1) normal, (2) inflammatory/infectious, (3) pleomorphic adenoma, (4) Warthin's tumor, (5) cystic, (6) small epithelial cells, (7) large epithelial cells, and (8) spindle cells. Benign mixed tumor and Warthin's tumor are included not only because they are common, but also for their occasional diagnostic difficulties in differentiating them from other tumors. The most common salivary gland masses will be covered in this fashion, and the rare entities will be mentioned briefly.

The USG-FNA in our outpatient clinic is performed with a 25-gauge needle without suction (Zajdela technique), as mentioned in the aspiration procedure section, early in this book. If the material obtained is limited, the use of an aspiration device may be indicated for applying moderate suction (3–4 mL of negative pressure). Rapid on-site evaluation (ROSE) is recommended to assess adequacy of the sample and need to harvest additional cellular material. USG-FNA with a 23-gauge applying moderate suction may be used for obtaining a bloody specimen, which is useful for preparation of a cell block for histologic evaluation and for ancillary tests including flow cytometry, immunohistochemistry, and molecular studies; salivary gland tumors have significant and highly prevalent translocations. USG-FNA has 87%, 98%, and 95% sensitivity, specificity, and accuracy, respectively, in the evaluation of salivary gland masses. USG-core needle biopsy (CNB) may be considered in rare, selected cases, solely when USG-FNA is non-diagnostic and the patient's risk for surgery is high. Facial nerve injury is a potential complication of CNB.

Air-dried and 95% ethanol-fixed preparations for Romanowsky (highlights extracellular matrix, mucin, and cytoplasmic detail including vacuolization) and Papanicolaou (or hematoxylin-eosin, highlights nuclear details) stains, respectively, are complementary and should be used in the cytologic evaluation of salivary gland samples.

The final cytopathology report should be issued using the Milan System for Reporting Salivary gland Cytopathology (MSRSGC) as published in the 2023 second edition (Tables 5.2 and 5.3).

The cytopathology report should include (1) satisfactoriness of the specimen, (2) one of the general diagnostic cate-

Table 5.2 The Milan System for Reporting Salivary gland Cytopathology (MSRSGC): diagnostic categories, definitions, and explanatory notes

Diagnostic category and definitions	Explanatory notes
I. Non-diagnostic Insufficient for cytologic diagnosis	Exceptions: cyst contents with crystals, matrix material, and mucinous cyst contents
II. Non-neoplastic Chronic sialadenitis, reactive lymph node, inflammation/infection	Inflammatory, metaplastic, and reactive changes, and infectious processes Flow cytometry is recommended in a reactive lymphoid cell pattern if clinically indicated
III. Atypia of Undetermined Significance (AUS) Atypia indefinite for a neoplasm	Most cases represent reactive cellular changes or a poorly sampled mass
IV. Neoplasm	
A. Benign Diagnosed based on established cytologic criteria	Classic examples include benign mixed tumor (pleomorphic adenoma), Warthin's tumor, etc.
B. Salivary Gland Neoplasm of Uncertain Malignant Potential (SUMP) Neoplasm but a specific diagnosis cannot be made	Most cases include benign cellular neoplasms, neoplasms with atypical features, and low-grade carcinomas
V. Suspicious for malignancy Suggestive but not unequivocal for malignancy	Provide a differential diagnosis and specify which type of malignant tumor is suspected Most cases are high-grade carcinomas
VI. Malignant Diagnostic of malignancy	Give a specific diagnosis (e.g., lymphoma, sarcoma, metastases). Attempt to provide the type and grade of carcinoma (i.e., low-grade mucoepidermoid carcinoma, high-grade salivary duct carcinoma)

Modified from Faquin WC, Rossi ED. The Milan System for Reporting Salivary Gland Cytopathology, 2nd. Ed 2023 Springer Nature Switzerland AG

Table 5.3 The Milan System for Reporting Salivary gland Cytopathology (MSRSGC): implied risk of malignancy and recommended clinical management

Diagnostic category	ROM (%)	Management
I. Non-diagnostic	15	Clinical and radiologic correlation. Repeat FNA
II. Non-neoplastic	11	Clinical follow-up and radiologic correlation.
III. AUS	30	Repeat FNA or surgery
IV. Neoplasm		
IVA. Benign	<3	Clinical follow-up or surgery
IVB. SUMP	35	Surgery
V. Suspicious	83	Surgery
VI. Malignant	98	Surgery

FNA fine needle aspiration, *ROM* risk of malignancy, *AUS* atypia of undetermined significance, *SUMP* salivary gland neoplasm of uncertain malignant potential
Modified from Faquin WC, Rossi ED. The Milan System for Reporting Salivary Gland Cytopathology, 2nd. Ed 2023 Springer Nature Switzerland AG

gories, (3) associated risk of malignancy (ROM), and (4) a specific diagnosis. The inclusion of the ROM is optional and left at the discretion of the cytopathologist. If a specific diagnosis cannot be made, a comment on the reason and a differential diagnosis based on clinical, imaging studies, and cytologic findings should be included.

FNA Findings of Salivary Gland Lesions and Tumors

Pattern I. Normal Salivary Gland Pattern

This pattern may be present in up to 20% of salivary gland FNAs in some series. Cytologic smears are cellular and show predominantly acinar and less common ductal elements as well as variable amounts of adipose tissue. Acinar elements are arranged in small, round aggregates of cells with large granulovacuolar cytoplasm, eccentric round nuclei, and small inconspicuous nucleoli. Acinar cells have a fragile cytoplasm; as a result, the smear background is granular and exhibits variable numbers of stripped nuclei that need to be distinguished from lymphocytes, which have a scant rim of basophilic cytoplasm. The ductal elements may be branching and show tubular structures and cell sheets with honeycomb architecture (Fig. 5.12a, b).

Sialosis

Sialosis or sialadenosis is a non-neoplastic, asymptomatic salivary gland enlargement that affects principally the parotid gland and less commonly the submandibular gland. It is the result of acinar hypertrophy and is usually bilateral. A related underlying cause is usually identified, i.e., diabetes mellitus, malnutrition, alcoholism, cirrhosis, obesity, hypothyroidism, HIV, drugs, etc.; however, it may be idiopathic. FNA smears show a normal salivary gland pattern (Fig. 5.12a, b, f). It has been suggested that the cellular yield is greater than that of normal gland, and acinar cells are 20% larger than normal cells, features that are difficult to evaluate even in a high-quality FNA smear. The aspirates may contain variable amounts of adipose tissue, but they are devoid of inflammatory cells. The differential diagnosis includes failure to sample the target and, depending on the amount of adipose tissue present, a lipoma or a lipomatous salivary gland should be considered, all of which require clinical correlation, including imaging studies. The diagnostic accuracy is improved when the cytopathologist performs USG-FNA to reduce the sampling error.

US features: There is bilateral gland enlargement with normal echogenicity (hyperechoic in comparison to adjacent musculature) and no focal lesions or increased blood flow; however, the glands may be brightly hyperechoic due to fat infiltration. The features are non-specific (Fig. 5.12c–e).

Pattern II. Inflammatory/Infectious Pattern and Similar Processes

Acute Inflammation

Acute inflammatory processes most commonly affect the parotid gland but are rarely subject to FNA. Viral sialadenitis (e.g., mumps, cytomegalovirus) is usually bilateral and is more common in children. Bacterial sialadenitis is usually unilateral, occurs at any age, and is commonly associated with poor oral hygiene, oral neoplasms, or systemic processes. Suspicion of an associated neoplastic process, abscess formation that needs drainage, a poor response to antibiotic therapy, or a clinically suspected infectious process in a setting of immunosuppression may prompt an FNA, best if done under US guidance. The FNA smear pattern is purulent and shows neutrophils, fibrin strands, and variable numbers of acinar and ductal cells, which may have marked reactive changes (Fig. 5.13a–c). Granulation tissue and squamous metaplasia may be identified in later stages (Fig. 5.13d, e). The most common agents are bacterial organisms, e.g., *Staphylococcus aureus* or *Streptococcus sp.* and FNA material must be submitted for cultures. High-grade malignant neoplasms, either primary or secondary may show a background of neutrophils and necrosis. Caution should be exercised in diagnosing malignancy, particularly of low grade, in the presence of acute inflammation. A residual mass present after the inflammation is controlled should be sampled by USG-FNA to rule-out a neoplasm.

US features: The enlarged gland is hypoechogenic with a heterogenous pattern due to duct and cyst dilatation and microabscess formation (Fig. 5.13f). The gland is hypervas-

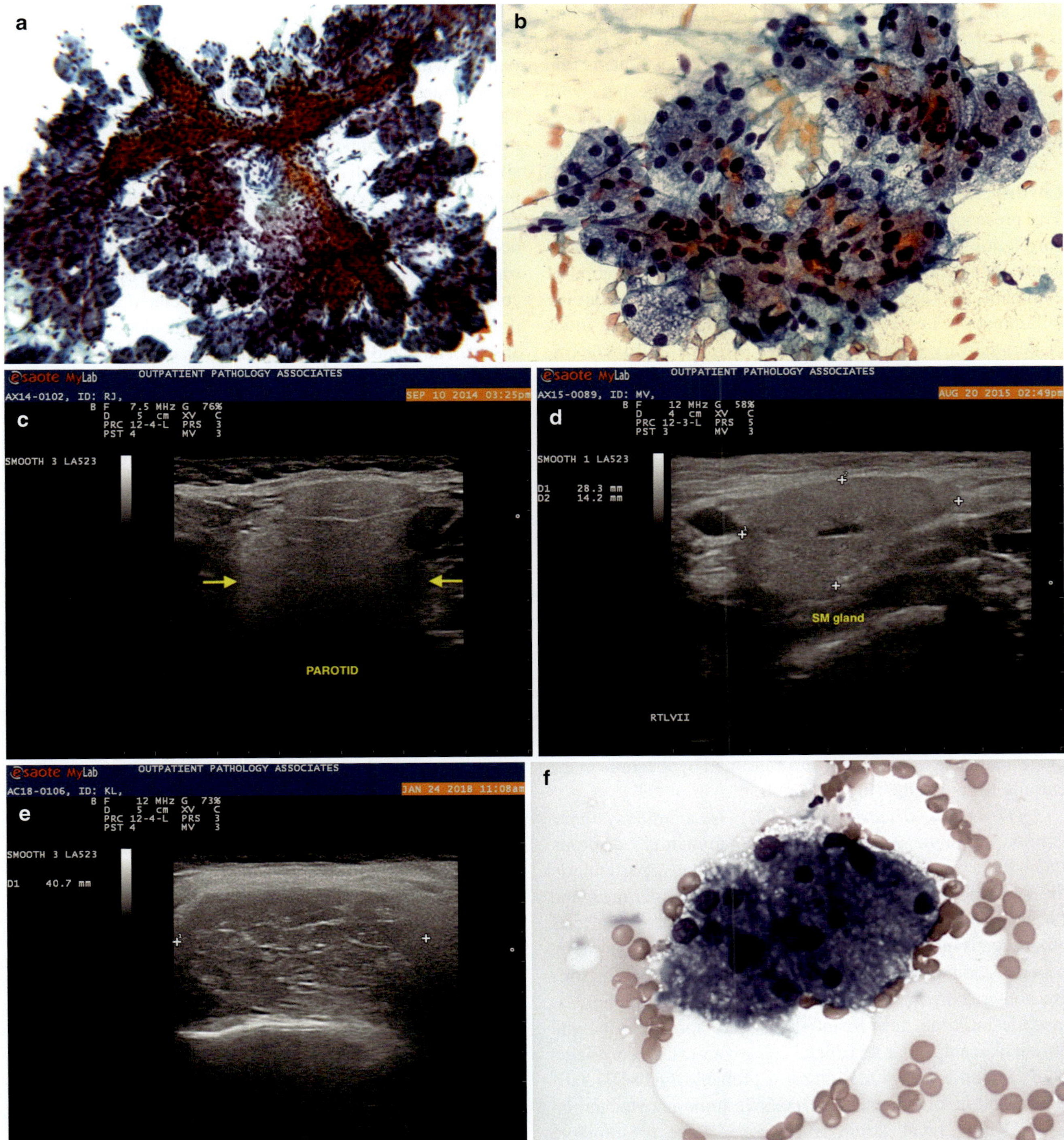

Fig. 5.12 Normal salivary gland cytology showing cohesive branching ducts and acini (**a**, **b**). US imaging of the left parotid (**a**, arrows) and right submandibular (**b**) gland enlargement (sialosis) in a patient with type II Diabetes mellitus show both glands with diffuse homogeneous echo texture and no hyper- or hypoechoic masses. There is a slight hyperechogenicity in the parotid gland compared with the submandibular gland (**c**, **d**). Thin hyperechogenic lines are seen in the US images in adipose tissue infiltration that may be present in sialosis (**e**). Cytology shows benign acini with adipose tissue metaplasia surrounded by lipid vacuoles (**f**). (**a**, **b** Papanicolaou stain, low and high magnification; **e**, MGG stain, high magnification)

cular, and intraparotid gland and regional lymphadenopathy is often present. A hypoechoic, ill-defined mass may be seen in early abscess formation (Fig. 5.13g); when liquefaction occurs, the mass becomes well-defined and anechoic with distinct or ill-defined borders and posterior acoustic enhancement (Fig. 5.13h).

Chronic Inflammatory Processes

The presence of chronic inflammatory cells needs clinical correlation because the majority of masses with this pattern represent salivary gland tumors with scant representation of epithelial cells and various degrees of non-specific chronic inflammation, i.e., Warthin's tumor or, in some cases, intra- or peri-salivary gland lymph nodes (Fig. 5.14a, b). On US, the gland is of normal size or small, heterogeneous, and hypoechoic with multiple round hypoechoic foci representing ectatic ducts. In general, the heterogeneity and hypoechogenicity of the glandular tissue is more prominent as the disease progresses. The vascularity of the glandular tissue is variably increased; however, branching blood vessels and calcification may be present (Fig. 5.14c–f).

Postradiation sialadenitis produces a firm nodular and often tender salivary gland with fibrosis, acinar atrophy, and preservation of the ductal epithelial system. Smears are sparsely cellular and show fibrosis, chronic inflammatory cells, and epithelial and stromal elements with variable cytologic atypia that may pose difficulty in distinguishing this from a neoplastic process (Fig. 5.15a, b). The clinical history helps in the distinction. The gland is enlarged and hypoechoic in the acute phase, and small, atrophic, and hypoechoic in the chronic fibrous stage (Fig. 5.15c, d).

IgG4-related disease (IgG4-RD) is a multisystemic chronic immune mediated fibroinflammatory disorder. IgG4-RD commonly involves salivary glands, particularly the submandibular gland of middle-aged and older men, and can present as a firm mass simulating a neoplasm. It affects other organs including, thyroid, lymph nodes, biliary system, pancreas, and retroperitoneum among others. Smear findings are non-specific and include sparse cellularity, lymphoplasmacytic infiltrate, few eosinophiles, rare spindle cells, and absent or scant acinar and ductal cells that must be correlated with clinical findings to suggest a probable IgG4-RD salivary gland involvement. IgG4-positive immunocytochemistry and high IgG4 serum levels support the presumptive diagnosis that must be proven histologically. Serum IgG4 levels are elevated with a cutoff level of >135 mg/dL to be a reliable marker predictive of IgG4-RD. IgG4-positive salivary gland lymphoplasmacytic infiltrate can be associated with autoimmune disorders and primary or metastatic malignancies. US findings are non-specific. Salivary glands are enlarged, hypoechoic, heterogeneous, with mottled appearance, multiple small foci, and smooth or ill-defined borders.

Benign lymphoepithelial lesions (lymphoepithelial sialadenitis) present as bilateral salivary gland enlargement in patients with Miculicz's disease or Sjögren's syndrome. This autoimmune disease is more common in women and often involves the parotid gland. Smears show a polymorphous population of lymphoid cells, rare or absent acinar cells, rare sheets of ductal cells with reactive changes, and epimyoepithelial islands or groups of myoepithelial cells, which may be inconspicuous (Fig. 5.16a, b). Clinical correlation is needed for consideration or support of the diagnosis. In contrast to the AIDS-related lymphoepithelial cyst, the cystic component seen in the autoimmune-related lesion is not prominent, and the normal salivary elements are almost absent. The gland is enlarged and shows normal echogenicity in the early stages. A gland with heterogeneous echotexture and multiple round hypoechoic areas without posterior acoustic enhancement, or even cysts with classic US features of cysts is seen in late stages (Fig. 5.16c, d). The incidence of lymphoma and primary parotid gland neoplasms is greatly increased in patients with Sjögren's syndrome.

Lymphomas

The lymphomas rarely affect the salivary glands (Fig. 5.17a–c); more often is the involvement of the parotid or submandibular space lymph nodes (Fig. 5.17d). The immunophenotype of NHL as determined by flow cytometry is helpful for the diagnosis in these cases. Hodgkin lymphoma rarely involves the salivary glands, and if diagnostic Hodgkin and / or Reed-Sternberg cells are not identified, these cases may be diagnosed as inflammatory process or reactive lymphoid hyperplasia. NHL of low grade may be confused with reactive processes and vice versa. Occasionally, NHL of high grade, although often recognized as malignant may be confused with poorly differentiated carcinoma or even small-cell carcinoma.

US features: Lymphomatous deposits are markedly hypoechoic and may show through acoustic transmission with posterior acoustic enhancement, the so-called "pseudocystic" appearance. Multiple coalescent lymph nodes may be seen within and outside the parotid gland. The vascular pattern is variable (Fig. 5.17e–h).

Granulomatous Processes

This pattern may be seen as a part of infectious, nonneoplastic, and neoplastic processes. Sarcoidosis, a commonly non-necrotizing granulomatous process, may involve salivary glands or intragland lymph nodes (Fig. 5.18a, b). Necrotizing granulomatous inflammation, as in other body sites, is commonly associated with mycobacterial and fungal infections. Clinical correlation including cultures for organisms is always important. Of note, FNA material is perfectly suitable for ancillary studies, including cultures.

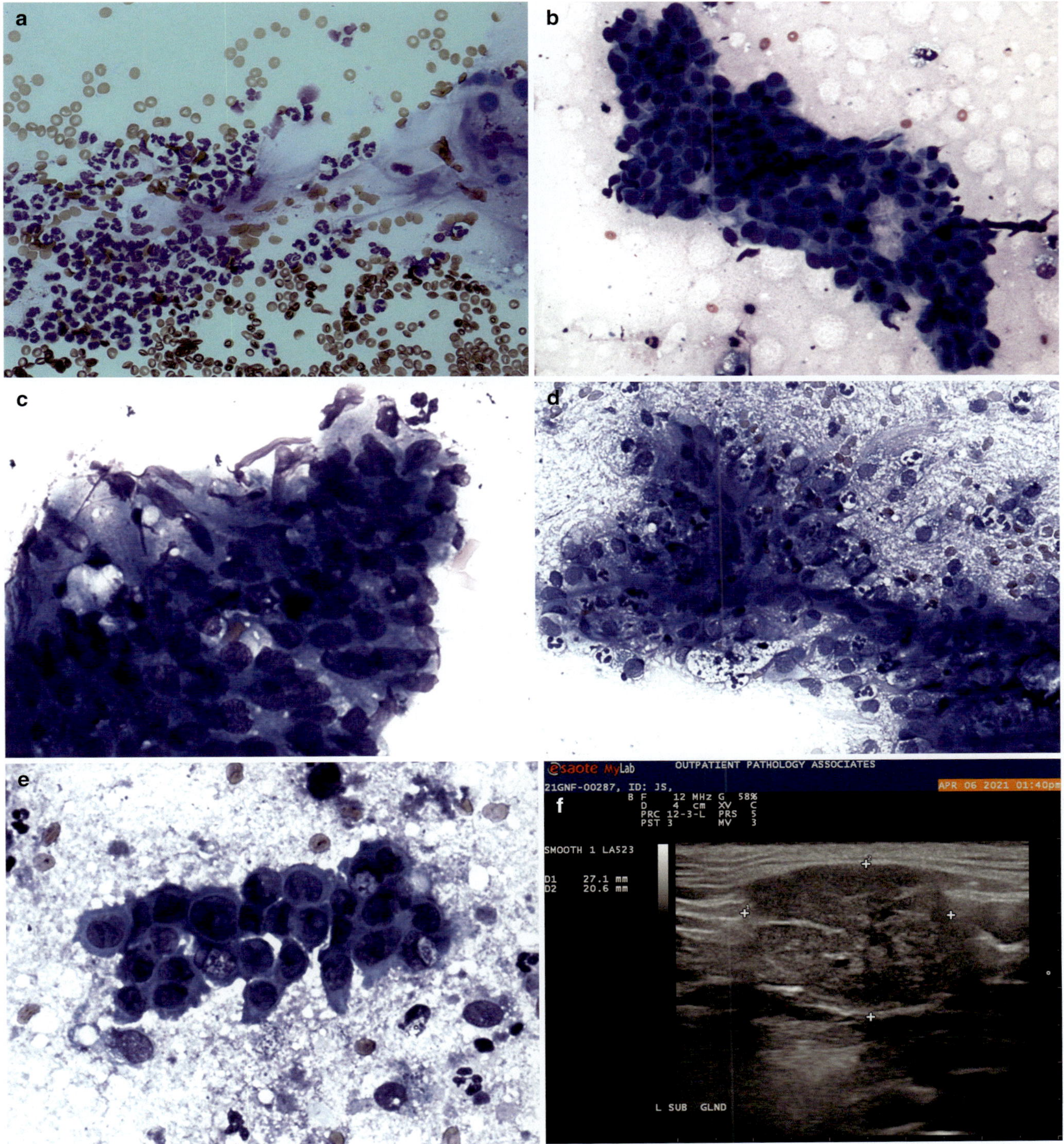

Fig. 5.13 Parotid abscess. These patients had an episode of acute sialadenitis and developed an abscess after antibiotic therapy. A purulent pattern (**a**) and rare sheets of ductal cells with squamous metaplasia (**b**) are seen. Reactive inflammatory changes (**c**), early granulation tissue (**d**), and more prominent squamous metaplasia that may be interpreted as atypia of unknown significance (**e**) may be seen in a later phase of acute inflammation. US imaging shows heterogeneity, slightly irregular hypo- or anechoic lesions with posterior acoustic enhancement, and variable vascularity (**f**–**h**). (**a**, **b**, **d**, MGG stain, medium magnification; **c**, **e**, MGG stain, high magnification)

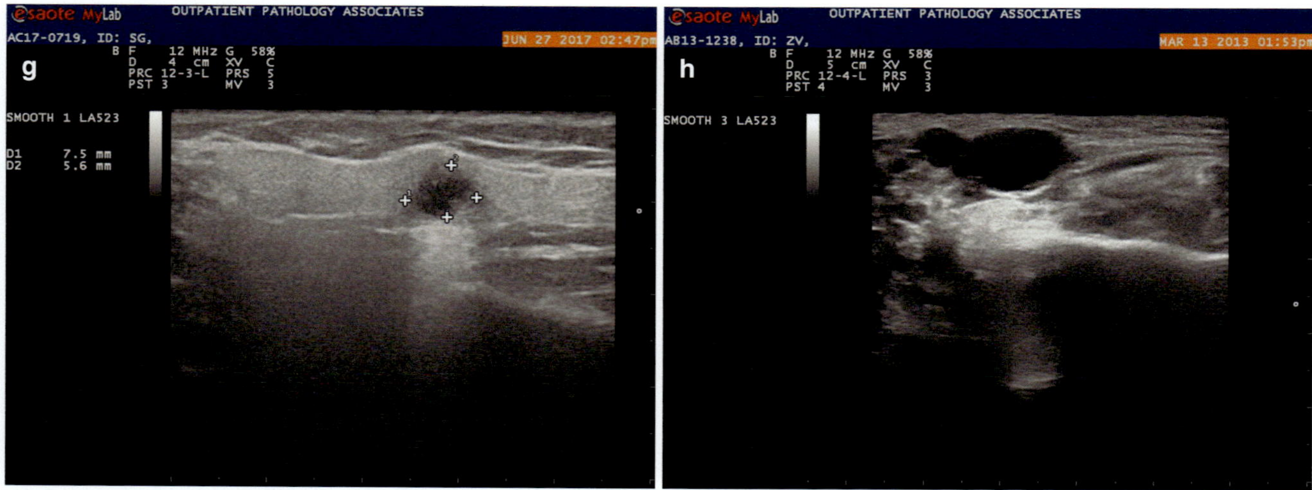

Fig. 5.13 (continued)

US features: The findings are non-specific and may show a normal or enlarged gland with diffuse hypoechogenicity or heterogeneous echotexture and lobulated gland borders. Vascularity may be increased in some granulomatous processes, such as sarcoidosis (Fig. 5.18c, d).

Pattern III. Pleomorphic Adenoma (Benign Mixed Tumor), Variants, and Similar Processes

Pleomorphic Adenoma

Pleomorphic adenoma or benign mixed tumor is composed of epithelial and stromal elements. Some tumors are cellular, and others exhibit various architectural patterns that may challenge the diagnosis. Complete surgical excision with preservation of the facial nerve is the treatment of choice. Local recurrence is rare and is often the result of incomplete resection or "spillage" of myxochondroid matrix. Complications include malignant transformation, particularly in large and long-standing tumors.

Clinical Findings Pleomorphic adenoma is the most common tumor of the salivary glands and occurs predominantly in the tail of the parotid gland. It is rare in the sublingual glands. It is the most frequent tumor of the parapharyngeal space, followed by peripheral nerve sheath tumors. It has a slight female predominance, with variable age presentation, usually occurring in adults and the elderly. Familial occurrence is rare. Bilateral or multiple tumors are uncommon. Tumors are slowly growing over years, and except for compressive mechanical symptoms, patients are almost always asymptomatic. Tumors are firm, well-circumscribed, with regular and lobulated borders, and of variable size.

Histopathology All tumors have a capsule of variable thickness and may be non-visible, particularly in cases with abundant myxoid matrix.

Typical pleomorphic adenomas have a mixture of ductal epithelial, myoepithelial, and stromal elements. The epithelial component may show variable architectural patterns including trabecular, papillary, tubular, solid or cystic, even within the same tumor. The islands and tubules have an inner layer of cuboidal/columnar/flattened epithelial cells and outer myoepithelial cell layer(s). The stromal component is myxoid, chondroid, or fibro-osseous alone or mixed (Fig. 5.19a, b). Crystalloids may also be present in the background. Squamous elements in the form of pearls or squamous cells as well as mucous cells, clear cells, spindle cells, plasmacytoid cells, sebaceous cells, oncocytic cells, calcification, and adipose tissue may be seen. Degenerative changes may be seen spontaneously or after FNA and include squamous metaplasia, reactive cellular changes, necrosis, and infarction.

Cellular pleomorphic adenomas may be rich in epithelial or myoepithelial cells, but every case shows the typical component described above, although it may be limited. There may be large atypical cells and rare non-atypical mitoses; as long as these features are focally present, they do not signify malignancy.

Most tumors are diagnosed without difficulty; however, those with a predominant cellular epithelial or myoepithelial component or those with variable architectural patterns must be recognized and distinguished from other tumors such as polymorphous adenocarcinoma when involving minor salivary glands or adenoid cystic carcinoma in the major salivary glands. Pleomorphic adenomas with predominant rich myxoid stroma must be distinguished from mesenchymal tumors,

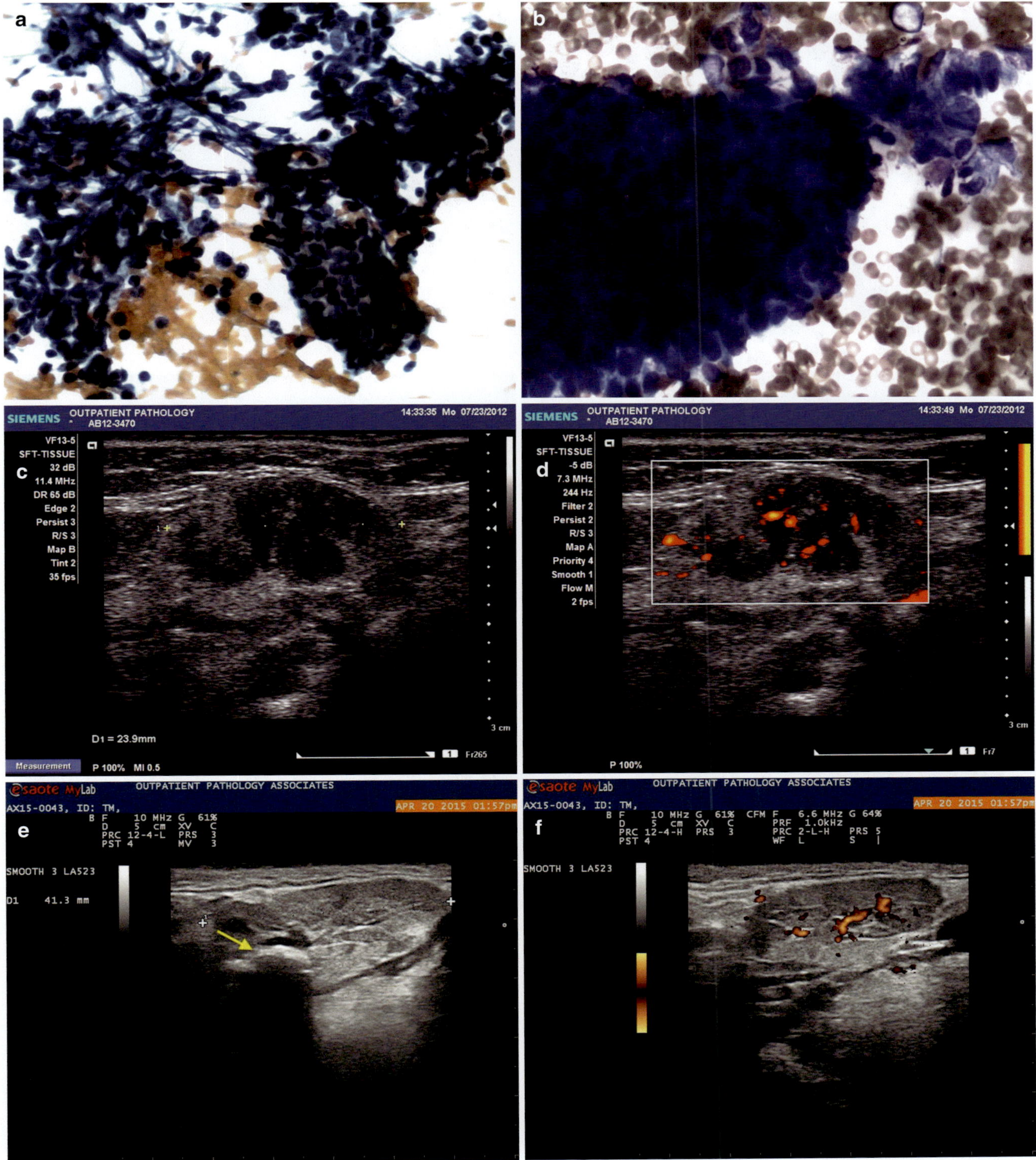

Fig. 5.14 Chronic sialadenitis. Chronic inflammatory cells, predominantly entangled with benign salivary gland elements (**a**) and reactive aggregates of ductal cells with squamous metaplasia (**b**). Ultrasound shows a complex mass with anechoic foci, septae of slightly hyperechoic bands, and mild internal blood flow by Doppler examination (**c**, **d**). A different case shows a submandibular gland with heterogeneous echotexture, macrocalcification (**e**, arrow) with posterior acoustic shadowing, and prominent vascular blood flow with branching vessels by Doppler exam (**f**). **a**, **b**, MGG stain, medium and high magnification

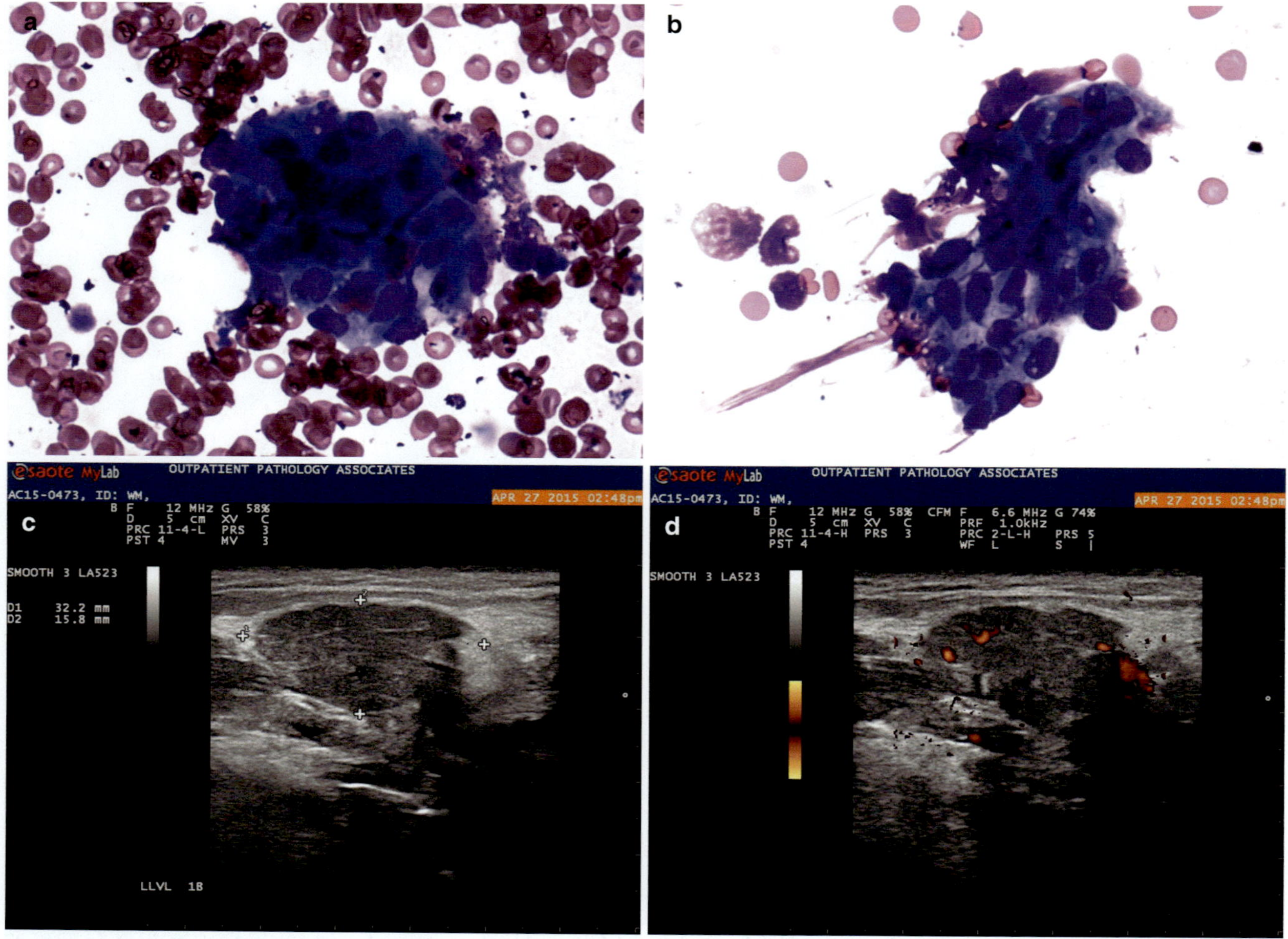

Fig. 5.15 Postradiation sialadenitis. Variable cytologic atypia is present (**a, b**). US imaging shows an enlarged hypoechoic gland, slight heterogeneous echotexture, and internal vascular blood flow (**c, d**). (**a, b**, MGG stain, high magnification)

including but not limited to myxoid lipoma, myxoid neurofibroma, and myxoma.

Immuno-Profile Epithelial cells show keratin, CEA, and EMA positivity. Myoepithelial cells are positive for calponin, p63, p40, actin, vimentin, SOX10, CD117, PLAG1 (Fig. 5.19c), HAMG2, LEF1, S100 protein, CD10, glial fibrillary acid protein, and keratin, but are CEA- and EMA-negative. Podoplanin, a myoepithelial cell marker, has been shown to be positive on the cell border and in the external periphery of the cells in pleomorphic adenoma and other salivary gland tumors with myoepithelial differentiation. Myoepithelioma and myoepithelial carcinoma are positive for PLAG1. Carcinoma ex-pleomorphic adenoma is positive for PLAG1 and HAMG2.

Molecular Profile Most pleomorphic adenomas have karyotypic abnormalities including 8q12 rearrangements, 12q14–15 rearrangements, or sporadic clonal changes. The 8q12 and the 12q14–15 abnormalities activate the target genes *PLAG1* and *HMGA2,* respectively, producing fusions that are highly specific and diagnostic for these tumors.

FNA Findings Ductal cells are small, cuboidal, and bland-appearing and can be single or form sheets, acini, tubules, or branching aggregates (Fig. 5.19d). Cells show round, regular nuclei with fine chromatin and inconspicuous nucleoli and may have mild to moderate pleomorphism (Fig. 5.19e); occasional intranuclear inclusions may be present. The epithelial component may have cystic change and squamous, clear cell, mucinous, oncocytic, and sebaceous metaplasia (Fig. 5.19f–h. Myoepithelial cells are usually dissociated or in small aggregates and show plasmacytoid or spindle shapes and may have moderate pleomorphism; they may be mistaken for hematopoietic and mesenchymal cells (Fig. 5.19i–k). Myoepithelial cells appear faint with poorly defined cell borders when admixed with the stroma (Fig. 5.19l). The chondromyxoid matrix, in air-dried Romanowsky-stained

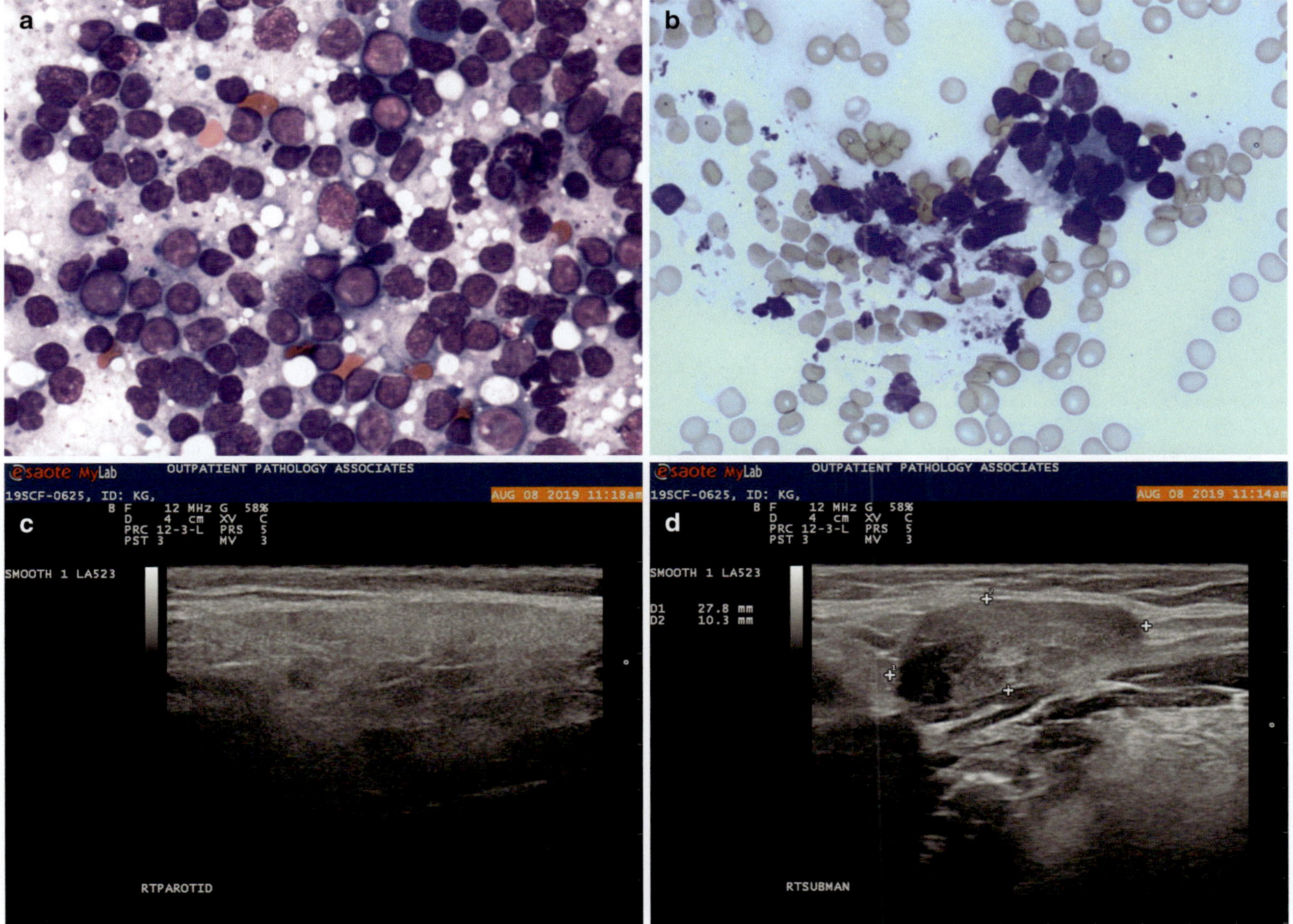

Fig. 5.16 Lymphoepithelial sialadenitis. Involvement of the parotid and submandibular glands is seen in this patient with history of Sjögren's syndrome. Smears show a polymorphous population of lymphoid cells (**a**) and rare acinar cells (**b**). Both glands show a heterogeneous echotexture and multiple round hypoechoic areas without posterior acoustic enhancement (**c, d**). (**a, b,** MGG stain, high magnification)

slides, is characteristic and appears metachromatic, dense, and fibrillary; the last feature is particularly visible in the frayed edges (Fig. 5.19l, m). The matrix is less conspicuous with Papanicolaou stain and appears pale and gray; and myoepithelial cells may appear stellate or spindle. Thus, Romanowsky-stained slides are advantageous for detection of small amounts of stromal elements, and they lower the possibility of an incorrect diagnosis. Cell block is invaluable to refine the diagnosis by using H&E and immunohistochemical stains (Fig. 5.19a–c). Necrosis and cellular atypia secondary to infarction may rarely be associated with prior FNA.

It should be emphasized that finding fibrillary stroma overrides any ductal or myoepithelial cell atypia that may suggest malignancy including carcinoma ex-pleomorphic adenoma, which should be carefully considered due to its rarity particularly in the absence of rapid tumor growth and

facial nerve-related clinical findings. Some cases may be categorized as salivary gland neoplasm of uncertain malignant potential (SUMP).

Myoepithelioma should be considered when myoepithelial cells predominate (Fig. 5.19k). However, because the stroma is the most conspicuous element in the pleomorphic adenoma pattern, the differential FNA diagnosis includes mucoepidermoid carcinoma, polymorphous adenocarcinoma, and adenoid cystic carcinoma. Pleomorphic adenoma may resemble mucoepidermoid carcinoma based on the presence of marked mucinous metaplasia, foam cells secondary to cystic change, and metaplastic squamous cells (Fig. 5.19h). Finding less dense stroma that, on careful examination appears fibrillary is helpful for reaching the correct diagnosis.

Cellular pleomorphic adenoma with a cilindromatous pattern and limited stromal elements should be distinguished from adenoid cystic carcinoma and will be discussed in the

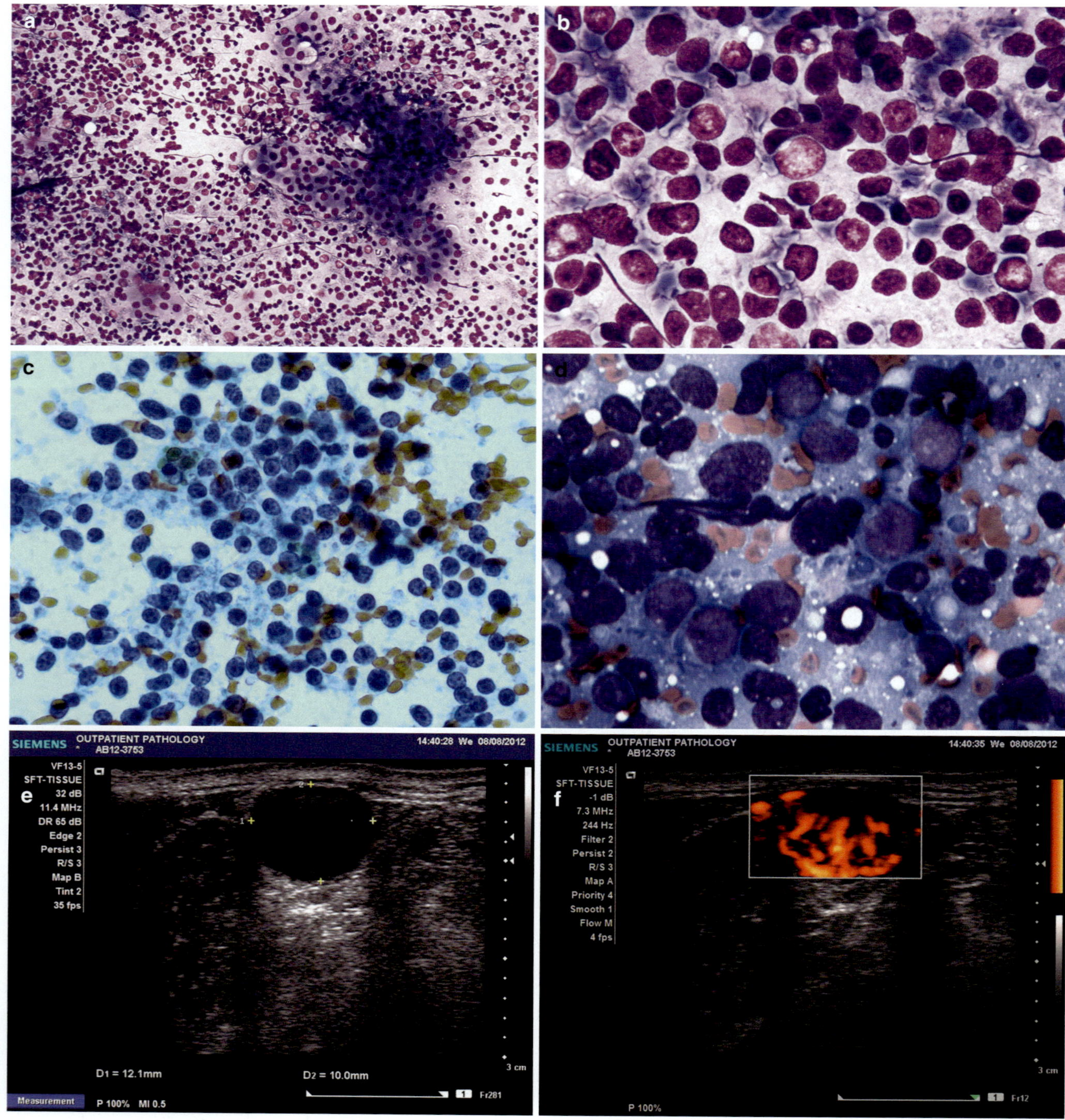

Fig. 5.17 Mixed cell follicular lymphoma and Warthin's tumor of the parotid gland (**a**, **b**). Follicular lymphoma of parotid gland (**c**). Large B-cell lymphoma involving submandibular space lymph node (**d**); US shows a round markedly hypoechoic lymph node with well-circumscribed margins, posterior acoustic enhancement, and chaotic internal blood flow by Doppler examination (**e**, **f**). US imaging of the parotid follicular lymphoma shows coalescing intraglandular nodes (**g**, **h**). (**a**, **b**, DiffQuik stain, medium and high magnification; **c**, MGG stain, high magnification; **d**, Papanicolaou stain, high magnification)

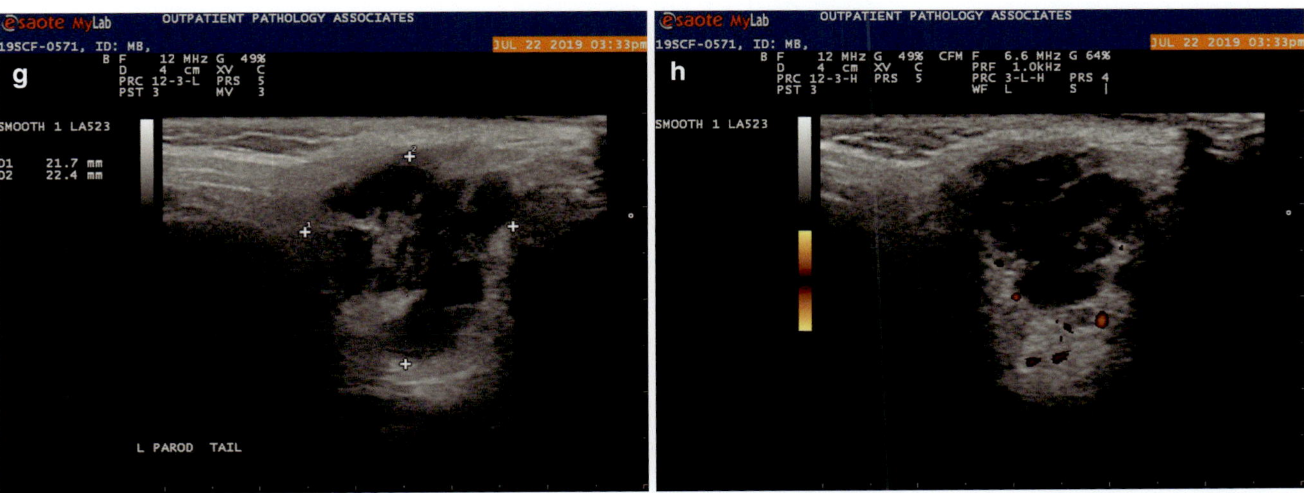

Fig. 5.17 (continued)

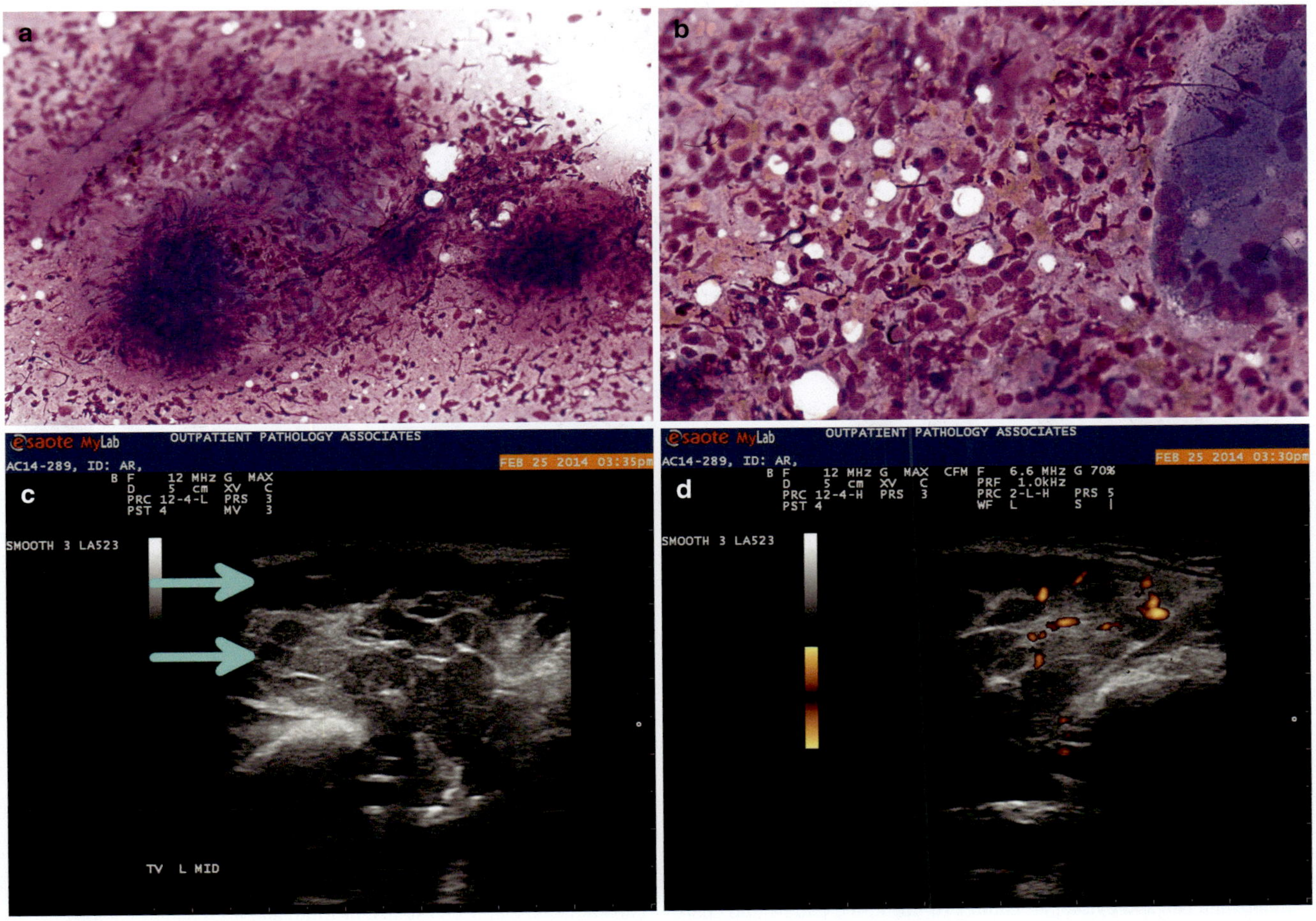

Fig. 5.18 Sarcoidosis. Non-necrotizing granulomatous inflammation. Granulomas, chronic inflammation, and tissue damage (**a**) and multinucleated giant cells are present (**b**). Ultrasound shows heterogeneous salivary gland echotexture with vascularized septae (**c**, **d**) (DiffQuik stain, medium and high magnification)

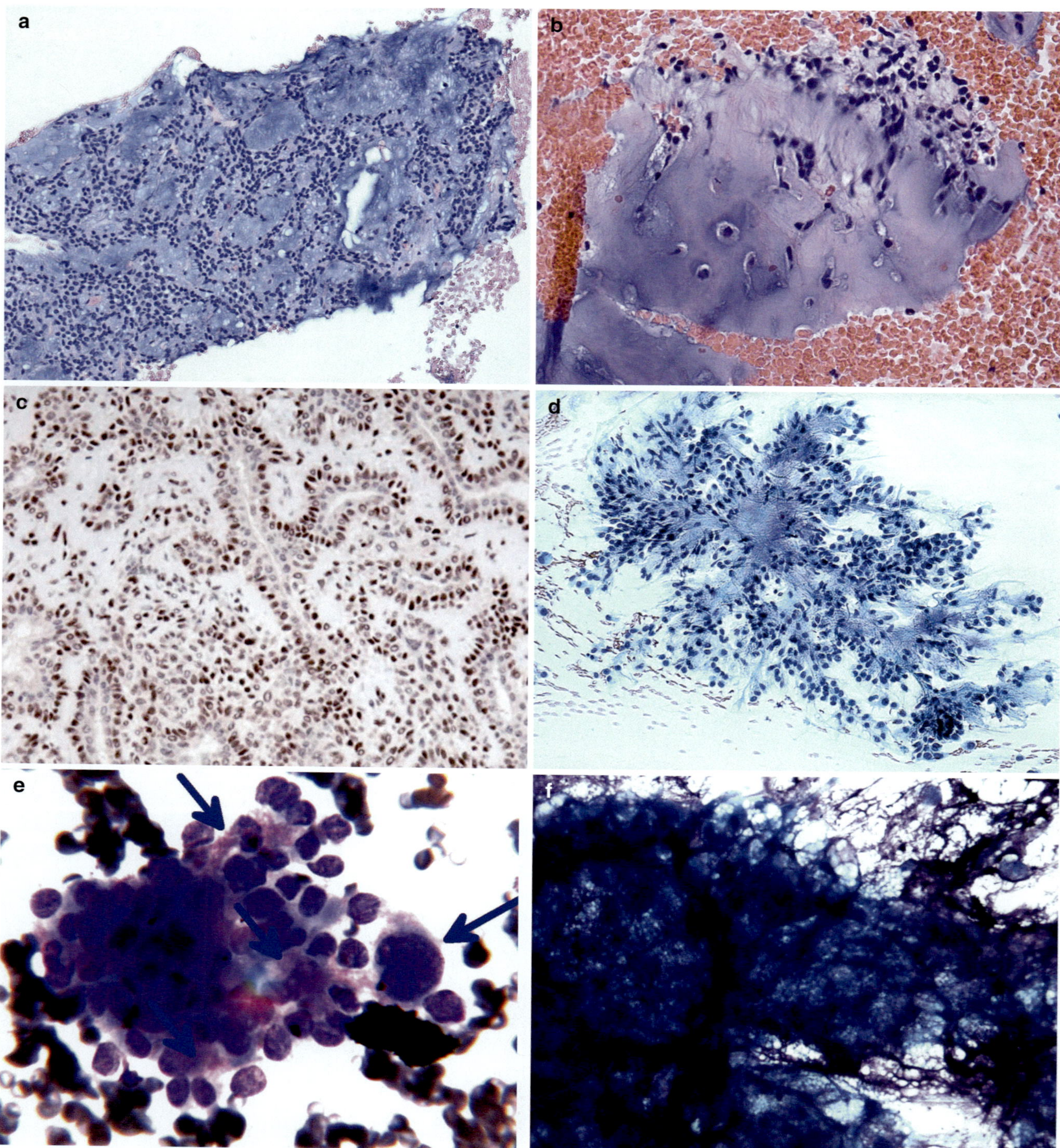

Fig. 5.19 Benign mixed tumor. Histologic features (**a**, **b**), PLAG-1 immunostain (**c**), and cytologic features (**d–m**, **v**, **w**). Ultrasound characteristics (**n–u**, **x**, **y**). (**a**, **b**, H&E stain, medium magnification; **c**, immunoperoxidase stain, low magnification; **a–m** and **v**, **w**, Papanicolaou and MGG stains, medium and high magnification)

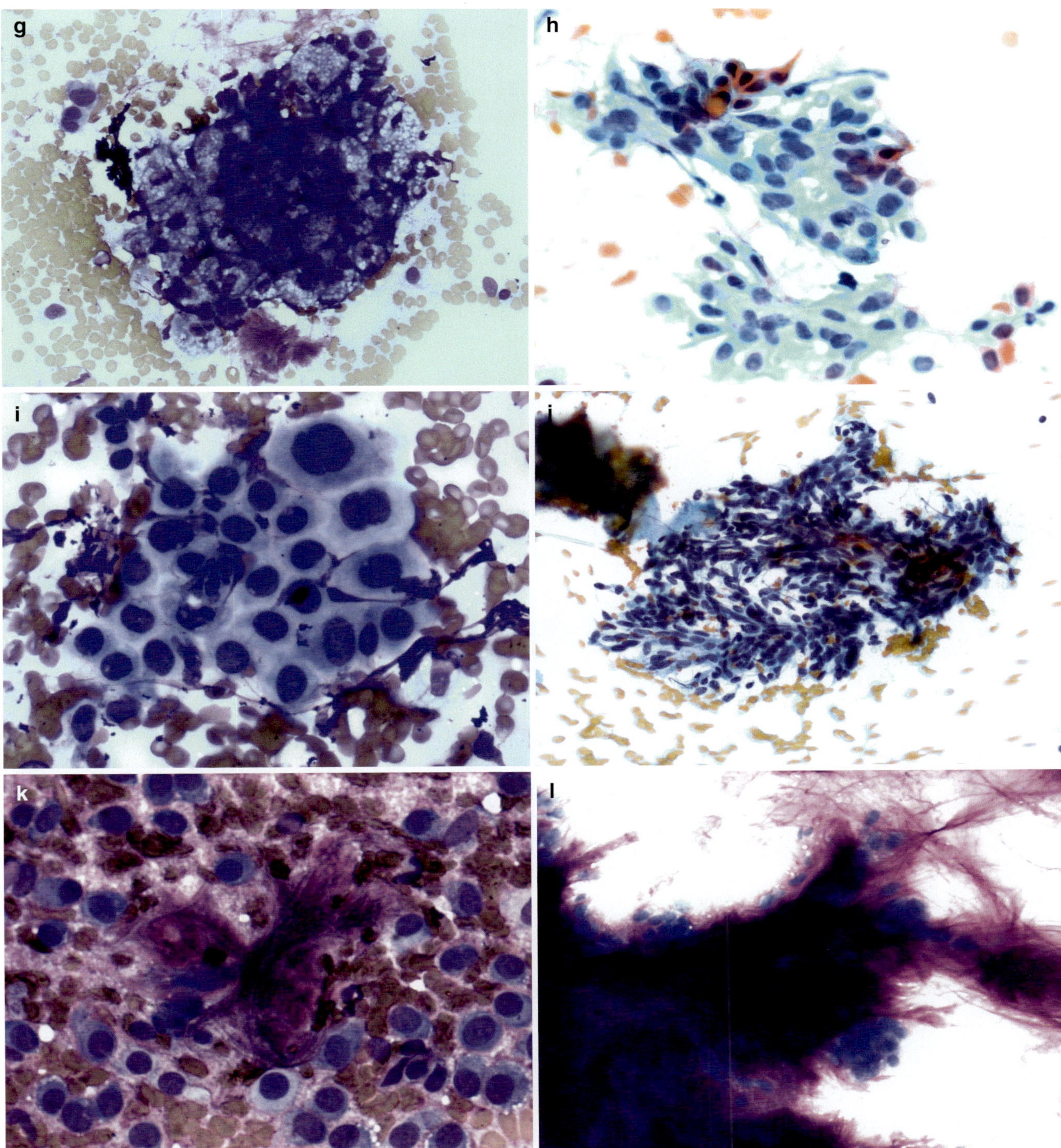

Fig. 5.19 (continued)

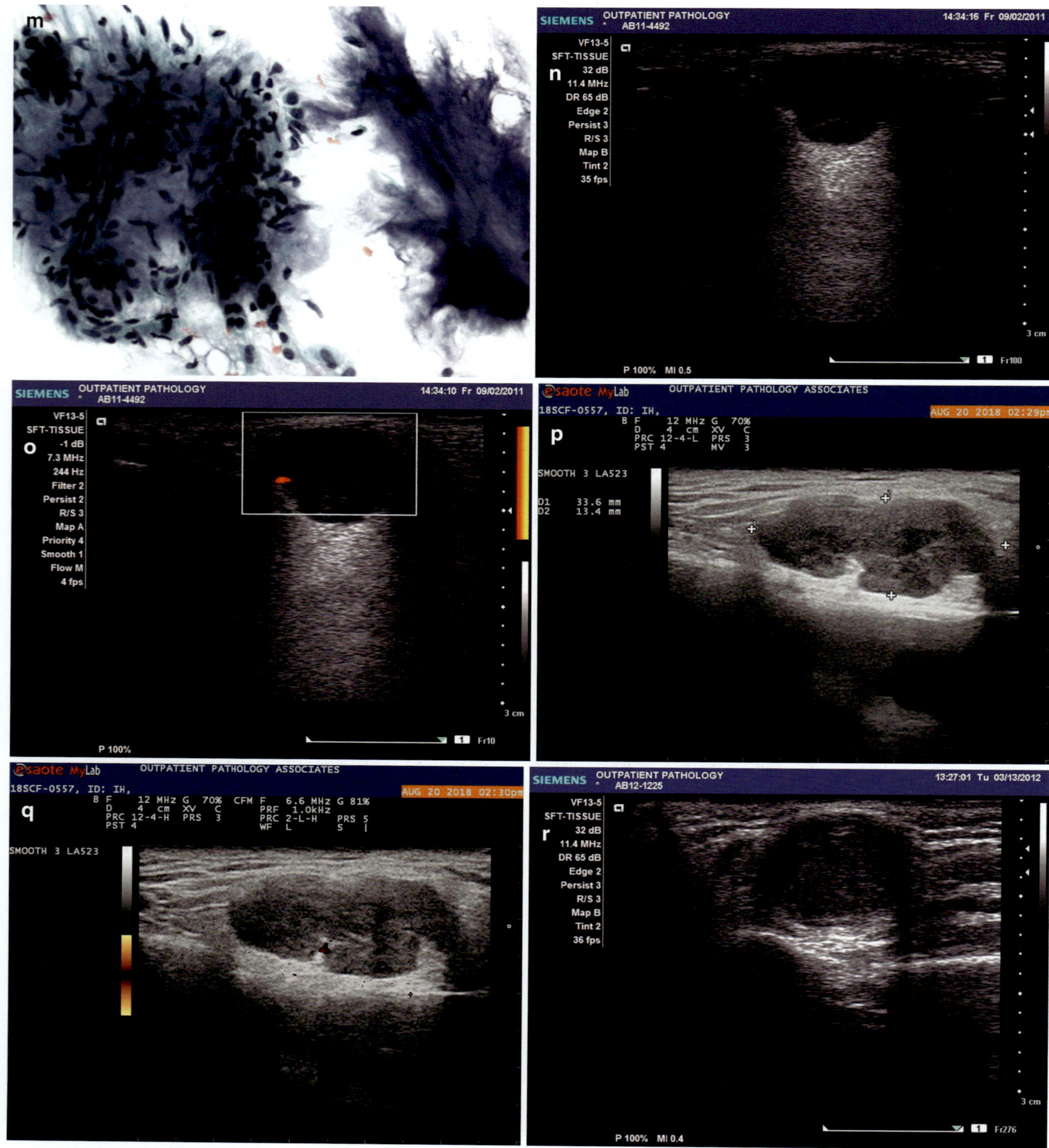

Fig. 5.19 (continued)

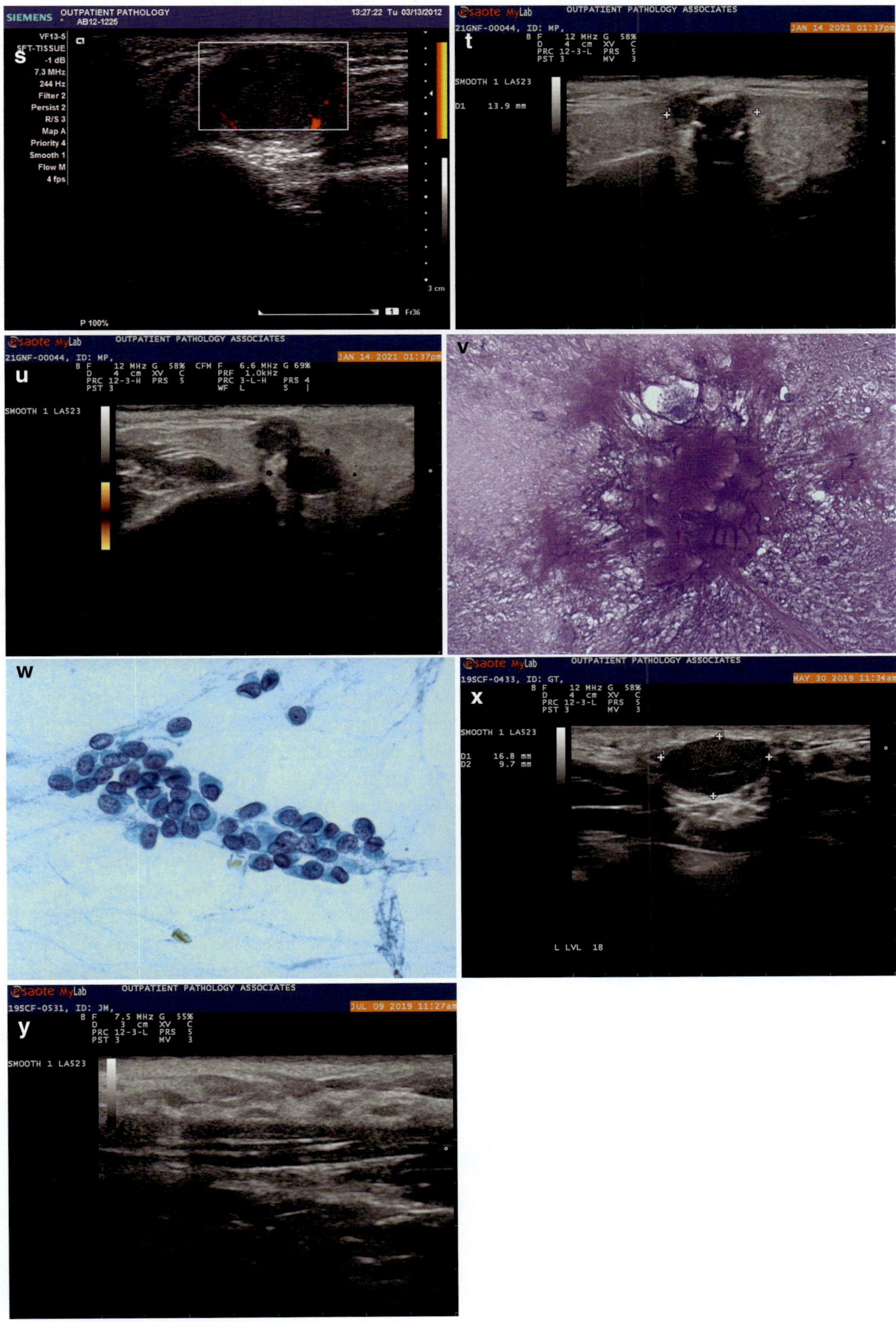

Fig. 5.19 (continued)

section "small epithelial cell pattern." Except for the proclivity to affect minor salivary glands instead of the parotid gland, and the perineural invasion seen in polymorphous adenocarcinoma, both polymorphous adenocarcinoma and pleomorphic adenoma have stromal and epithelial cell similarities that make FNA distinction difficult. Some cases may be categorized as salivary gland neoplasm of uncertain malignant potential (SUMP).

US Features A round or oval well-defined hypoechoic solid mass with a lobulated or bosselated surface is usually located in the superficial portion of the parotid gland. The mass is homogeneous and often displays a "through" transmission with posterior acoustic enhancement ("pseudocystic" appearance). Power Doppler demonstrates peripheral intratumor blood flow. Irregular ill-defined margins and heterogeneity raise the possibility of malignancy. Cystic and hemorrhagic degeneration is usually not seen; however, it may be observed in tumors larger than 3 cm. Calcifications may occur in long-standing tumors (Fig. 5.19n–u).

Recurrent pleomorphic adenoma almost always occurs in or around the surgical excision site. Single or multiple nodules with smooth and well-defined borders, homogeneous echotexture, posterior acoustic enhancement, and peripheral vascularity may be present within the salivary gland bed in these recurrent tumors (Fig. 5.19v–y).

Atypical Pleomorphic Adenoma

The atypical features of this tumor include high cellularity, cellular pleomorphism, increased mitoses, and / or necrosis. These features may suggest malignancy and should prompt extensive tissue sampling; however, they should not be mistaken for malignancy (Fig. 5.20). The atypical features identified in the smears of an otherwise benign mixed tumor must be correlated with clinical findings including US and other imaging studies. Atypia of undetermined significance (AUS) or salivary gland neoplasm of uncertain malignant potential (SUMP) may be the diagnostic categorization in these instances.

Pleomorphic Adenoma-like Distant Deposits

Deposits of otherwise typical pleomorphic adenoma may be seen occasionally in the lungs, mimicking pulmonary hamartoma, or in bone, mimicking chondrosarcoma or myxoid malignant fibrous histiocytoma. Clinical, radiographic, immunohistochemistry, and molecular studies are required for adequate interpretation of the FNA findings. A mixed tumor of the skin (i.e., chondroid syringoma described in Chap. 6) can be excluded based on dermal location and clinical findings. Such distant deposits are described in this chapter to help in the differential diagnosis of masses with such features outside the area of prior resection.

Polymorphous Adenocarcinoma

Characteristically, this tumor shows bland cyto- and histomorphology, variable histologic patterns, and has low metastatic potential. The recently described cribriform adenocarcinoma is included under polymorphous adenocarcinoma in the fifth WHO classification of salivary gland tumors.

Clinical Findings This tumor originates almost exclusively in the minor salivary glands of the oral cavity, particularly the palate. It is more common in women and frequently occurs in the sixth to eighth decade of life. The patient has a non-tender mass that can last for months to years.

Histopathology This well-circumscribed unencapsulated tumor shows various growth patterns, including a solid, cribriform, glandular, tubular, cystic, papillary, trabecular, or single-cell linear pattern (Fig. 5.21a). Tumor cells are bland-appearing cuboidal, and of medium size with round to elon-

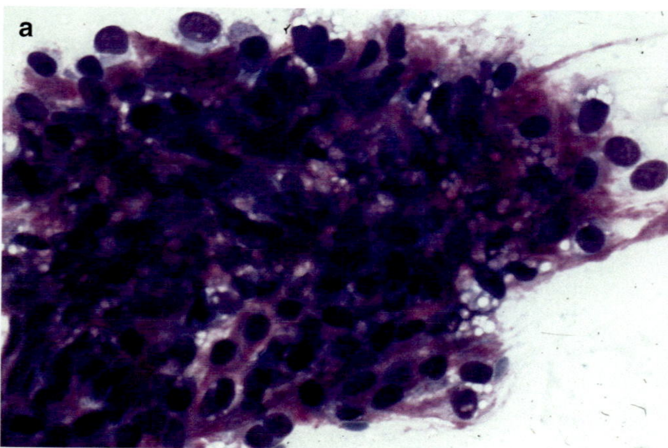 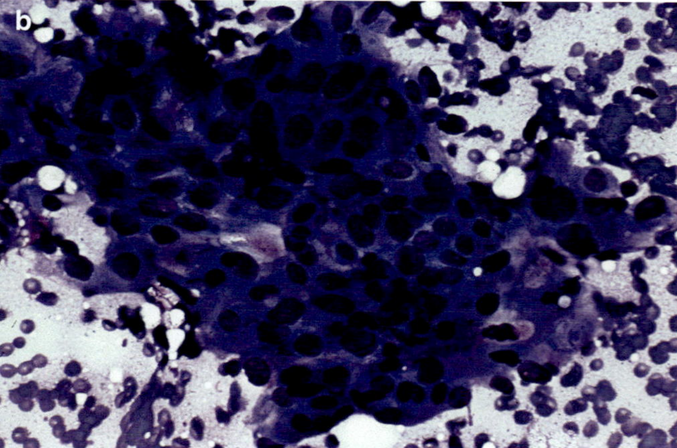

Fig. 5.20 Benign mixed tumor with atypia and sebaceous (**a**) and squamous (**b**) metaplasia. (DiffQuik stain, high magnification)

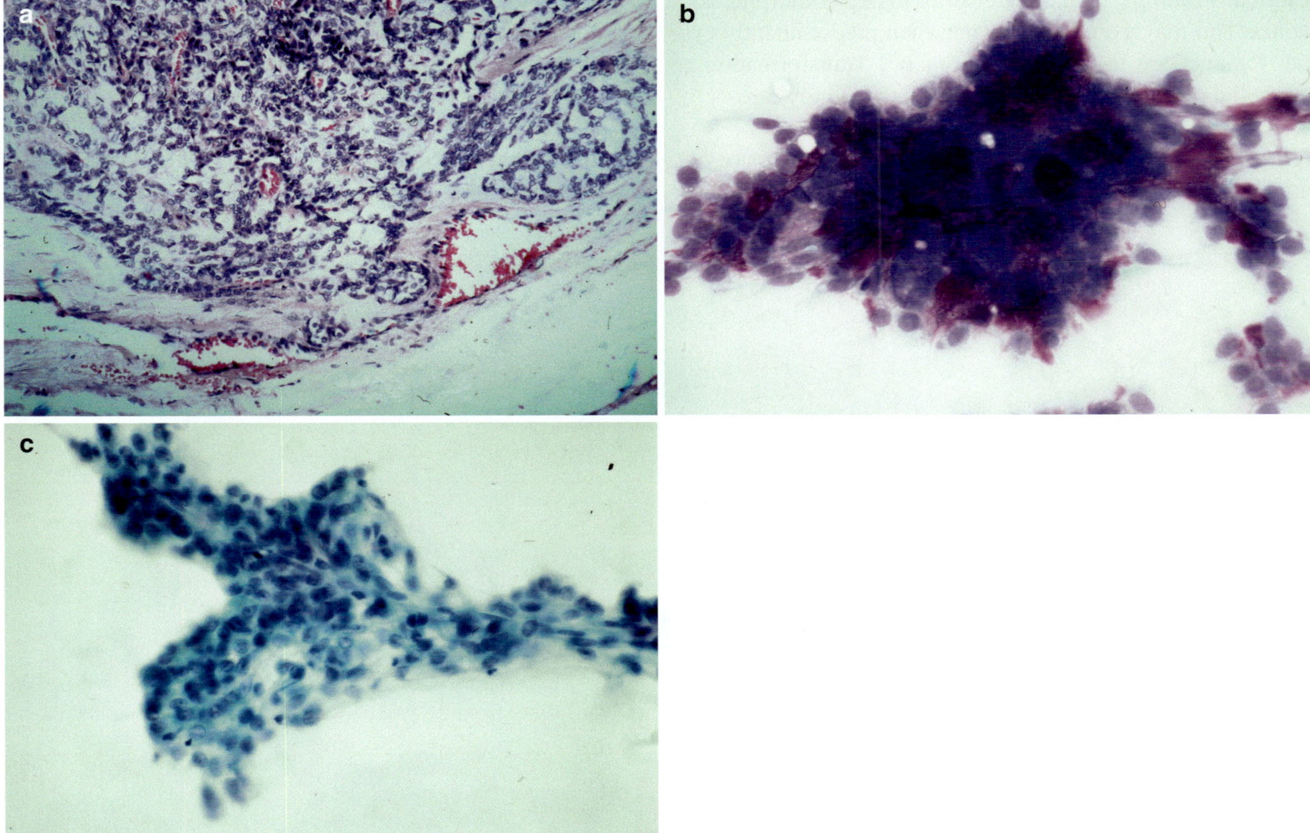

Fig. 5.21 Polymorphous adenocarcinoma. Histology shows glandular, cribriform, and trabecular patterns (**a**). Pseudopapillary aggregates with myxoid matrix are present (**b**). There are fine capillaries surrounded by bland-appearing epithelial cells (**c**). (**a**, H&E stain medium magnification; **b**, MGG stain high magnification; **c**, Papanicolaou stain medium magnification)

gated nuclei, granular fine chromatin, and inconspicuous nucleoli. Nuclear pleomorphism, necrosis, and mitoses are rare. The stroma is hyaline or mucoid and may have areas of hemorrhage. Squamous, oncocytic, or mucinous metaplasia may be seen as well as intratubular calcifications. Pseudoepitheliomatous hyperplasia of the overlying epithelium may be present.

Immuno-Profile Neoplastic cells show positive immunoreactivity for CEA, keratin, p63, S100 protein, vimentin, EMA, actin, SOX10, CD117, Bcl-2, and galectin-3. Immunochemistry for actin, calponin, b-catenin, GFAP, LEF1, HMGA2, and p40 is negative.

Molecular Profile Alterations of the 8q12 chromosome band, 12q rearrangements, and clonal t(6:9)(p21;p22) have been observed.

FNA Findings Smears are often of high cellularity and show epithelial cells, myoepithelial cells, and myxoid and metachromatic globular matrix admixed with epithelial aggregates. The epithelial cells are seen in aggregates, acinar arrangements, or sheets and occasionally as branching pseudopapillary aggregates. Cells are cuboidal to spindle-shaped with round to oval uniform nuclei, fine chromatin, inconspicuous nucleoli, and dense cytoplasm (Fig. 5.21b, c). Nuclear grooves and rare intranuclear inclusions can be seen. The cell features are important for distinguishing this tumor from pleomorphic adenoma that has plasmacytoid myoepithelial cells or adenoid cystic carcinoma that shows more basaloid hyperchromatic cells and lacks cell pleomorphism or necrosis.

Pattern IV. Warthin's Tumor and Similar Processes

Warthin's Tumor

Warthin's tumor is the second most common salivary gland tumor, has cigarette smoking as the main risk factor, is more prevalent after the fourth decade of life, involves almost exclusively the parotid gland (often the tail), is bilateral in 10% of cases, and is slightly more common in men. Complete surgical excision is the treatment of choice.

Clinical Findings Tumors are softer than pleomorphic adenomas and may even be fluctuant when predominantly cystic. Patients are usually asymptomatic. Transformation to epithelial or lymphoid malignancy is exceedingly rare.

Histopathology The epithelial component is oncocytic, arranged as a double layer with inner columnar and outer smaller cuboidal cells that decorate cystic, glandular, or papillary projections. The lymphoid elements are predominantly mature and may exhibit germinal centers (Fig. 5.22a, b). Mucus and goblet cells as well as sebaceous glands may be seen.

Immuno-Profile Epithelial cells show positivity for keratin and EMA and are negative for S100 protein, p63, calponin,

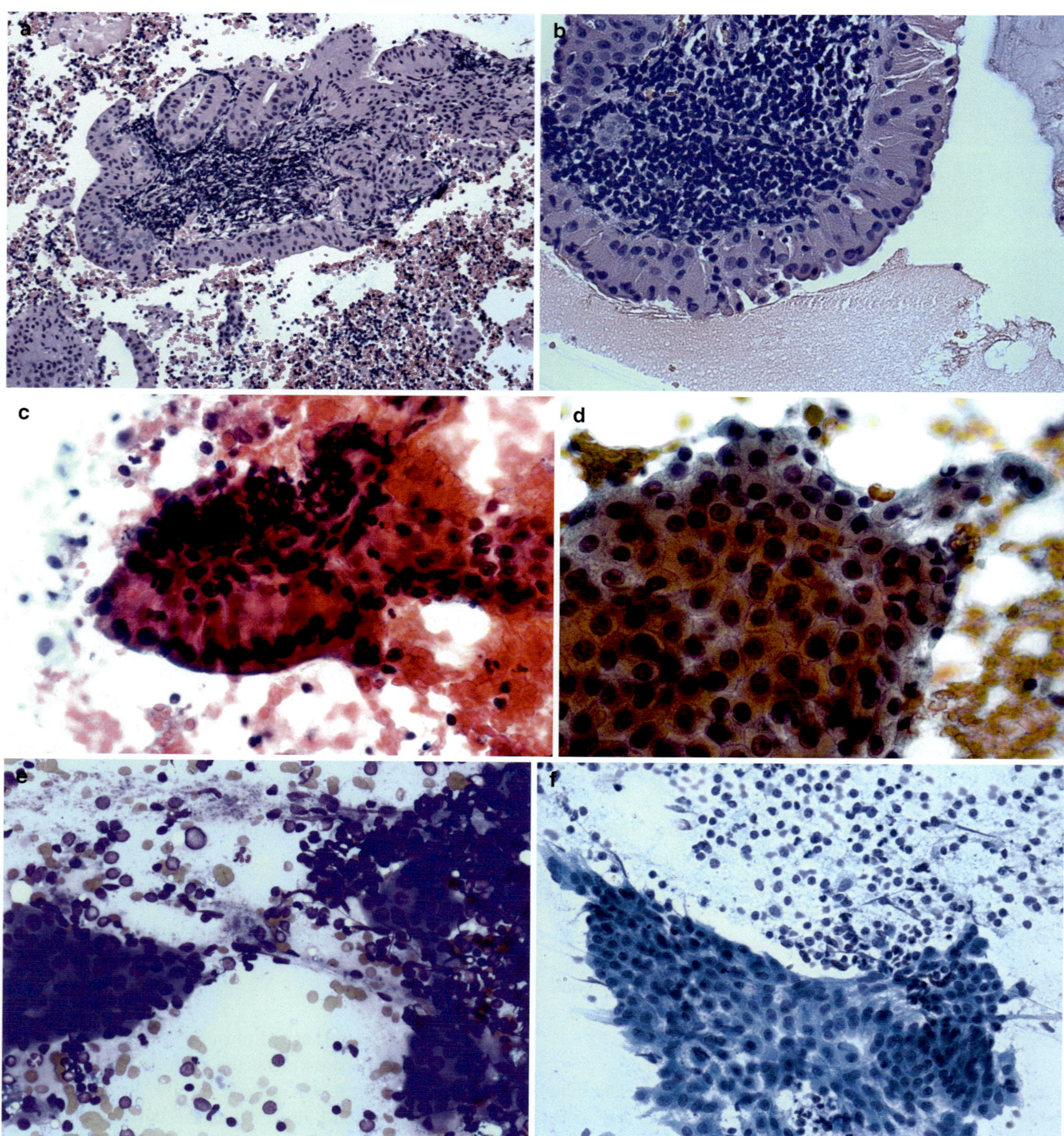

Fig. 5.22 Warthin's tumor. Histologic (**a**, **b**) and cytologic features (**c–j**). Ultrasound characteristics (**k–p**). (**a**, **b**, H&E stain, low and medium magnification; **c–j**, Papanicolaou and MGG stains, medium and high magnification)

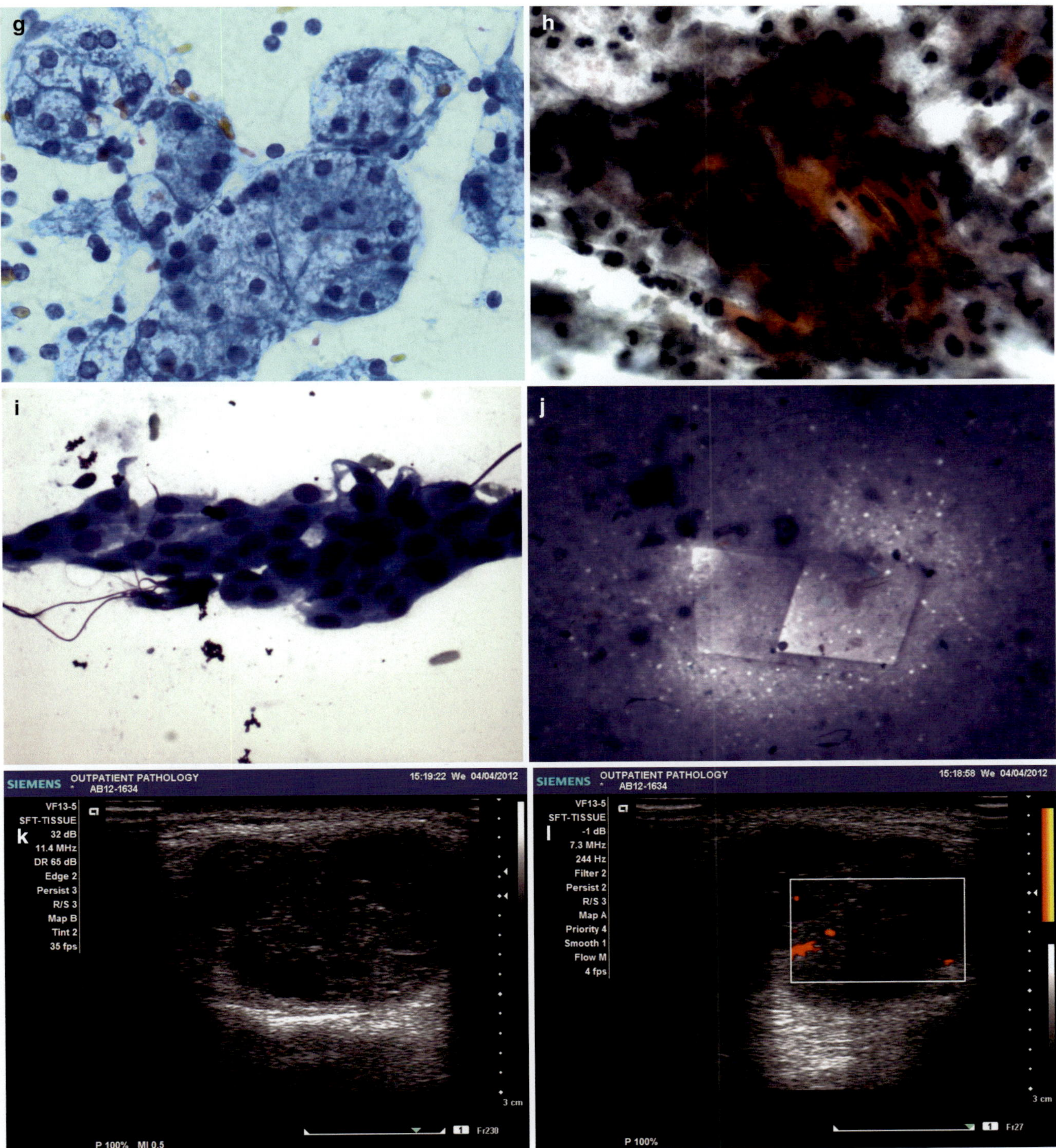

Fig. 5.22 (continued)

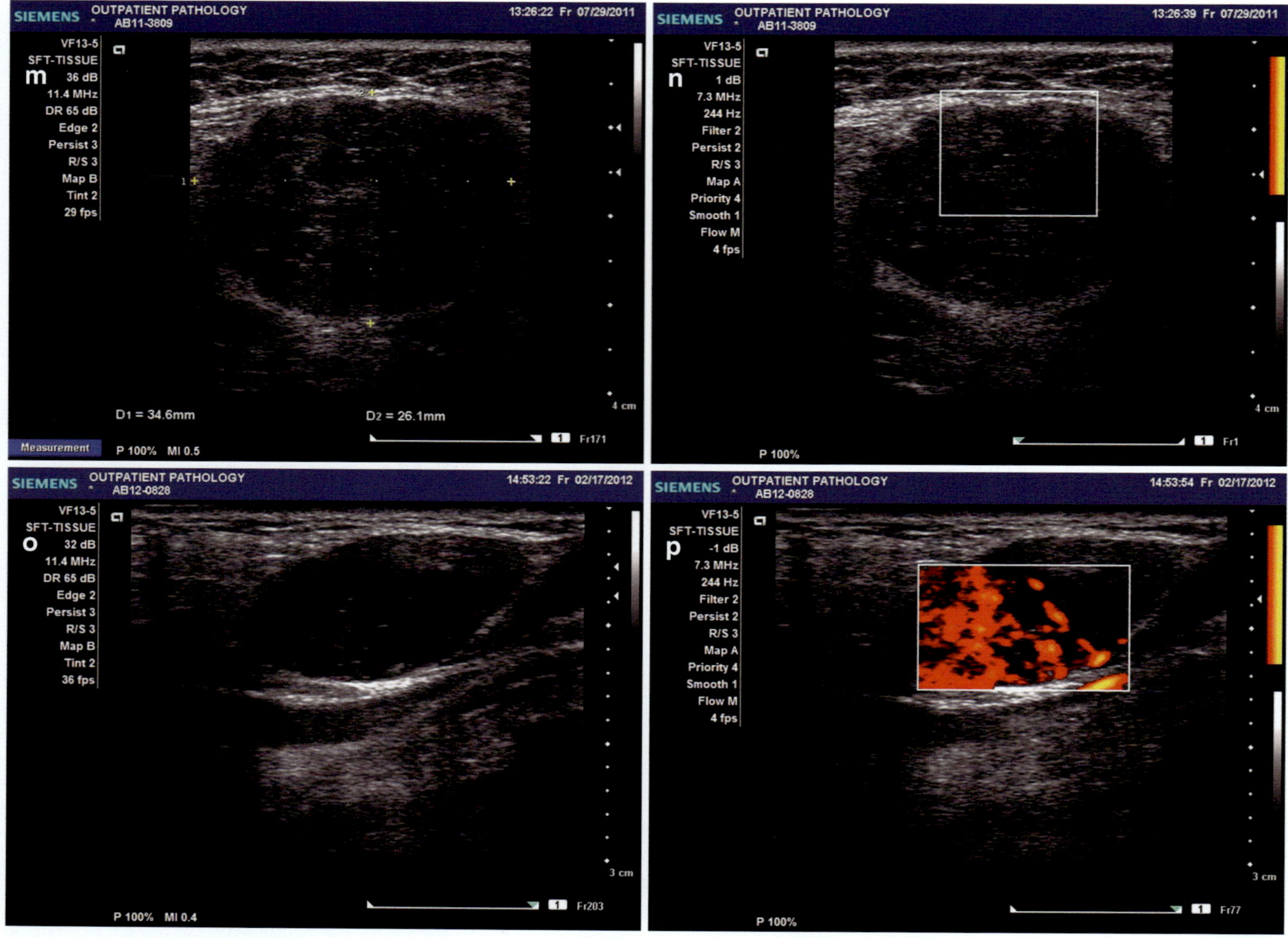

Fig. 5.22 (continued)

actin, and GFAP. Nuclear positivity for p40 and p63 is seen in the basal cells. Lymphoid cells lack light-chain restriction and are positive for mature B- and T-cell markers.

Molecular Profile The majority of these tumors show a normal karyotype. Approximately 10% of tumors have cytogenetic abnormalities; 6p rearrangement and 11q;19p translocations are the most common and consistent abnormalities in this tumor.

FNA Findings Smears may show three components in various proportions: oncocytic cells, lymphocytes, and cyst fluid. Oncocytic cells often occur in cohesive flat sheets showing abundant cytoplasm, well-defined cytoplasmic borders, round nuclei, and conspicuous nucleoli. The cytoplasm is granular and eosinophilic when stained with Papanicolaou stain or dense in air-dried Romanowsky-stained preparations. The lymphoid cells are usually small and may be scattered in the smear background or tangled among themselves or with the epithelial elements (Fig. 5.22c–e). The cystic component shows debris admixed with variable numbers of macrophages, and lymphocytes (Fig. 5.22f). Sebaceous, mucinous, or squamous metaplasia may be seen (Fig. 5.22g–i). Cholesterol crystals may be seen (Fig. 5.22j).

In the presence of a lymphoid-rich FNA, chronic inflammation, reactive lymphoid hyperplasia, or even small-cell-type non-Hodgkin lymphoma may be differential diagnostic considerations. Flow cytometry is helpful in questionable cases. Cyst content characteristics are highly suggestive of Warthin's tumor; however, the diagnosis cannot be made without the presence of oncocytic cells; then repeat FNA under US guidance should be performed for sampling of the solid component. Mucoepidermoid carcinoma may be considered when the oncocytic epithelium is not prominent, and squamous metaplasia is identified in a background of cyst fluid that may be mistaken for mucin (Fig. 5.22i). Cystic squamous cell carcinoma may be considered when atypical squamous metaplasia is apparent in a background of cystic elements (Fig. 5.22h). When oncocytic cells predominate and the cyst fluid is not prominent, the differential diagnosis includes oncocytosis and oncocytic neoplasms, i.e., oncocytoma or oncocytic papillary cystadenoma among others. Oncocytosis is a hyperplastic process of ductal and acinar epithelia with variable degrees of oncocytic metaplasia, that on smears exhibit ample granular eosinophilic cytoplasm. Cells of acinic cell carcinoma may be difficult to differentiate from those of oncocytic neoplasms, particularly Warthin's tumor, because both lymphocytes and cystic fluid may be present in these tumors. In contrast to the fine granularity of Warthin's tumor, the coarse cytoplasmic zymogen granules of acinic cell carcinoma are more prominent in cell block slides. Smears from acinic cell carcinoma, secretory carcinoma, and oncocytic and Warthin-like variants of mucoepidermoid carcinoma (mostly affect young nonsmoker females) may show lymphoid cells and cystic change similar to Warthin's tumor, and ancillary tests may be needed in the differential diagnosis. *MAML2* fusion is positive in mucoepidermoid carcinoma and negative in Warthin's tumor. Necrosis, infarction, reactive changes, and hemorrhagic and granulation tissue may be encountered as a result of previous FNA sampling.

US Features This tumor is usually a well-circumscribed round or ovoid hypoechoic mass which is heterogeneous with solid and cystic areas or multiseptated with spongiform cystic architecture. This US pattern is highly suspicious, but is not common. Power Doppler may show vascularity, particularly in the septa of the tumor and may be central, peripheral, or both (Fig. 5.22k–p).

Pattern V. Cystic Pattern and Similar Processes

The cyst contents obtained by FNA may be broadly classified as non-mucinous and mucinous. Each of these categories has a broad differential diagnosis that includes primary non-neoplastic and neoplastic benign or malignant lesions. It should be remembered that cystic change may also be the result of degeneration in solid tumors. The differential diagnosis is narrowed when other cellular or non-cellular elements are visualized.

US features: Regardless of the etiology, cysts have similar characteristics, including well-defined edges, thin walls, anechoic pattern, posterior acoustic enhancement, and no vascularity (Fig. 5.23a, b). If the cyst becomes infected, the wall becomes thick and there is internal debris.

Non-Mucinous Cystic Lesions

Crystals in Cystic Lesions
Cysts may contain crystals, i.e., α-amylase, tyrosine.

Alpha-amylase crystals are not associated with malignant processes. Smears show polyhedral and multifaceted structures of variable size and thickness commonly associated with scant epithelial elements, predominantly oncocytic cells (Fig. 5.24a). These crystals have been observed predominantly in cystic spaces lined with metaplastic oncocytic cells in Warthin's tumor, oncocytic papillary cystadenoma, pleomorphic adenoma, sialadenitis, and sialolithiasis. The crystals may be a product of oncocytic cell secretion.

Tyrosine crystals, on the contrary, have been found in malignant and non-malignant neoplastic processes, more frequently in black patients (Fig. 5.24b).

Lymphoepithelial Cyst
This AIDS-related process affects principally the parotid gland, unilaterally or bilaterally, and shows hyperplastic lymphoid tissue lining cystic structures, which may show squamous, columnar ciliated or non-ciliated, or mucinous

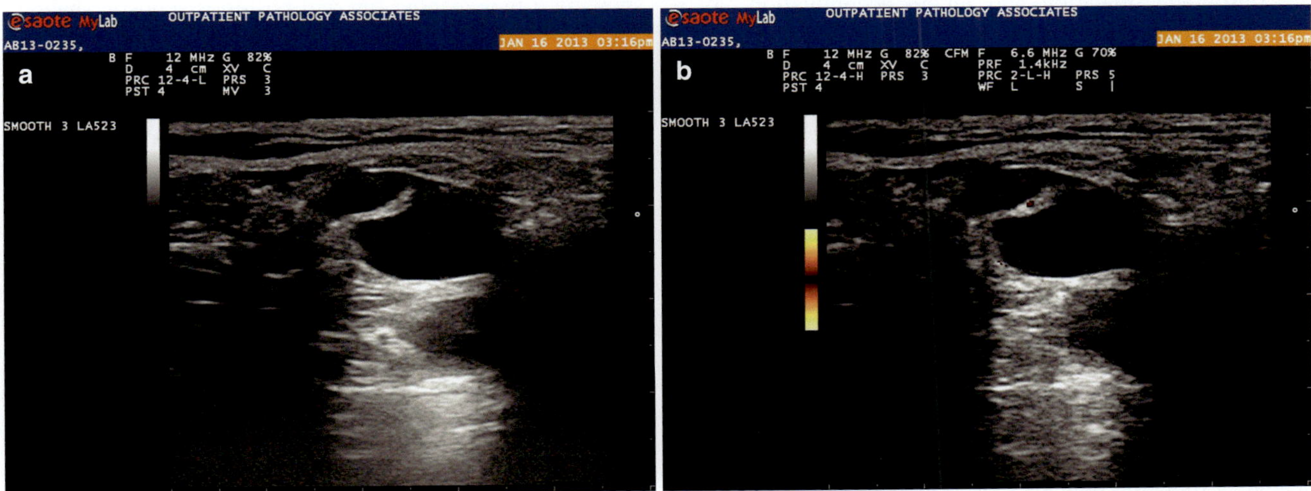

Fig. 5.23 Parotid gland cyst. US shows a round anechoic nodule with well-defined margins, posterior acoustic enhancement, and no vascularity by Doppler exam

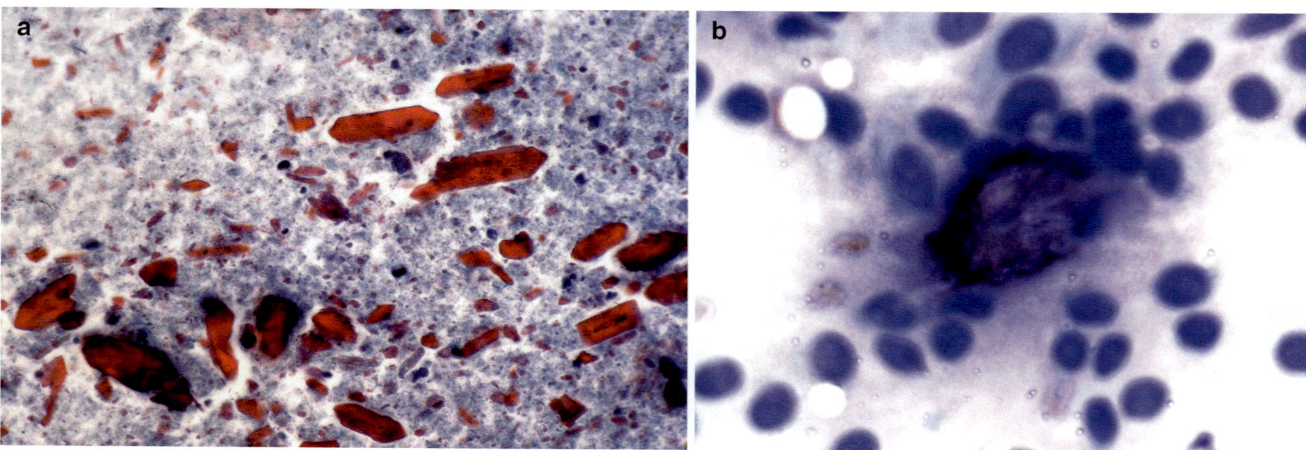

Fig. 5.24 Alpha-amylase (**a**) and tyrosine (**b**) crystals. (**a**, SurePath preparation, high magnification; **b**, MGG stain, high magnification)

epithelium or even sebaceous glands (Fig. 5.25a). Cytologic findings include epithelial cells of the types described, polymorphous lymphoid cells, and a cystic background (Fig. 5.25b, c). The differential diagnosis depends on the predominant elements identified; however clinical correlation is important, considering that reactive lymphoid hyperplasia and lymphoepithelial cysts are more common than primary neoplasms in patients with AIDS, malignant lymphoma and Kaposi's sarcoma, the most common malignancies in these patients. Some lymphoepithelial cysts may have a complex echotexture with solid and cystic areas resembling tumors.

Mucinous Cystic Lesions

Obstructive Sialopathy

These processes may be the result of fibrosis, adjacent masses, or sialolithiasis obstructing the ductal system, causing retrograde dilatation and mucin accumulation. As a result, acinar atrophy, chronic inflammation, and occasionally acute inflammation may occur. The lining epithelium of the dilated ducts is usually flattened or may show squamous, mucinous, or ciliated metaplasia. Foreign body reaction and stromal reactive changes may occur if there is rupture of the dilated duct. Cytology preparations are similar, if not identical to those of a low-grade mucoepidermoid carcinoma (Fig. 5.26).

Sialolithiasis

This process is more common in women than in men and affects predominantly the submandibular gland, mainly as a unilateral lesion. Most calculi are single; 90% of submandibular gland and 10% of parotid-gland stones are radiopaque. Clinically, patients classically present with pain at mealtime; however, they may be asymptomatic and have a firm mass suggestive of malignancy.

The FNA diagnosis can be made in the presence of stone fragments that may be associated with cell metaplasia, including ciliated columnar cells, which may be interpreted as a congenital cyst when stone fragments are not evident. The background is mucinous, with debris, and may be sparsely cellular (Fig. 5.27a–d).

The main differential diagnosis is low-grade mucoepidermoid carcinoma in the absence of stone fragments and ciliated metaplasia, and in the presence of squamous metaplasia, foam cells, and reactive, bland ductal cells. In cases where mucus is only present, the FNA diagnosis of "Mucinous smear pattern" is suggested, followed by a comment addressing the differential diagnosis.

US Features The gland appears enlarged due to ectasia and has variably dilated ducts. The lesion may be hypoechoic and heterogeneous with ill-defined and lobulated borders. Duct dilatation may be usually seen, with the duct stone showing a hyperechoic rim and posterior acoustic shadowing. Parenchymal stones can also be identified. Cyst and abscess formation may also be seen (Fig. 5.27e, f).

Low-Grade Mucoepidermoid Carcinoma

Mucoepidermoid carcinoma (MEC) is a malignant tumor composed of mucin-producing epithelium, squamous cells, intermediate cells, and mucus. Wide local surgical excision with preservation of the facial nerve is the treatment of choice.

Clinical Findings This is the most common salivary gland malignant neoplasm in both adults and children. It is more common in women than in men and occurs principally in the fifth decade of life, although it may occur in children in the second decade of life. It affects predominantly the parotid gland, the palate being the most frequent minor salivary site. The low-grade tumors are slowly growing and usually are

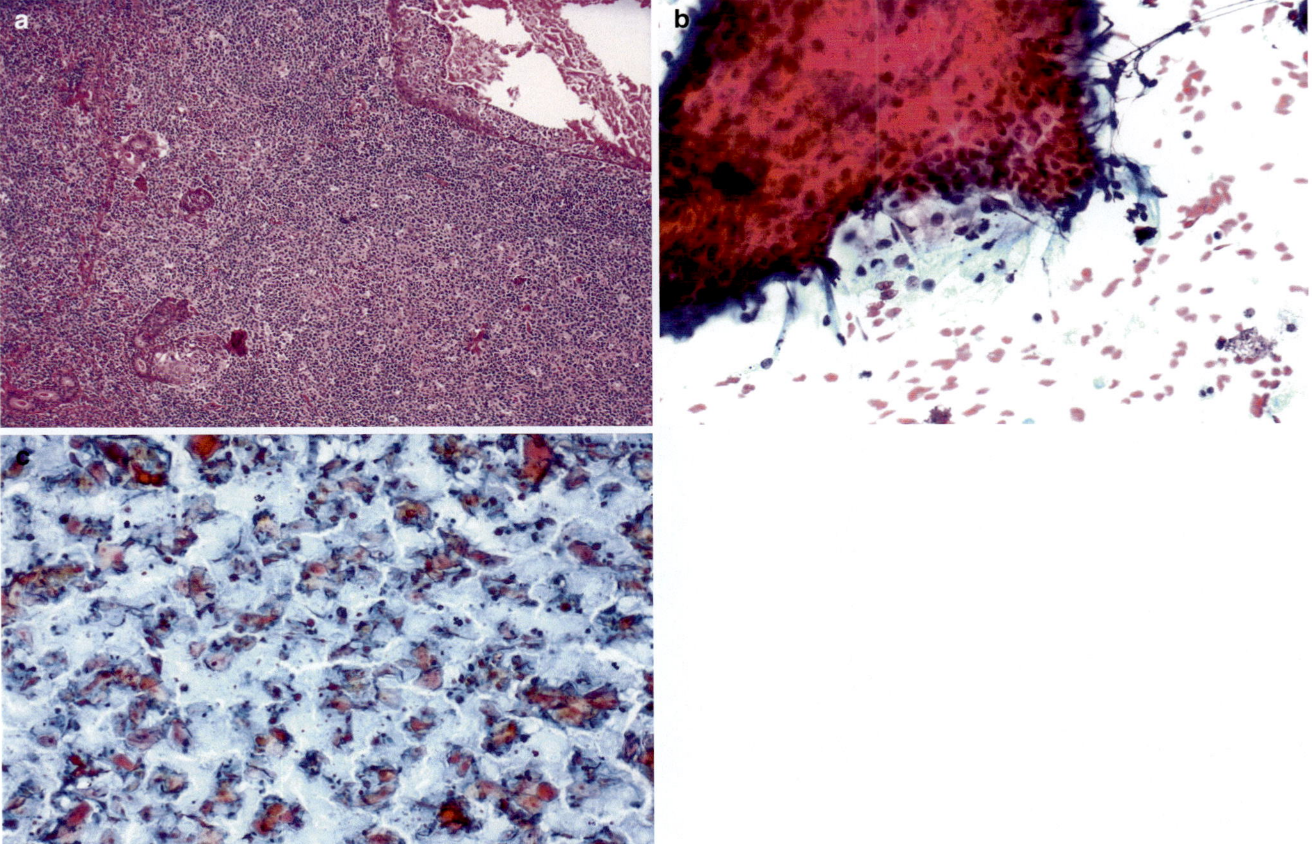

Fig. 5.25 Lymphoepithelial cyst. Histologic section showing reactive follicular hyperplasia and a cyst lined with benign squamous epithelium (**a**). Squamous cells in complex aggregates and single are seen along with lymphocytes (**b**, **c**). (**a**, hematoxylin eosin stain, low magnification; **b**, **c**, Papanicolaou stain, low and medium magnification)

asymptomatic, in contrast to the high-grade type, which are fast-growing and cause local pain. Low-grade tumors have an excellent prognosis, whereas high-grade ones have a poor prognosis.

Histopathology The tumors are often cystic. Mucus cells usually compose <10% of the tumor and are round, large, and show well-defined cytoplasmic borders, clear or foamy cytoplasm, and small, dark eccentric nuclei. Epidermoid cells have a polygonal shape, dense eosinophilic cytoplasm, well-defined cytoplasmic borders, and vesicular nuclei. Keratinization is rare except in inflamed tumors. Intermediate cells may be small basal or large polygonal cells. Basal cells have round/oval nuclei and scant eosinophilic cytoplasm. Large polygonal cells are round to oval with more abundant cytoplasm. Clear cells may be present and are occasionally prominent, as in the rare clear-cell variant of MEC. Oncocytic cells are seen in the oncocytic variant of MEC. Hyalinized or sclerosed stroma is seen in sclerosing MEC. Psammomatous MEC is another variant.

The histologic grading is fundamentally based on the predominance of the cystic component (low-grade MEC) or the solid component (high-grade MEC). Cellular pleomorphism, necrosis, mitosis, and hemorrhage are usually absent in low-grade tumors. The differential diagnosis depends on the tumor grade and includes obstructive sialopathy, necrotizing sialometaplasia, cystadenoma, and carcinomas including metastasis.

Immuno-Profile Epidermoid, intermediate, and columnar cells are cytokeratin- and EMA-positive. Mucus cells are cytokeratin- and EMA-negative. CK5/6 and p63 highlight squamous derivation and PAS demonstrate mucus. Oncocytic variant is strongly positive for p63. Nuclear immunostaining

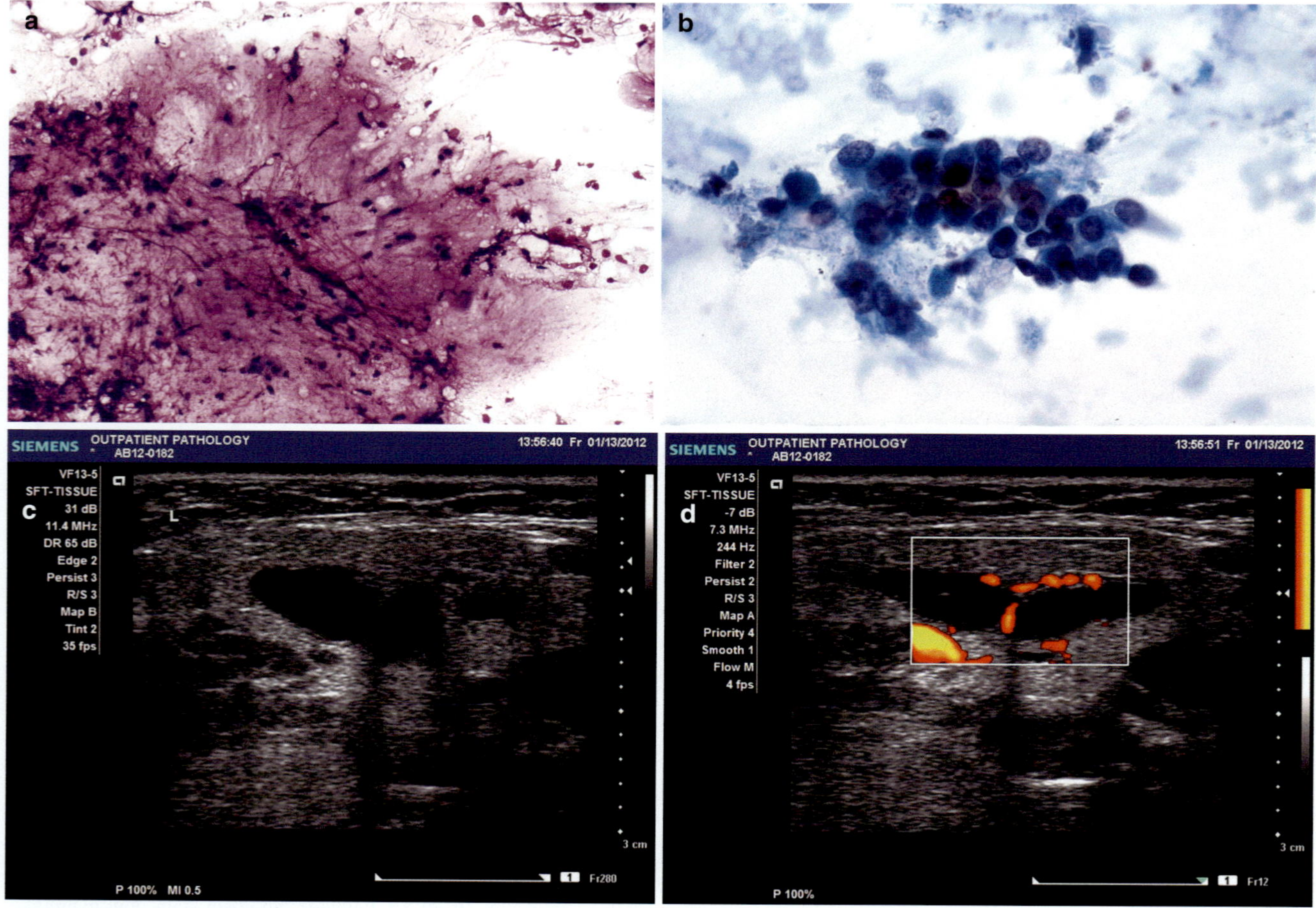

Fig. 5.26 Obstructive sialopathy. Squamous metaplasia, chronic inflammation, and cyst contents were the findings in this submandibular gland lesion (**a**, **b**). US shows cystic cavity surrounded by a thick wall, vascular by Doppler examination (**c**, **d**). (**a**, **b**, Papanicolaou stain, high magnification)

with Areg (amphiregulin), an epidermal growth factor receptor reveals the presence of MECT1-MAML2 fusion (see molecular profile).

Molecular Profile Mutations are found mainly in high-grade tumors. The t(11;19)(q21;p13) in MEC is highly specific and results in fusion of the MEC translocated gene-1 or *MECT1* gene and the mastermind-like gene family or *MAML2* gene. The MECT1-MAML2 fusion transcript, which is present in more than half of all MECs, is associated with lower histologic grades and improved survival, suggesting both diagnostic and prognostic roles. The translocation has not been seen in other salivary gland malignancies and can potentially be of diagnostic value using a FISH-based approach in FNA material, when MEC particularly of low-grade is suspected.

FNA Findings The smear pattern is similar to that seen in obstructive sialopathy. Smears are acellular or hypocellular, and the background shows abundant mucin that, in contrast to pleomorphic adenoma, does not appear fibrillary and does not stain as intensely. Cellular elements appear singly or in aggregates (Fig. 5.28a, b). The epidermoid cells are bland-appearing, and the mucus cells are plump with vacuolated cytoplasm indistinguishable from macrophages, well-defined cytoplasmic borders, and eccentric nuclei displaced by the cytoplasmic mucin (Fig. 5.28c). The mucus cells are fewer than the epidermoid cells. Intermediate cells are bland-appearing and have moderate amounts of cytoplasm. The oncocytic cells in the oncocytic variant have ample dense cytoplasm with well-defined cytoplasmic borders; a mucinous background and cellular degeneration may be present (Fig. 5.28d, e). High-grade MEC may be indistinguishable from other high-grade salivary gland carcinomas including metastases (Fig. 5.28h–j).

US Features Low-grade MEC is usually hypoechoic and well-defined, and it shares US features with benign salivary gland tumors (Fig. 5.28f, g). In contrast, high-grade malignancies may be frankly infiltrative and have a more solid

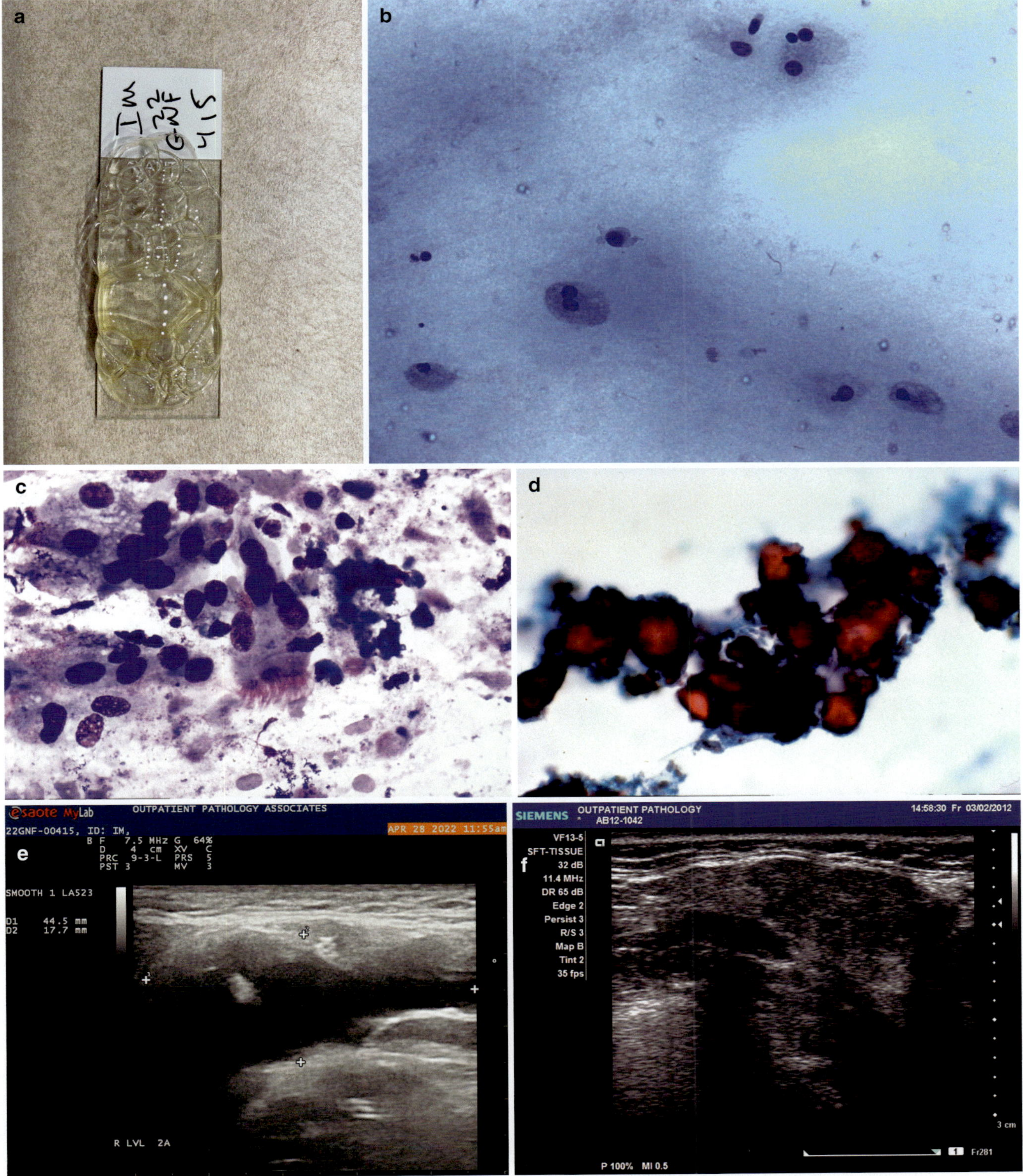

Fig. 5.27 Sialolithiasis. Aspirated thick mucus from a dilated submandibular gland duct (**a**). Smear shows a dense mucoid background (**b**). Ciliated metaplasia and crystals are present in a mucoid background aspirated from a submandibular gland mass (**c**, **d**). US shows a hypoechoic dilated submandibular gland duct (**e**) that corresponds to figures **a**, **b**. A mass with lobulated edges (**f**) and high vascular blood flow by Doppler exam (not shown) that corresponds to figures **c**, **d**. (**b**, MGG stain, medium magnification; **c**, **d**, Papanicolaou stain, high magnification)

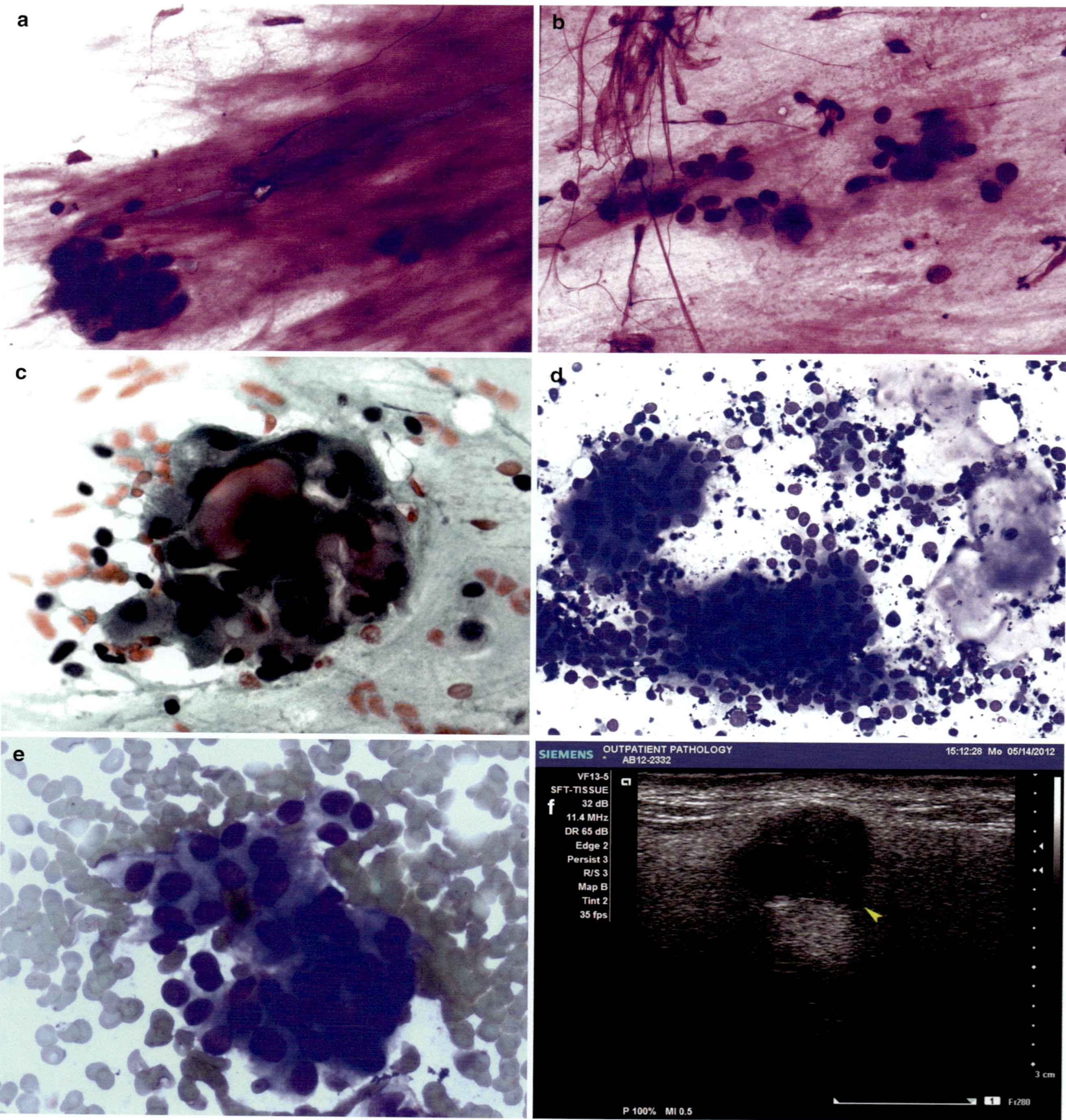

Fig. 5.28 Low-grade mucoepidermoid carcinoma. The cytomorphology is characteristic, although not diagnostic of this tumor (**a–e, h–j**). US features are not specific and overlap with those of benign cysts and tumors including marked hypoechogenicity and well-defined borders (**f, g**). The arrowhead points to an area of extracapsular invasion. Intermediate- and high-grade mucoepidermoid carcinomas may show US features of malignancy (**k, l**). (**a, b, d, e, h, i**, DiffQuik stain low, medium, and high magnification; **c, j**, Papanicolaou stain, high magnification)

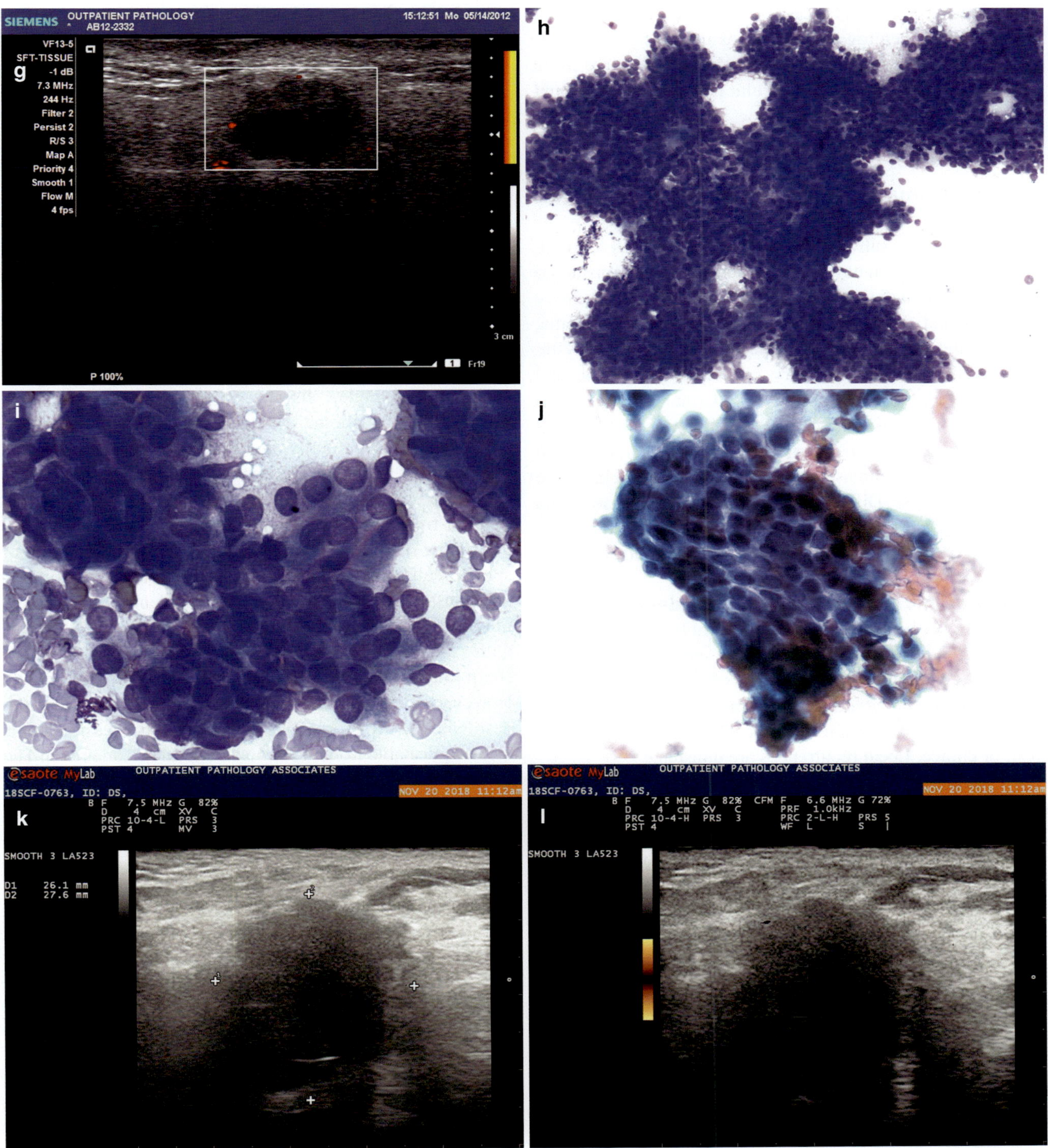

Fig. 5.28 (continued)

appearance (Fig. 5.28k, l). Large tumors are hypoechoic and have a complex heterogeneous echotexture reflecting intratumoral necrosis or hemorrhage. Malignant tumors are more likely to have a disorganized vascular flow and have regional neck lymph node metastases.

Pattern VI. Small Epithelial Cell Pattern

Various primary salivary neoplasms as well as dermal, adnexal, and even metastatic deposits should be considered in the differential diagnosis of this cytologic pattern. Primary salivary gland neoplasms include monomorphic adenoma, pleomorphic adenoma with scanty stroma, adenoid cystic carcinoma, and rarely, primary small-cell carcinoma, and lymphoepithelioma-like carcinoma. Dermal eccrine cylindroma and pilomatrixoma, infiltrative or metastatic basal cell carcinoma, metastatic neuroendocrine carcinoma of the skin or lung, and lymphomas must be considered in light of the clinical findings. Differentiating monomorphic adenoma from adenoid cystic carcinoma may be one of the most difficult diagnostic problems in salivary gland cytology.

Monomorphic Adenoma (Basal Cell Adenoma)

This tumor is composed of small, uniform basaloid cells and absence of the myxochondroid stroma seen in pleomorphic adenoma. Cytologically, this tumor is often indistinguishable from pleomorphic adenoma with scant stroma and adenoid cystic carcinoma. Complete surgical excision is the treatment of choice. Local recurrences are unusual.

Clinical Findings This rare tumor affects predominantly the parotid gland of adults, with no sex predilection. Patients often have an asymptomatic mass present for a variable period ranging from months to years. Superficial-lobe tumors are detected earlier; thus, the size usually is <3 cm. Larger tumors are located in the deep lobe and tend to have cystic degeneration.

Histopathology Tumors of major glands are encapsulated, whereas those of minor glands are often unencapsulated, although well-circumscribed. Cells are columnar or cuboidal and are arranged in tubular, solid, trabecular or membranous patterns of growth. All patterns but in particular the solid pattern, may show squamous horns or eddies, and the membranous pattern shows thick eosinophilic hyaline membranes, which are reduplicated basement lamina similar to those of dermal cylindroma. The differential diagnosis includes basal cell adenocarcinoma, adenoid cystic carcinoma, and basaloid squamous cell carcinoma (Fig. 5.29a).

Immuno-Profile In the tubular component, epithelial cells are CK7-, CK8-, CK18-, EMA-, and CEA-positive (Fig. 5.29b). The myoepithelial cells are CD10-, calponin-, p63-, actin-, and S100 protein-positive (Fig. 5.29c). Lymphoid enhancer bindings factor 1 (LEF1) immunohistochemical marker is positive in basal cell adenoma and distinguishes it from adenoid cystic carcinoma that is negative (97% positive predictive value).

Molecular Profile Loss of heterozygosity 16q12–13, a region related to the cylindromatosis gene *CYLD*, has been found. Trisomy of chromosome 8 and t(7;13) have also been reported.

FNA Findings Smears are cellular and show numerous blue cells and variable amounts of collagenous stroma that appears metachromatic on Romanowsky stains. Cellular dissociation and single cells may be numerous. The membranous basal cell adenoma shows features identical to those of adenoid cystic carcinoma, and the distinction between the two is almost impossible. When cellular complex aggregates with little or no stroma are the predominant pattern, the distinction from the solid (anaplastic) type of adenoid cystic carcinoma may be extremely difficult. The identification of spindle cells and capillaries within the arborizing collagenous stroma is useful for the correct identification of the tumor. Also, the stroma-cell interface is fuzzy and fibrillary, with a subtle interconnection between the two instead of the sharp interface often seen in adenoid cystic carcinoma. However, adenoid cystic carcinoma may show a fibrillary desmoplastic stroma produced in the areas of invasion that is indistinguishable from the stroma of basal cell adenoma. The difficulty of the distinction is even more difficult in the solid type of adenoid cystic carcinoma that shows limited amounts of the characteristic globular cilindromatous metachromatic extracellular matrix. The well-demarcated cylinder-cell interface may not be prominent in this type. In the absence of stroma and presence of cellular atypia, the distinction from basal cell adenocarcinoma or metastatic basal cell carcinoma with or without clinical history is essentially impossible (Fig. 5.29d–g).

US Features Superficial tumors are solid and often round or oval, well-circumscribed, hypoechoic, with a homogeneous echotexture (Fig. 5.29h, i). Deep tumors are larger, often round, and well-circumscribed, and hypoechoic, with a variably heterogeneous echotexture due to cystic change, particularly in tumors measuring >3 cm (Fig. 5.29j, k).

Adenoid Cystic Carcinoma

This basaloid malignant tumor is composed of epithelial and modified myoepithelial cells, and varying amounts of globular cylindromatous matrix. Surgery is the treatment of choice and radiation therapy may be considered in unresectable and/or deeply invasive tumors.

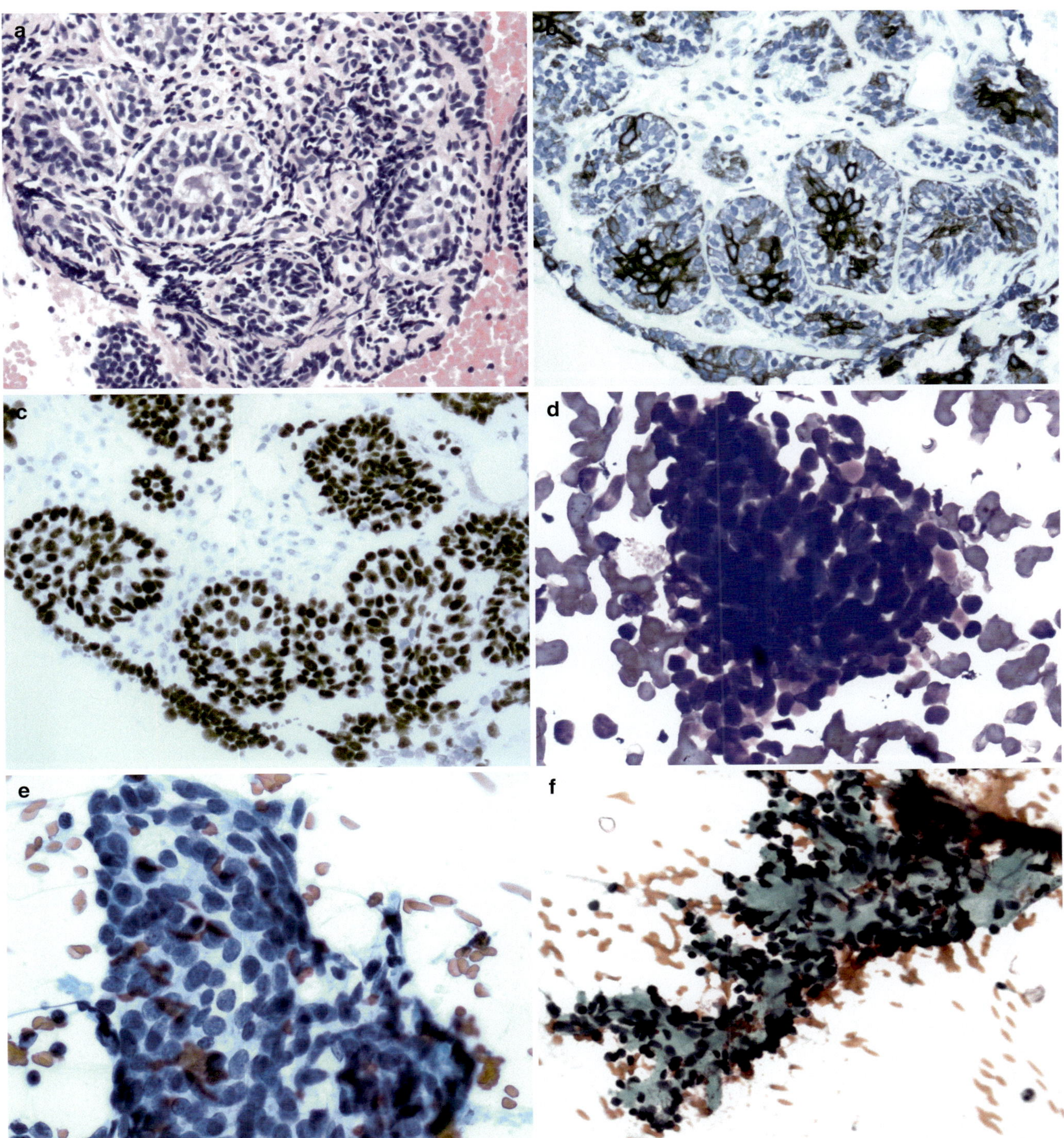

Fig. 5.29 Monomorphic (basal cell) adenoma. Histopathology (**a**) and positive immunostains for cytokeratin (**b**) and p63 (**c**). Cytologic findings (**d–g**). Ultrasound features are not specific and overlap with those seen in benign mixed tumors including lobulated margins, hypoechogenicity with posterior acoustic enhancement (**h, i**), and slightly heterogeneous echotexture in larger tumors (**j, k**). (**a**, H&E stain, cell block, low magnification; **b, c**, immunoperoxidase stain, medium magnification; **d, g**, DiffQuik stain medium and high magnification; **e, f**, Papanicolaou stain, medium and high magnification)

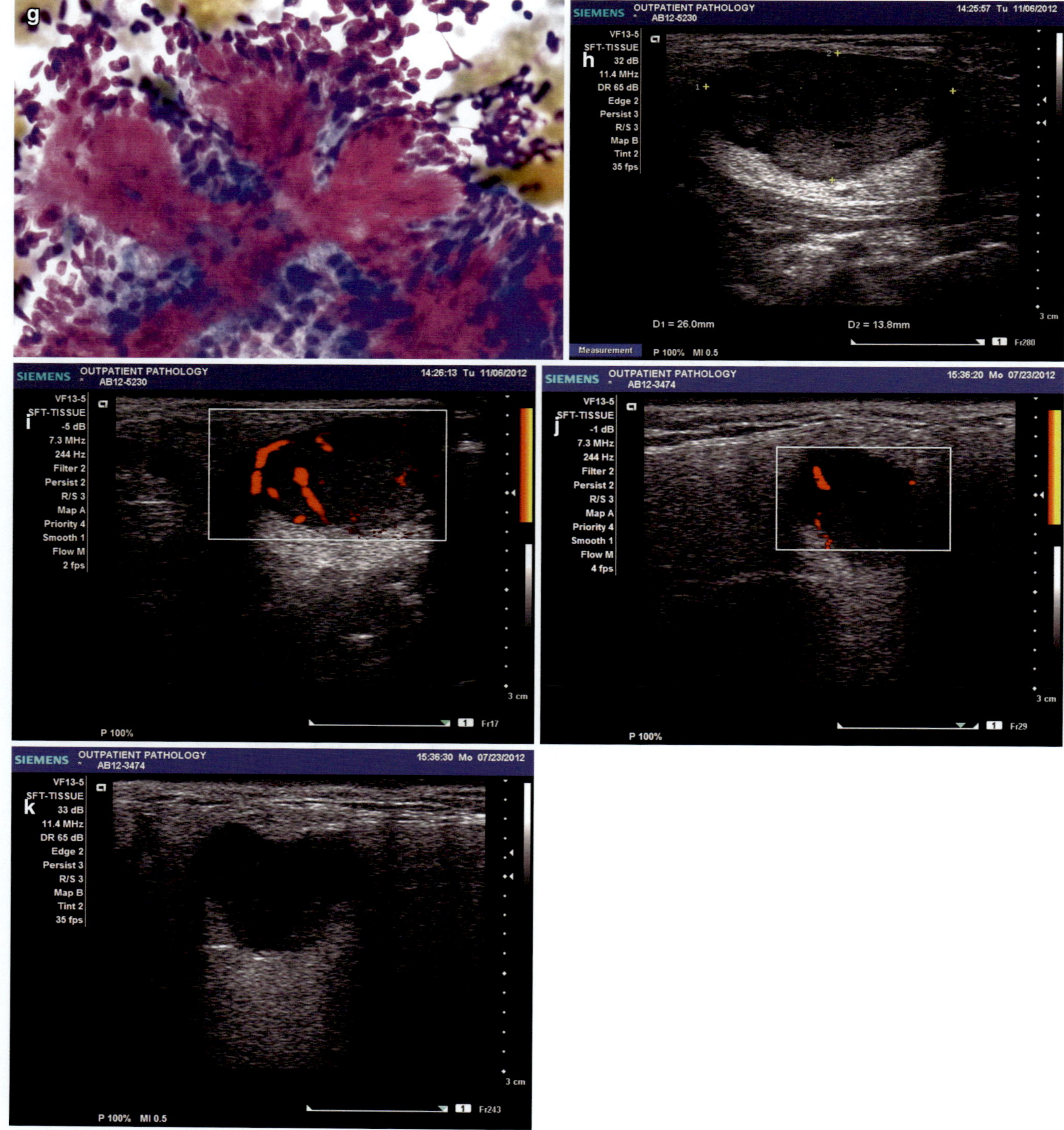

Fig. 5.29 (continued)

Clinical Findings This tumor comprises 10% of salivary gland neoplasms and affects mayor and minor salivary glands. It occurs predominantly in adult and old individuals who present with a slow-growing mass with associated local pain, paresthesia, or even facial nerve paralysis. The prognosis is poor, and the outcome is usually fatal.

Histopathology This infiltrative unencapsulated tumor has cells arranged in tubular, cribriform, and solid architectural patterns that are present in various proportions in the tumor. The lumens are filled with hyaline mucoid material (Fig. 5.30a). Perineural invasion is commonly seen.

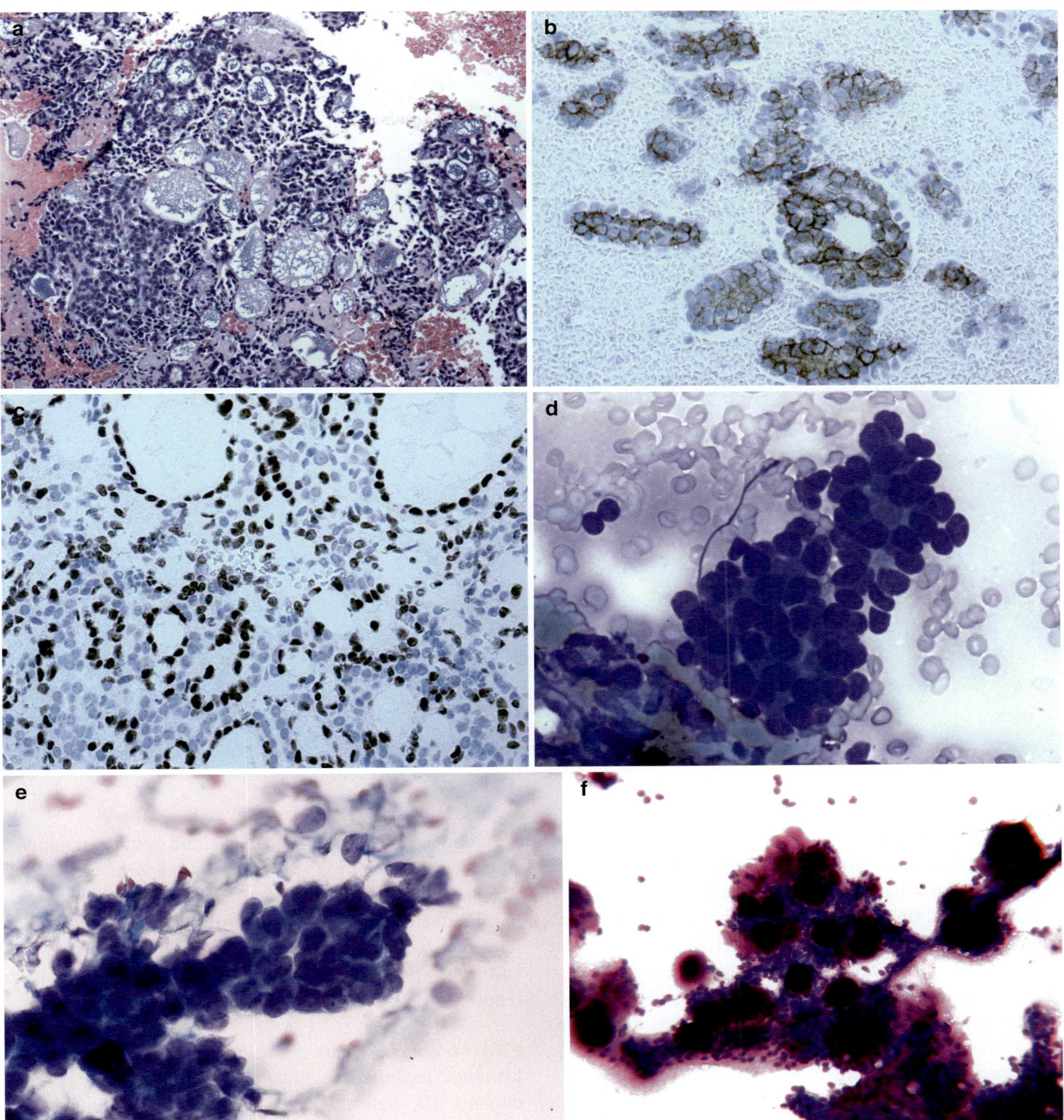

Fig. 5.30 Adenoid cystic carcinoma. Histopathology (**a**) and positive immunostains for CD117 (**b**) and p63 (**c**). Cytologic findings (**d**–**h**). Ultrasound images show a mass with ill-defined margins, heterogeneous echo texture and infiltrating borders (arrowheads) (**i, j**); the needle length is seen emerging from the left upper corner (**i**). (**a**, H&E stain, cell block, low magnification; **b**, **c**, immunoperoxidase stain, cell block, medium magnification; **d**, **f**, **g**, MGG stain, medium and high magnification; **e**, **h**, Papanicolaou stain, medium and high magnification)

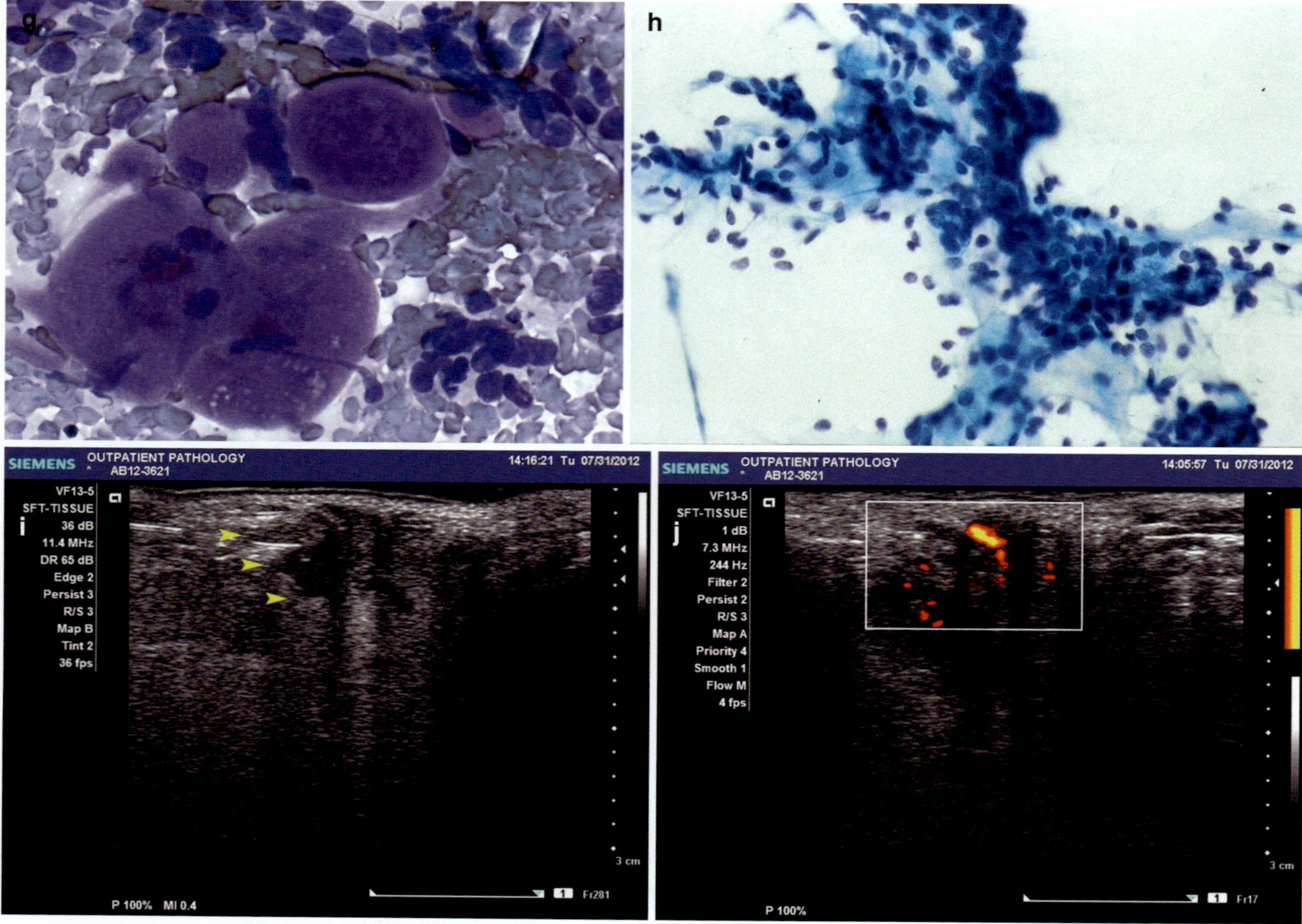

Fig. 5.30 (continued)

Immuno-Profile No markers are specific for this tumor. Two cell populations with distinct immunphenotypes are seen. Epithelial cells are keratin-, CD117, CEA-, and EMA-positive (Fig. 5.30b). The myoepithelial cells are CD10-, calponin-, p63-, actin-, vimentin, and S100 protein-positive (Fig. 5.30c). The extracellular material is PAS- and mucicarmine-positive. The tumor also is positive for bcl-2. Ki-67 immunostain may be helpful for distinguishing this tumor from polymorphous adenocarcinoma. Other biomarkers expressed in adenoid cystic carcinoma include p53, EGFR, and MYB that is positive in almost all cases. MYB is not observed in normal salivary gland tissue. Most adenoid cystic carcinomas, especially the solid subtype show cytoplasmic expression of the NOTCH oncogene. LEF1 immunostain is negative in adenoid cystic carcinoma and helps to differentiate it from basal cell adenoma that is positive.

Molecular Profile The t(6;9)(q22–23;p23–24) translocation in adenoid cystic carcinoma results in fusion and activation of the *MYB* gene at 6q22–23 and the *NFIB* gene at 9p23–24. The *MYB-NFIB* fusion transcript, present in at least one third of salivary gland adenoid cystic carcinomas, can be detected by FISH analysis of next generation sequencing, and has emerged as a potential therapeutic target. Frequently, there is overexpression of the C-KIT protein; however, no *c-kit* gene mutations have been shown and no response to imatinib mesylate therapy has been reported.

FNA Findings Smears are cellular and, depending on the histologic pattern, the cellular elements may be complex tridimensional, glandular, trabecular, and solid, composed of small blue cells (Fig. 5.30d). Cell dissociation is usually prominent, and numerous stripped nuclei are present in the background. The cells are uniform, and nuclear features are usually bland-appearing with small nucleoli and do not show features of malignancy (Fig. 5.30e).

The stroma seen in adenoid cystic carcinoma is of two types: (1) the classic cylindromatous globular stroma resulting from basal membrane reduplication is acellular, avascular, and has a sharp separating edge from the surrounding blue cells (Fig. 5.30f, g), and (2) the desmoplastic tumor stroma seen in the areas of invasion is fibrillary with fuzzy borders and interdigitates with the surrounding blue epithelial cells in a fashion similar to that seen in basal cell adenoma (Fig. 5.30h).

Two important features that may be seen in smears are necrosis and atypical mitoses that would favor the diagnosis of adenoid cystic carcinoma over basal cell adenoma; however, these features are found infrequently. Thus, considering the overlapping FNA cytology between these two tumors, the Swedish school of cytology recommends, based on its vast experience, that even in the presence of classical cytologic features of adenoid cystic carcinoma, such a conclusive diagnosis should be made only in the presence of symptoms and signs of facial nerve damage.

Neoplasms that have a cylindromatous pattern and mimic adenoid cystic carcinoma include pleomorphic adenoma, basal cell adenoma, epithelial myoepithelial carcinoma, and polymorphous adenocarcinoma. Pilomatrixoma with prominent basaloid cell representation and scanty squamous ghost cells and calcific matter is another tumor that resembles solid adenoid cystic carcinoma and basal cell adenoma. Clinical features and careful search for additional cytologic features are helpful for reaching the diagnosis. Likewise, basal cell adenocarcinoma primary to the salivary gland and basal cell carcinoma of skin origin show cytologic features very similar to those of solid adenoid cystic carcinoma and basal cell adenoma. Mitoses and necrosis, when present, help in the distinction of a malignant process from basal cell adenoma. Cytologic diagnosis of the specific type of malignancy is often less than impossible. Metastasis from Merkel cell and small cell carcinoma should also be considered in the diagnosis.

US Features Small tumors are encapsulated, well-defined, and hypoechoic, and mimic benign tumors. Large tumors are often infiltrative, hypoechoic, and heterogeneous with a complex echotexture reflecting areas of necrosis and hemorrhage (Fig. 5.30i, j).

Pattern VII. Large Epithelial Cell Pattern

These neoplasms can be arbitrarily divided into low-grade and high-grade types. The large-cell low-grade tumors include acinic cell carcinoma, secretory carcinoma, oncocytic neoplasms, epithelial-myoepithelial carcinoma, clear cell adenocarcinoma, and metastasis. Those with a high-grade pattern include high-grade mucoepidermoid carcinoma, carcinoma ex pleomorphic adenoma, high-grade carcinoma NOS, e.g., "dedifferentiation" from acinic cell carcinoma, squamous cell carcinoma, salivary duct carcinoma, and metastasis including, but not limited to melanoma.

Acinic Cell Carcinoma

This is a malignant salivary gland neoplasm showing differentiation from intercalated duct / serous acinar cells. It contains cytoplasmic zymogen granules and forms various histologic patterns. Complete surgical excision is the treatment of choice; however, there is 35% recurrence rate and 15% metastatic rate.

Clinical Findings Acinic cell carcinoma represents approximately 20% of salivary gland malignancies, often arises in the parotid gland, and is slightly more common in women, with a peak incidence in the seventh decade of life, but may occur at all ages, including in children, in whom it is the second frequent malignancy after mucoepidermoid carcinoma. In adults, it is the third frequent malignancy after mucoepidermoid carcinoma and adenoid cystic carcinoma. Patients have a slow-growing mass that may be present for months or even years and are commonly asymptomatic, although some masses may cause vague and intermittent pain.

Histopathology The tumor cells grow forming solid, microcystic, papillary-cystic, and follicular patterns, the first two being the most common. Papillary projections supported by thin fibrovascular cores are present in the papillary-cystic pattern. The tumor is similar to thyroid parenchyma in the follicular-patterned tumor and has eosinophilic proteinaceous material lined by columnar or cuboidal cells (Fig. 5.31a).

The cellular elements may have variable proportions of *acinar cells* with polyhedral shape, eccentric round nuclei, and granular cytoplasm with zymogen granules that are characteristic of this tumor and are predominant in well-differentiated tumors. The granules are identified by electron microscopy as round electron-dense cytoplasmic secretory granules. Variable numbers of <u>intercalated ductal cells</u> with columnar or cuboidal shape, eosinophilic cytoplasm, and central nuclei, <u>clear cells</u>, and <u>vacuolated cells</u> may also be present. In summary, this tumor show different architectural patterns and cytologic findings within the same tumor. Chronic inflammation and hemorrhage may be seen. Cell pleomorphism and mitoses are usually absent.

Immuno-Profile Immunostains are not specific and show keratin-, E-cadherin-, SOX10-, and DOG1-positivity (Fig. 5.31b–d). Myoepithelial markers like calponin, actin, and p63 are negative, with high expression for p53, COX2, and bcl-2. Moderate to strong immunoreaction for NR4A3 helps in the diagnosis of acinic cell carcinoma, and is not expressed in normal salivary gland tissues. However, overexpression od NR4A3 is seen in secretory carcinoma, mucoepidermoid carcinoma, polymorphous adenocarcinoma, and

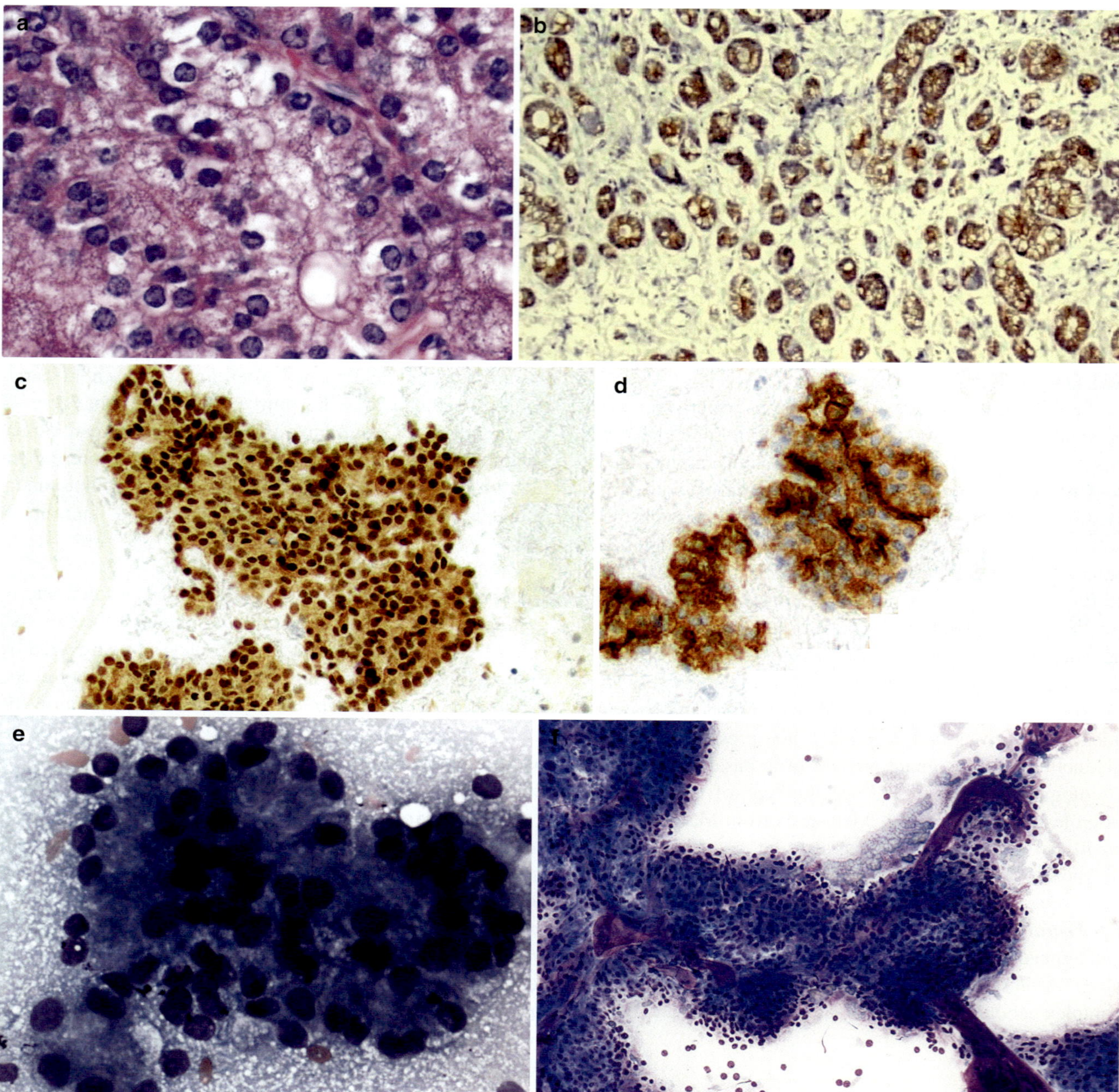

Fig. 5.31 Acinic cell carcinoma. Histopathology (**a**) and positive immunostains for E-cadherin (**b**), SOX-10 (**c**), and DOG-1 (**d**). Cytologic findings (**e–m**). The US images show an irregularly shaped hypoechoic mass with slight heterogeneous echo texture and no vascularity by Doppler examination (**n**, **o**). (**a**, **h**, H&E stain, cell block, medium and high magnification; **b–d**, immunoperoxidase stain, cell block, medium and high magnification; **e**, **f**, **j**, **l**, MGG stain, medium and high magnification; **g**, **k**, **m**, Papanicolaou stain, medium magnification). Courtesy, Dr. Eugenio Leonardo, San Lazzaro Hospital, Alba, Italy (**a–d**)

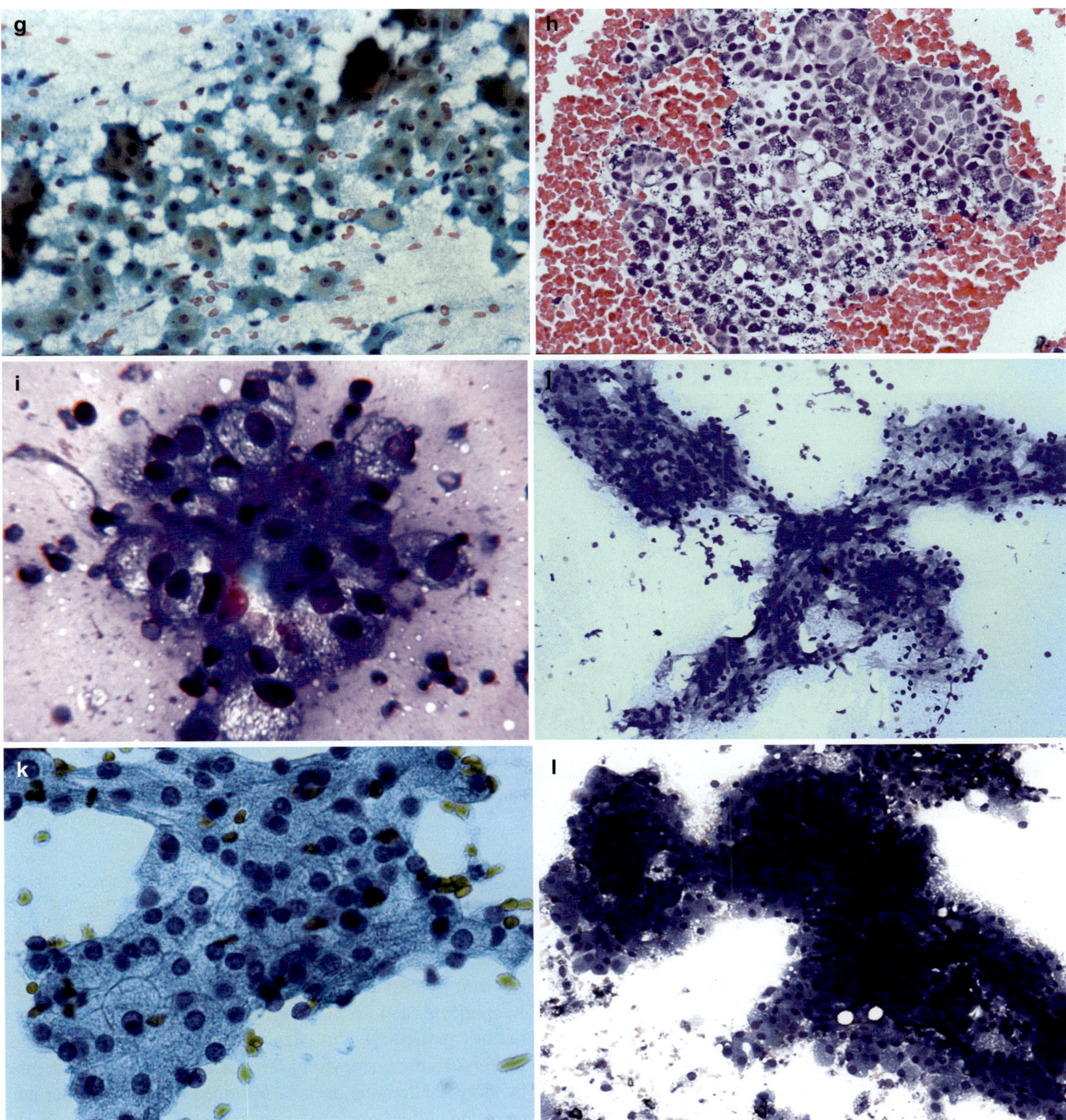

Fig. 5.31 (continued)

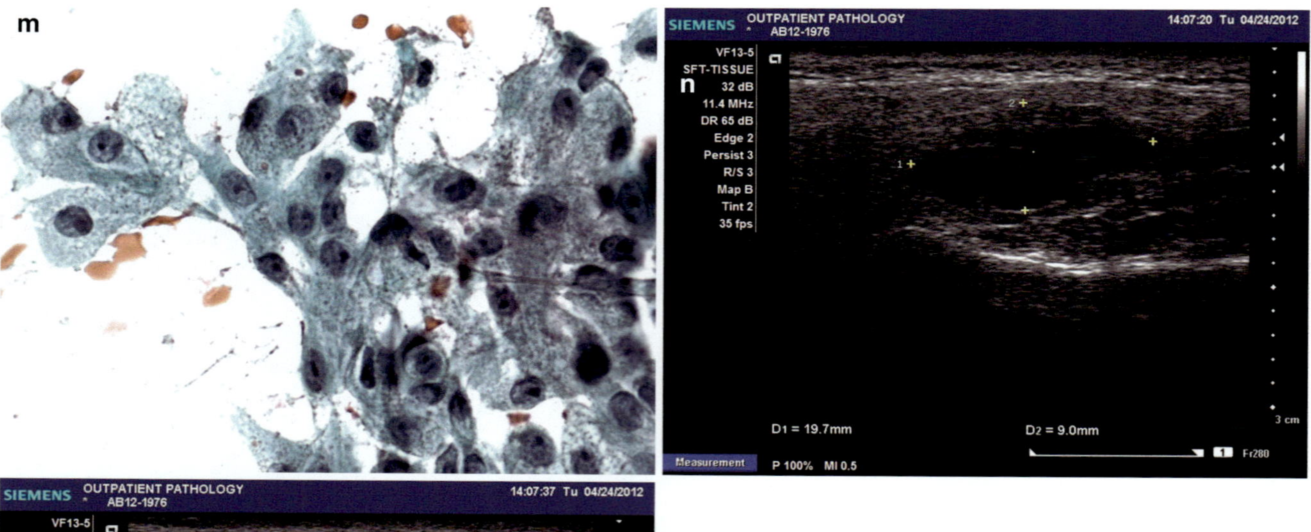

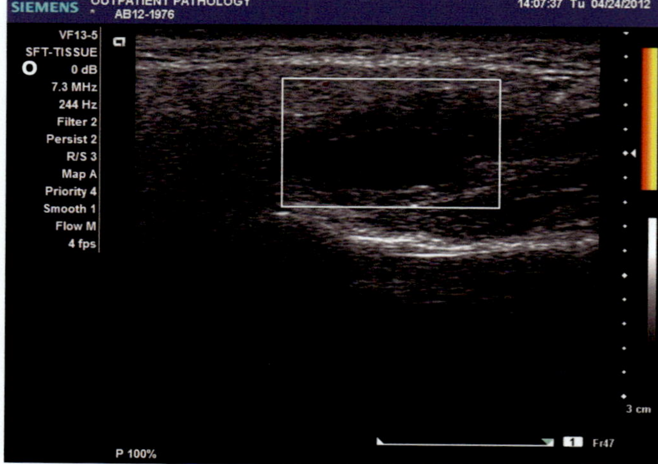

Fig. 5.31 (continued)

pleomorphic adenoma. Acinar and intercalated cells are PAS+ diastase-resistant and mucicarmine-negative. All other cells are PAS (−).

Molecular Profile Recurrent (t[4;9][q13;q31]) genomic rearrangement leading to NR4A3 overexpression has been described.

FNA Findings Aspirates are usually cellular with cells both single and grouped, including formation of acinar arrangements (Fig. 5.31e). Thin vascular structures decorated with cellular elements of variable size and complexities are often present (Fig. 5.31f). The cytoplasmic membrane is friable, and the cells are easily damaged during the smear process, resulting in the presence of numerous naked nuclei and a granular background. Detached small fragments of vascular elements may also be found in the background. Macrophages are identified when cystic change is present.

In contrast to benign salivary gland tissue, well-differentiated acinic cell carcinoma often lacks ductal cells and adipose tissue, unless surrounding benign salivary gland tissue is inadvertently sampled. Lack of the narrow cytoplasmic rim permits the distinction of naked nuclei from small lymphocytes and avoids an erroneous diagnosis of Warthin's tumor, particularly in the presence of cystic change. Distinguishing oncocytoma from acinic cell carcinoma may be more challenging because the smear pattern, cellular features including nuclear characteristics, and smear background are almost identical (Fig. 5.31g). When cell-block slides stained with H&E are available, the basophilic, coarse cytoplasmic granules are more conspicuous than the uniform eosinophilic granules of oncocytoma (Fig. 5.31h). Of note, clear-cell change may be seen in both acinic cell carcinoma and oncocytoma, and even the possibility of epithelial-myoepithelial carcinoma, clear cell adenocarcinoma, and metastatic renal cell carcinoma may be entertained

(Fig. 5.31i). Cystic acinic cell carcinoma may show vacuolated cells resembling low-grade mucoepidermoid carcinoma. Differential diagnosis includes other low-grade salivary gland neoplasms such as mucoepidermoid carcinoma and secretory carcinoma; mammaglobin is negative and helpful to distinguish it from secretory carcinoma. Chronic sialadenitis with clear cell metaplasia may resemble acinic cell carcinoma with clear cell changes (Fig. 5.31j, k). Benign mixed tumor with oncocytic change may resemble acinic cell carcinoma (Fig. 5.31l, m).

US Features The features are not specific, and the tumor is well-demarcated, hypoechoic, heterogeneous, with lobulated borders, and areas of cystic degeneration and necrosis (Fig. 5.31n, o).

Secretory Carcinoma

This tumor was described in 2010 and is strikingly similar to the secretory breast carcinoma not only morphologically but also at the molecular level with identical translocation.

Clinical Findings The tumor appears to be more common in men than in women with an average age of presentation of 45 years and predominantly affects major salivary glands. The tumor is considered of low-grade, has a disease-free survival of 90 months, and may involve regional neck lymph nodes.

Histopathology The architectural pattern is often microcystic; however, macrocystic and solid patterns have been described. Cytologically, the tumor often shows monomorphic large cells with finely vacuolated cytoplasm with bland-appearing round nuclei and small nucleoli. Few mitoses may be present. Hobnailing, eosinophilic vacuolated cytoplasm, and variable mucin production have been described. This tumor must be distinguished from oncocytic tumors, acinic cell carcinoma, low-grade mucoepidermoid carcinoma, and salivary gland duct carcinoma (Fig. 5.32a, b). The histo- and cytomorphology may be similar and the final diagnosis rests upon the molecular detection of the specific and unique translocation.

Immuno-Profile The tumor is strongly positive for S100 protein, mammaglobin, and pan-TRK. High molecular weight keratin, vimentin, EMA, vimentin, MUC1, MUC4, GATA3, STAT5a, GCDFP15, adipophilin, and cytokeratin 19 are also positive (Fig. 5.32c, d). DOG1 and myoepithelial immunostains are negative.

Molecular Profile The translocation between the *ETV6* gene and the *NTRK3* gene located on chromosomes 12p13 and 15q25 is identical to its counterpart in the breast, and seen in almost 100% of tumors, and can be detected by FISH

analysis in paraffin-embedded tissue or FNA cytology material.

FNA Findings Smears are cellular showing cell aggregates and single cells. Cell aggregates may have acinar, tight, small, tubular, or arborizing papillary patterns with transgressing capillaries (Fig. 5.32e, f). Cells have abundant finely granular and variably vacuolated cytoplasm, eccentrically placed round nuclei, and nucleoli of variable size (Fig. 5.32g–i). Ample eosinophilic cytoplasm, binucleation, signet-ring cell-like cells, and mild to moderate nuclear atypia may be seen (Fig. 5.32j–l). Amorphous aggregates of mucin and stripped tumor cell nuclei may be seen in the background (Fig. 5.32m, n).

US Features The features are not specific. Small tumors may be hypoechoic, solid, and homogeneous with irregular borders. Large tumors may have a heterogeneous echotexture with of hypo- and hyperechogenic areas, and ill-defined and infiltrative borders. Vascular blood flow is variable and is inversely proportional to the cystic component of the tumor (Fig 5.32o, r).

Oncocytoma

This rare benign tumor that comprises <1% of salivary gland neoplasms is composed of large cells with granular mitochondria-rich eosinophilic cytoplasm. Complete surgical excision is the treatment of choice.

Clinical Findings The tumor often occurs in the parotid gland, has no gender preference, and occurs in the 6th–eighth decade of life. Patients have a painless mass and are asymptomatic.

Histopathology The tumor is encapsulated with a solid, organoid, and trabecular pattern composed of enlarged, polyhedral oncocytic cells with central round nuclei and conspicuous nucleoli (Fig. 5.33a). Cellular pleomorphism, necrosis, or mitoses are absent. A clear-cell variant, in part due to accumulation of cytoplasmic glycogen, with variable transitional-cell areas may occur.

Immuno-Profile The epithelial elements show an immune-profile similar to that of Warthin's tumor.

Molecular Profile Alterations in mitochondrial DNA mutations have not been consistently found.

FNA Findings The oncocytic cells are arranged in flat sheets, papillary clusters, and as individual cells (Fig. 5.33b, d). Cytologic atypia is focal or absent, bare nuclei and scattered lymphoid cells may be present (Fig. 5.33e, f). Cystic changes may occur. The differential diagnosis includes

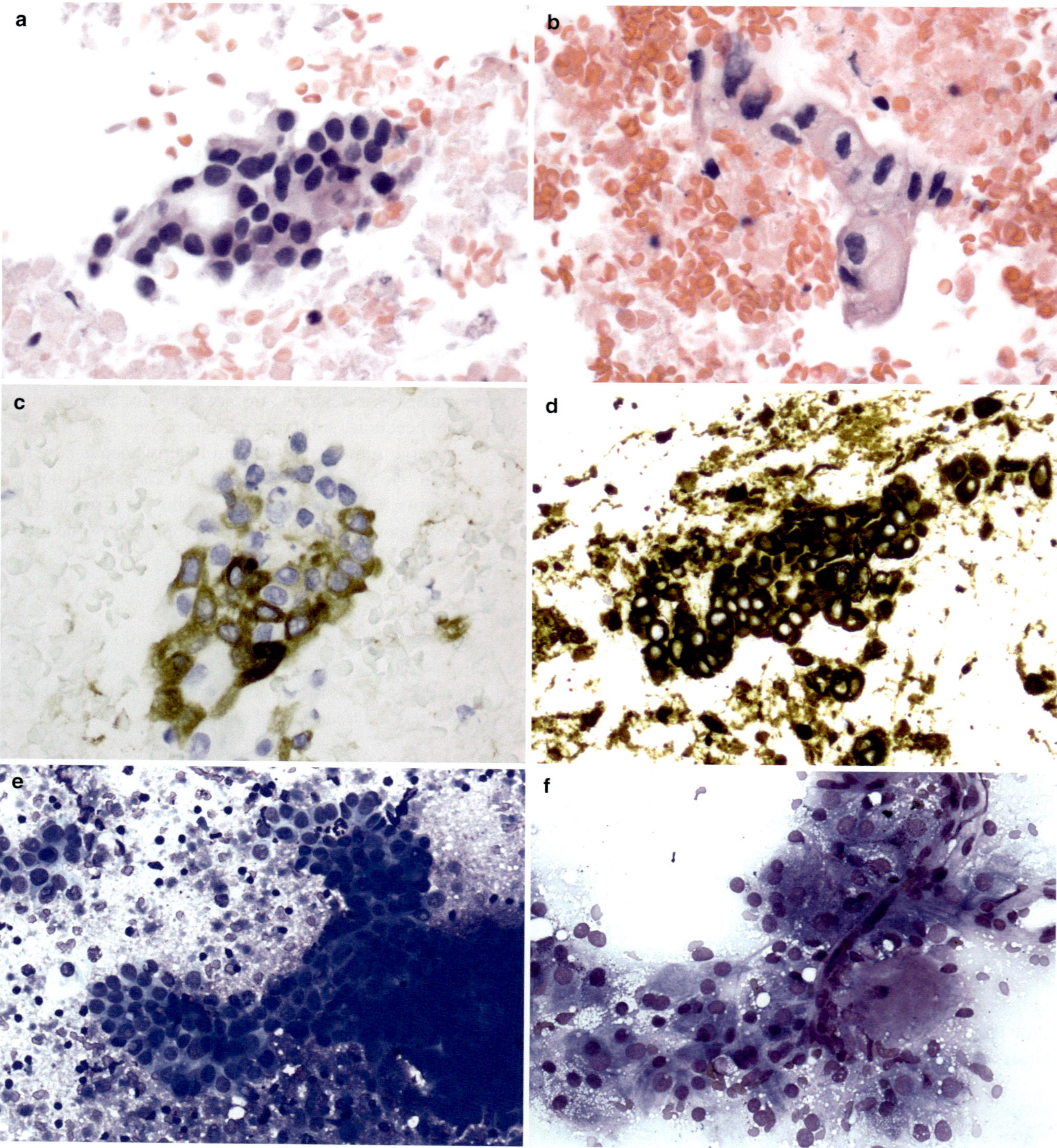

Fig. 5.32 Secretory carcinoma. Histopathology (**a**, **b**) and positive immunostains for mammaglobin (**c**) and CK-7 (**d**). Smears are cellular and show cells with ample eosinophilic dense cytoplasm, granular background and scattered stripped nuclei; large cytoplasmic vacuoles displacing the nucleus to the periphery ("signet ring-like" cells) are also noted. Papanicolaou stained smears show sheets of large cells with eosinophilic cytoplasm, round central and eccentrically placed nuclei, and small inconspicuous nucleoli. Occasional cells with variable cytoplasmic vacuolization are also seen. Note the striking similarity with oncocytic neoplasms, low-grade mucoepidermoid carcinoma, and acinic cell carcinoma (**e–n**). The US shows a large ill-defined parotid mass with heterogeneous echotexture, hyper- and hypoechoic areas, and minimal vascular blood flow (**o**, **p**). A small hypoechoic 11 mm parotid mass with irregular and slightly spiculated borders, and minimal vascular blood flow as seen in a different case (**q**, **r**). (**a**, **b**, H&E stain, cell block, high magnification; **c**, **d**, immunoperoxidase stain, cell block, medium and high magnification; **e,f**, **i**, **m-n**, MGG stain, medium and high magnification; **g-h**, **j-l**, Papanicolaou stain, high magnification)

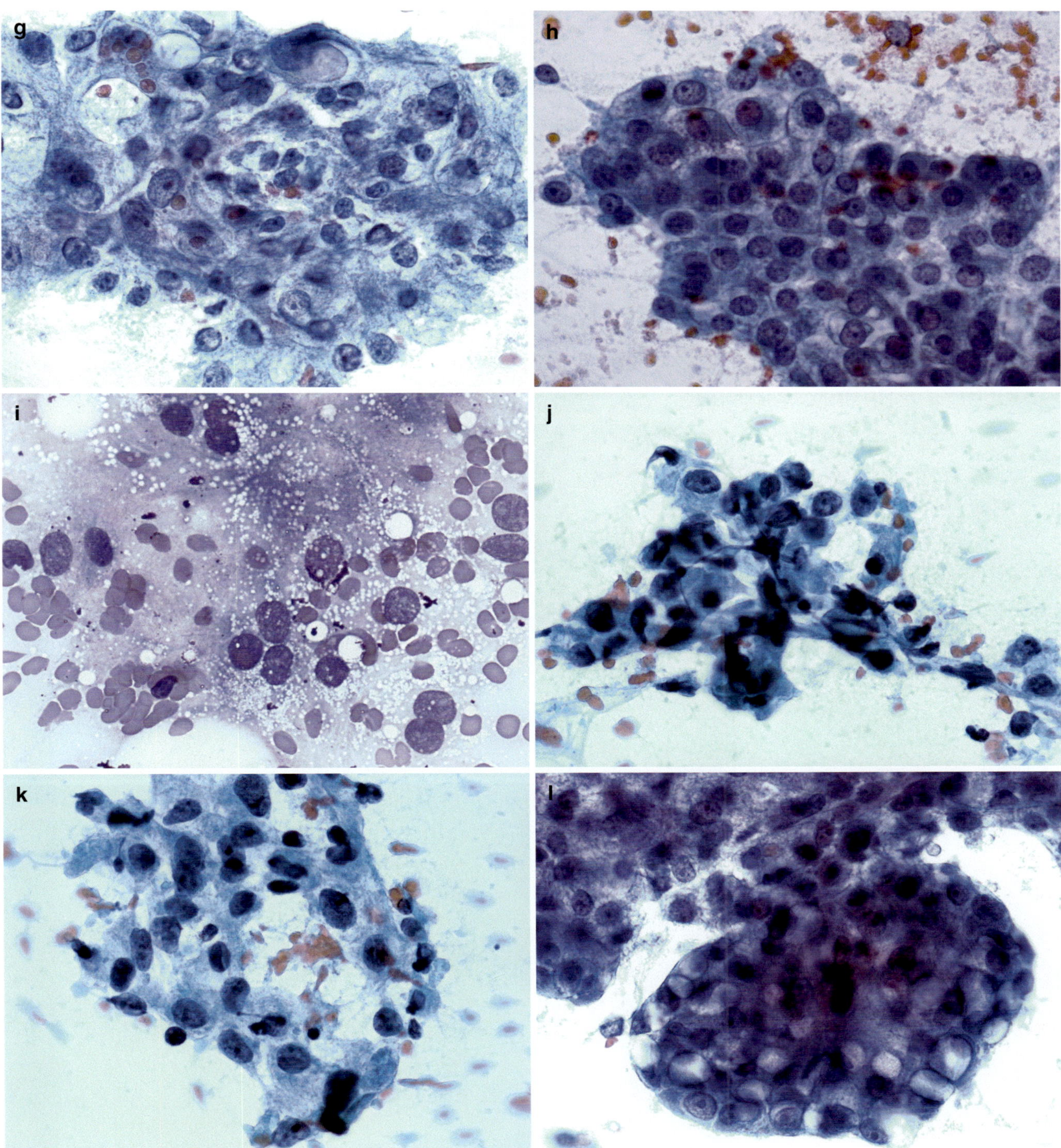

Fig. 5.32 (continued)

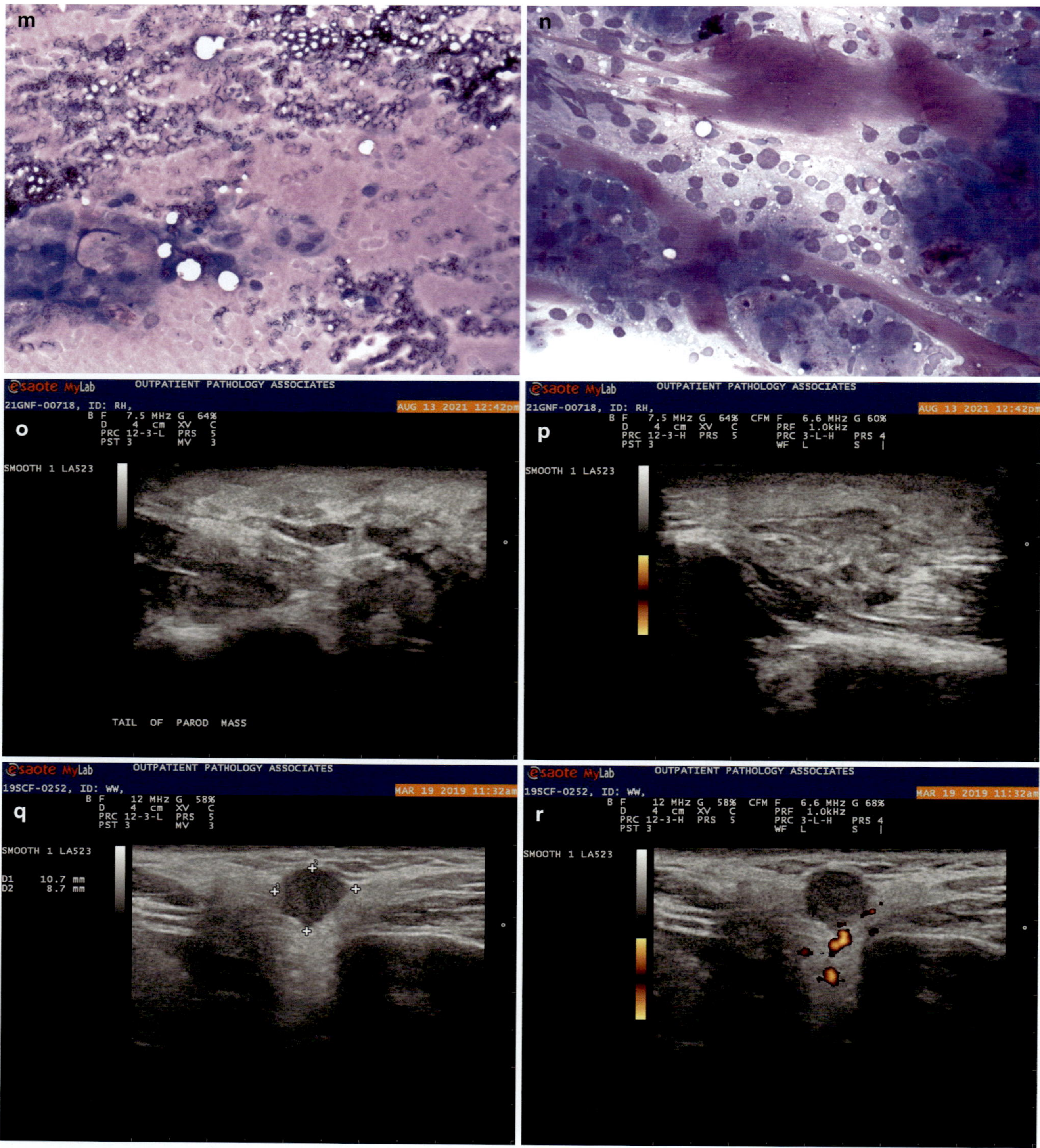

Fig. 5.32 (continued)

oncocytosis or adenomatous hyperplasia, Warthin's tumor, pleomorphic adenoma, and salivary gland carcinoma with oncocytic cells such as mucoepidermoid carcinoma, acinic cell carcinoma, adenoid cystic carcinoma, or oncocytic carcinoma. When clear cells predominate, one should consider clear variants of epithelial-myoepithelial carcinoma, primary salivary gland adenocarcinoma, myoepithelioma, mucoepidermoid carcinoma, and metastatic renal cell carcinoma.

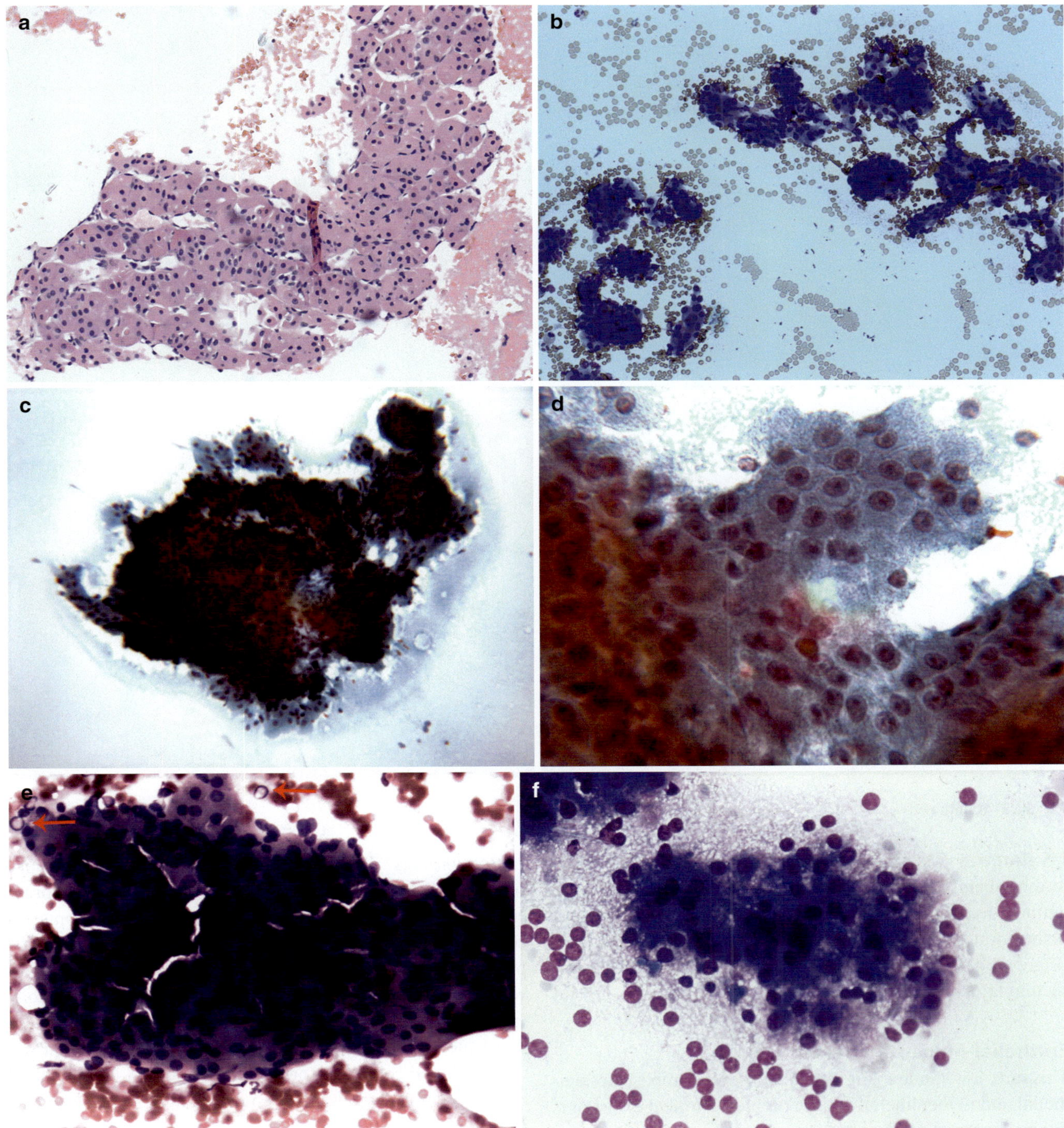

Fig. 5.33 Oncocytoma. Histopathology (**a**). Cytologic features (**b–f**). The red arrows (**e**) point to rare lymphoid cells that may be found in oncocytoma. The US findings are not specific (**g–j**). (**a**, H&E stain, cell block, medium magnification; **b**, **e**, MGG stain, high magnification; **c**, **d**, Papanicolaou stain low and medium magnification; **f**, DiffQuik stain, high magnification)

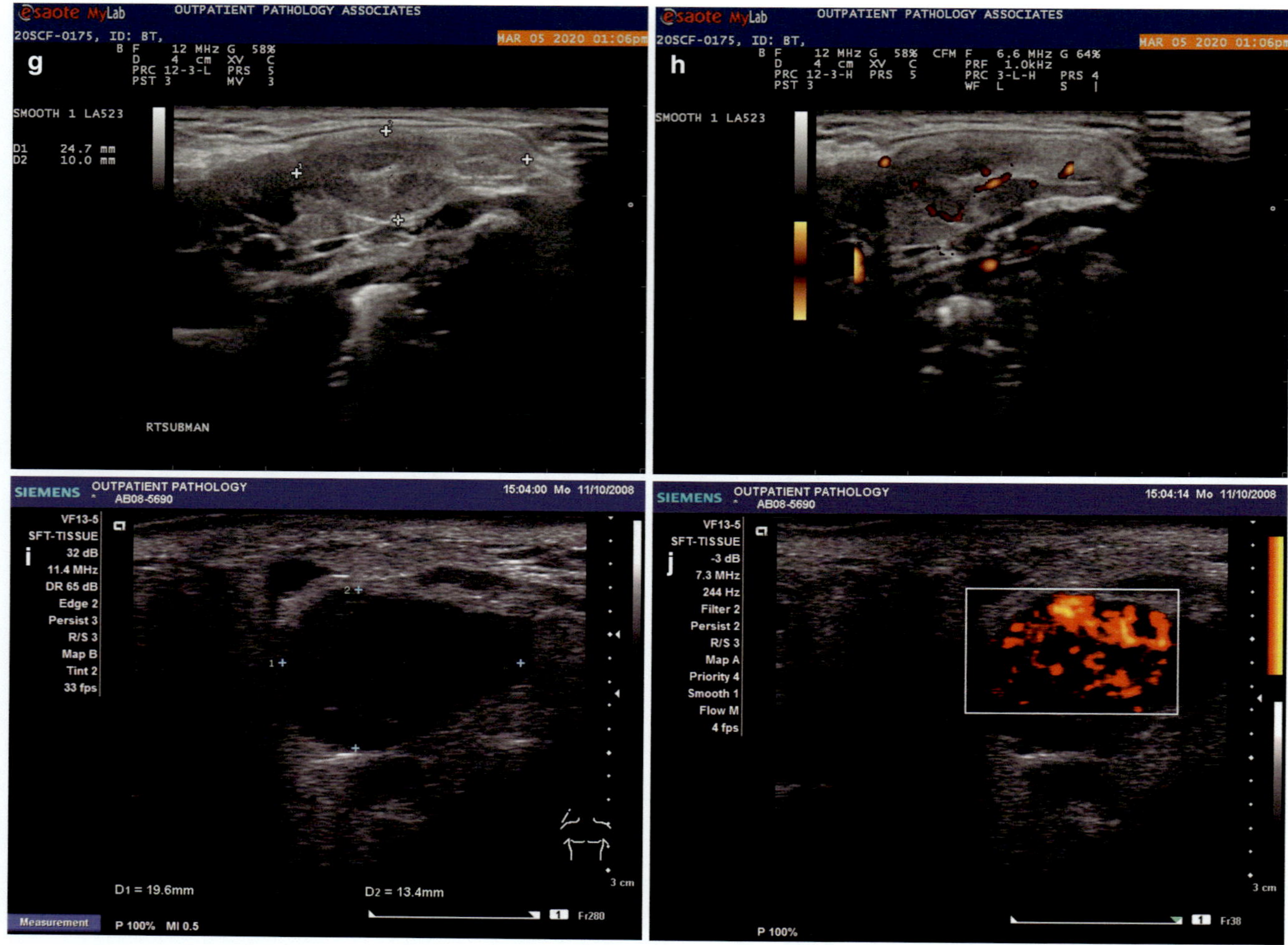

Fig. 5.33 (continued)

US Features There is no typical US pattern; this is similar to other benign lesions. The tumor is a round or oval, well-defined hypoechoic homogeneous mass. Power Doppler demonstrates peripheral and intratumor blood flow (Fig. 5.33g–j). Cystic and hemorrhagic degeneration may be seen in tumors >3 cm.

Epithelial-Myoepithelial Carcinoma

This rare, low-grade malignant neoplasm is composed of epithelial and myoepithelial cells. Complete surgical excision is the treatment of choice; however, there is a 30–50% recurrence rate and 20% metastatic rate. High-grade transformation or dedifferentiation to other salivary gland tumors can occur.

Clinical Findings The tumor often develops in the parotid gland, is slightly more common in women, and occurs in the sixth and seventh decade of life. Patients have a slow-growing, often painless mass. Facial nerve paralysis is infrequent.

Histopathology Tumor cells often show tubular, cystic, solid, papillary, and trabecular growth patterns that are present in various proportions within the tumor. The neoplastic cells are of two types: epithelial cuboidal with scant eosinophilic cytoplasm and myoepithelial polyhedral, large cells with vacuolated clear cytoplasm. Epithelial cells are inconspicuous in solid tumors, where the myoepithelial cells predominate. Of note, the epithelial-cell layer is single, but the myoepithelial cells may form several layers. A dual layer of inner epithelial and outer myoepithelial lining cells is visualized in tumors that have cystic and tubular components. The separating stroma may be fibrovascular, myxoid, hyaline, or dense and is PAS-positive. Mitoses, necrosis, or marked cellular anaplasia are not typically present. Oncocytic, apocrine, and sebaceous differentiation may occur.

Immuno-Profile The epithelial cells are positive for cytokeratin, CEA, CD117, and EMA. Myoepithelial cells are p63-, CK5/6-, calponin-, actin-, vimentin-, SOX10, and S100 protein-positive. Bcl-2 is frequently positive.

Molecular Profile *HRAS* mutations are present in 82% of epithelial myoepithelial carcinomas and help in the distinction from adenoid cystic carcinoma, basal cell adenoma, basal cell adenocarcinoma, and myoepithelial carcinoma that lack *HRAS* mutations. However, these mutations can be found in other salivary gland tumors including salivary duct carcinoma.

FNA Findings Smears are usually cellular and show two patterns, small dark epithelial cells with scant dense cytoplasm and large myoepithelial cells with distinct borders and ample and clear glycogen-rich cytoplasm (Fig. 5.34a–d). However, myoepithelial cells have a fragile cytoplasm and may be present as naked nuclei or cells without much cytoplasm. This may be the predominant pattern. Fragments of acellular hyaline material, which may be globular and laminated, may be present, suggesting adenoid cystic carcinoma (Fig. 5.34e, f). When clear cells predominate, alternate diagnoses to consider include hyalinizing clear cell adenocarcinoma, clear cell acinic cell carcinoma, sebaceous carcinoma, or metastatic renal cell carcinoma; however, these tumors do not exhibit a dual cell population. Likewise, myoepithelioma, myoepithelial carcinoma, and cellular pleomorphic adenoma lack the biphasic pattern and the prominent presence of clear myoepithelial cells seen in epithelial myoepithelial carcinoma. Thus, a thorough sampling is required for a correct diagnosis.

US Features Features of epithelial-myoepithelial carcinoma mimic those of a benign salivary gland tumor. Our case images show a mass with prominent cystic component. The solid component is isoechoic, homogeneous, and well circumscribed with smooth borders. The cystic component was substantially drained (not shown) (Fig. 5.34g–h).

Hyalinizing Clear Cell Adenocarcinoma

This is a rare malignant epithelial neoplasm composed of monotonous clear cells. The tumor has ductal, but not myoepithelial cell differentiation. Complete surgical resection is the treatment of choice for this low-grade neoplasm. Prognosis is good; however, local recurrence and lymph node metastases may be seen.

Clinical Findings The tumor often develops in the intraoral minor salivary glands and occurs mostly in females. There is no age preference. Patients present with swelling and may have pain and mucosal ulceration.

Histopathology Polygonal to round cells with clear glycogen-rich cytoplasm, eccentric round nuclei and small nucleoli are arranged in sheets, nests, and cords. Ductal structures are absent. There is mild to moderate nuclear pleomorphism, and mitoses are rare. The stroma is usually thin and fibrous, but may be broad and thick, hyalinized or loose. The differential diagnosis includes clear cell mucoepidermoid carcinoma, myoepithelial neoplasms, epithelial myoepithelial carcinoma (when clear cells predominate), and metastatic renal cell carcinoma.

Immuno-Profile Tumors are strongly positive for cytokeratin, p63, CEA, and EMA. There is variable positivity with p16, vimentin and GFAP. However, myoepithelial markers such as, S100 protein, calponin, and smooth muscle actin are usually negative. SOX10, DOG1 and CD117 immunostains are negative.

Molecular Profile Tumors show a consistent translocation t(12;22) involving the *EWSR1* (Ewing sarcoma breakpoint region *1*) gene and the *ATF1* gene. This marker may be used to differentiate this tumor from other salivary gland tumors that do not harbor this translocation such as myoepithelioma, acinic cell carcinoma, pleomorphic adenoma, mucoepidermoid carcinoma, oncocytic neoplasms, salivary duct carcinoma, adenoid cystic carcinoma, and polymorphous adenocarcinoma.

FNA Findings Smears are cellular and show groups and sheets of cells with well-defined cytoplasmic borders, uniform round nuclei, small nucleoli, and abundant clear cytoplasm. Hyaline globules are absent, although fragments of hyalinized stroma may be present.

Salivary Duct Carcinoma

This high-grade malignancy arises from the excretory ducts and resembles breast carcinoma on histology. Treatment of choice includes complete excision with radical neck dissection, and postoperative radiotherapy. There is a 30–40% recurrence rate, 50–60% metastatic rate, and 60–80% mortality rate.

Clinical Findings This rare tumor is more common in men, often occurs after the age of 50 years, represent 10% of malignant salivary gland tumors, and commonly affects the parotid gland. When the parotid gland is affected, patients have a rapidly growing mass, with or without local pain and / or facial nerve paralysis. Most cases represent malignant transformation from an existing pleomorphic adenoma (carcinoma ex-pleomorphic adenoma).

Histopathology The tumor resembles the pathologic findings of intraductal and infiltrating ductal breast carcinoma, including comedo necrosis and cribriform, solid, cystic, and papillary patterns. Neoplastic cells are large with large hyperchromatic nuclei, prominent nucleoli, and slightly eosinophilic cytoplasm. Necrosis and mitosis are often present. Squamous metaplasia, oncocytic changes, chronic

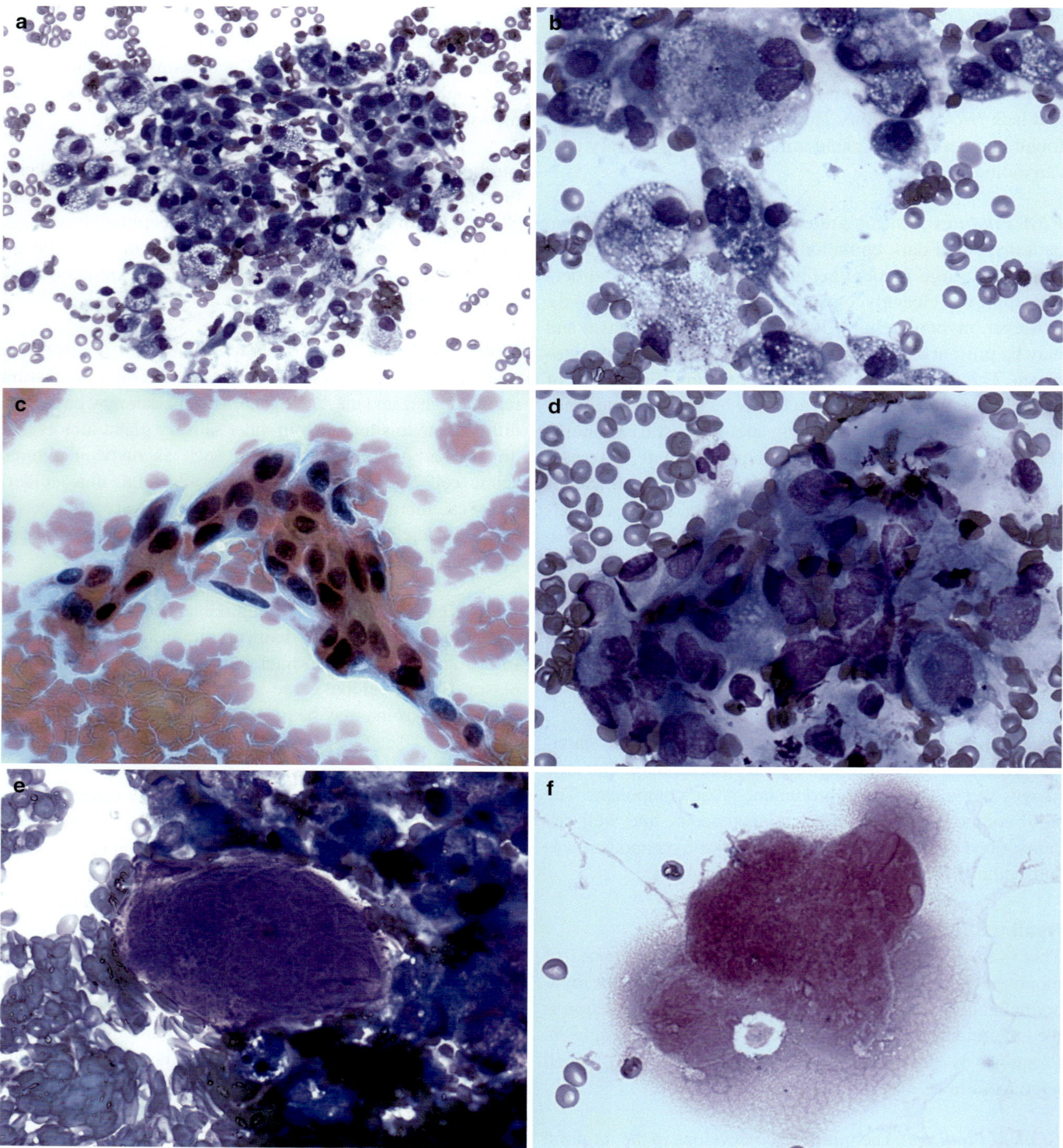

Fig. 5.34 Epithelial-myoepithelial carcinoma. Cytologic features (**a–f**). Note the globular laminated extracellular material that is characteristic of this tumor (**e**, **f**). The US showed a mixed cystic and solid (isoechoic to the parotid tissue) mass (**g**, **h**). (**a**, **b**, **d**, **e**, MGG stain, medium and high magnification; **c**, **f**, Papanicolaou stain, high magnification)

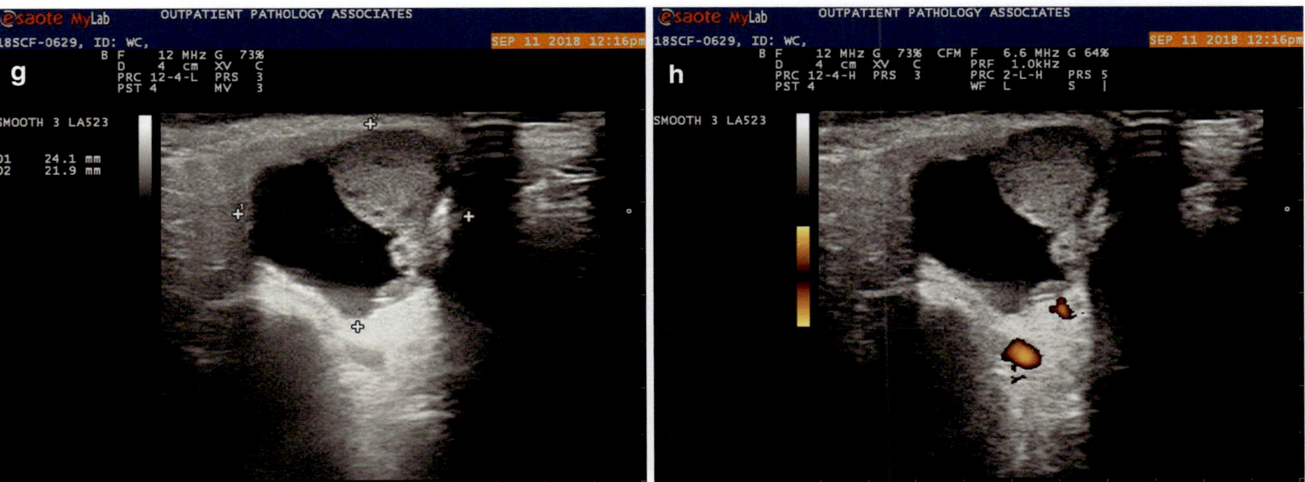

Fig. 5.34 (continued)

inflammation, and psammoma-like bodies may be present. Histologic variants including sarcomatoid, papillary, micropapillary, oncocytic, mucin-rich, and osteoclast-like giant cell may occur, as in breast carcinoma (Fig. 5.35a).

Immuno-Profile Salivary duct carcinoma expresses some markers also found in breast carcinoma. Gross cystic disease fluid protein-15 (GCDFP-15) is found in 80% of cases (Fig. 5.35b). HER-2/neu is positive in 90% of cases; however, it depends on the antibody clone used and scoring system (Fig. 5.35c). ER and PR expression is exceptional; in contrast, androgen receptor (AR) positivity is seen in 67–83% of cases (Fig. 5.35d). Cytokeratin, EMA, and CEA are also positive. Myoepithelial differentiation markers including p63, calponin, smooth-muscle actin, and vimentin may be positive, particularly in carcinoma ex-pleomorphic adenoma.

Molecular Profile There is loss of heterozygosity of polymorphic markers of chromosome locus 9p21 containing the tumor suppressor gene *p16*(INK4a/CDKN2/MTS1). The apoptosis-related genes *CASP10* and *MMP11* are overexpressed.

FNA Findings Smears are cellular and show a high-grade carcinoma pattern. Complex tri-dimensional aggregates and flat sheets are present arranged in cribriform, solid, and papillary patterns. Occasional psammoma bodies, squamous metaplastic cells, and comedo-like necrosis may be seen. Cells are large and polyhedral with granular or vacuolated cytoplasm, large hyperchromatic nuclei, prominent nucleoli, and increased mitotic activity (Fig. 5.35e–j). Differential diagnosis includes high-grade mucoepidermoid carcinoma, metastatic adenocarcinoma mainly of breast and lung origins, and metastatic squamous cell carcinoma. Intracellular

mucin and keratinization are exceedingly rare in salivary duct carcinoma and help in the diagnosis of metastases. Clinical history and judicious use of immunohistochemical stains are essential and complement the FNA findings.

US Features Features are not specific and include hypoechoic and heterogeneous echotexture, ill-defined irregular and spiculated margins, and variable vascular blood flow (Fig. 5.35k–n). Regional lymph node metastases are present in some cases.

Metastases

Malignant neoplasms showing large cells and a high nuclear grade, including metastases, are rare, and a specific FNA diagnosis based on cytomorphology only cannot be made in most cases. In such cases, it is sufficient to state the diagnosis of a high-grade malignancy and exclude direct extension of a head and neck tumor or metastasis to the salivary gland or intraparotid lymph node to avoid unnecessary surgery. A clinical history of previous malignancy, comparison of the histo- and/or cytomorphologic features, and the use of immunostains are of extreme importance to render a precise diagnosis (Fig. 5.36a–f). In general, a metastatic deposit must be suggested when the smear pattern is different from that of known salivary gland malignancies.

Pattern VIII. Spindle Cell Pattern

Processes showing this pattern can be divided into low grade and high grade. Myoepithelioma is the typical example of low-nuclear-grade lesions and primary or secondary sarcomas, myoepithelial carcinoma, and malignancies with spindle cell morphology including metastatic melanoma, should be considered in the high-grade group. These tumors are

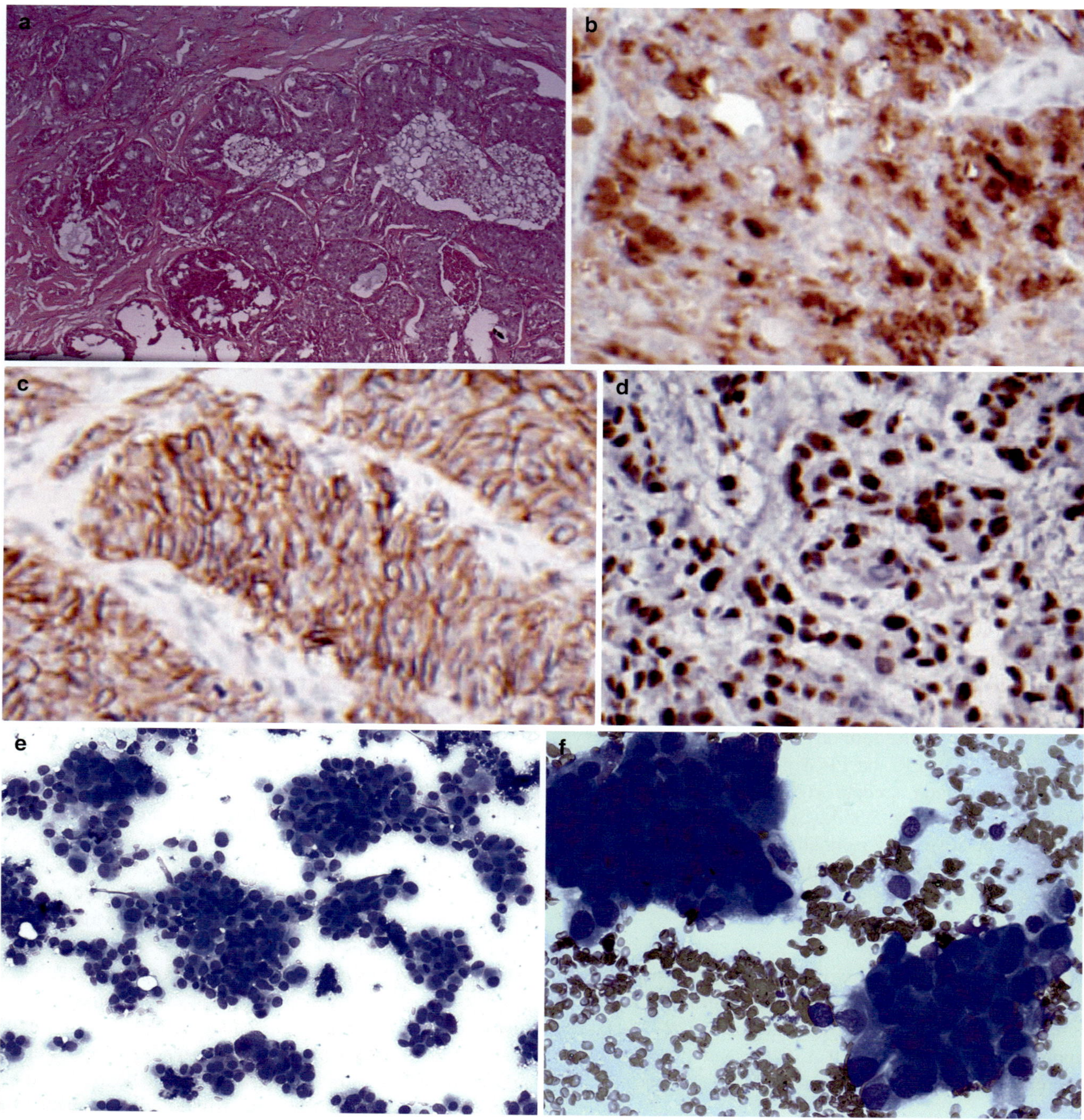

Fig. 5.35 Salivary duct carcinoma. Histopathology (**a**) and positive immnunostains for GCDFP, HER-2, and androgen receptor (**b–d**). Cytologic features (**e–j**). Cytologically and histologically this tumor is almost indistinguishable from ductal breast carcinoma. The US from two different cases shows a large hypoechoic heterogeneous parotid mass with spiculated, irregular, and ill-defined borders (**k**, **l**, arrows) and a 13 mm hypoechoic submandibular gland mass with irregular borders (**m**, **n**). (**a**, H&E stain, low magnification; **b–d**, immunoperoxidase stain, medium and high magnification; **e–h**, MGG stain, medium and high magnification; **i-j**, Papanicolaou stain, medium and high magnification). Courtesy, Dr. Eugenio Leonardo, San Lazzaro Hospital, Alba, Italy (**b-d**)

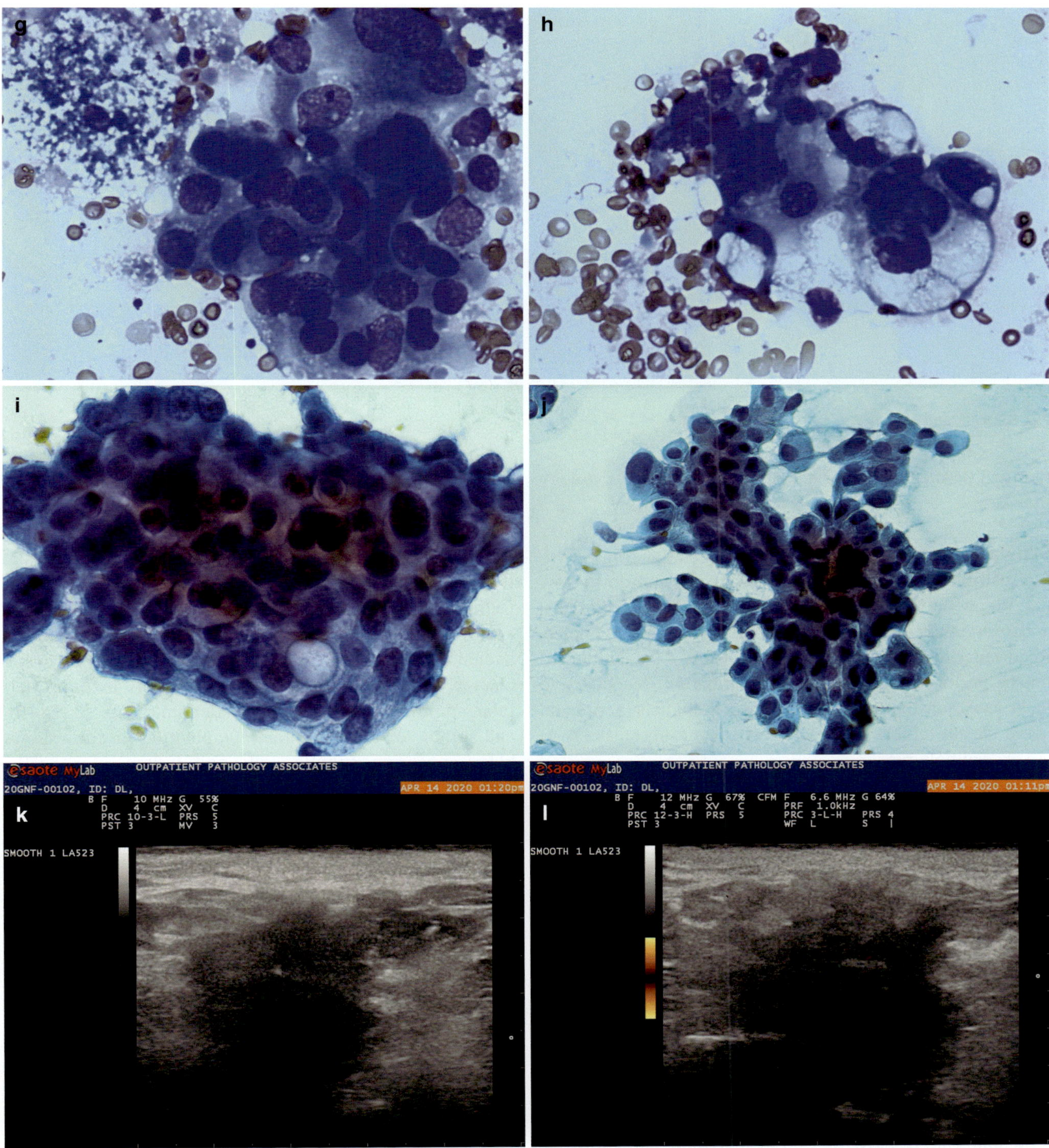

Fig. 5.35 (continued)

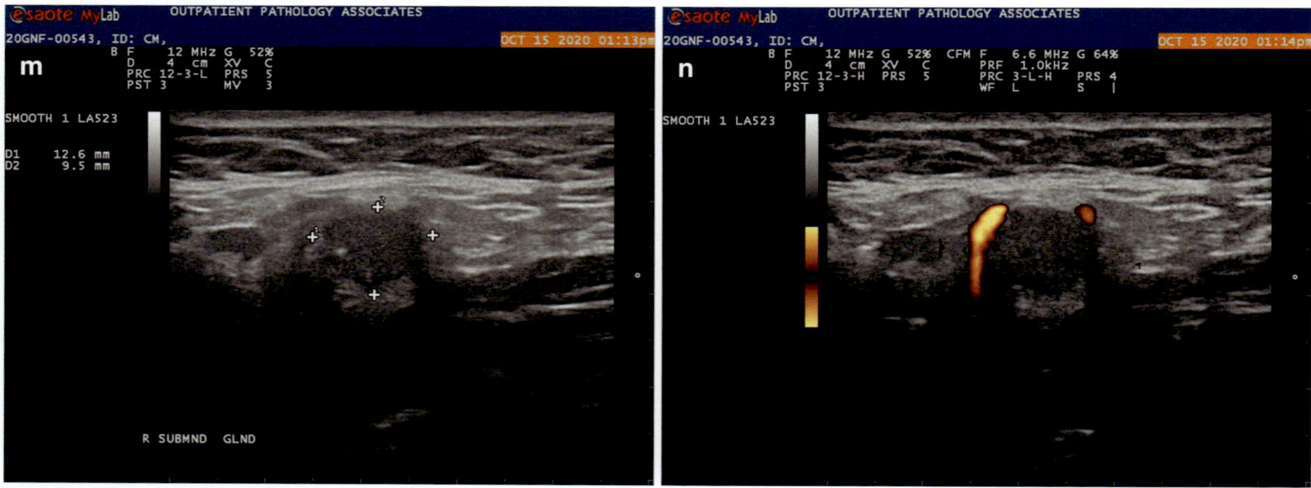

Fig. 5.35 (continued)

rarely described in either the histopathology or cytology literature.

Schwannoma

Intraparotid facial nerve Schwannoma is rare and slow growing. Preoperative diagnosis is difficult, and if made by FNA, a conservative management can be treatment of choice. Recurrence may occur if complete excision of the tumor cannot be performed. Malignant transformation, secondary to local radiation exposure, or de novo malignant peripheral nerve sheath tumors (associated with neurofibromatosis 1) are exceedingly rare.

Clinical Findings Parotid Schwannomas are slightly more common in men in the third to fourth decades, are usually painless, and without facial nerve dysfunction.

Histopathology Cellular Anthony A areas with cell palisading (Verocay bodies), and myxoid hypocellular Anthony B (may not be evident in small tumors) patterns are seen along with a lymphoid cell cuff (Fig. 5.37a). Cystic change may be identified, particularly in long-standing Schwannomas.

Immuno-Profile Cells are positive for S100 protein (Fig. 5.37b), calretinin, SOX-10 (Fig. 5.37c), CD56, podoplanin, and vimentin. Keratin, desmin, and smooth muscle actin stains are negative as well as myoepithelial and melanoma markers (except melanocytic Schwannoma).

Molecular Profile Loss of function of the tumor suppressor gene, *merlin.*

FNA Findings An intense pain may be elicited at the time of needle insertion into the mass resulting in a nondiagnostic smear pattern; however, interlacing fascicles of bland-appearing spindle cells pointy ends, fibrillary cytoplasm, elongated "twisted" nuclei, and a fibrillary myxoid stroma may be identified when sampling is adequate. Scattered benign small lymphocytes are also present and their identification may require a diligent search. Cellularity is variable (Fig. 5.37d, e). Anisocytosis and anisonucleosis with bizarre appearing nuclei are seen in ancient Schwannoma, usually with associated cystic change (Fig. 5.37f). Differential diagnosis includes cellular spindle cell pleomorphic adenoma (Fig. 5.37g, h), and spindle cell myoepithelioma. Nodular fasciitis shows bland-appearing spindle cells and inflammatory cells. Spindle cell malignancies, e.g., carcinoma, melanoma, and sarcoma exhibit cellular pleomorphism and mitoses and are excluded based on clinical history and a judicious use of ancillary studies.

US Features The sonographic features are non-specific and similar to those of other benign parotid tumors. Features include a well-circumscribed mass of variable size, smooth borders, solid, hypoechoic, and homogeneous, or slightly heterogeneous echotexture (Fig. 5.37i, j). Masses are anechoic when cystic change is present (Fig. 5.37k, l).

Myoepithelioma

This tumor is a benign neoplasm composed of spindle, epithelioid, plasmacytoid, or clear cells. Complete surgical excision is the treatment of choice. Recurrence is related to incomplete excision.

Clinical Findings This slow-growing tumor is rare, has no gender predilection, often occurs in adults with an average age of 44 years, and develops preferentially in the parotid gland.

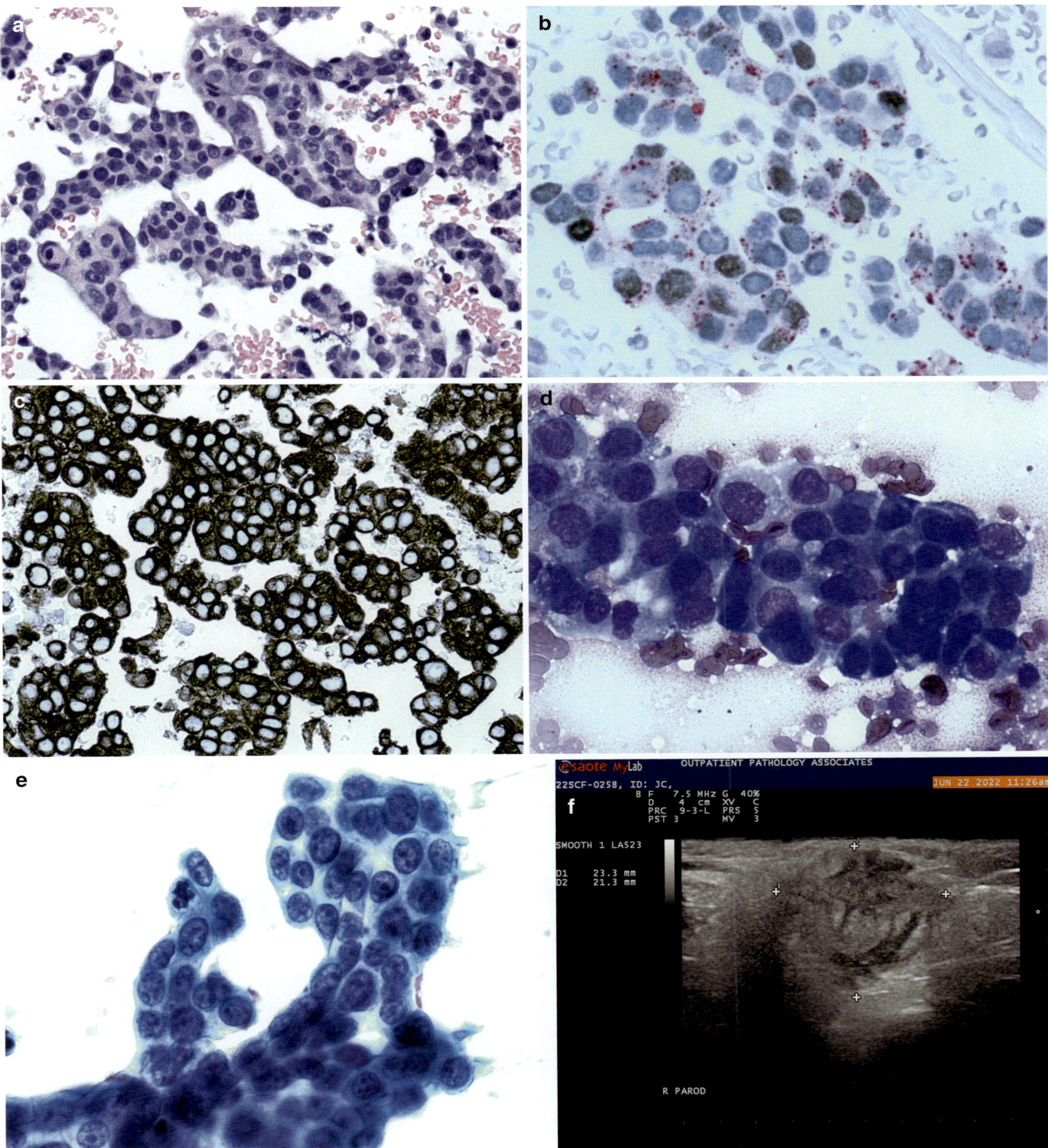

Fig. 5.36 Metastatic adenocarcinoma from pulmonary origin. Histopathology (**a**) and positive immnunostains for TTF-1 / NapsinA (**b**) and CK7 (**c**). Cytologic features (**d, e**). The US shows a large ill-defined parotid mass with heterogeneous echotexture and hyper- and hypoechoic areas (**f**). (**a**, H&E stain, cell block, medium magnification; **b, c**, immunoperoxidase stain, medium and high magnification; **d**, MGG stain, high magnification; **e**, Papanicolaou stain, high magnification)

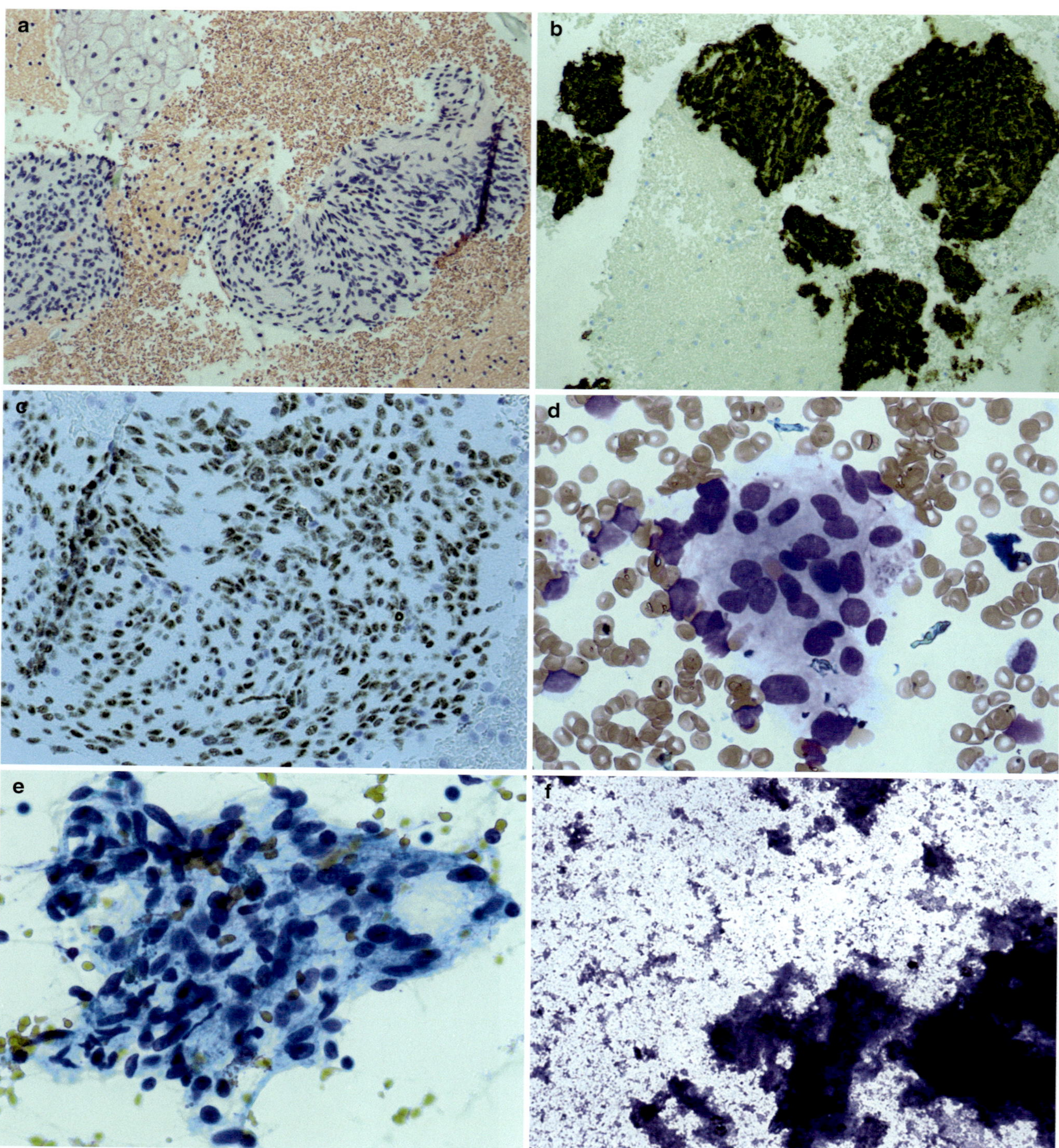

Fig. 5.37 Schwannoma. Histopathology (**a**) and positive stains for S-100 protein (**b**) and SOX-10 (**c**). Cytologic features (**d**, **e**). A cystic change may be present in ancient Schwannomas (**f**). A benign mixed tumor (pleomorphic adenoma) showing a spindle cell pattern that is similar to that of Schwannoma (**g**, **h**). The US shows a solid, homogeneous, hypoechoic mass with loculated borders (**i**, **j**). A cystic anechoic mass with lobulated borders and prominent posterior acoustic enhancement is seen in a cystic Schwannoma (**k**, **l**). The vascular blood flow is minimal or absent. (**a**, H&E stain, cell block, low magnification; **b**, immunostain, medium magnification; **c**, immunoperoxidase stain, medium magnification; **d**, **f**–**h**, MGG stain, medium and high magnification; **e**, Papanicolaou stain, high magnification)

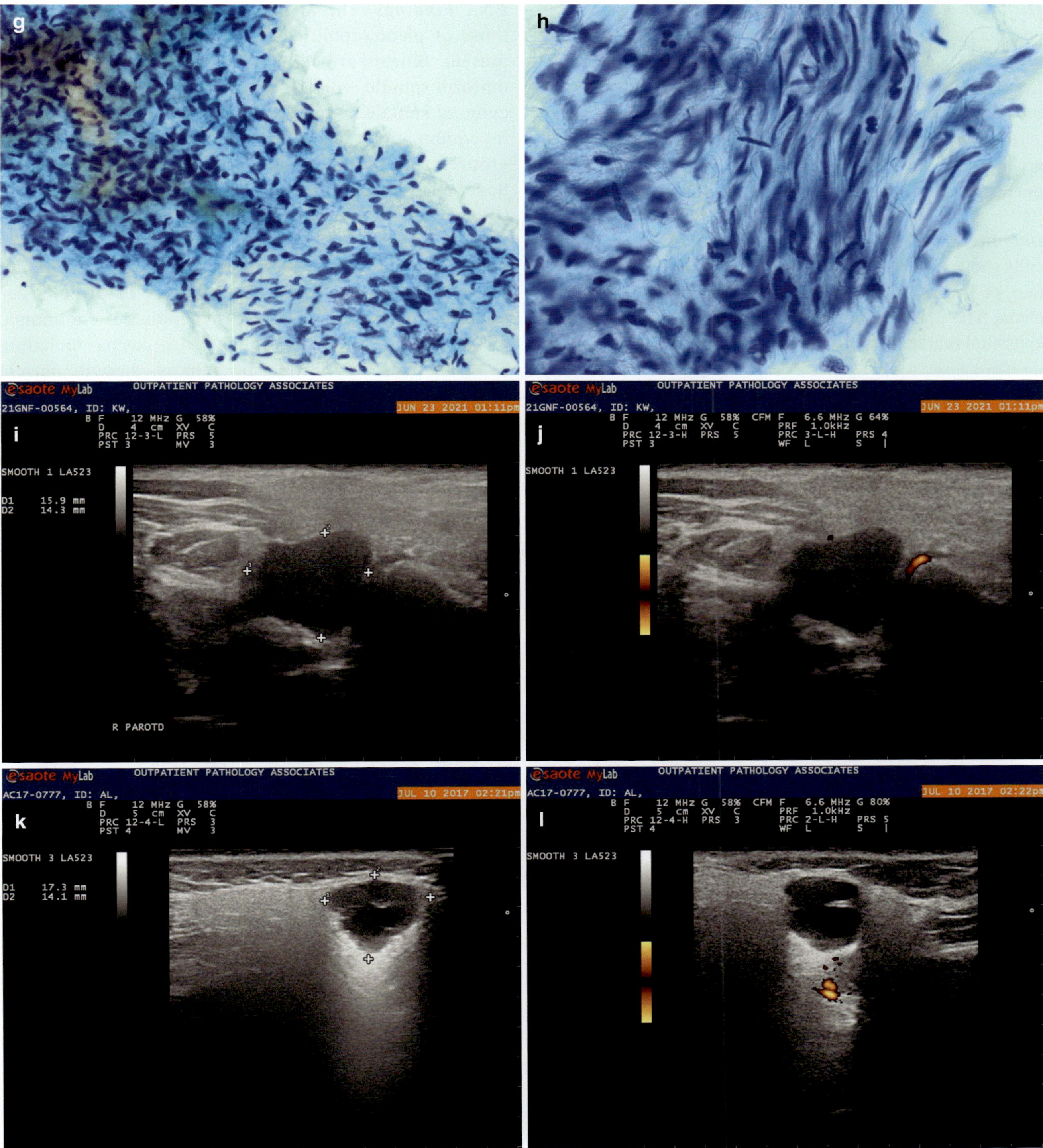

Fig. 5.37 (continued)

Histopathology Spindle, epithelioid, clear, plasmacytoid, and oncocytic variants are described; a combination of cell types may occur. Spindle cells are arranged in interlacing fascicles resembling stroma. The stroma is collagenous, hyalinized, myxoid, or mucoid.

Plasmacytoid cells are often seen in myoepitheliomas arising in the minor salivary glands and are often unencapsulated.

Immuno-Profile Cells are positive for cytokeratins. Spindle cells show variable reactivity with actin, calponin, S100 protein, p63, SOX10, GFAP, and smooth-muscle myosin heavy chain. The plasmacytoid variant may be negative for myoepithelial markers.

Molecular Profile *NTF3-PLAG1*, *FBXO32-PLAG1,* and *GEM-PLAG1* fusions have been detected in the oncocytic variant. Alterations of chromosomes 1, 9, 12, and 13 have been detected.

FNA Findings The myoepithelial cells are identical to those of pleomorphic adenoma. Epithelial cells are not present. Smears are cellular and show bland-appearing, uniform spindle, epithelioid / plasmacytoid, clear, oncocytic, or stellate myoepithelial cells. Cells can be present in combination, but often one predominates. Nuclear grooves and intranuclear inclusions may be present. Scant mucoid, myxoid, and fibrillary matrix may be seen (Fig. 5.38a, b). The stroma may have a globular appearance in some cases, resembling adenoid cystic carcinoma. Marked nuclear pleomorphism or mitoses are not present. Differential diagnosis includes basal cell adenoma, pleomorphic adenoma, myoepithelial carcinoma, plasmacytoma, and spindle cell neoplasms including Schwannoma, myofibroblastic tumors, smooth muscle tumors, nodular fasciitis, melanoma, sarcomas, and spindle cell carcinomas. A pattern of large clear cells in a mucinous background must be distinguished from adenocarcinoma.

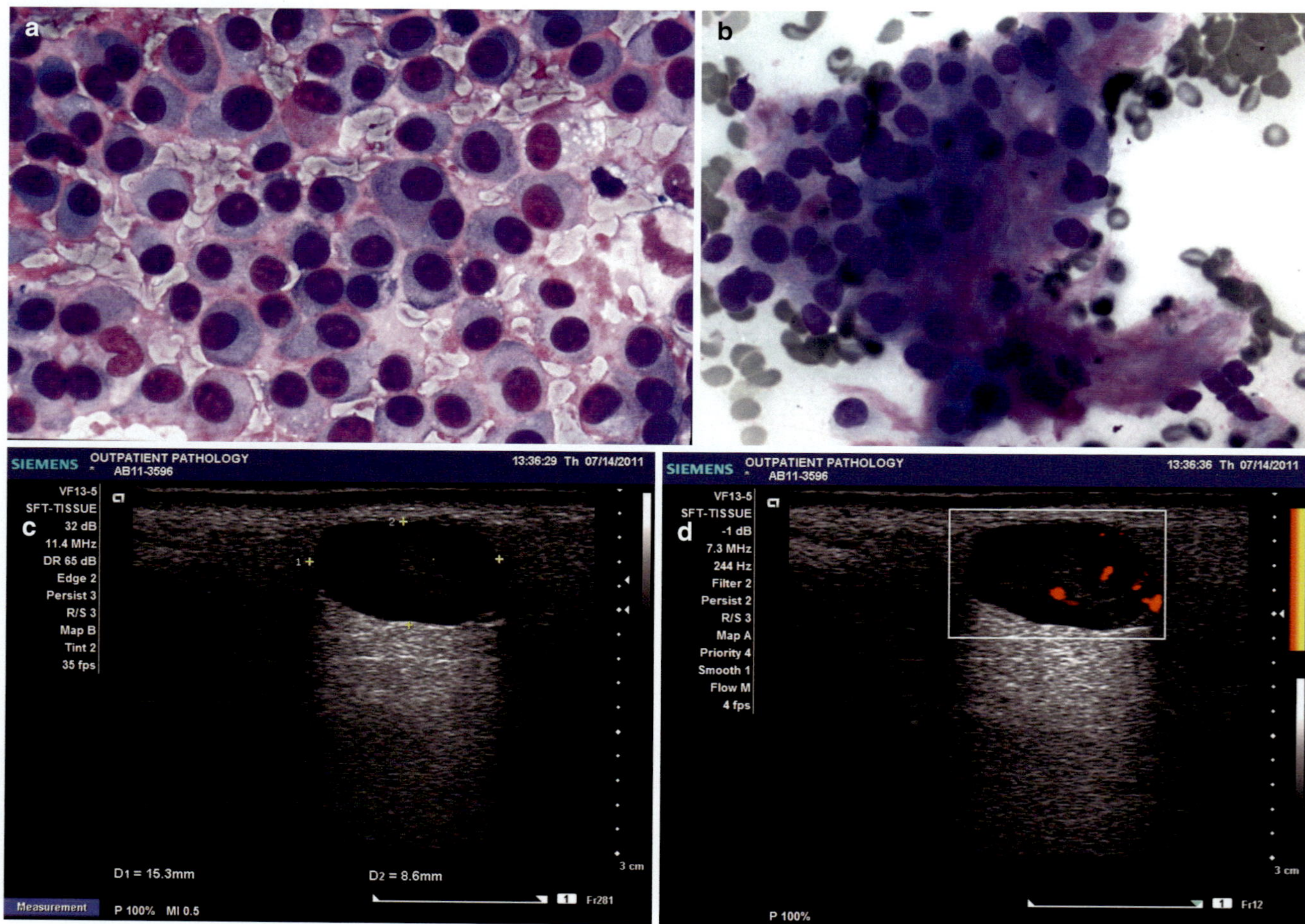

Fig. 5.38 Myoepithelioma. Numerous myoepithelial cells are present both single and supported by a collagenous stroma with lack of fibrillary magenta features (**a, b**). The US findings are non-specific including oval, slightly lobulated well-defined tumor edges, marked hypoechogenicity, and minimal internal vascularity by Doppler examination (**c, d**). (**a**, DiffQuik stain, high magnification; **b**, MGG stain, high magnification)

US Features The sonographic characteristics of benign and malignant neoplasms have no significant differences. Thus, US cannot differentiate with certainty between benign and malignant cases, particularly in low-grade neoplasms (Fig. 5.38c, d). US findings reported in a 7.8 cm tumor included a well-circumscribed mass with solid and cystic components and posterior acoustic enhancement.

Myoepithelial Carcinoma

This tumor is the malignant counterpart of myoepithelioma.

Clinical Findings Myoepithelial carcinoma is rare, has no gender predilection, occurs in adults, and commonly affects the parotid gland. Patients often have a slow-growing, asymptomatic mass. It can arise de novo or ex pleomorphic adenoma.

Histopathology Myoepithelial carcinoma can range from low to high grade. Various proportions of spindle, plasmacytoid, epithelioid, and clear cells with variable nuclear pleomorphism are seen. Variable amounts of myxoid or mucoid stroma may be seen and, in some areas, may appear globular and eosinophilic resembling adenoid cystic carcinoma (Fig. 5.39a). Cystic changes may be present. In the absence of malignant cytomorphology, invasion into surrounding tissue is the only indication of malignancy.

Immuno-Profile Neoplastic cells exhibit the myoepithelial phenotype, and show reactivity for CK5, CK6, CK14, CK17, CD10, calponin, p63, actin, S100 protein, SOX10, and vimentin. CAM5.2 and AE1 / AE3 are also positive.

Molecular Profile One fourth of clear cell myoepithelial carcinomas harbor PLAG1 gene rearrangements, supporting its relationship with pleomorphic adenoma. Infrequent cytogenetic alterations have been seen.

FNA Findings Smears are cellular with plasmacytoid, spindle, clear, or epithelioid cells similar to those of myoepithelioma; however, marked nuclear pleomorphism, atypical mitosis, and necrosis may be present depending on the tumor grade. Metachromatic stroma is seen forming globules and bands of variable sizes. Low-grade myoepithelial carcinoma is almost impossible to diagnose by cytology only since it is indistinguishable from myoepithelial cell-rich pleomorphic adenoma and myoepithelioma (Fig. 5.39b–e). High-grade myoepithelial carcinoma is difficult to distinguish from other high-grade malignancies, e.g., melanoma, mucoepidermoid carcinoma, and epithelial myoepithelial carcinoma, without the help of ancillary studies (Fig. 5.39f–h).

US Features A recurrent submandibular gland myoepithelial carcinoma showed a homogeneous, hypoechoic solid mass, lobulated and focally infiltrative fuzzy borders, and minimal vascular blood flow (Fig. 5.39i, j). The second case showed a solid, slightly heterogeneous hypoechoic parotid mass with posterior acoustic enhancement, well-defined slightly lobulated margins, and minimal peripheral vascular blood flow by Doppler exam (Fig. 5.39k, l). One additional reported case describes a hypoechogenic and heterogeneous 2 cm tumor with irregular borders, invading the surrounding soft tissue including the masseter muscle and subcutaneous tissue; Doppler examination showed a hilar vascular pattern.

In summary, USG-FNA should be considered in the diagnostic evaluation of a patient with a salivary gland mass, allowing for optimal surgical planning and preoperative patient counseling. It has >90% sensitivity and specificity, modifies or avoids surgery in 30% of cases, and procures material for ancillary tests, including molecular studies potentially useful for targeted therapy.

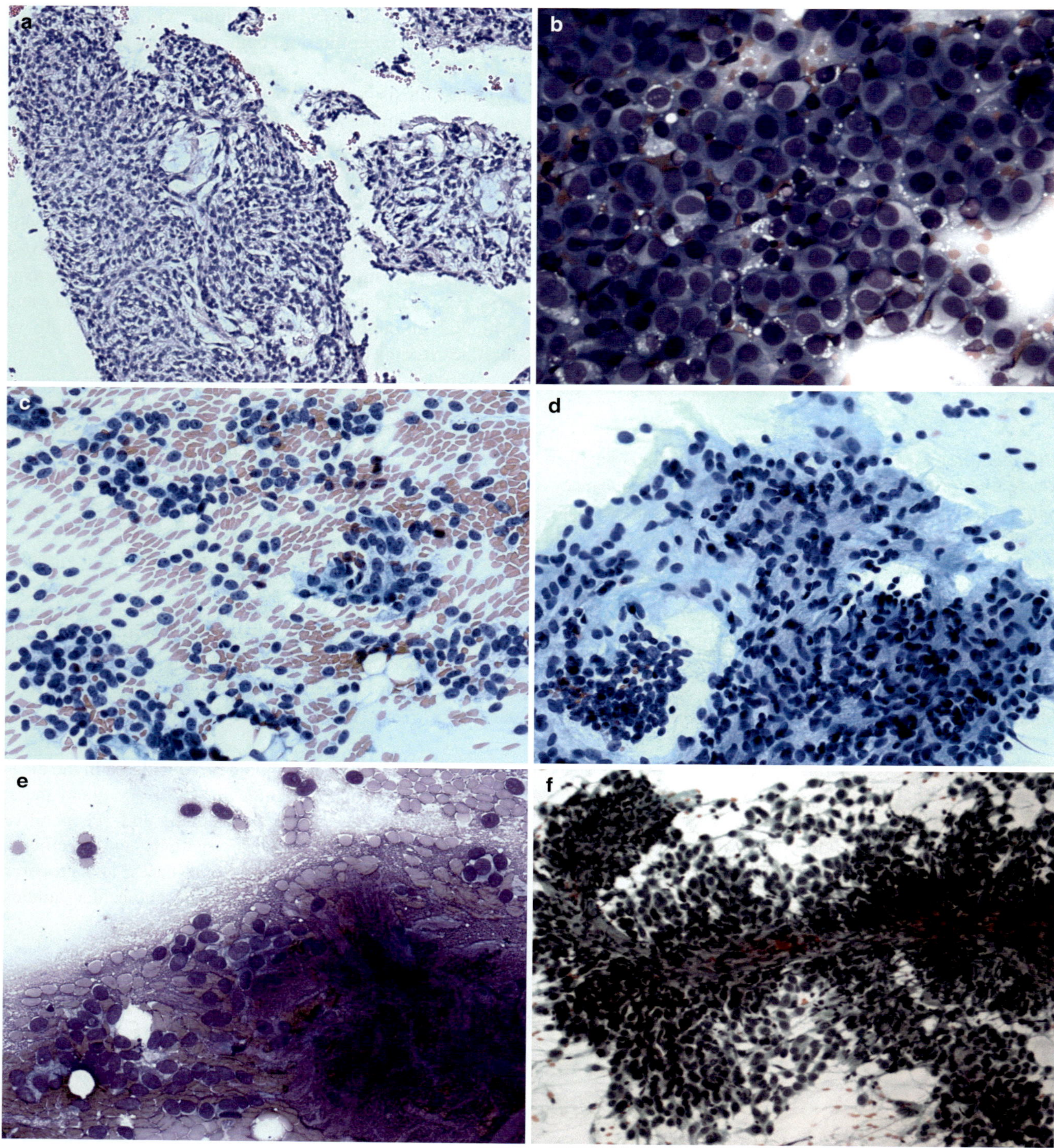

Fig. 5.39 Myoepithelial carcinoma. Histopathology (**a**). Smears show high cellularity, branching complex pseudopapillary aggregates, plasmacytoid and spindle cell features and variably nuclear atypia (**b–h**). The US of these two cases show homogeneous hypoechoic masses with posterior acoustic enhancement and minimal vascularity by Doppler examination (**i–l**). (**a**, H&E stain, cell block, medium magnification; **b–e**, MGG stain, medium and high magnification; **f–h**, Papanicolaou stain, medium and high magnification)

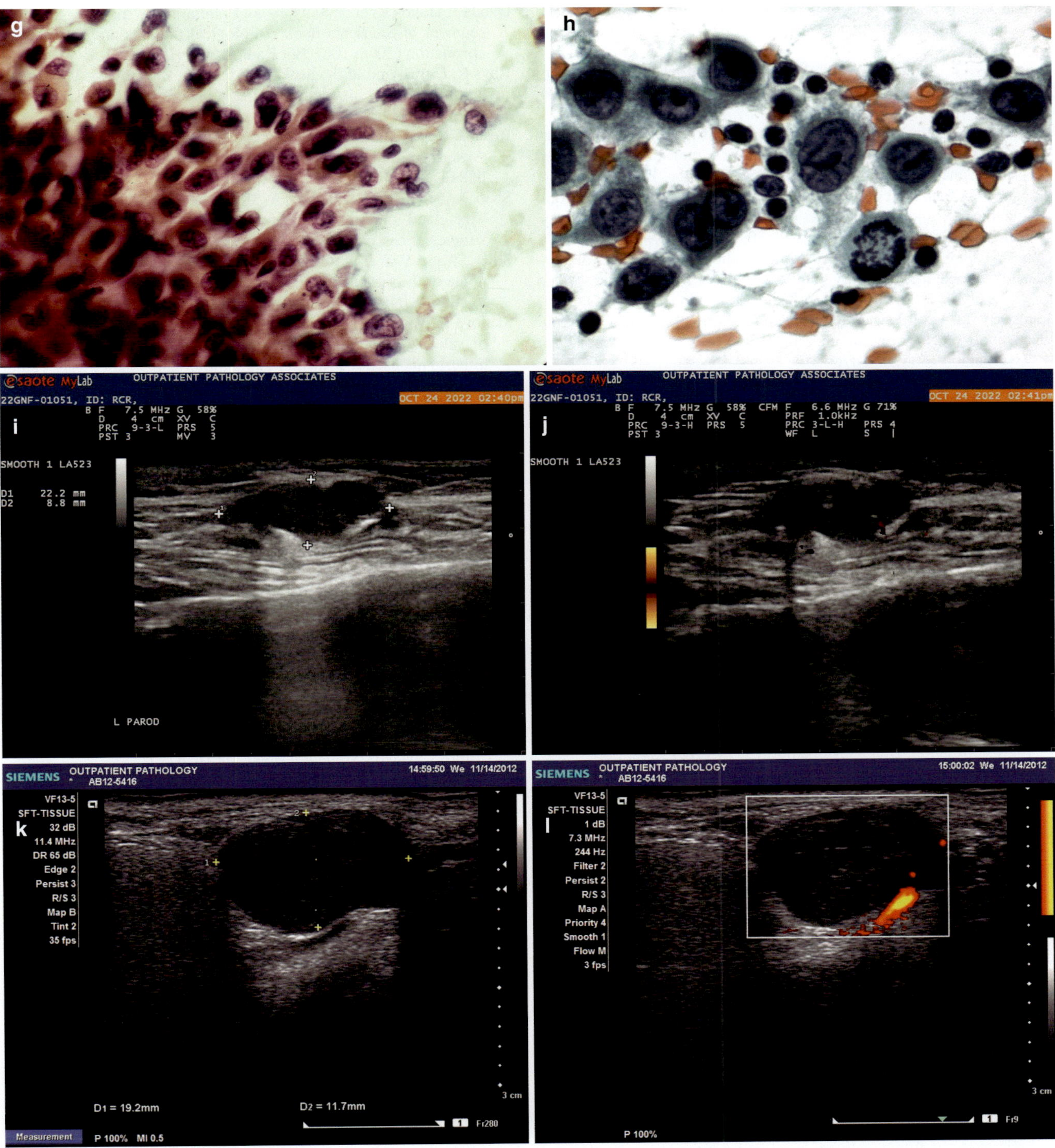

Fig. 5.39 (continued)

Further Reading

Bardales R. The invasive cytopathologist. In: Ultrasound guided fine-needle aspiration of superficial masses. New York: Springer; 2014.

Barnes L, Eveson JW, et al. Salivary glands. In: Barnes L, Eveson JW, Reichart P, Sidransky D, editors. Pathology and genetics of head and neck tumors. IARC: Lyon; 2005. p. 209–81.

Brill LB 2nd, Kanner WA, et al. Analysis of MYB expression and MYB-NFIB gene fusions in adenoid cystic carcinoma and other salivary neoplasms. Mod Pathol. 2011;24(9):1169–76.

Di Palma S, Simpson RH, et al. Salivary duct carcinomas can be classified into luminal androgen receptor-positive, HER2 and basal-like phenotypes*. Histopathology. 2012;61(4):629–43.

El-Naggar AK. Cellular and molecular pathology of head and neck tumors. In: Bernier J, editor. Head and neck cancer: multimodality management. New York: Springer; 2011. p. 57–79.

Faquin WC, Rossi ED. The Milan system for reporting salivary gland cytopathology. 2nd ed. Cham: Springer Nature Switzerland AG; 2023.

Geisinger KR, Stanley MW, et al. Salivary gland masses. In: Modern cytopathology. Philadelphia: Churchill Livingstone; 2004. p. 781–811.

Griffith CC, Stelow EB, et al. The cytological features of mammary analogue secretory carcinoma: a series of 6 molecularly confirmed cases. Cancer Cytopathol. 2013;121(5):234–41.

Gupta S, Sodhani P, et al. Oncocytic papillary cystadenoma of parotid gland: a diagnostic challenge on fine-needle aspiration cytology. Diagn Cytopathol. 2011;39(8):627–30.

Henry-Stanley MJ, Beneke J, et al. Fine-needle aspiration of normal tissue from enlarged salivary glands: sialosis or missed target? Diagn Cytopathol. 1995;13(4):300–3.

Johnson FB, Oertel YC, et al. Sialadenitis with crystalloid formation: a report of six cases diagnosed by fine-needle aspiration. Diagn Cytopathol. 1995;12(1):76–80.

Kim J, Kim EK, et al. Characteristic sonographic findings of Warthin's tumor in the parotid gland. J Clin Ultrasound. 2004;32(2):78–81.

Klijanienko J, Vielh P. Fine-needle sampling of salivary gland lesions. I. Cytology and histology correlation of 412 cases of pleomorphic adenoma. Diagn Cytopathol. 1996;14(3):195–200.

Klijanienko J, Vielh P. Fine-needle sample of salivary gland lesions. V: cytology of 22 cases of acinic cell carcinoma with histologic correlation. Diagn Cytopathol. 1997a;17(5):347–52.

Klijanienko J, Vielh P. Fine-needle sampling of salivary gland lesions. II. Cytology and histology correlation of 71 cases of Warthin's tumor (adenolymphoma). Diagn Cytopathol. 1997b;16(3):221–5.

Klijanienko J, Vielh P. Fine-needle sampling of salivary gland lesions. III. Cytologic and histologic correlation of 75 cases of adenoid cystic carcinoma: review and experience at the Institut curie with emphasis on cytologic pitfalls. Diagn Cytopathol. 1997c;17(1):36–41.

Klijanienko J, Vielh P. Fine-needle sampling of salivary gland lesions. IV. Review of 50 cases of mucoepidermoid carcinoma with histologic correlation. Diagn Cytopathol. 1997d;17(2):92–8.

Klijanienko J, Vielh P. Cytologic characteristics and histomorphologic correlations of 21 salivary duct carcinomas. Diagn Cytopathol. 1998a;19(5):333–7.

Klijanienko J, Vielh P. Fine-needle sampling of salivary gland lesions. VI. Cytological review of 44 cases of primary salivary squamous-cell carcinoma with histological correlation. Diagn Cytopathol. 1998b;18(3):174–8.

Klijanienko J, Vielh P. Fine-needle sampling of salivary gland lesions. VII. Cytology and histology correlation of five cases of epithelial-myoepithelial carcinoma. Diagn Cytopathol. 1998c;19(6):405–9.

Klijanienko J, Vielh P. Salivary carcinomas with papillae: cytology and histology analysis of polymorphous low-grade adenocarcinoma and papillary cystadenocarcinoma. Diagn Cytopathol. 1998d;19(4):244–9.

Klijanienko J, El-Naggar AK, et al. Fine-needle sampling findings in 26 carcinoma ex pleomorphic adenomas: diagnostic pitfalls and clinical considerations. Diagn Cytopathol. 1999a;21(3):163–6.

Klijanienko J, El-Naggar AK, et al. Comparative cytologic and histologic study of fifteen salivary basal-cell tumors: differential diagnostic considerations. Diagn Cytopathol. 1999b;21(1):30–4.

Klijanienko J, Lagace R, et al. Fine-needle sampling of primary neuroendocrine carcinomas of salivary glands: cytohistological correlations and clinical analysis. Diagn Cytopathol. 2001;24(3):163–6.

Lee YYP, Wong KT, et al. Ultrasound investigations in head and neck cancer patients. In: Bernier J, editor. Head and neck cancer: multimodality management. New York: Springer; 2011. p. 221–33.

Leonardo E, Bardales R. Practical immunocytochemistry in diagnostic cytology. Cham: Springer; 2020.

Mukunyadzi P. Review of fine-needle aspiration cytology of salivary gland neoplasms, with emphasis on differential diagnosis. Am J Clin Pathol. 2002;118(Suppl):S100–15.

Okada F, Honda K, et al. Salivary duct carcinoma of the extra-glandular segment of Stensen's duct: radiological findings and pathological correlation (2008: 10b). Eur Radiol. 2009;19(1):254–7.

Rhys R. Ultrasound of the neck. In: Allan PL, Baxter GM, Weston MJ, editors. Clinical ultrasound, vol. 2. London: Churchill Livingstone Elsevier; 2011. p. 890–919.

Rosai J. Major and minor salivary glands. In: Rosai J, editor. Rosai and Ackerman's surgical pathology. Elsevier: Edinburgh, Mosby; 2011. p. 817–56.

Shah AA, LeGallo RD, et al. EWSR1 genetic rearrangements in salivary gland tumors: a specific and very common feature of hyalinizing clear cell carcinoma. Am J Surg Pathol. 2013;37(4):571–8.

Shi L, Wang YX, et al. CT and ultrasound features of basal cell adenoma of the parotid gland: a report of 22 cases with pathologic correlation. AJNR Am J Neuroradiol. 2012;33(3):434–8.

Skalova A, Vanecek T, et al. Mammary analogue secretory carcinoma of salivary glands, containing the ETV6-NTRK3 fusion gene: a hitherto undescribed salivary gland tumor entity. Am J Surg Pathol. 2010;34(5):599–608.

Stanley MW. Selected problems in fine needle aspiration of head and neck masses. Mod Pathol. 2002;15(3):342–50.

Stanley MW, Horwitz CA, et al. Basal-cell adenoma of the salivary gland: a benign adenoma that cytologically mimics adenoid cystic carcinoma. Diagn Cytopathol. 1988;4(4):342–6.

Stanley MW, Bardales RH, et al. Primary and metastatic high-grade carcinomas of the salivary glands: a cytologic-histologic correlation study of twenty cases. Diagn Cytopathol. 1995;13(1):37–43.

Stanley MW, Bardales RH, et al. Sialolithiasis. Differential diagnostic problems in fine-needle aspiration cytology. Am J Clin Pathol. 1996a;106(2):229–33.

Stanley MW, Horwitz CA, et al. Basal cell (monomorphic) and minimally pleomorphic adenomas of the salivary glands. Distinction from the solid (anaplastic) type of adenoid cystic carcinoma in fine-needle aspiration. Am J Clin Pathol. 1996b;106(1):35–41.

Stanley MW, Horwitz CA, et al. Basal cell carcinoma metastatic to the salivary glands: differential diagnosis in fine-needle aspiration cytology. Diagn Cytopathol. 1997;16(3):247–52.

Swid MA, Li L, Drahnak EM, Idom H, Quinones W. Updated salivary gland immunohistochemistry: a review. Arch Pathol Lab Med. 2023;147(12):1383–9. https://doi.org/10.5858/arpa.2022-0461-RA.

Topuz MF, Genç O, Kadioglu N, et al. Intraparotid facial nerve schwannoma: a report of two cases. Int J Otorhinolaryngol Clin. 2020;12(1):4–7.

Tsuneki M, Maruyama S, et al. Podoplanin is a novel myoepithelial cell marker in pleomorphic adenoma and other salivary gland tumors with myoepithelial differentiation. Virchows Arch. 2013;462(3):297–305.

Urano M, Nakaguro M, Yamamoto Y, et al. Diagnostic significance of HRAS mutations in epithelial-myoepithelial carcinomas exhibiting a broad histopathologic spectrum. Am J Surg Pathol. 2019;43(7):984–94. https://doi.org/10.1097/PAS.0000000000001258.

Wenig BM. Major and minor salivary glands. In: Atlas of head and neck pathology. Philadephia: Saunders Elsevier; 2008. p. 536–702.

Yuan WH, Hsu HC, et al. Gray-scale and color Doppler ultrasonographic features of pleomorphic adenoma and Warthin's tumor in major salivary glands. Clin Imaging. 2009;33(5):348–53.

Zhang C, Cohen JM, et al. Fine-needle aspiration of secondary neoplasms involving the salivary glands. A report of 36 cases. Am J Clin Pathol. 2000;113(1):21–8.

Zhao X, Wei S. Myoepithelioma. PathologyOutlines.com website 2024. . https://www.pathologyoutlines.com/topic/salivaryglandsmyoepithelioma.html. Accessed 24 Jan 2024.

Żurek M, Fus Ł, Niemczyk K, et al. Salivary gland pathologies: evolution in classification and association with unique genetic alterations. Eur Arch Otorhinolaryngol. 2023;280:4739–50. https://doi.org/10.1007/s00405-023-08110-w.

Miscellaneous Masses of Head and Neck and Other Body Sites

Ricardo H. Bardales

This chapter will cover USG-FNA of masses found in the head and neck, with exception of the thyroid, major salivary glands, and lymph nodes, which are described in other chapters of this book. Common and uncommon palpable and/ or US-visible masses of skin and soft tissue of the head and neck and other body sites are also described, with emphasis on their cytology and US features.

The neck is divided into regions to facilitate the clinical and US localization of these masses and their subsequent follow-up for therapy, including surgical interventions. Based on the tissue of origin or on embryologic development, most masses of the head and neck are found in foreseeable areas, and their location helps to narrow the differential diagnosis.

The Neck by Regions

I will topographically address masses found in the following regions when they are evaluated by US and USG-FNA. The regions included are sublingual (Fig. 6.1), submental (Fig. 6.2a, b), anterior infrahyoid, submandibular (Fig. 6.3), parotid, lateral superior (Fig. 6.4), lateral mid (Fig. 6.5), supraclavicular medial (Fig. 6.6), supraclavicular lateral (Fig. 6.7), posterior (Fig. 6.8), and suprasternal.

Solid masses of the head and neck are sampled by USG-FNA by use of a 25- or 27-G needle without suction (Zajdela technique), following the directions given in Chap. 2. Suction can be applied to solid lesions for harvesting of material for a cell block for performance of ancillary tests. Large cystic lesions of the head and neck are also approached by USG-FNA under suction for drainage of the cyst contents with use of cyst-drainage supplies as mentioned in Chap. 2. When

cyst fluid is obtained, it should be processed by centrifugation, and smears should be made from the pellet or processed by liquid-based techniques. Most important is the US evaluation of the lesion after fluid drainage, looking for a residual solid component, which must be sampled preferably by USG-FNA with 27- or 25-G needles without suction.

Sublingual and Submental Region (Neck Level Ia)

Cysts of various types, including the thyroglossal duct cyst, lymph nodes, and solid masses including sublingual salivary gland tumors can be identified in this region.

Ranula

The ranula is a mucus retention cyst of the sublingual gland and is seen as a painless and cystic swelling in the floor of the mouth. A "simple ranula" is limited to the mucus membranes

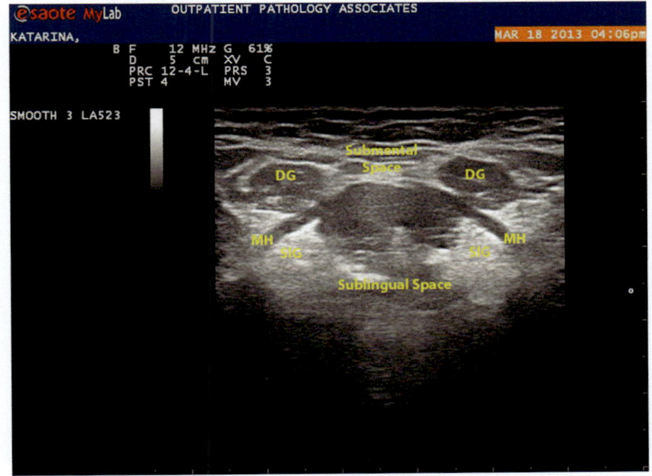

Fig. 6.1 Submental and sublingual regions, axial view. The transducer is held in a transverse position. *DG* digastric muscle, *MH* mylohyoid muscle, *SlG* sublingual gland

Supplementary Information The online version contains supplementary material available at https://doi.org/10.1007/978-3-031-73702-2_6.

R. H. Bardales (✉)
Precision Pathology, Outpatient Pathology Associates, Sacramento, CA, USA

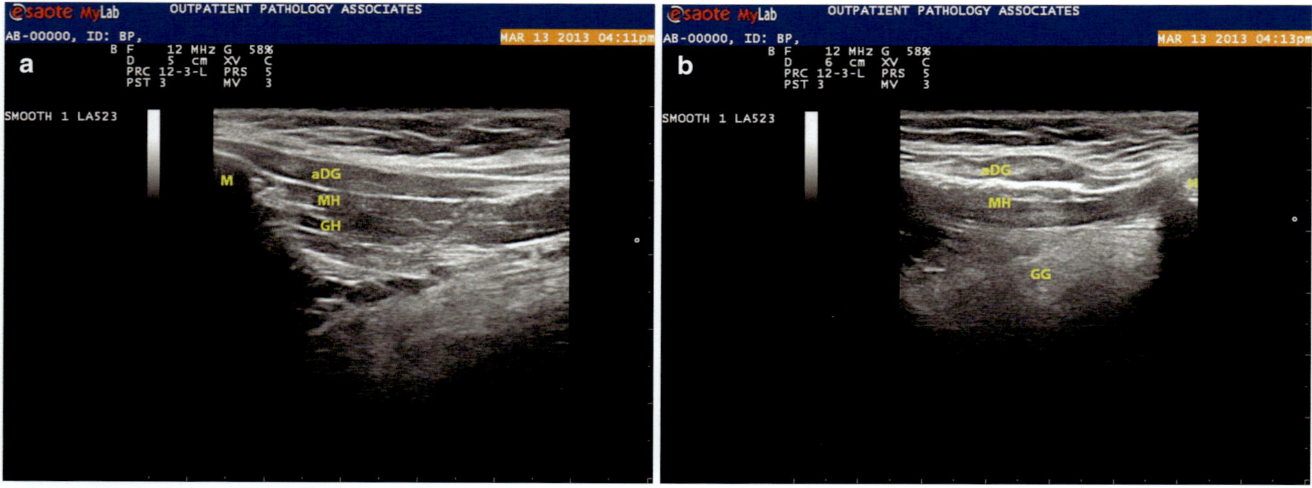

Fig. 6.2 (**a**, **b**) Submental region, sagittal view. The transducer is held parallel to the midline below the mandible (**a**) and superior to the hyoid bone (**b**). *M* mandible, *aDG* anterior belly of digastric muscle, *MH* mylohyoid muscle, *GH* geniohyoid muscle, *GG* genioglossus, *H* hyoid bone

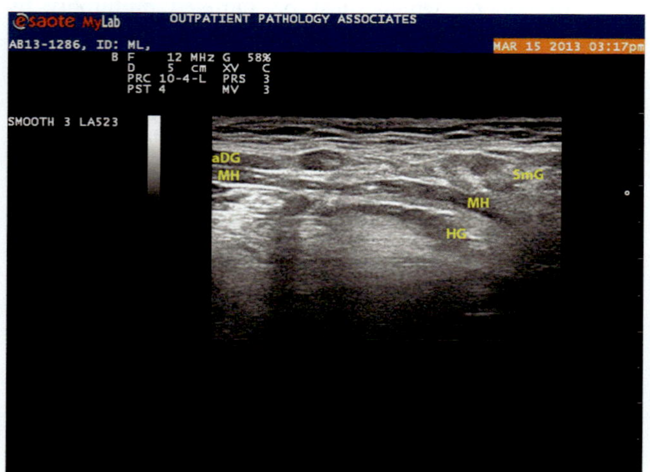

Fig. 6.3 Left submandibular region. The transducer is held parallel to the mandible. *aDG* anterior belly of digastric muscle, *SmG* submandibular gland, *MH* mylohyoid muscle, *HG* hyoglossus muscle

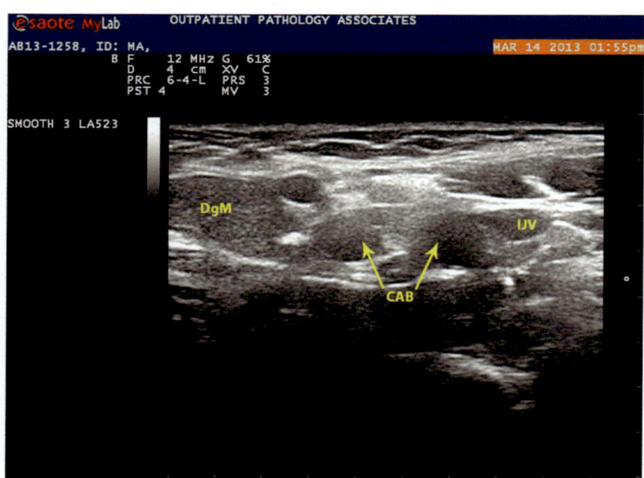

Fig. 6.4 Left level II neck (lateral superior) region. The transducer is held in a transverse position at the level of the common carotid artery bifurcation. *DgM* posterior belly of digastric muscle, *CAB* carotid artery bifurcation, *IJV* internal jugular vein

above the mylohyoid muscle. A "plunging ranula" extends posterior to the mylohyoid muscle beyond the sublingual space into the neck and can be palpable.

Histopathology. The ranula epithelial lining may be cuboidal, columnar, or squamous of non-keratinizing type. The so-called "plunging ranula" or pseudocyst lacks a lining epithelium.

FNA findings. Smears from a plunging ranula show variably dense mucin and macrophages (Fig. 6.9a). Aspirates from the ranula show a granular precipitate, crystals, macrophages, columnar cells, and occasionally metaplastic squamous cells. Differentiation of foamy histiocytes from mucin-producing malignant cells may be difficult, and separation from low-grade mucoepidermoid carcinoma may be

impossible (Fig. 6.9c–e). The reader is referred to the salivary gland chapter of this book for further discussion.

US features. The cyst is situated offline in the sublingual space, well-defined, anechoic, uninoculated, and shows posterior acoustic enhancement. The large lesion is called a "plunging or diving ranula" (Fig. 6.9b) and is seen off-midline in the medial submandibular space.

Choristomas (Dermoid and Epidermoid Cysts)

Dermoid and epidermoid cysts are choristomas. Epidermoid cysts that develop in other body sites frequently occur later in life and are also known as epidermal inclusion cysts or sebaceous cysts.

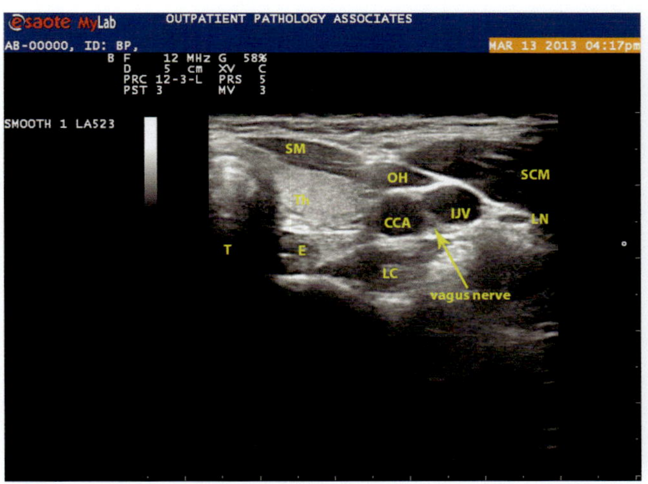

Fig. 6.5 Left level III neck (lateral mid) region. The transducer is held in a transverse position in the mid-neck at the level of the omohyoid muscle, which is seen crossing from medial to lateral over the common carotid artery. *T* trachea, *SM* strap muscles (sternohyoid, sternothyroid), *Th* thyroid, *E* esophagus, *OH* omohyoid, *SCM* sternocleidomastoid muscle, *LC* longus colli, *CCA* common carotid artery, *IJV* internal jugular vein, *LN* lymph node

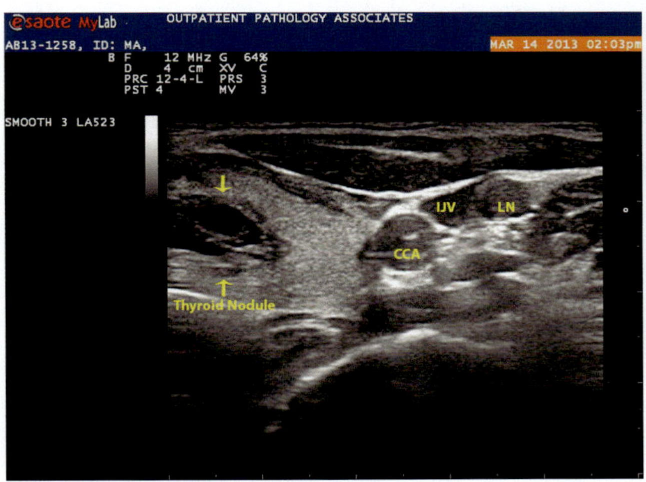

Fig. 6.6 Left level IV neck (supraclavicular medial) region. The transducer is placed transverse parallel to the clavicle in the upper and lower portions of level IV. *CCA* common carotid artery, *IJV* internal jugular vein, *LN* lymph node

Clinical Findings They occur frequently close to the midline in the head and neck during infancy and early childhood and have no gender preference. Patients often have a subcutaneous lesion in the orbit, nose, and less commonly in the anterior, lateral, or upper neck. Dermoid cysts also arise in the anterior portion of the floor of the mouth, particularly in the sublingual space, and epidermoid cysts develop in the midline of the submental space. They do not move with swallowing or tongue protrusion. A congenital syndrome is suspected when numerous epidermoid cysts develop in unusual locations of the head and neck and before puberty.

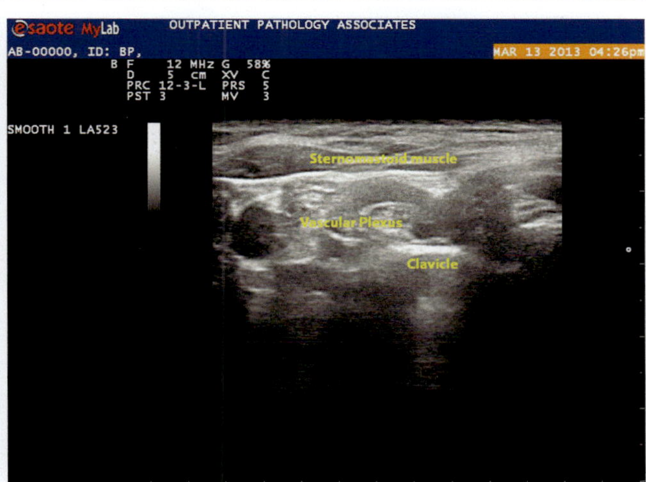

Fig. 6.7 Left level Vb neck (supraclavicular lateral) region. The transducer is placed parallel to the clavicle in the mid- and lateral supraclavicular regions

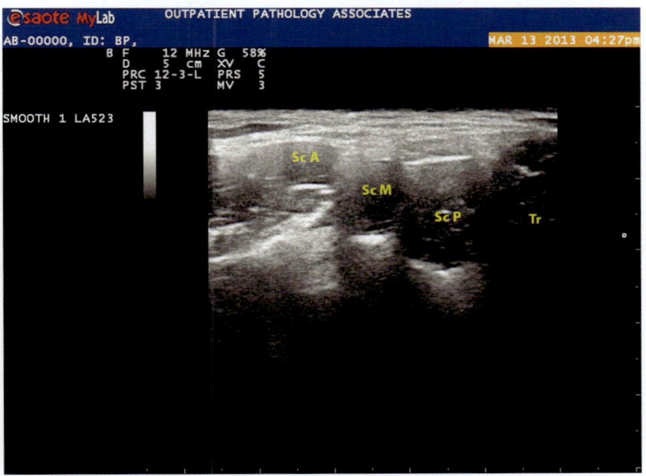

Fig. 6.8 Left mid-level Va neck region. The transducer is placed transverse in the mid-posterior neck region. *ScA* scalene muscle anterior, *ScM* scalene muscle medius, *ScM* scalene muscle posterior, *Tr* trapezius muscle

Histopathology The dermoid cyst wall is lined with keratinized squamous epithelium and contains skin appendages. Epidermoid cysts are squamous-lined cysts and lack skin appendages. The cyst cavity contains keratin and sebaceous material. When there is rupture into the surrounding soft tissue, a foreign-body tissue reaction occurs.

FNA Findings The material obtained from both dermoid and epidermoid cysts is "cheesy," with a peculiar odor. Smears show numerous anucleated squamous cells and keratinaceous debris (Fig. 6.10a). Skin appendages and occasionally columnar ciliated epithelium are findings that are of diagnostic significance and may be present in smears of dermoid cysts. The presence of acute inflammatory cells and

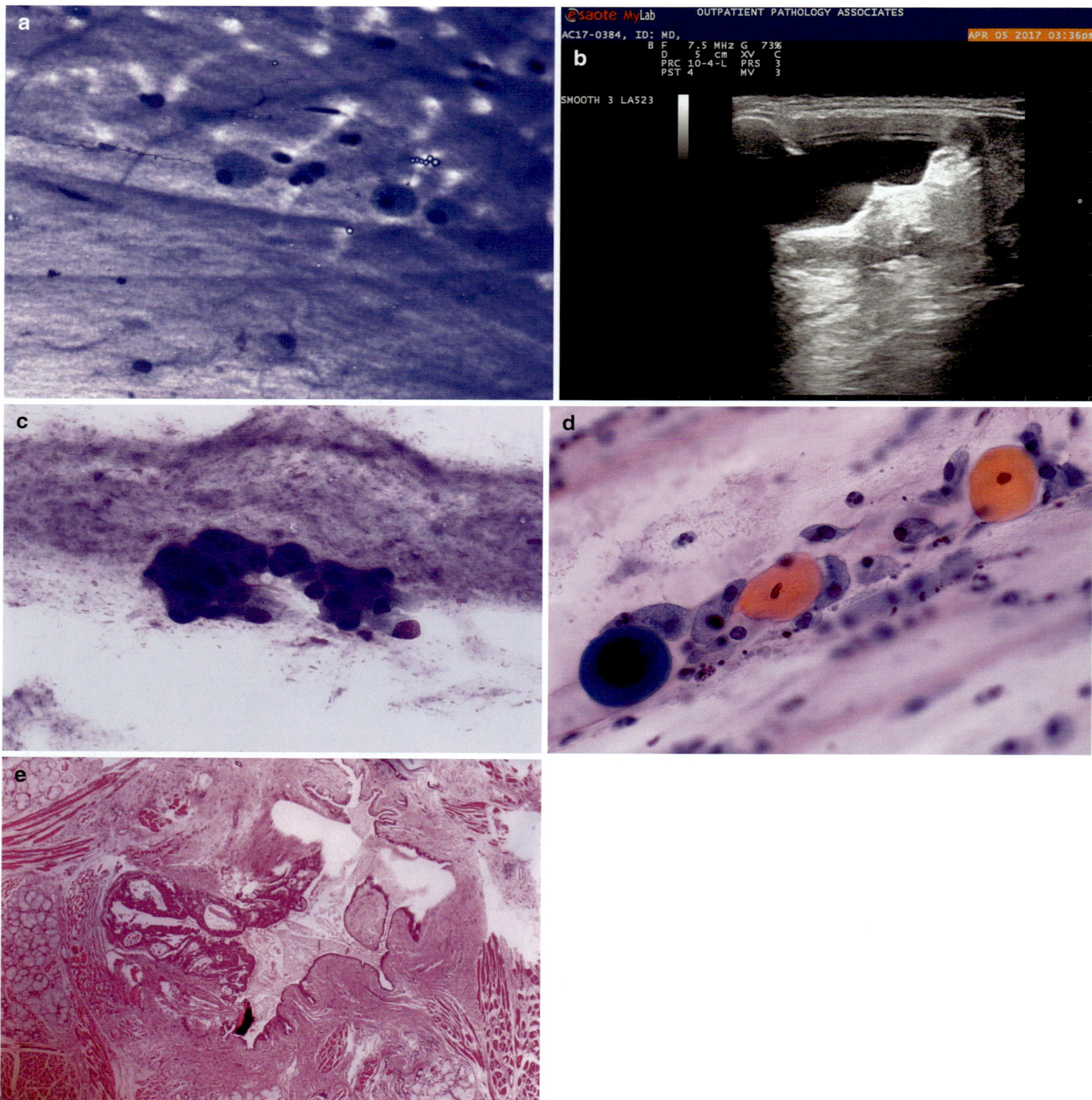

Fig. 6.9 (**a–e**) Ranula. Smears of a "diving ranula" show abundant mucin and rare macrophages (**a**). Epithelial cells may be present in the smears from a ranula. By US, ranula and diving ranula are anechoic with posterior acoustic enhancement, uniform, thin and lobulated borders, and no solid mural nodules (**b**). Cytologic features of mucocele include scattered small aggregates of bland-appearing epithelial cells, squamous metaplastic cells, mucinophages, and mucus (**c**, **d**). The cytologic pattern is very similar, if not identical, to that of low-grade mucoepidermoid carcinoma, and surgical excision is necessary (**e**). (**a**, MGG stain, high magnification; **b**, ultrasound, high frequency, sagittal view; **c**, DiffQuik stain, high magnification; **d**, Papanicolaou stain, high magnification; **e**, H&E stain, low magnification)

foreign-body-type multinucleated giant cells indicates cyst rupture. Stromal cells may show prominent reactive changes that may suggest squamous cell carcinoma. Nucleated squamous cells with anaplastic nuclei are seen in squamous cell carcinoma; this is a consideration in older patients.

US Features Cysts are round to oval of variable size, well-defined, smooth, isoechoic or hypoechoic, with a thin wall, and with posterior acoustic enhancement (Fig. 6.10b–d). The borders are irregular in the presence of cyst rupture. Dermoid cysts may be more heterogeneous than epidermoid and may

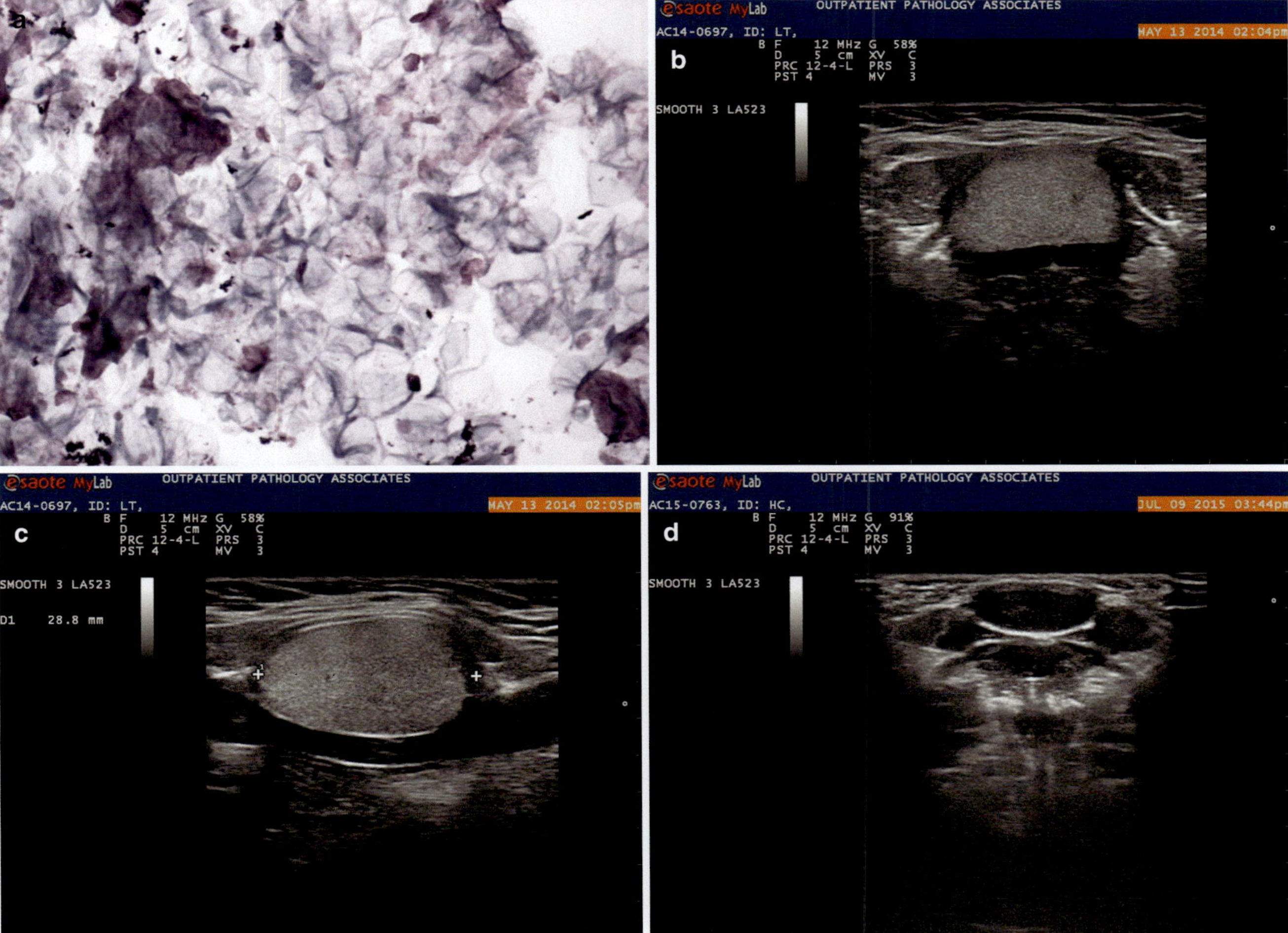

Fig. 6.10 (**a–d**) Dermoid cysts. These two submental masses, identified in two children, were sampled by USG-FNA, and smears showed anucleated squamous cells (**a**). By US, round hyperechoic and oval anechoic masses with smooth, well-defined borders were identified (**b–d**). Both anterior bellies of the digastric muscles are seen on the sides (**b**, **d**). (**a**, Papanicolaou stain, medium magnification; **b–d**, ultrasound, high frequency; **b**, **d**, transverse view; **c**, sagittal view)

have hyperechogenic streaks due to the presence of adipose tissue and skin appendages. Echogenic foci with posterior shadowing may be seen in the presence of bone or teeth.

Thyroglossal Duct Cyst

Occasionally, an off-midline hyoid or suprahyoid thyroglossal-duct cyst may develop and should be considered in the differential diagnosis of submental lesions. A comet tail artifact is seen in these cases (Fig. 6.11a–c). Cytology smears in these cases show mucoid fluid with cholesterol crystals and rare macrophages (Fig. 6.11d).

Undescended Thyroid

Clinical Findings An undescended thyroid gland is often located in the base of the tongue; however, it may occur along the thyroglossal tract and may be present as an anterior midline neck mass, which is often mistaken as a thyroglossal-duct cyst.

Histopathology Benign thyroid parenchyma is present.

FNA Findings Aspirates show sheets of benign follicular cells and colloid (Fig. 6.12b).

US Features This is a well-circumscribed, round, solid, and isoechoic mass with homogeneous echotexture (Fig. 6.12a).

Tongue Tumors

The precise location and depth of tongue tumors may be assessed by US imaging of the submental region by placement of the probe in a longitudinal position from the hyoid bone to the chin. The sample is harvested by USG-FNA via a submental approach or palpation guidance, depending on the location and clinical setting. Malignancies and infectious processes can be accurately diagnosed by use of FNA (Fig. 6.13a–e)

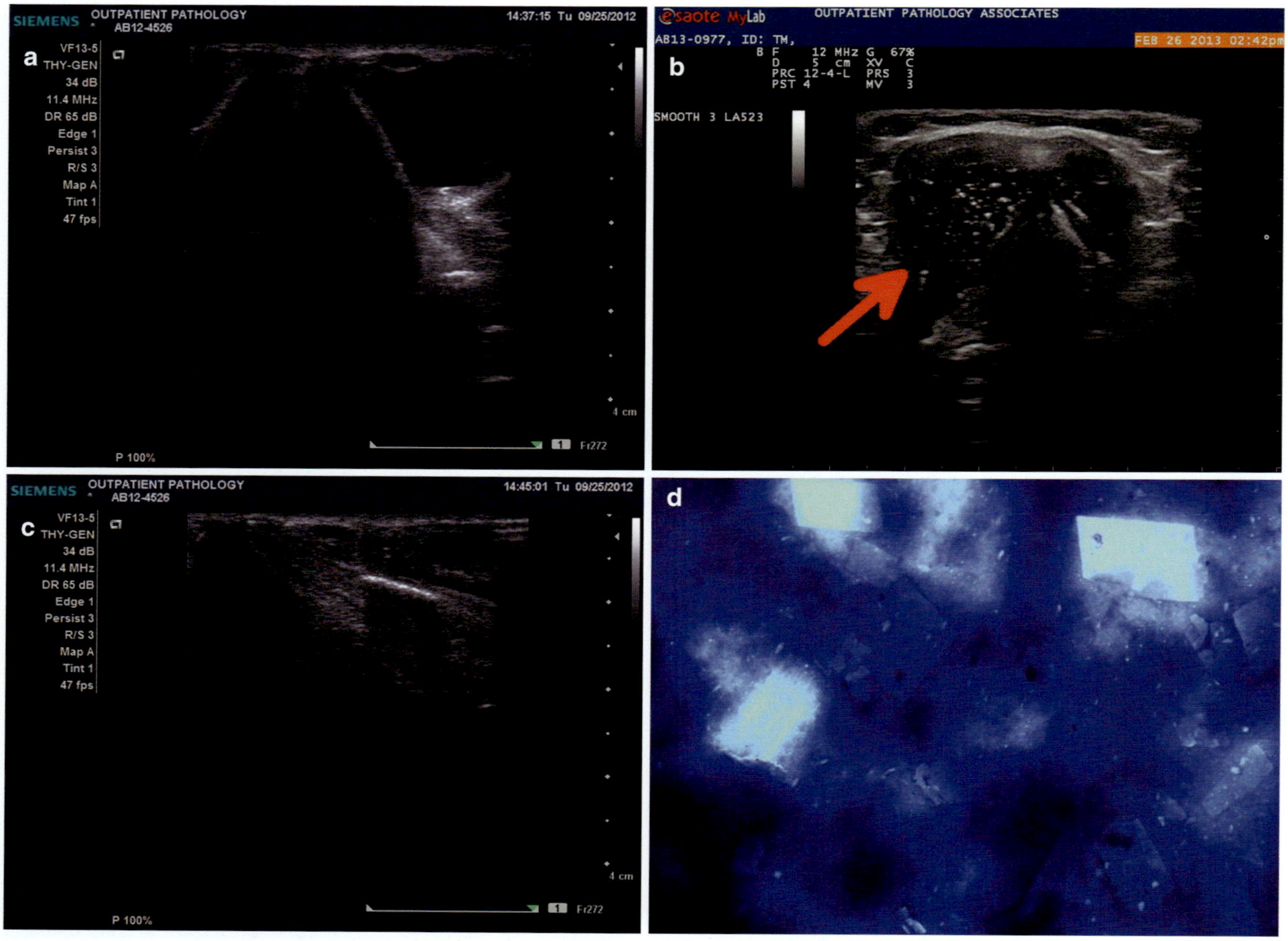

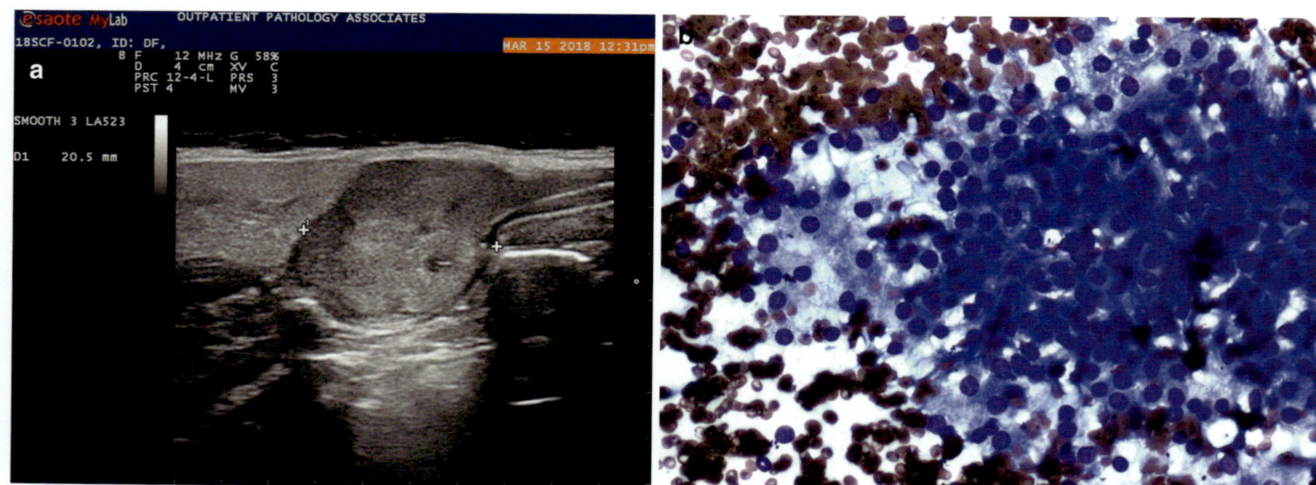

Fig. 6.11 (**a**, **b**) Thyroglossal-duct cyst. Left and right off-midline unilocular, well-defined cysts at the level of the hyoid bone and laryngeal cartilage show "comet tails," regular borders, and posterior acoustic enhancement (**a**, **b**) in these two cases. The left off-midline cyst collapsed totally after fluid drainage (**c**). Smears showed cholesterol crystals, mucin, and rare macrophages (**d**). (**a–c**, Ultrasound, high frequency, transverse view; **d**, MGG stain, high magnification)

Fig. 6.12 (**a**, **b**) Undescended thyroid gland. By US, the ectopic thyroid is well-circumscribed, isoechoic, solid, homogeneous with posterior acoustic enhancement, and is present at the level of the hyoid bone (**a**) in this case. Cytology shows a sheet of benign follicular epithelial cells (**b**). (**a**, US, high frequency, sagittal view; **b**, MGG stain, medium magnification)

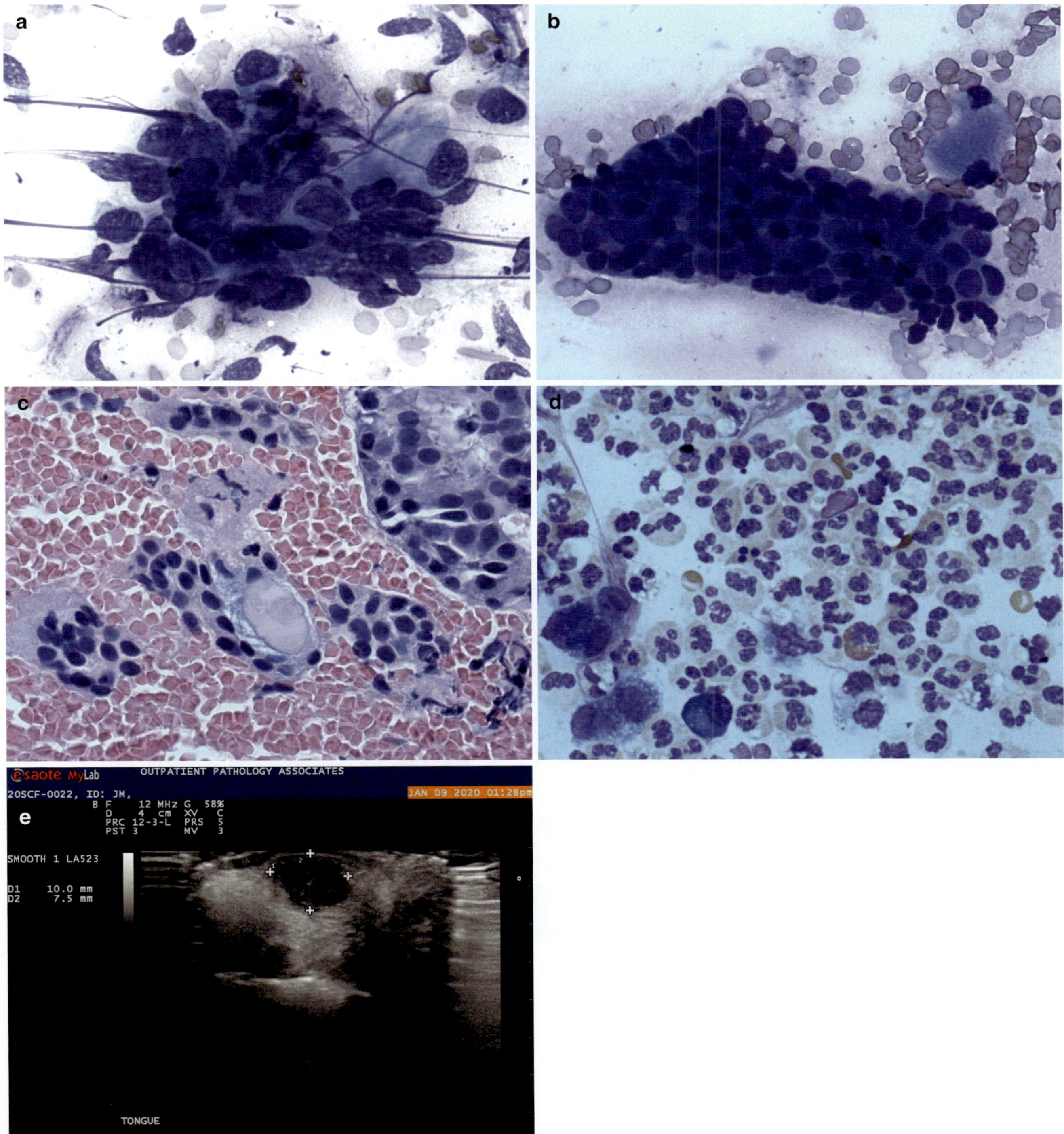

Fig. 6.13 (**a–e**) Tongue tumors. A large, ulcerated tongue mass was sampled by palpation guidance and diagnosed as p16+ squamous cell carcinoma (**a**). An adenoid cystic carcinoma was present as a large submucosal tongue mass with no ulceration. It was also sampled by palpation guidance, and smears showed predominantly basaloid cells with scant globular stroma (**b**), which was more evident in the cell block slide (**c**). Immunohistochemistry confirmed the diagnosis in both cases. A tongue abscess yielded a purulent smear pattern when it was sampled by USG-FNA (**d**). US showed a hypoechoic mass with heterogeneous echotexture and ill-defined borders (**e**). (**a, b, d**, MGG stain, high magnification; **c**, H&E, medium magnification; **d**, ultrasound, high frequency, transverse view)

Oral Cavity Tumors

Squamous cell carcinoma, sinonasal carcinomas extending through the roof of mouth, and minor salivary gland tumors, i.e., adenoid cystic carcinoma and mucoepidermoid carcinoma, are the most common neoplasms of the oral cavity (Fig. 6.14a–c). Occasionally, tumors arising in the sublingual gland, i.e., adenoid cystic carcinoma, may reach a large size and extend into the submental and submandibular spaces.

Submandibular Region (Neck Level Ib)

Primary benign and malignant tumors identified in the submandibular region are mostly of submandibular-gland and lymph node origin. Squamous cysts, lipomas, and recurrent benign and malignant submandibular gland neoplasms are less common (Fig. 6.15a–d).

The US image of a lipoma is characteristic and shows a hypoechoic mass with fine, bright, echogenic striations producing a "feathery" appearance, characteristic, if not pathognomonic of this tumor. The mass is in the deep subcutaneous tissue, and the striations remain parallel to the probe regardless of the direction of the scan.

Parotid Region (Neck Level IIb)

Pilomatrixoma

This lesion is seen predominantly in children and affects mainly the pre-auricular region and proximal upper extremities. It is a slow-growing tumor that arises from the hair follicles and is a hard subcutaneous nodule. The US image shows a skin-based, well-defined, irregular, hypoechoic nodule with inner echogenic foci (fibrosis and calcifications) and a peripheral hypoechoic rim. The mass may be completely echogenic, with strong posterior acoustic shadowing suggestive of calcification (Fig. 6.16a, b).

Branchial-Cleft Cyst

Branchial-cleft cyst derived from the first branchial-cleft anomaly is located in the pre-, post-, or infra-auricular region and may be mistaken as a parotid gland tumor. This lesion is rare; histo-

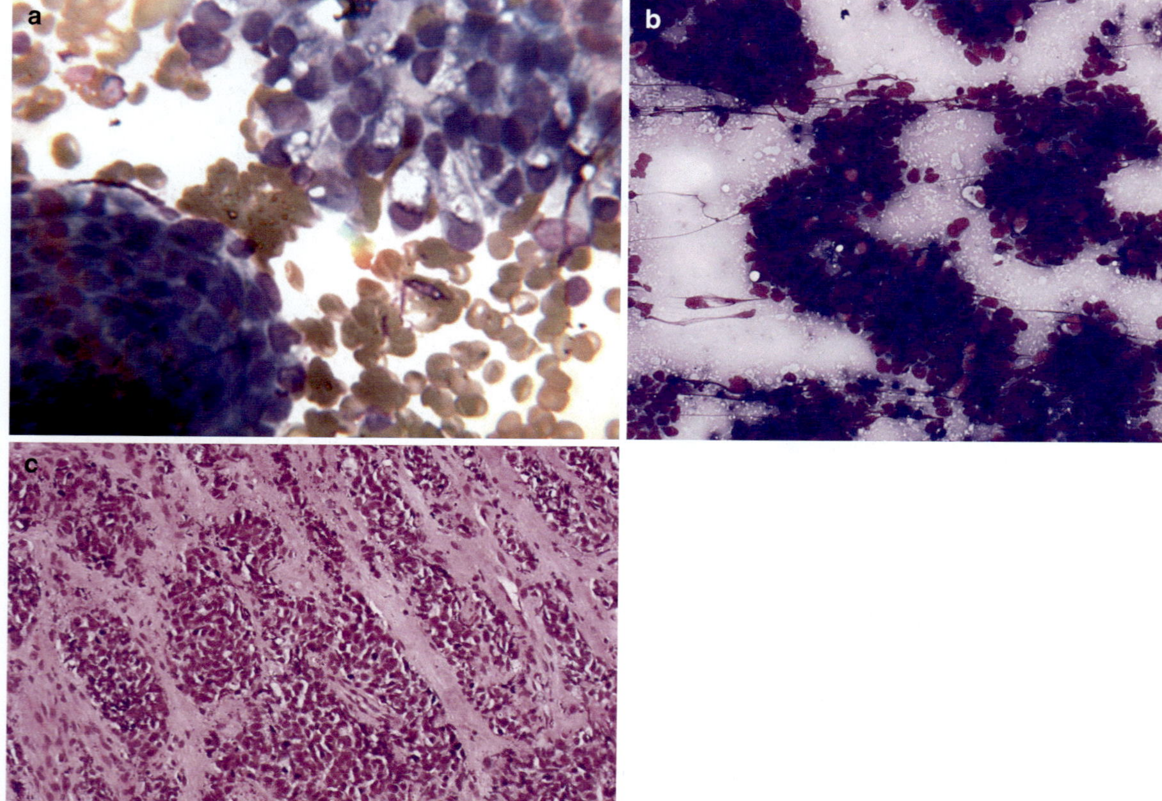

Fig. 6.14 (**a–c**) Oral cavity tumors. These two masses, which were sampled by palpation guidance, showed mucoepidermoid carcinoma (**a**, squamous and glandular components toward the left and right of the frame, respectively) identified as a large soft-palate mass, and sinonasal carcinoma extending through the roof of mouth (**b–c**). Immunohistochemistry confirmed the diagnoses. (**a**, MGG stain, high magnification; **b**, DiffQuik, medium magnification; **d**, H&E stain, low magnification) (**a**, courtesy Dr. John S. Abele, Sacramento, Ca)

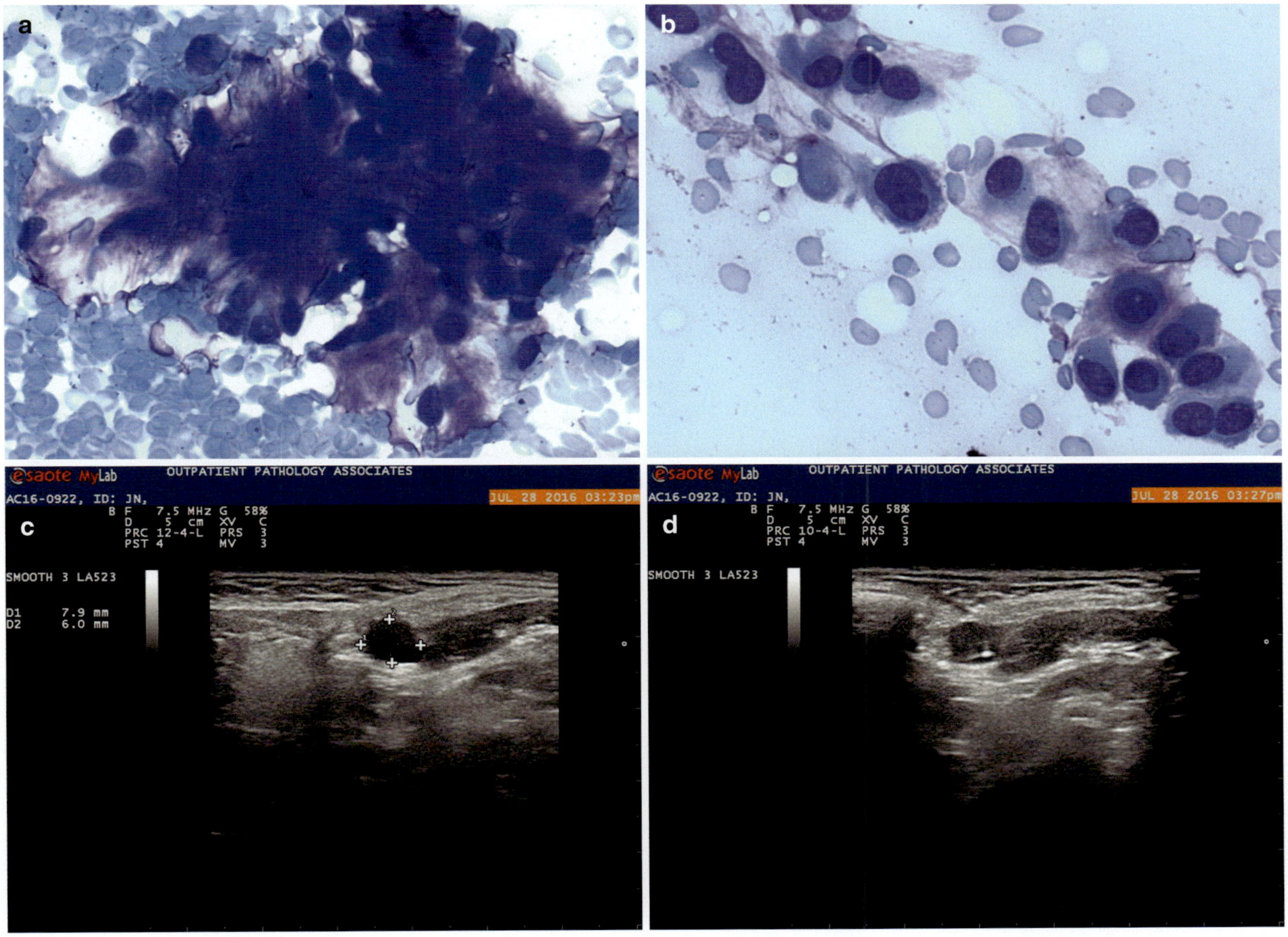

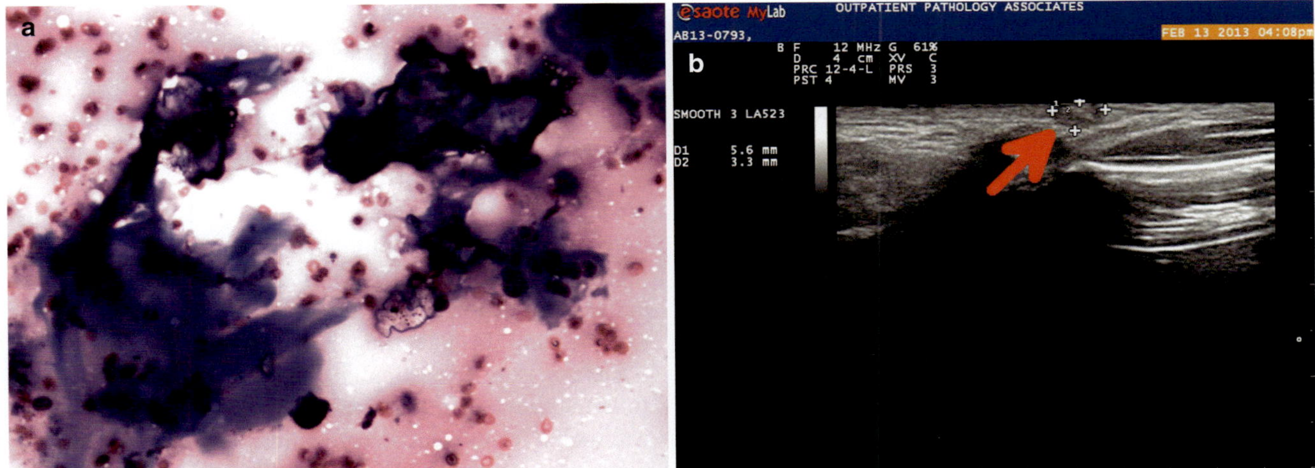

Fig. 6.15 (**a–d**) Submandibular space. Smears showed fibrillary stroma (**a**) and myoepithelial cells (**b**) diagnostic of a submandibular gland recurrent benign mixed tumor. A hypoechoic nodular mass is present at neck level Ib (**c**). The sampling needle tip is identified within the target lesion (**d**). (**a**, MGG stain, medium magnification; **b**, MGG stain, high magnification; **c**, **d**, ultrasound, high frequency, transverse view)

Fig. 6.16 (**a**, **b**) Parotid-region pilomatrixoma. Predominantly anucleated squamous cells and calcific material were seen in the smears of this 7-year-old child (**a**). Ultrasound shows a superficial small skin lesion with internal hyperechoic foci suggestive of microcalcifications (**b**). (**a**, MGG stain, medium magnification; **b**, ultrasound, high frequency, transverse view)

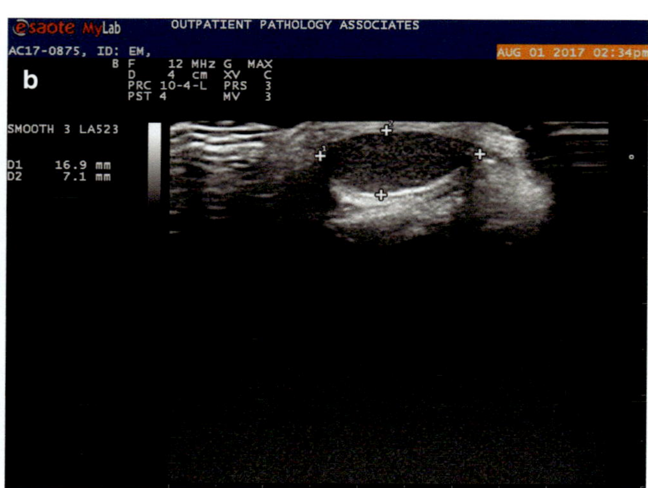

Fig. 6.17 (**a**, **b**) Branchial cleft cyst, retroauricular. USG-FNA of this cystic mass in a 5-year-old boy yielded anucleated squamous cells (**a**). Ultrasound showed a hypoechoic, oval, well-defined mass with poste-rior acoustic enhancement, and homogeneous echotexture (**b**). (**a**, MGG stain, medium magnification; **b**, ultrasound, high frequency, longitudinal view)

logically it may or may not have adnexal elements in addition to the keratinizing squamous epithelium. However, in contrast to the findings in branchial-cleft cysts derived from the second branchial-cleft anomaly, the inflammatory component is not prominent unless the cyst becomes infected (Fig. 6.17a, b).

Myxoid/Mucinous/Synovial Cyst

Clinical Findings Myxoid or mucinous cysts are found anterior to the parotid gland around the temporomandibular joint, where they may develop in association with a temporo-mandibular-joint (TMJ) syndrome. On examination, this cyst appears as a small, firm, well-circumscribed, and variably tender nodule.

FNA Findings USG-FNA is done by use of a 25-G needle with or without suction. The aspirated fluid is thick, mucoid, and transparent. Smears are essentially acellular; a few mac-rophages may be present (Fig. 6.18a, b).

Ultrasound Features By US, they are commonly unilocu-lar, anechoic with posterior acoustic enhancement, and sur-rounded by a thin echogenic rim (Fig. 6.18c, d).

Other lesions that occur predominantly in the masticator space/masseter regions include dental abscesses, vascular malformations, lipomas, an ectopic salivary gland, and mus-cle hypertrophy because of bruxism.

Anterior Infrahyoid (Neck Level VI) and Suprasternal (Neck Level VII) Regions

The most common pathology of the area superior to the thy-roid gland (level VI) is the thyroglossal-duct cyst, and less frequently, laryngocele and chondroid tumors of the laryn-geal cartilages (most commonly the cricoid), and a pharyn-geal pouch. The thymus and soft-tissue masses may be seen in the suprasternal region (neck level VII).

Thyroglossal-Duct Cyst and Thyroglossal-Duct Carcinoma

The thyroglossal duct involutes at the 8th gestational week; failure to involute results in the presence of a thyroglossal-duct cyst or of ectopic thyroid tissue. A thyroglossal-duct cyst is the most common congenital mass and is located below the hyoid bone (65%), at the level of the hyoid bone (20%), and suprahyoid in 15%. The cysts are often located in the midline, particularly when suprahyoid, and off the mid-line and surrounded by the strap muscles when they are infrahyoid. When located off midline, they are always located medial to the jugular vein.

Clinical Findings Most patients are less than 10 years old, but the cysts may also occur in adults as a slowly growing, painless mass that moves vertically with swallowing or tongue protrusion, due to attachment to the hyoid bone.

Histopathology The lining epithelium is columnar and may have a squamous component. The wall may contain thyroid tissue in various proportions, commonly in the sub-epithelial location. Both benign and malignant neoplasms can develop in a setting of a thyroglossal-duct cyst. Neoplasms are of follicular derivation, i.e., they may be follicular adenoma, follicular carcinoma, papillary thyroid carcinoma, or anaplastic carcinoma. Squamous cell carci-noma occurs rarely and, in all likelihood, it arises from the squamous epithelium and not from the follicular epithe-lium. Papillary thyroid carcinoma is the most common form. Medullary carcinoma does not occur; C cells have a different embryologic origin.

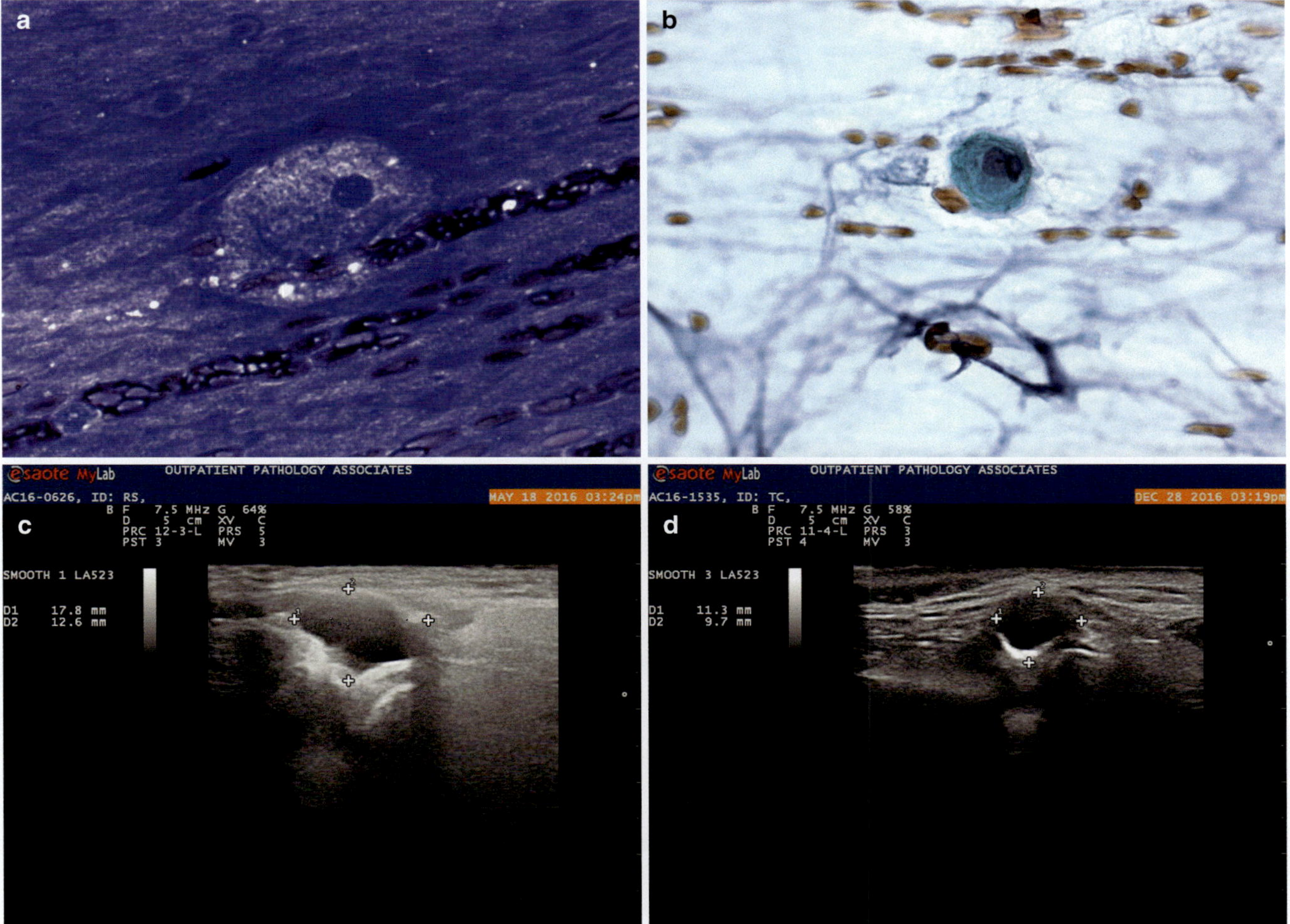

Fig. 6.18 (**a–d**) Temporo-mandibular synovial cyst. USG-FNA yields a dense mucinous fluid, and smears show rare macrophages and no epithelial cells (**a**). A rare cell may resemble a chondrocyte (**b**). Ultrasound shows an anechoic, round to oval, well-defined cyst with variable posterior acoustic enhancement and may resemble a lymph node (**c, d**). (**a**, MGG stain, high magnification; **b**, Papanicoloau stain, high magnification; **c, d**, ultrasound, high frequency, transverse view)

FNA Findings Smears are sparsely cellular and show scattered degenerated columnar, ciliated, or squamous cells, macrophages, a few inflammatory cells, proteinaceous fluid, and debris. Squamous metaplastic cells may be seen in the presence of infection or inflammation (Fig. 6.19a–c). In cases of papillary thyroid carcinoma, the smear findings are similar to those seen in the cystic variant of papillary thyroid carcinoma, including sheets of degenerated malignant cells, metaplastic cells, and psammoma bodies; the cytomorphology is described in the thyroid chapter of this book (Fig. 6.19d–i).

US Features The US image of the thyroglossal-duct cyst shows a well-defined, smooth, unilocular cystic mass with a thin wall. The relationship to the hyoid bone in the sagittal or longitudinal midline view helps in the US identification. The cystic mass may be anechoic with posterior acoustic enhancement when purely cystic, hypoechoic when it contains debris, hypoechoic and heterogeneous when there is infection or hemorrhage, or "pseudosolid" when there is dense proteinaceous content (Fig. 6.20a, b). A diagnosis of malignancy is suspected when there is a variably vascular and solid component within the cyst wall, i.e., when nodules or excrescences are seen on US imaging (Fig. 6.20c, d; Video 6.1).

Thymus

The normal thymus gland may be seen in children and is located deep in the suprasternal notch (neck level VII). By US, the thymus is hypoechoic with well-defined and smooth borders. The gland may have a sparkly appearance due to the presence of comet-tail-like artifacts. A thymic cyst may be identified in the sternal notch.

Dermoid cysts may be identified in the suprasternal region (neck level VII) of children as exemplified in Fig. 6.21a, b.

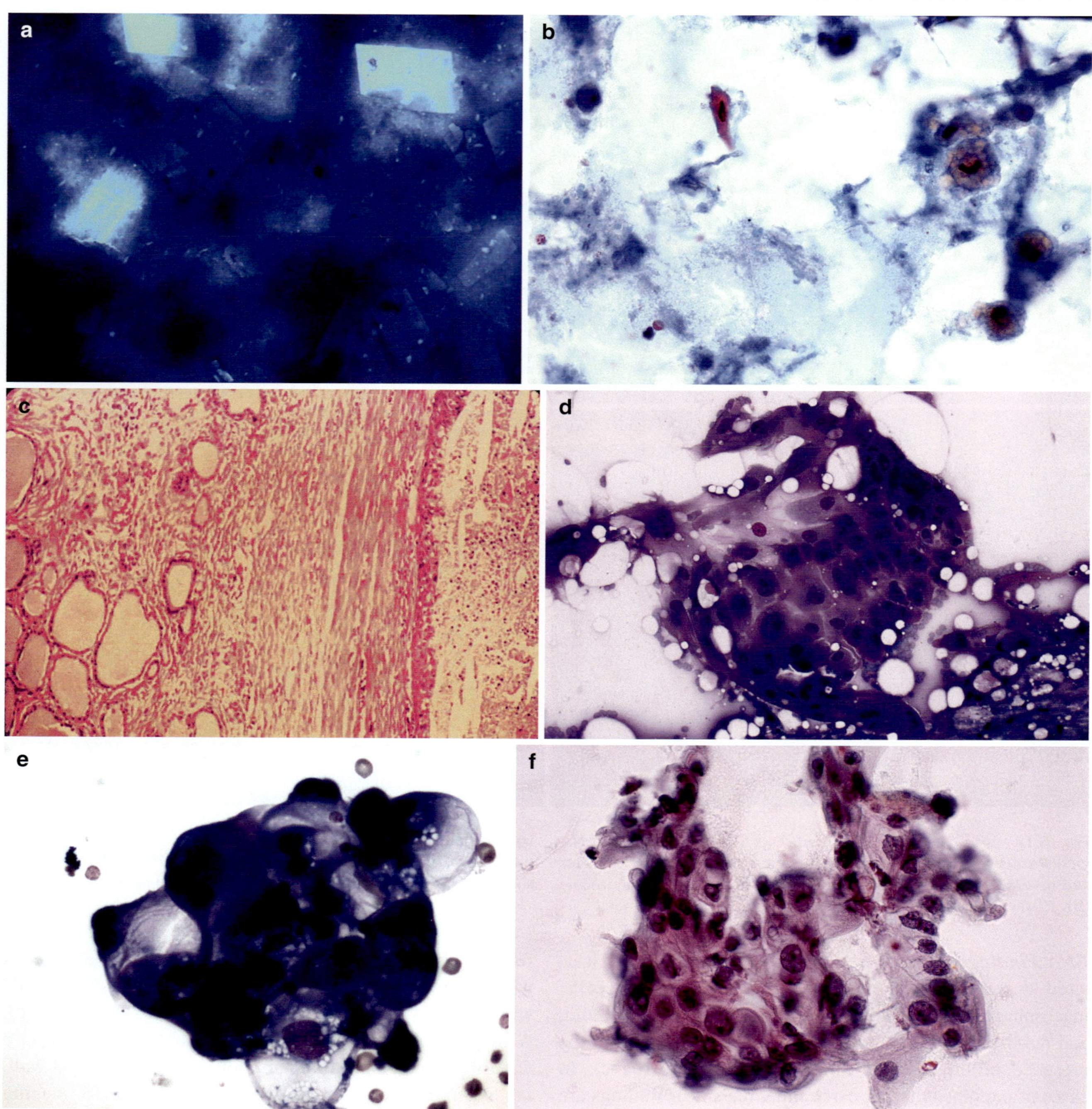

Fig. 6.19 (**a–i**) Thyroglossal-duct cyst shows scattered macrophages, squamous cells, cholesterol crystals, and colloid (**a**, **b**). Tissue sections show lining squamous epithelium and subepithelial thyroid parenchyma toward the left side of the frame (**c**). This thyroglossal duct papillary carcinoma shows complex aggregates of large squamous metaplastic cells (**d**), "histiocytoid" cells (**e**), atypical cells (**f**), and psammoma bodies (**g**). Histology confirms the cytologic diagnosis (**h**). A different case of thyroglossal duct squamous carcinoma is shown in figure (**i**). (**a**, **d**, DiffQuik stain high magnification; **b**, **f**, **g**, **i**, Papanicolaou stain, high magnification; **c**, **h**, H&E stain, low magnification; **e**, MGG stain, high magnification)

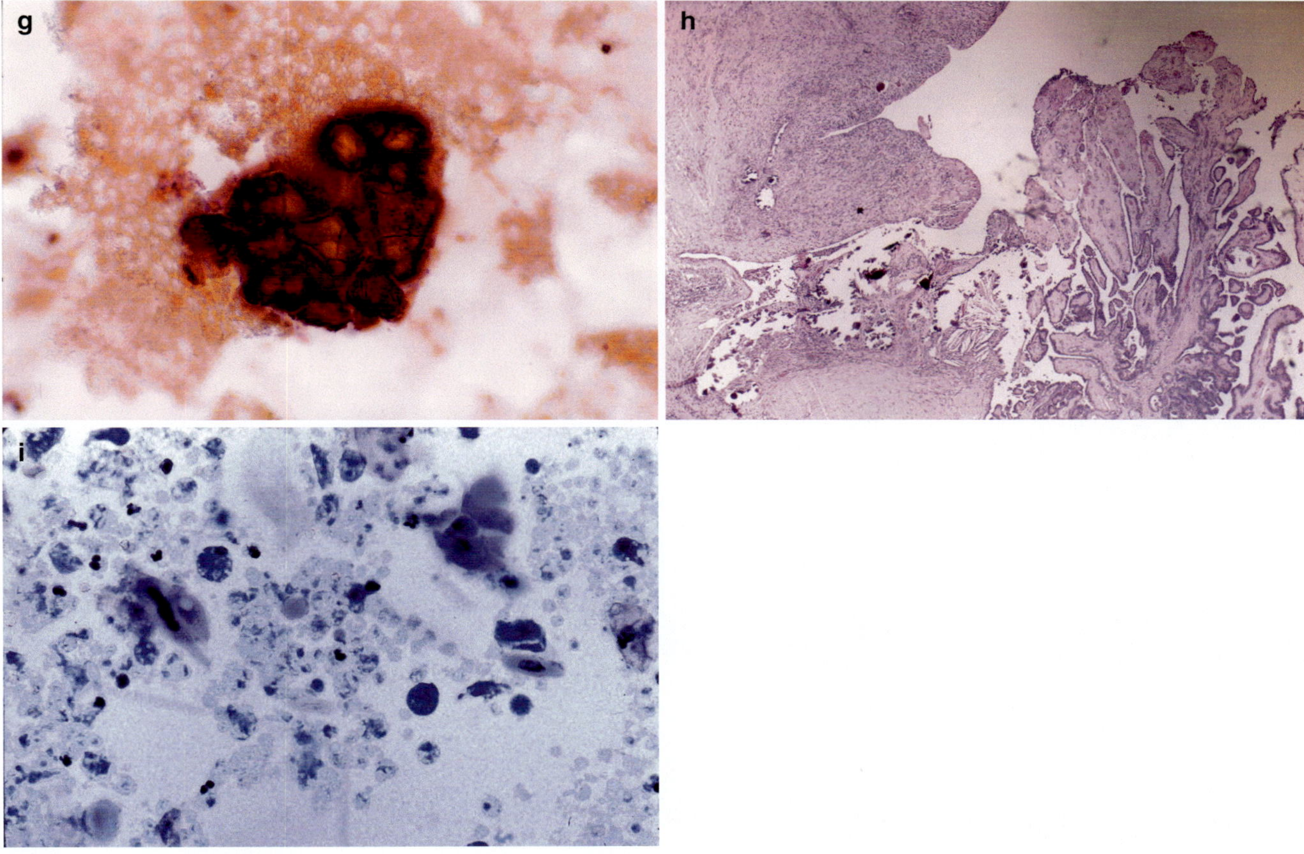

Fig. 6.19 (continued)

Lateral Region (Neck Levels IIb and III)

Carotid-Body Paraganglioma/Tumor

Parasympathetic paragangliomas can occur in various locations in the head and neck: glomus jugulare in the skull base, glomus vagale below the skull base, glomus tympanicum in the middle ear, and carotid-body tumor in the carotid bifurcation. Carotid-body tumor or carotid-body paraganglioma is a neuroendocrine tumor that arises from the carotid-body paraganglia.

Clinical Findings The carotid-body tumor usually affects adults, commonly women in the 4th–5th decade of life, and occurs as a painless and progressively growing lateral neck pulsatile mass deep to the anterior border of the sternocleido-mastoid muscle below the angle of the mandible at the level of the hyoid bone. It is frequent especially in patients living >2000 m above sea level. About 10% of these tumors are multiple and may be familial, and 10% are malignant. The familial form is autosomal dominant and is associated with MEN syndromes, the Carney triad, and others.

Histopathology There is a cell nest or organoid growth pattern surrounded by fibrovascular stroma. Chief cells are round or oval, with abundant eosinophilic cytoplasm, granular uniform chromatin, and variable anisonucleosis. The sustentacular cells are spindle and basophilic cells, are located surrounding the nests of chief cells, and are difficult to identify on tissue sections (Fig. 6.22d). Cellular pleomorphism may be present; necrosis and mitosis are exceedingly rare and do not indicate malignancy. Metastasis is the only true criterion for a malignant paraganglioma.

Immuno-profile Chief cells are neuron-specific enolase-, chromogranin-, and synaptophysin-positive (Fig. 6.22k). Sustentacular cells are S100-protein-positive. CD56 is positive, and INSM1 and Gata3 show diffuse nuclear positivity. Calcitonin, epithelial, and melanoma markers are negative.

FNA Findings Most aspirates are bloody and show tumor cell aggregates and single cells of variable nuclear size. A nesting pattern is seen at low magnification. Microfollicular architecture may be present. The nuclear to cytoplasmic ratio, chromatin clumping, and nucleolar prominence are variable. Most nuclei are round or oval, eccentric, and may show intranuclear inclusions. The cytoplasm is cyanophilic with Papanicolaou stain and finely granular with

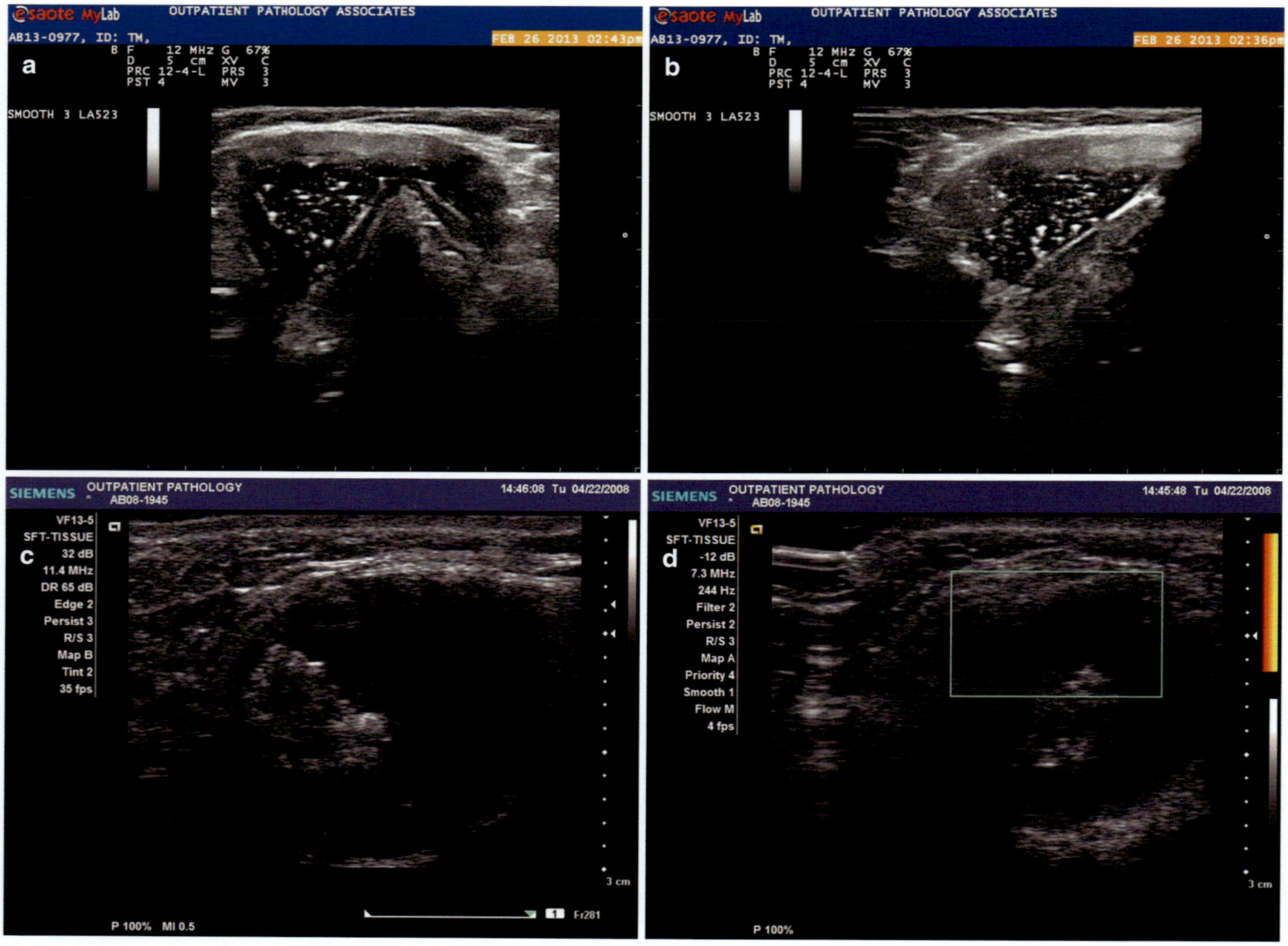

Fig. 6.20 (**a**–**d**) Ultrasound findings in thyroglossal duct cyst (**a**, **b**) and thyroglossal duct papillary carcinoma (**c**, **d**). Prominent "comet tails" are seen in the thyroglossal cyst and microcalcifications in the solid component of the papillary carcinoma. Vascularity by Doppler examination is not prominent in the carcinoma (**d**). (Ultrasound, high frequency, transverse views)

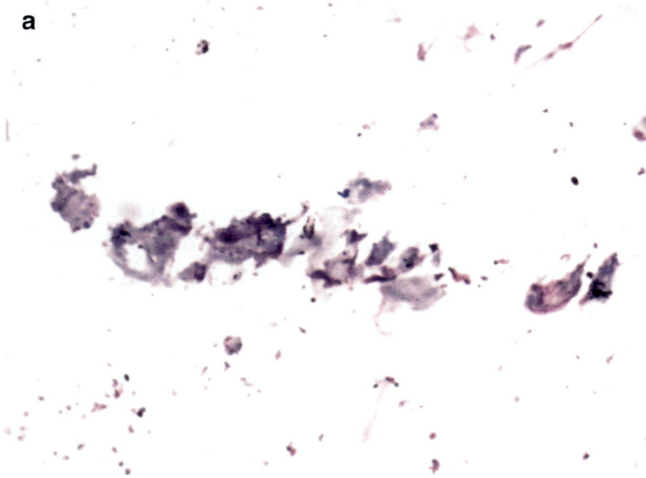

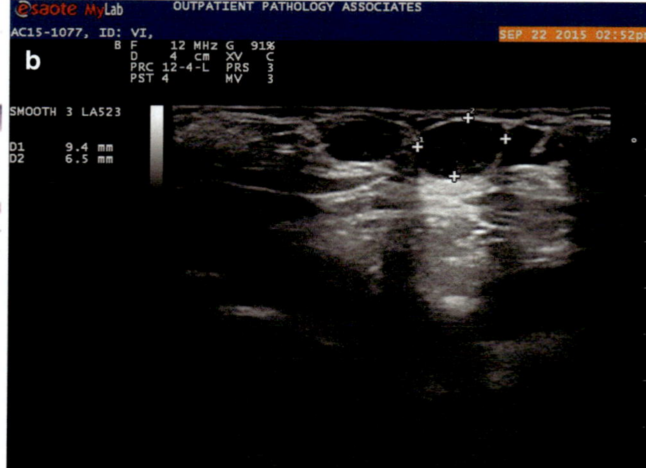

Fig. 6.21 (**a**, **b**) Dermoid cyst at neck level VII. USG-FNA yields anucleated squamous cells (**a**), and ultrasound shows an oval, anechoic, well-defined cystic mass, with posterior acoustic enhancement between the sternoclavicular joints (**b**). (**a**, Papanicolaou stain, medium magnification; **b**, ultrasound, high frequency, transverse view)

Romanowsky stains. Cells may show interlacing cytoplasmic processes. Cellular pleomorphism may be present, but necrosis or mitosis is absent (Fig. 6.22a–c, g, j).

The differential diagnosis includes neuroendocrine carcinomas, metastatic follicular and medullary carcinomas of the thyroid, and metastatic renal-cell carcinoma. Carefully obtained clinical findings, identification of cell clusters and single cells with fine cytoplasmic granules, and variations in size and shape are helpful. Special stains and electron microscopy are also contributory. Cells are seen to contain cytoplasmic neurosecretory granules by electron microscopy.

US Features The tumor can be reliably visualized by US imaging. The tumor is well-defined, heterogeneous, and hypoechoic. It has multiple anechoic foci that light up on Doppler examination and correspond to blood vessels. Doppler examination shows a vascular pattern usually originating from the external carotid artery (Figs. 6.22e, f, h, i, l, m; Video 6.2).

Peripheral-Nerve-Sheath Tumor

Schwannomas and neurofibromas and their variants are included in the WHO Classification of Soft Tissue and Bone Tumors, 5th edition, under "peripheral nerve sheath tumors." In general, these tumors are rare, Schwannomas occurring most commonly in the head and neck. Local resection is curative, and local recurrences are infrequent.

Clinical Findings Schwannoma is a benign tumor. Patients commonly have a non-painful, slowly growing mass that can be displaced horizontally and not vertically, as in carotid-body tumors. Schwannomas most commonly affect the lateral aspect of the neck, often of adult patients, and there is no gender preference. At times, insertion of a needle into the mass elicits an intense pain that is an almost pathognomonic indicator for the diagnosis.

Histopathology The tumor originates in the Schwann cells and is usually encapsulated. It has alternating Antony A (cellular) and Antony B (loose) areas. The cells have spindle and hyperchromatic nuclei, and they are embedded in a fibrillary stroma with scattered lymphoid cells. Whorling and palisading of nuclei may be seen. Rare mitosis and necrosis may be present; they are not indicative of malignancy. Histologic variants include plexiform, epithelioid, glandular, and neuroblastoma-like forms. The "melanotic Schwannoma" has been renamed "malignant melanocytic nerve sheath tumor."

FNA Findings Smears show scant to moderate cellularity with uniform spindle cells held within glassy, dense, collagenous tissue fragments. The cells show slender and twisted nuclei and indistinct cytoplasmic borders and may have elongated fibrillary processes. The amount of matrix predominates over the cellular elements in most cases, and the tissue fragments are sharply defined. The cell clusters may show compact (Antony A) and loose hypocellular (Antony B) areas. Verrocay bodies are uncommon, but diagnostic; there is a zone of palisading nuclei separated by a zone of fibrillary substance. High cellularity, sparse mitoses, and pleomorphism are not indicative of malignancy; pleomorphism is a feature of ancient schwannomas. Moderate numbers of free-lying, twisted nuclei with pointy ends are present in the background. Scattered lymphoid cells may be seen admixed in the tissue fragments. Cystic degeneration, necrosis, hemorrhage, and calcification are considered retrogressive changes (Fig. 6.23a–d).

The differential diagnosis includes neurofibromas of the head and neck that may have FNA cytomorphology that is similar to that of Schwannoma (Fig. 6.23g). Diagnostic keys include the cutaneous-subcutaneous location, non-twisted spindle-cell shape, cellular arrangement, and stromal features that distinguish them from Schwannomas. An organized thrombus can be sizable and show a cytomorphology similar to that of Schwannoma (Fig. 6.23i).

US Features Characteristically, the tumors are oval with well-defined edges, homogeneous, and markedly hypoechoic with a "pseudocystic" appearance showing posterior enhancement. These features are seen particularly in small tumors. These tumors can be confused clinically with lymph nodes; however, they lack fatty hilum and, when scanned longitudinally, they have tapered ends that merge with the echogenic fibrillary nerve bundles. The tumors tend to be hypervascular, although less so than are carotid-body tumors. The US of Schwannoma is similar to that of an organized thrombus and fibromatosis, with the exception that the mass is related to the subcutaneous tissue in the latter. When occurring in the parotid area, Schwannoma is difficult to distinguish from pleomorphic adenoma (Fig. 6.23e–f, h, j–m).

Branchial-Cleft Cyst

Branchial cleft cyst is the most common congenital anomaly of the second branchial cleft and can occur anywhere along a tract that passes inferiorly from the junction of the middle and lower thirds of the sternocleidomastoid muscle (anterior border) to the tonsilar fossa, passing between the internal and external carotid arteries. The position in the neck is identical to that of the jugulo-digastric lymph node.

Clinical Findings The most common location of the cyst is at the level of the angle of the mandible, posterior to the submandibular gland, anterior to the sternocleidomastoid muscle, and superficial to the great vessels. Patients are usually less than 40 years and have a fluctuant, painless mass. The

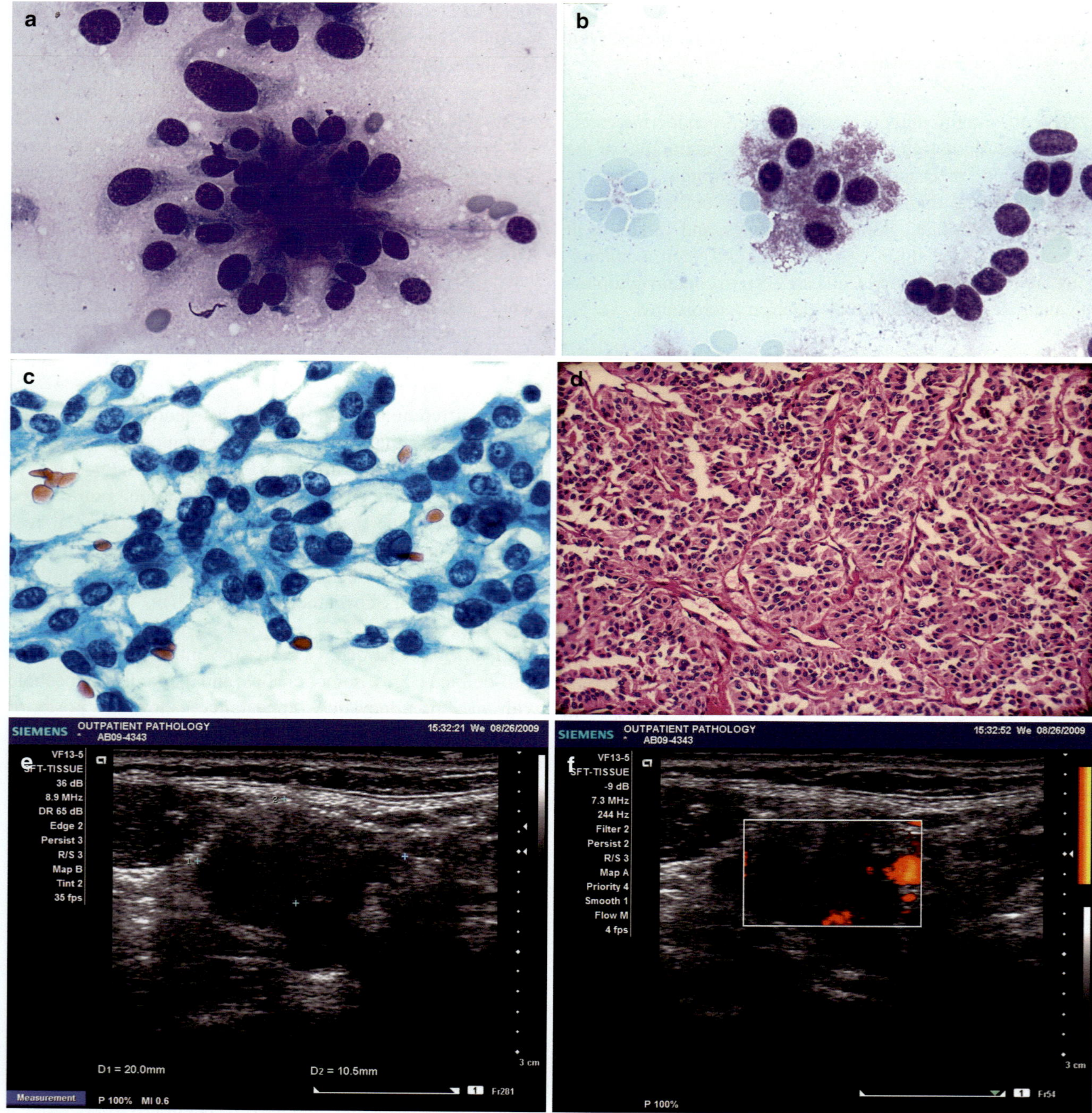

Fig. 6.22 (**a–m**) Carotid body paraganglioma. Smears are cellular and show moderate to marked cell pleomorphism, microfollicular architecture (**a**), red cytoplasmic granules (**b**), nuclear inclusions (**c**), and "salt and pepper" chromatin with inconspicuous nucleoli. An organoid/trabecular pattern is evident in the resected tumor (**d**). Ultrasound shows an ill-defined hypoechoic mass with subtle merging of the normal vessels and the tumor mass (**e**, **f**). The following three images correspond to a 9 cm paraganglioma occupying the left neck levels II and III diagnosed in a 14-year-old female. The smear shows aggregates of pleomorphic cells with fine granular cytoplasm and ill-defined cytoplasmic borders, that are arranged in a nesting pattern (**g**). US shows a solid, hypoechoic mass encasing the carotid artery (**h**, **i**). The following four images correspond to a 2 cm neck paraganglioma adjacent to the right thyroid lobe (neck level III) diagnosed in a 49-year-old woman. Smears show a pleomorphic cell population that had a positive immunohistochemical stain for CD56 (**j**, **k**). US shows a solid vascular hypoechoic extra-thyroidal mass with well-circumscribed borders (**l**, **m**). (**a**, **b**, DiffQuik stain, high magnification; **c**, Papanicolaou stain, high magnification; **d**, H&E stain, low magnification; **g**, **j**, MGG stain, high magnification; **k**, cellblock, immunohistochemistry for CD56, medium magnification; **e**, **f**, **h**, **i**, **l**, **m**, ultrasound, high frequency, transverse view)

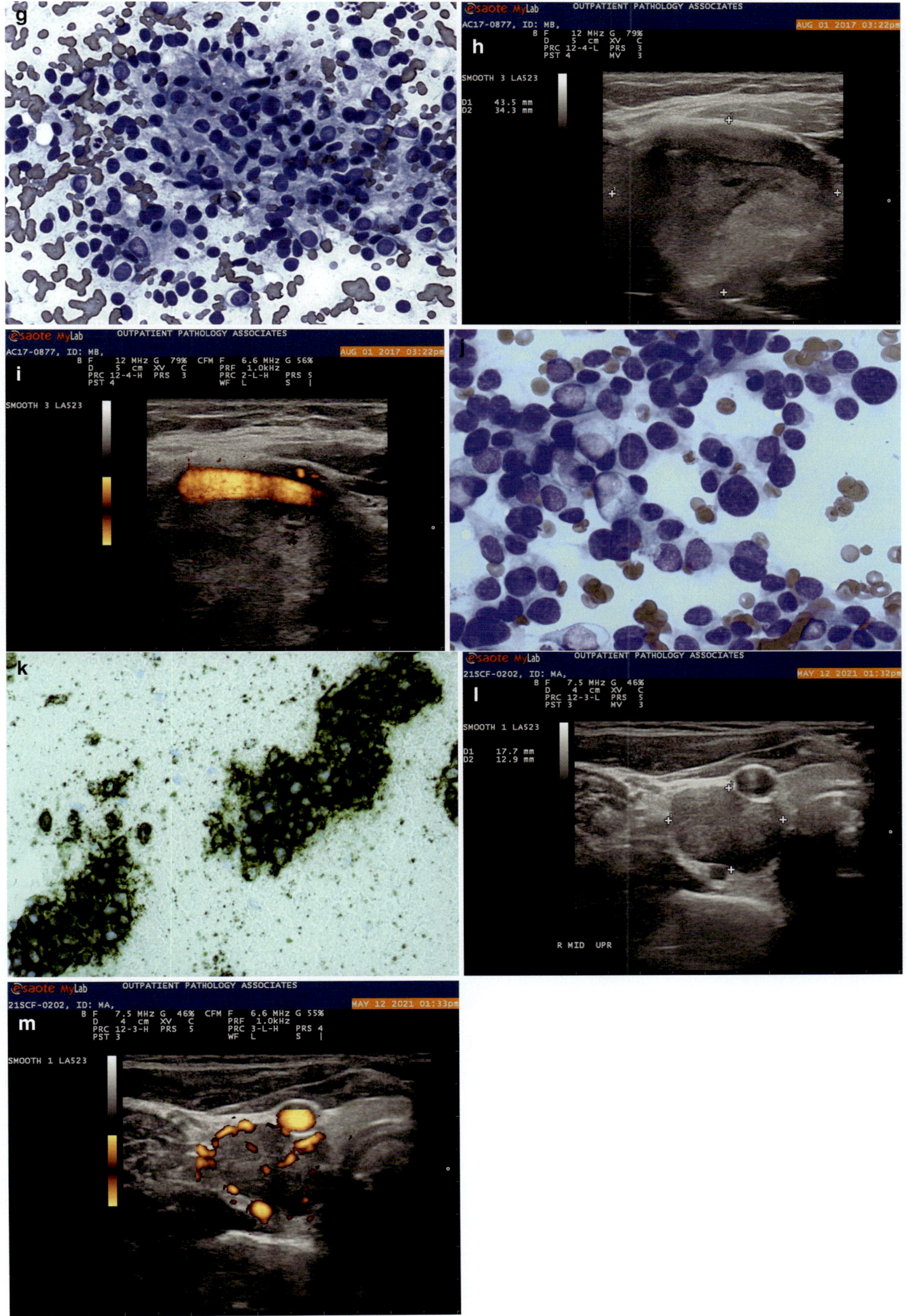

Fig. 6.22   (continued)

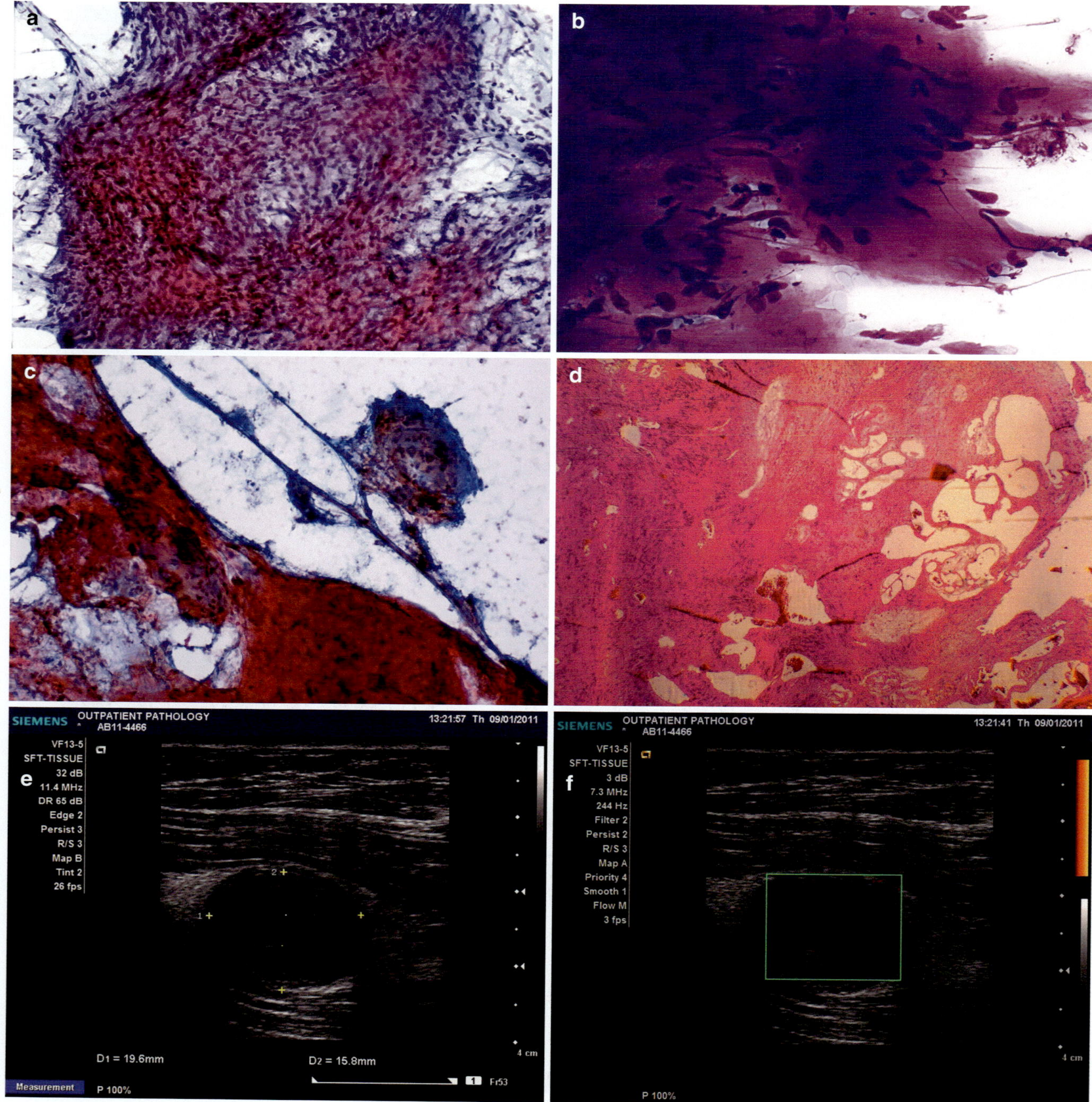

Fig. 6.23 (**a–m**) Schwannoma. Smear shows cellular fragments of spindle cells (**a**) supported by dense, slightly fibrillary stroma (**b**). Cellular and less cellular aggregates correspond to Antony A and B areas, respectively (**a**). Cystic degeneration is present in (**c**) and correlates with findings in a long-standing cystic Schwannoma (**d**). Cytomorphology is similar to that of fibromatosis (**g**) and an organized thrombus (**i**). US shows a hypoechoic, slightly heterogeneous, and slightly elongated mass with posterior acoustic enhancement and minimal, if any, vascular flow by Doppler examination (**e**, **f**). US of fibromatosis shows a hypoechoic mass that is situated in the subcutaneous tissue (**h**). US image of an organizing thrombus is similar to that of Schwannoma (**j**, **k**). The insertion of the needle into this Schwannoma located in level II of the neck elicited intense pain. The similarity to the US features of a lymph node is notable; however, the tapered ends of the mass merging with the nerve provides a suggestion to reconsider a Schwannoma (**l**, **m**). (**a**, **c**, Papanicolaou stain, medium magnification; **b**, DiffQuik stain, medium magnification; **d**, H&E stain, low magnification; **g**, **i**, MGG stain, high magnification; **e**, **f**, **h**, **j**, **k**, US high frequency, transverse views; **l**, **m**, US high frequency, transverse and sagittal views respectively)

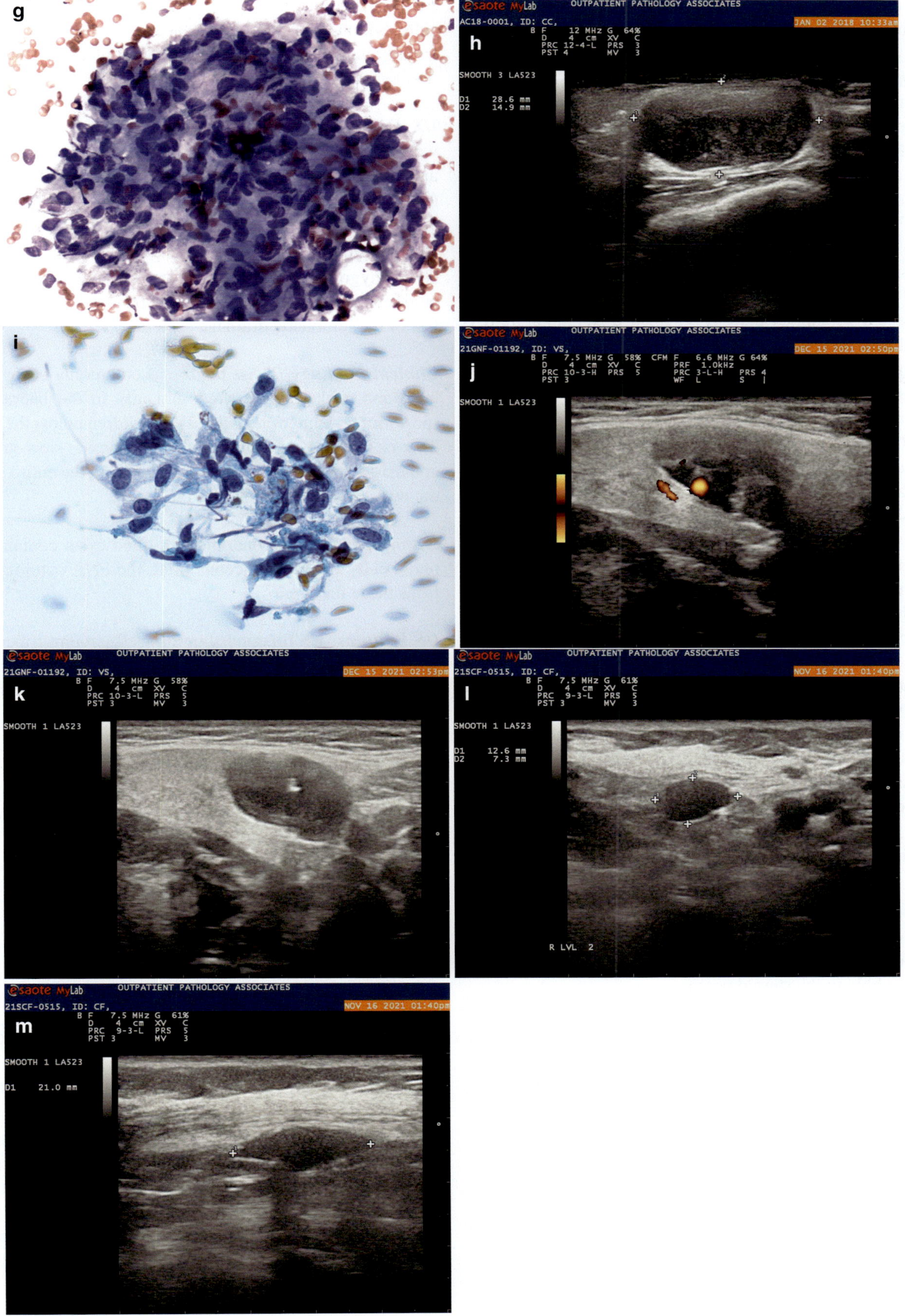

Fig. 6.23 (continued)

mass is of variable size and may become larger, and firmer at the time of an upper airway infection.

Histopathology The cyst lining is of the keratinized squamous type in 90% of cases, being columnar or mixed in the remaining 10%. The cyst wall contains nodular lymphoid tissue, often with germinal centers. The cyst fluid contains squamous cells, lymphocytes, and cholesterol crystals.

FNA Findings USG-FNA is done with a 25- or a 23-G-needle under suction and yields a turbid yellow fluid (Fig. 6.24a, b). Smears show numerous nucleated and anucleated squamous cells (Fig. 6.24c). Acellular fluid is occasionally encountered. Variable numbers of columnar, mucinous, and lymphoid cells in a background of debris and cholesterol crystals may be present. Inflamed cysts may show epithelial atypia, but frank anaplasia is absent (Fig. 6.24d, e). The differential diagnosis includes other congenital cysts, cystic squamous cell carcinoma (with nuclear anaplasia), and salivary gland cysts (which may contain crystalloids). Of note, diagnosis of a jugulo-digastric lymph node with cystic necrosis associated with metastasis from squamous cell or thyroid carcinoma should be kept in mind particularly in patients older than 40 years and from papillary thyroid carcinoma, before the diagnosis of a branchial-cleft cyst is made (Fig. 6.24f).

US Features The US image shows a well-defined anechoic or hypoechoic mass with regular borders, a thin and uniform wall, internal debris, and posterior acoustic enhancement. Occasionally, homogeneous internal echoes may be present and mimic a solid mass ("pseudosolid"). US of cystic masses, i.e., hematoma, cystic metastasis from squamous cell carcinoma, etc. should be kept in mind in the differential diagnosis (Fig. 6.24g–m; Videos 6.3 and 6.4).

Cervical Thymic Cyst

Solid or cystic remnants of thymic tissue may occur in the neck along the course of the carotid sheath from the angle of the mandible to the sternal notch.

Clinical Findings These remnants of thymic tissue are more common in men than in women. They occur in the first decade of life or less commonly, up to the third decade. Patients have a slow-growing, painless mass that increases in size with the Valsalva maneuver.

Histopathology The cysts are unilocular or multilocular, contain clear fluid, are lined with cuboidal, columnar, or squamous epithelium, and contain thymic tissue. Because of the common embryologic origin with the parathyroid glands, parathyroid tissue may be present in the wall.

FNA Findings Smears of thymic cysts show rare epithelial cells, lymphocytes, and proteinaceous fluid. The distinction from branchial-cleft cyst is based on clinical and histologic findings (Fig. 6.25a).

US Features The findings are not specific and include a well-defined, smooth, anechoic cystic mass with a thin wall and posterior acoustic enhancement (Fig. 6.25b–d; Video 6.5).

Cystic Hygroma

Cystic hygromas are the most common subtypes of lymphangiomas and are believed to result from congenital anomalies of the lymphatic drainage system.

Clinical Findings These hygromas commonly occur in the head and neck regions, predominantly in the lateral neck (posterior and anterior triangles) of children below the age of 2 years; they rarely occur in adults. The mass is slow-growing and may be of considerable size, occupying the entire side of the neck, and may extend into the thorax.

Histopathology The endothelium-lined cysts contain lymphoid cells and proteinaceous fluid; the FNA cytology confirms these findings.

US Features US imaging shows a well-circumscribed, uniform, solitary or multicystic anechoic mass with internal septations, a thin wall, and posterior acoustic enhancement.

Supraclavicular Region (Neck Level IV)

Lymphadenopathy is the most common finding in the supraclavicular region that comprises neck level IV to the lower portion of neck level Vb. Among the rare non-nodal lesions of this region, benign adipose tissue prominence and lipomas predominate. Occasionally, a palpable, prominent vertebral transverse process may be present and mimic a mass (Fig. 6.26).

Posterior Neck Region (Neck Levels Va and Vb)

The area posterior to the sternocleidomastoid and anterior to the trapezius muscles is designated as neck levels Va (superior) and Vb (inferior). Lymphadenopathy is most common in the posterior neck region. Non-nodal pathology is rare, and includes lipomas, peripheral-nerve-sheath tumors, and cystic hygroma (in children) predominant.

Lipomas are discussed in the section "common and uncommon superficial masses of the head and neck and other body sites," later in this chapter.

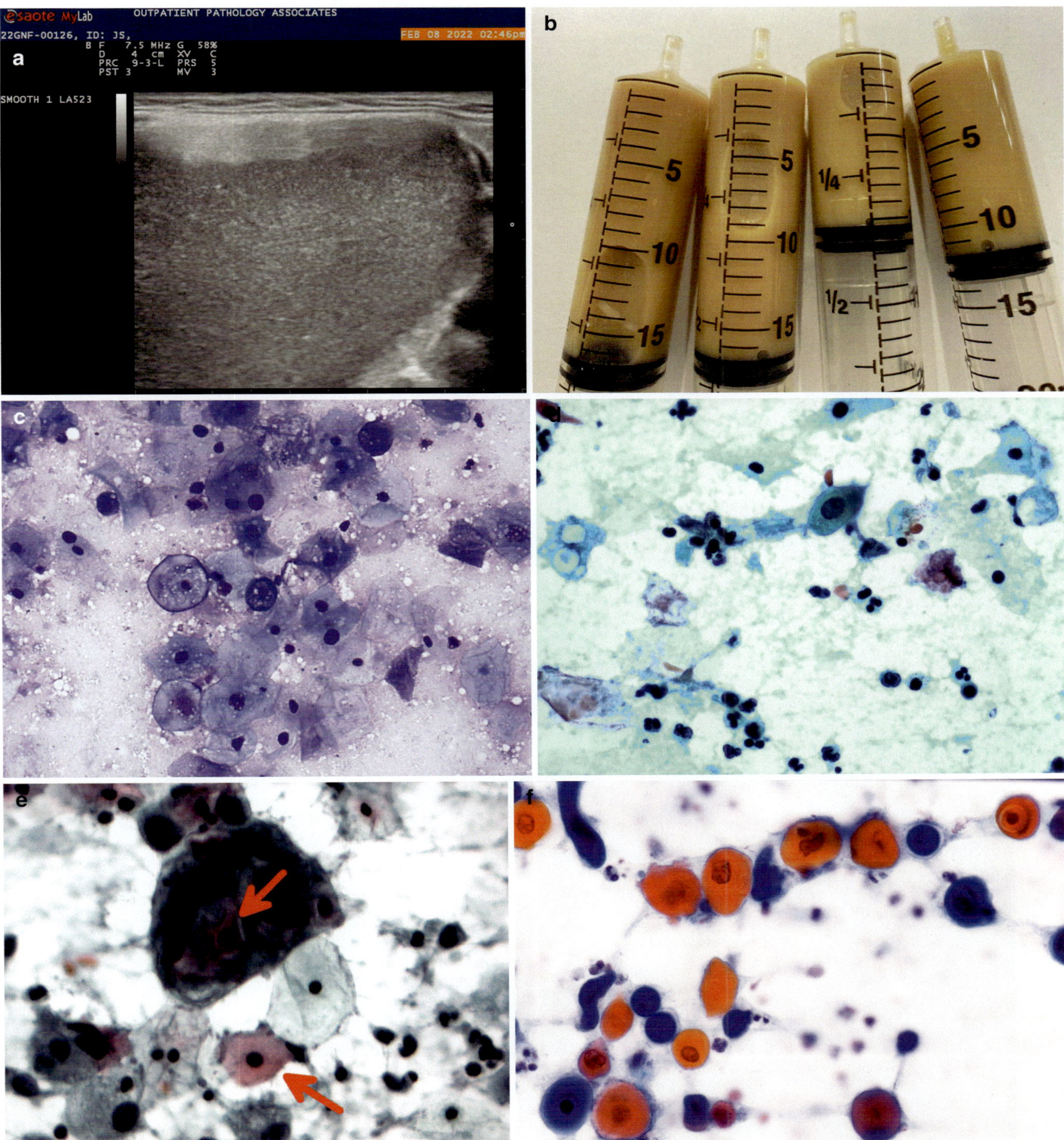

Fig. 6.24 (**a–m**) Branchial-cleft cyst. USG-FNA from this large branchial-cleft cyst yielded 55ml of fluid (**a, b**). Rare squamous cells and proteinaceous fluid are present when the cyst is not inflamed (**c**). Reactive cytologic changes are seen in the inflamed branchial cleft cyst (**d**) or in a ruptured epidermal inclusion cyst (**e**, arrows), but frank anaplasia is absent. Keratinized and non-keratinized anaplastic cells are seen in a cystic metastasis from squamous cell carcinoma (**f**). US imaging shows a well-circumscribed oval-shaped mass with posterior acoustic enhancement, thin wall, and no blood flow by Doppler examination (**g, h**). Cyst fluid drainage is done under US guidance as mentioned in Chap. 2. These images show the cyst pre- and post-fluid drainage (**i, j**). Ruptured epidermal inclusion cysts may have a heterogeneous echotexture, fuzzy borders, and Doppler exam shows increased blood flow in the area of rupture (**k, l**). Cystic degeneration in squamous carcinoma may show a thick-walled cyst, and USG-FNA from the wall yields viable malignant cells (**m**). (**c**, MGG stain, high magnification; **d–f**, Papanicolaou stain, high magnification; **a, g–m**, US high frequency, transverse view)

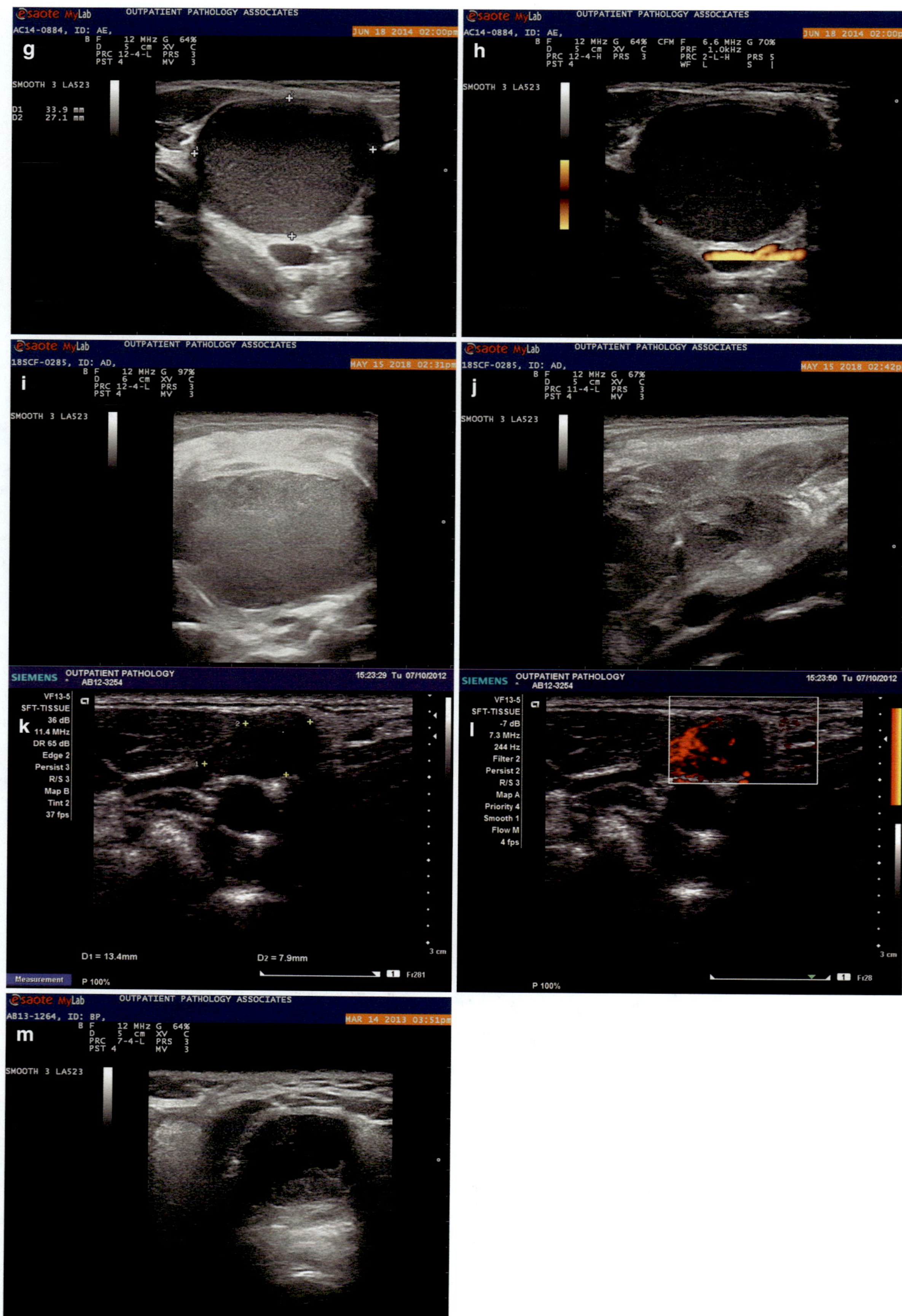

Fig. 6.24 (continued)

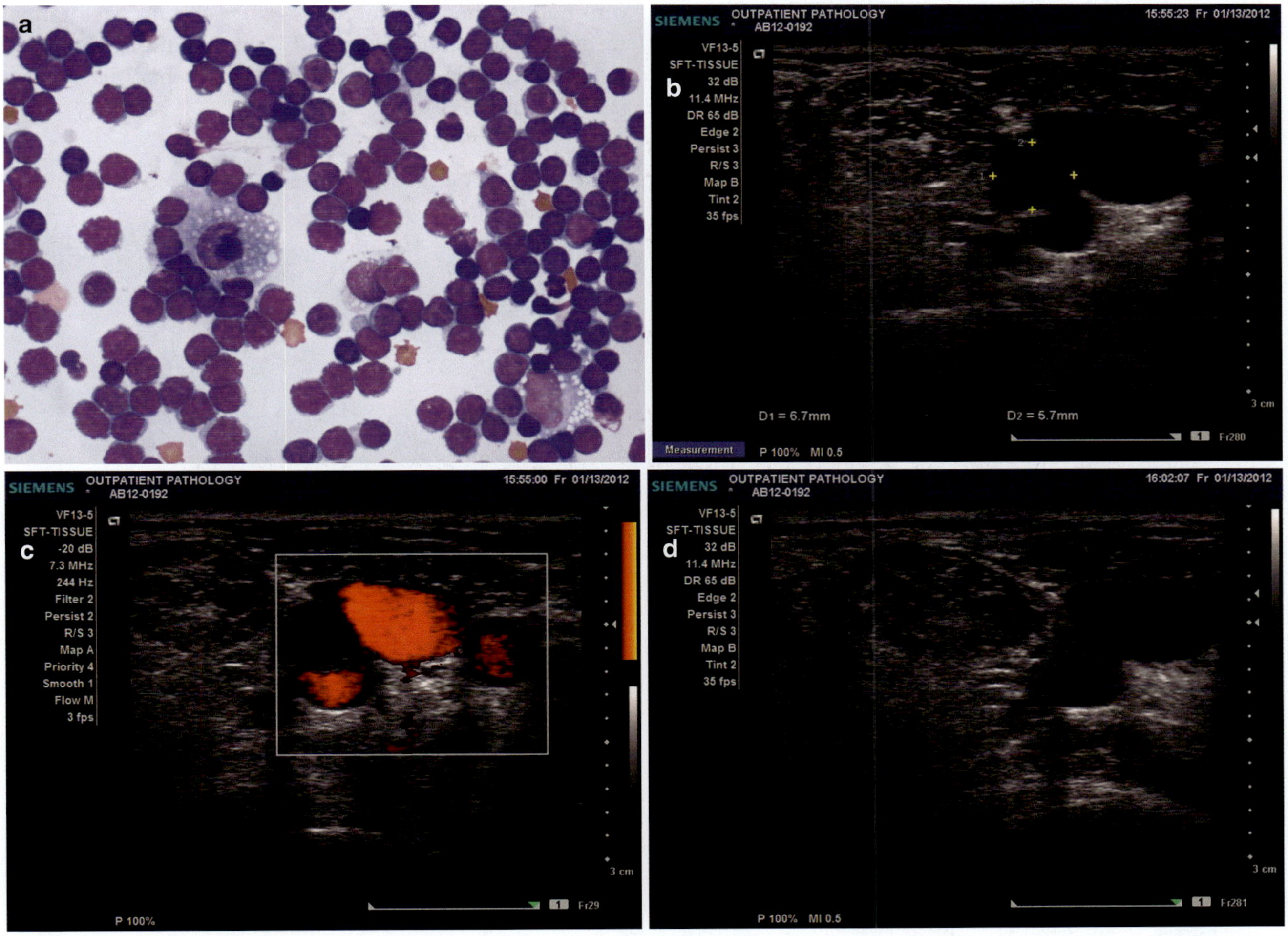

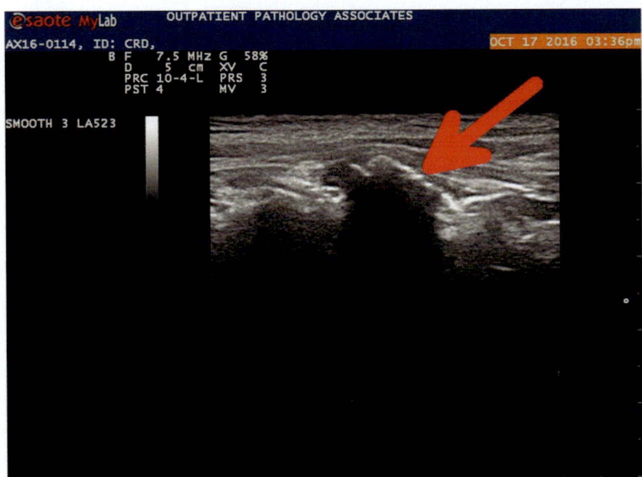

Fig. 6.25 (a–d) Cervical thymic cyst. Scattered small lymphoid cells and a rare macrophage are present in the smears from this small left neck level II cyst in a 9-year-old child (**a**). US images show an anechoic, avascular, cystic lesion with thin borders, situated supero-medial to the carotid and jugular vein (**b**, **c**). The cyst collapsed after fluid drainage (**d**). (**a**, MGG stain, high magnification; **b–d**, ultrasound, high frequency, transverse view)

Fig. 6.26 Ultrasound image of a palpable vertebral transverse prominence. The arrow shows the irregularly shaped echogenic cortical bone. No soft-tissue mass is identified by US

Skin and Scalp

FNA is rarely used for the diagnosis of skin tumors, mainly because of their size and accessibility to surgical biopsies. However, aspirates can be used successfully in the diagnosis of suspected metastatic disease, evaluation of recurrent skin neoplasms, or in the diagnosis of tumors of unclear nature.

Pilomatrixoma

Clinical Findings This benign adnexal (hair matrix) skin tumor is a hard subcutaneous tissue nodule often seen in the face, neck, and upper extremities, and identified mostly during the first two decades of life.

FNA Findings Smears show scattered single and dense groups of overlapping, degenerating basaloid cells mixed with a pink background substance (seen on MGG stain). The cells are usually stripped of cytoplasm and exhibit round to oval nuclei, regular nuclear contours, evenly distributed granular chromatin, and small, distinct nucle-oli. Foreign-body giant cells with absent or minimal inflammation, ghost cells with keratinization, elongated reactive fibroblasts, and calcium debris may be present (Fig. 6.27a–d).

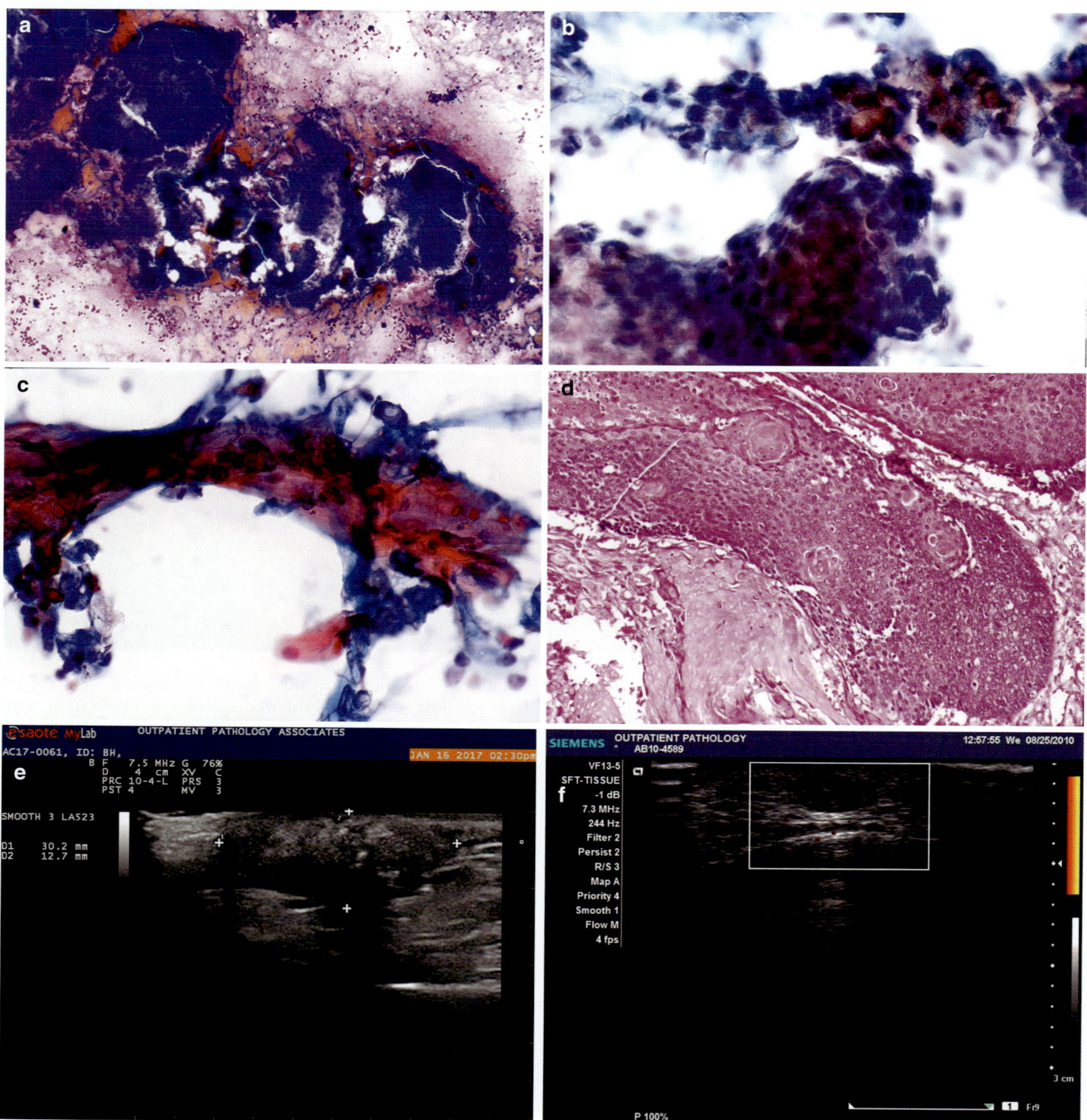

Fig. 6.27 (**a–d**) Pilomatrixoma. Smear shows complex 3-dimensional aggregates of basaloid cells (**a**), tight squamous pearls, anucleated squamous cells, calcific fragments admixed with the basaloid cells (**b**), and foreign-body-type giant cell reaction to keratin (**c**). Histologic section confirms the cytologic findings (**d**). The following US images correspond to two pilomatrixomas. The large mass shows a hypoechoic oval mass with ill-defined borders, heterogeneous echotexture, and echogenic foci with posterior acoustic shadowing suggestive of calcifi-cations. Doppler examination of the small mass shows a hypoechoic and homogeneous echotexture, posterior acoustic enhancement, and lack of vascularity. Both masses are present in the subcutaneous tissue (**e**, **f**). (**a**, DiffQuik stain, low magnification; **b**, **c**, Papanicolaou stain, medium magnification; **d**, H&E stain, medium magnification; **e**, **f**, US, high frequency, transverse views)

The differential diagnosis of pilomatrixoma includes carcinomas with basaloid cells (skin, salivary glands) and small blue-cell tumors. Diagnostic key features include the patient's age, clinical history, physical examination, and cytology findings of ghost squamous cells, basaloid cells, multinucleated cells, and calcium deposits.

US Features As mentioned in the section on parotid region masses, an ill-defined, irregular, hypoechoic subcutaneous nodule that may have calcifications is identified (Fig. 6.27e, f).

Cylindroma

Because of its multinodular and diffuse distribution, this tumor of skin appendage origin is called a "turban tumor of the scalp."

FNA Findings The features are identical to those of basal cell carcinoma, except for an occasional layer of hyaline material that surrounds the periphery of some cell clusters.

Apocrine Mixed Tumor

Synonyms: benign mixed tumor the the skin, chondroid syringoma, apocrine mixed tumor, eccrine mixed tumor.

Clinical Findings This is a nodular, circumscribed, slow-growing tumor of sweat gland derivation that commonly occurs in the head and neck of middle-aged men, particularly affecting the central region of the face. Malignant tumors characterized by rapid growth and ulceration are rare.

Histopathology This is morphologically similar to a benign mixed tumor (pleomorphic adenoma) of salivary glands and has epithelial, myoepithelial, and stromal (chondromyxoid and fibrous) components. The tumor often has follicular, sebaceous, and apocrine differentiation with prominent branching tubular structures.

FNA Findings Cytology smears show myoepithelial cells with varying degrees of anisocytosis and anisonucleosis, chondromyxoid fibrillary stroma, and "basaloid" epithelial cells. Marked cellular pleomorphism, nucleoli, mitosis, and necrosis are absent (Fig. 6.28a–c).

US Features This tumor is solid, hypoechoic, well-defined, heterogeneous, with echogenic foci, and is located in the deep dermis/subcutaneous tissue. Vascular blood flow is minimal or absent (Fig. 6.28d).

Basal Cell Carcinoma

Aspirates from basal cell carcinomas are usually performed for verification of recurrence of an excised primary tumor.

FNA Findings Smears show variable cellularity, complex aggregates, and single basaloid cells with hyperchromatic nuclei, mitosis, and necrosis (Fig. 6.29a, b). The differential diagnosis includes small-cell carcinoma, Merkel cell tumor, and tumors with predominance of the basaloid component as in pilomatrixoma.

Cutaneous Metastasis of Squamous Cell Carcinoma

The smears are cellular and show varying degrees of keratinization and cellular anaplasia (Fig. 6.30a, b). The differential diagnosis mainly includes ruptured epidermal inclusion cysts and pilomatrixoma. Ruptured branchial-cleft cysts may show acutely inflamed granulation tissue and reactive inflammatory changes of squamous cells; however, cellular anaplasia is absent. Clinical work-up including imaging studies together with FNA smear findings are important for making the correct diagnosis (Fig. 6.30c, d).

Merkel Cell Tumor

This uncommon malignant neoplasm occurs in the dermis of elderly patients and behaves aggressively, with frequent metastases to regional lymph nodes. Cytology and differential diagnosis are discussed in the section on metastatic tumors to lymph nodes of Chap. 7 (Fig. 6.31a–d).

Sebaceous Carcinoma

Aspirates from this neoplasm show two cell types and a necrotic background. Larger cells show vacuolated cytoplasm, vesicular nuclei, and prominent nucleoli. Smaller cells show basaloid to intermediate cell characteristics. When the former cells predominate, they must be differentiated from other clear-cell neoplasms; the latter can be confused with basal cell carcinoma and basaloid squamous cell carcinoma.

Kaposi Sarcoma

This vascular tumor may be classic (indolent tumor that affects the lower extremities of elderly individuals of Mediterranean ancestry), endemic (African form that affects children and

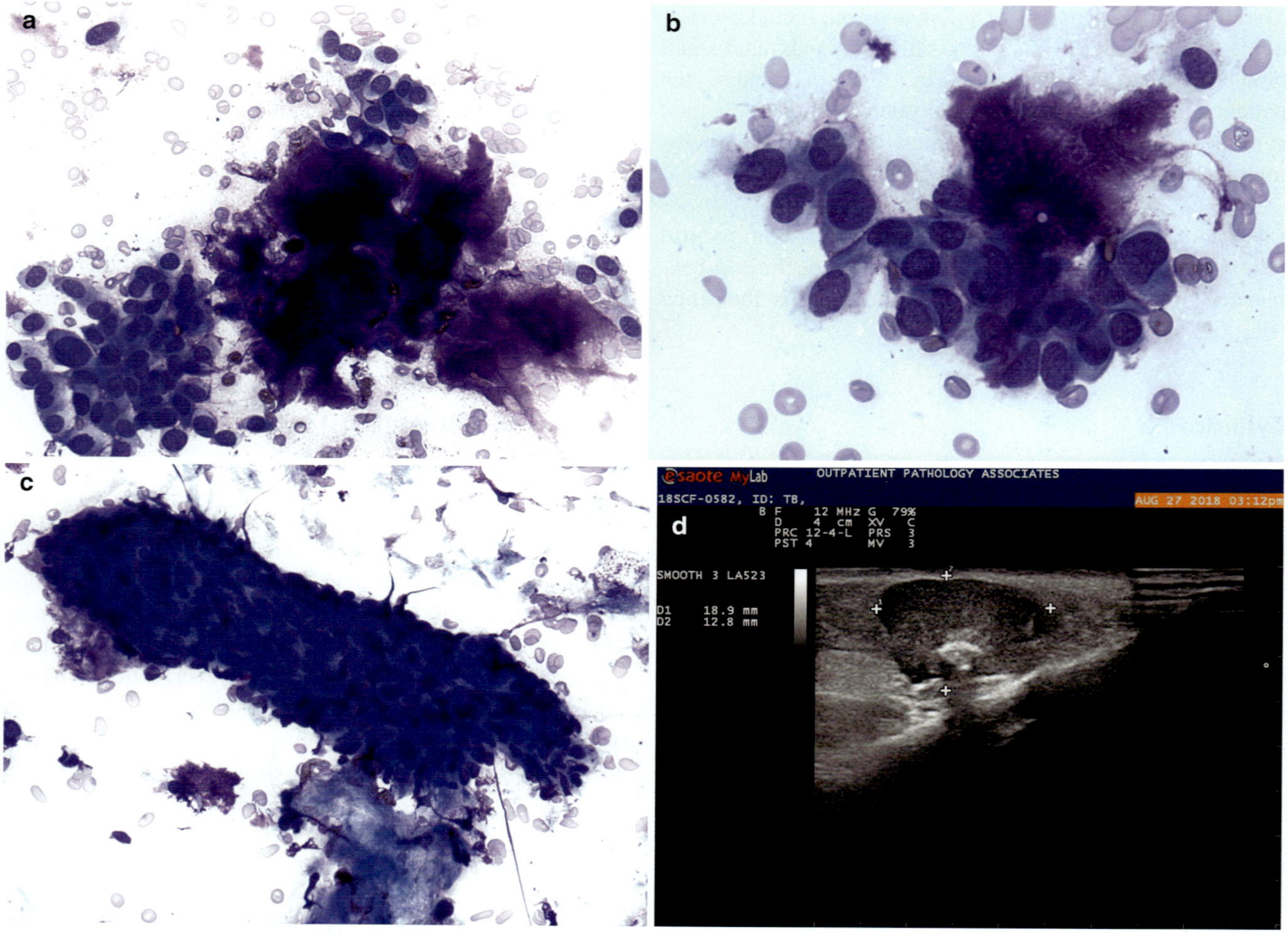

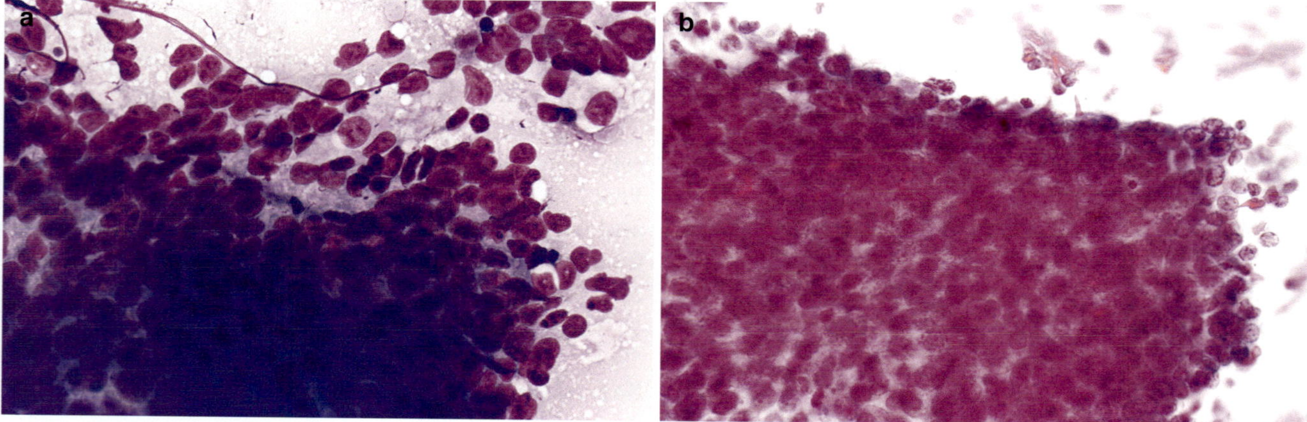

Fig. 6.28 (**a–d**) Apocrine mixed tumor. This 2 cm nasolabial-fold skin tumor was present for 2 years in a 49-year-old woman. Smears show a prominent fibrillary myxoid background and metaplastic myoepithelial cells with mild anisonucleosis and anisocytosis (**a, b**). Bland-appearing, well-organized "basaloid" epithelial cells forming a tubule are also present (**c**). Anucleated squamous cells and calcification may be present and pilomatrixoma must be considered as a diagnostic possibility, particularly in patients in the first and second decades of life. Ultrasound shows a deep subcutaneous tissue hypoechoic, well-circumscribed mass, with macrocalcification and posterior acoustic shadowing (**d**). (**a**, MGG stain, medium magnification; **d**, ultrasound, high frequency, transverse view)

Fig. 6.29 (**a, b**) Basal cell carcinoma. Recurrence in the site of prior surgery. (**a**, DiffQuik stain, high magnification; **b**, Papanicolaou stain, medium magnification)

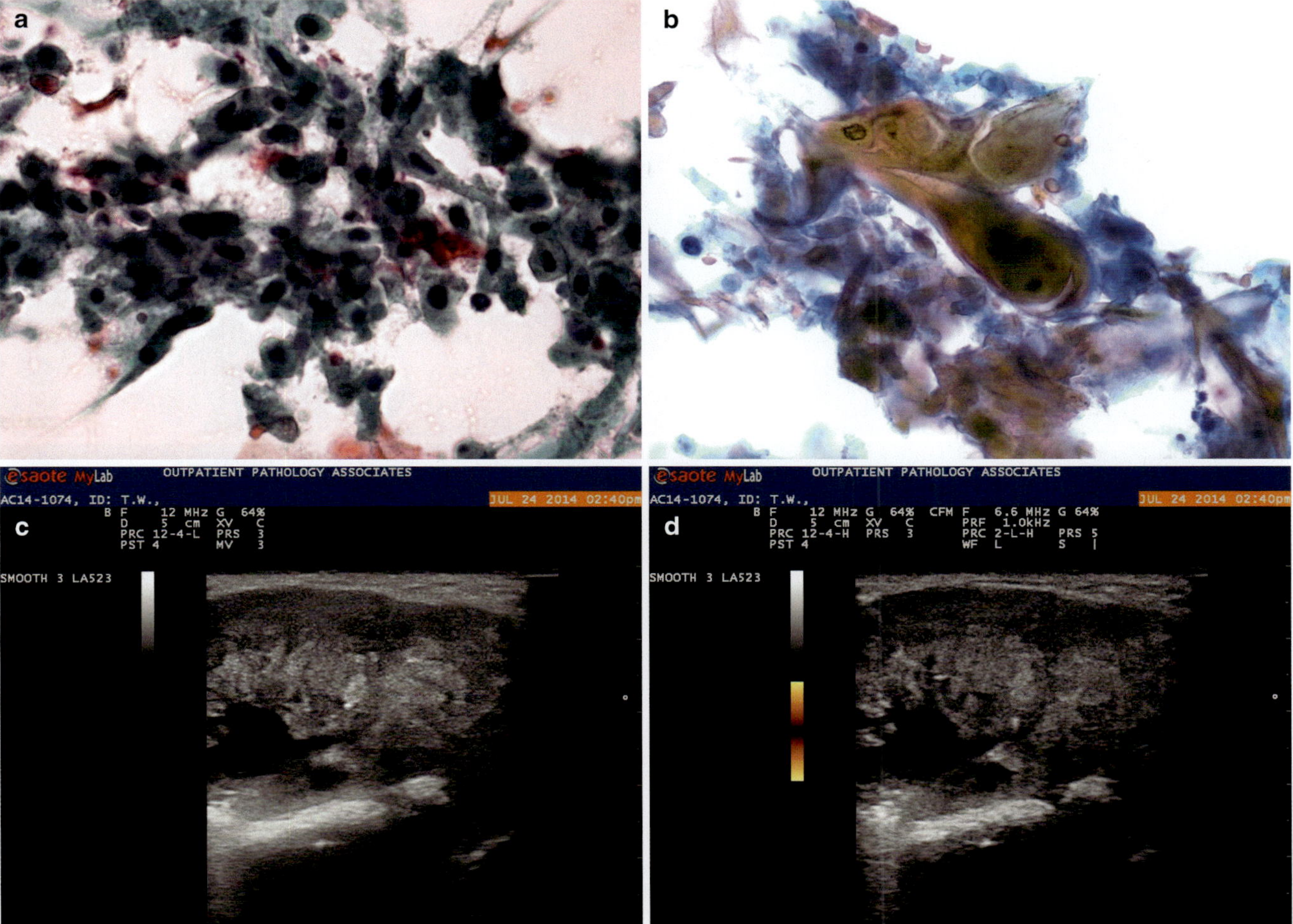

Fig. 6.30 (**a–c**) Cutaneous metastasis of squamous cell carcinoma. This 54-year-old man with history of hemi-glossectomy for squamous cell carcinoma noticed a progressive enlargement of a right-cheek mass. Examination showed a 6 × 6 cm fixed, nodular, and firm mass attached to the overlying skin. FNA shows extensive necrosis, cellular degeneration, anaplasia, and prominent keratinization (**a**, **b**). A hypoechoic, heterogeneous, minimally vascular, and well-demarcated mass involving the deep subcutaneous tissue is seen by US (**c**, **d**). (**a**, **b**, Papanicolaou stain, medium magnification; **c**, **d**, US, high frequency, transverse view)

middle-aged persons), iatrogenic (immunosuppression), and AIDS-associated. It may be present in the oral cavity and lymph nodes of patients with AIDS. Human herpesvirus-8 is involved in the pathogenesis of Kaposi sarcoma.

FNA Findings   There are cohesive clusters and single plump spindle cells in a bloody background. The cytoplasmic borders are ill-defined, and many of the single cells are stripped of cytoplasm. Slit-like spaces may be found in the cell clusters (Fig. 6.32a, b). The lesion resembles granulation tissue, and inflammatory cells including lymphocytes and plasma cells may be present.

The differential diagnosis includes other reactive and neoplastic spindle cell processes. The diagnostic key is the clinical history.

Metastatic Malignancies

Most malignancies metastasize late in the course of the disease process (Fig. 6.33a, d). However, scalp metastasis from renal cell carcinoma (Fig. 6.33b) or from small-cell carcinoma of the lung (Fig. 6.33c) may be the first evidence of malignancy. Diagnostic keys include a high grade of suspi-

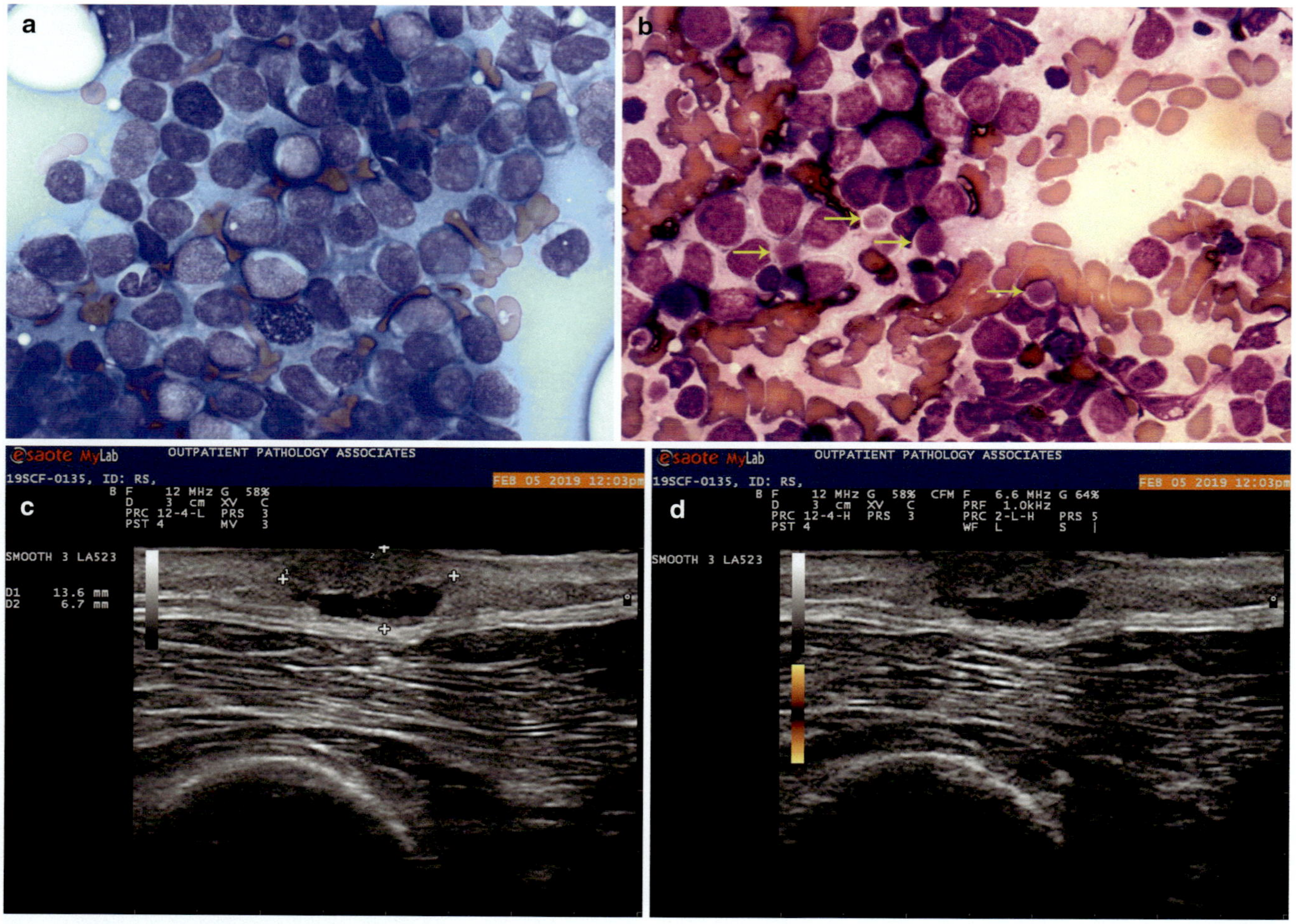

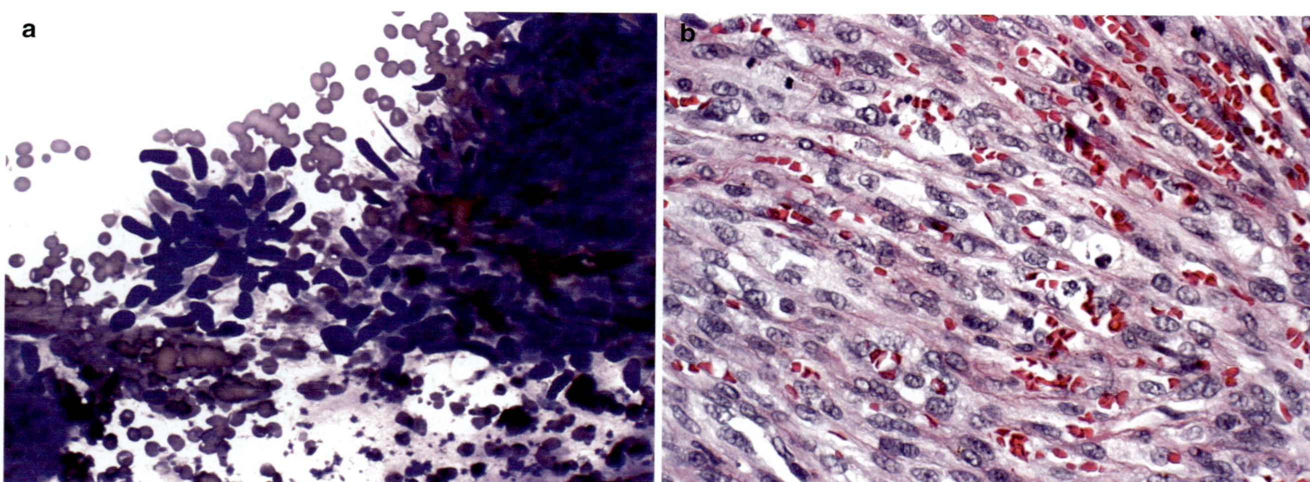

Fig. 6.31 (**a–d**) Merkel cell carcinoma. The smears of this skin-based tumor show a small/intermediate-size blue cell tumor (**a**). MGG stain shows a paranuclear condensation of intermediate filaments (keratin) (**b**, arrows). US shows a slightly hypoechoic deep dermis mass with an anechoic focus of necrosis, heterogeneous echotexture, irregular and fuzzy margins, and no identifiable vascular blood flow by Doppler examination (**c**, **d**). (**a**, **b**, MGG stain, high magnification; **c**, **d**, Ultrasound, high frequency, transverse views)

Fig. 6.32 (**a**, **b**) Kaposi's sarcoma. Spindle-cell pattern and red blood cells are noted (**a**). This cytologic pattern needs clinical correlation to support the diagnosis. Tissue section shows a poorly formed slit-like pattern filled with red blood cells (**b**). (**a**, DiffQuik stain, high magnification; **b**, H&E stain, medium magnification)

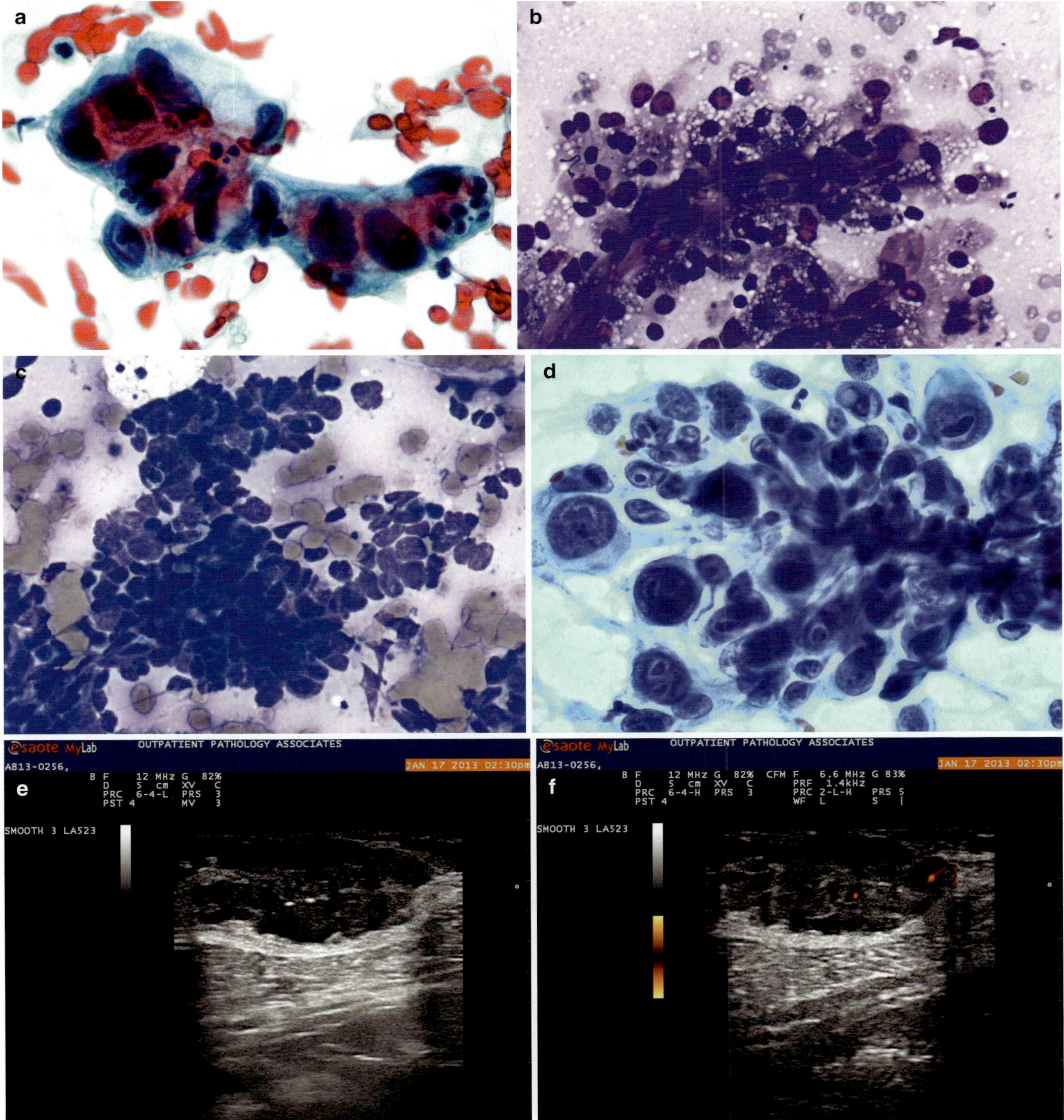

Fig. 6.33 (**a–e**) Skin metastases. Breast ductal carcinoma (**a**), renal cell clear-cell carcinoma (**b**), small-cell carcinoma of lung (**c**), and melanoma (**d**) metastases to subcutaneous tissue of the clavicular area (**a**) and scalp (**b–d**). Ultrasound findings are nonspecific; however, in the appropriate clinical history, a presumptive diagnosis of a metastatic deposit can be made. US shows a subcutaneous tissue mass with lobulated and fuzzy edges, as well as minimal vascular flow by Doppler examination (**e**, **f**). (**a**, **b**, Papanicolaou stain, high magnification; **b**, **c**, DiffQuik stain, medium magnification; **e**, **f**, ultrasound, high frequency, transverse view)

cion, clinical history, and careful evaluation of aspirate smears. US findings are not specific and usually show a hypoechoic mass with heterogeneous echotexture and irregular, indistinct margins; however, in the appropriate clinical history, a presumptive diagnosis of a metastatic deposit can be made by US (Fig. 6.33e, f).

Common and Uncommon Superficial Masses of the Head and Neck and Other Sites

Soft-tissue tumors including adipose tissue, vascular, fibroblastic, and myofibroblastic tumors, involving mainly the head and neck, are covered in this section. The clinical setting, FNA findings, and the judicious use of ancillary tests help to provide the correct diagnosis.

Abscesses and Superficial Soft-Tissue Infections/Inflammations

Infectious, inflammatory, and reactive conditions can involve the head and neck and any site of the body and can mimic neoplastic processes. A mass with classical clinical findings of infection or inflammation (swelling, redness, warmth, and tenderness) is rarely sampled by FNA, unless cultures or special studies are needed, or an inflammatory non-infectious etiology is entertained.

FNA Findings When FNA of an abscess is performed, the yellowish, thick material harvested grossly resembles the material that is commonly seen in a malignant mass with necrosis, i.e., squamous cell carcinoma. Thus, a preliminary interpretation of the smear provides information to submit material for culture studies or other ancillary tests. Smears show numerous acute inflammatory cells (purulent smear pattern) and necrosis. In the subacute or chronic phase, lymphocytes, histiocytes, and granulation tissue (capillaries surrounded by histiocytes) are present (Fig. 6.34a, b). Variable numbers of myofibroblasts and small fragments of fibrous tissue are seen during the healing phase. In addition to infectious processes, the finding of numerous histiocytes, multinucleated giant cells, and granulomas may be seen in the foreign-body reaction to injection of foreign substances such as hyaluronic acid or hydroxyapatite. Calcium deposits are present in long-standing scleroderma and calcinosis (Fig. 6.34e, f, 1–o). Always, malignancy must be carefully searched for in the presence of an inflammatory smear pattern. Malignant cells and reactive fibroblasts or myofibroblasts may be similar in their cytomorphology; however, malignant cells exhibit anaplasia and myofibroblasts show reactive features.

US Features The mass is oval or round and has ill-defined borders. It may be unilocular (anechoic or hypoechoic), or have a heterogeneous echotexture with hypoechoic or anechoic foci. Posterior acoustic enhancement is seen in some cases (Fig. 6.34c, d). The fluid collection may move within the abscess when pressure is applied with the US probe. The normal subcutaneous tissue is hypoechoic with hyperechoic bands of connective tissue. Panniculitis appears as a hyperechoic area finely dissected by anechoic bands of edematous stroma, forming a characteristic cobblestoning (Fig. 6.34g, h). Injectable material including hyaluronic acid and hydroxyapatite (polarizable crystals) used for cosmetic purposes shows no specific US features (Fig. 6.34k, m). Varying degrees of soft-tissue calcification may be seen in nodular or diffuse calcinosis, as seen in a case of scleroderma (Fig. 6.34p).

Epidermal Inclusion Cyst (Sebaceous Cyst)

Epidermal inclusion cysts are lined with squamous epithelium, lack adnexal appendages, occur in any part of the body, and are diagnosed late in life. They communicate with the skin through a keratin-filled orifice or punctum, which is more prominent in large than in small cysts (Fig. 6.35a).

FNA Findings The cyst contents are thick, grumous, cheesy, and "malodorous." These characteristics are helpful for making the diagnosis at the time of FNA. The smeared material may be lost during preparation and staining unless the smears are fixed in alcohol for a few hours. Smears show anucleated squamous cells and granular keratinaceous material (Fig. 6.35b). If rupture of the cyst wall occurs, the keratin is spread and elicits a foreign-body inflammatory reaction with multinucleated foreign body-type giant cells, acute inflammation, and granulation tissue (Fig. 6.35c, d). The differential diagnosis includes a well-differentiated squamous carcinoma, particularly when the cyst is in the upper lateral neck of patients who are in the 5th decade of life or older. Nucleated squamous cells with anaplastic nuclei are seen in squamous carcinoma.

US Features Epidermal inclusion cysts are located deep in the subcutaneous tissue of the skin. They are round to oval, well-circumscribed, hypoechoic with posterior acoustic enhancement, and avascular. Occasionally, they are isoechoic or hyperechoic with minimal or no posterior acoustic enhancement. Internal echogenic foci may be present. If the epidermoid cyst ruptures, its borders become ill-defined, cyst contents outside the cyst appear hypoechoic, and a slight vascular blood flow may be seen in the periphery of the cyst, around the rupture. Internal echoes may be seen; this vary with the amount of keratin present (Fig. 6.35e, f).

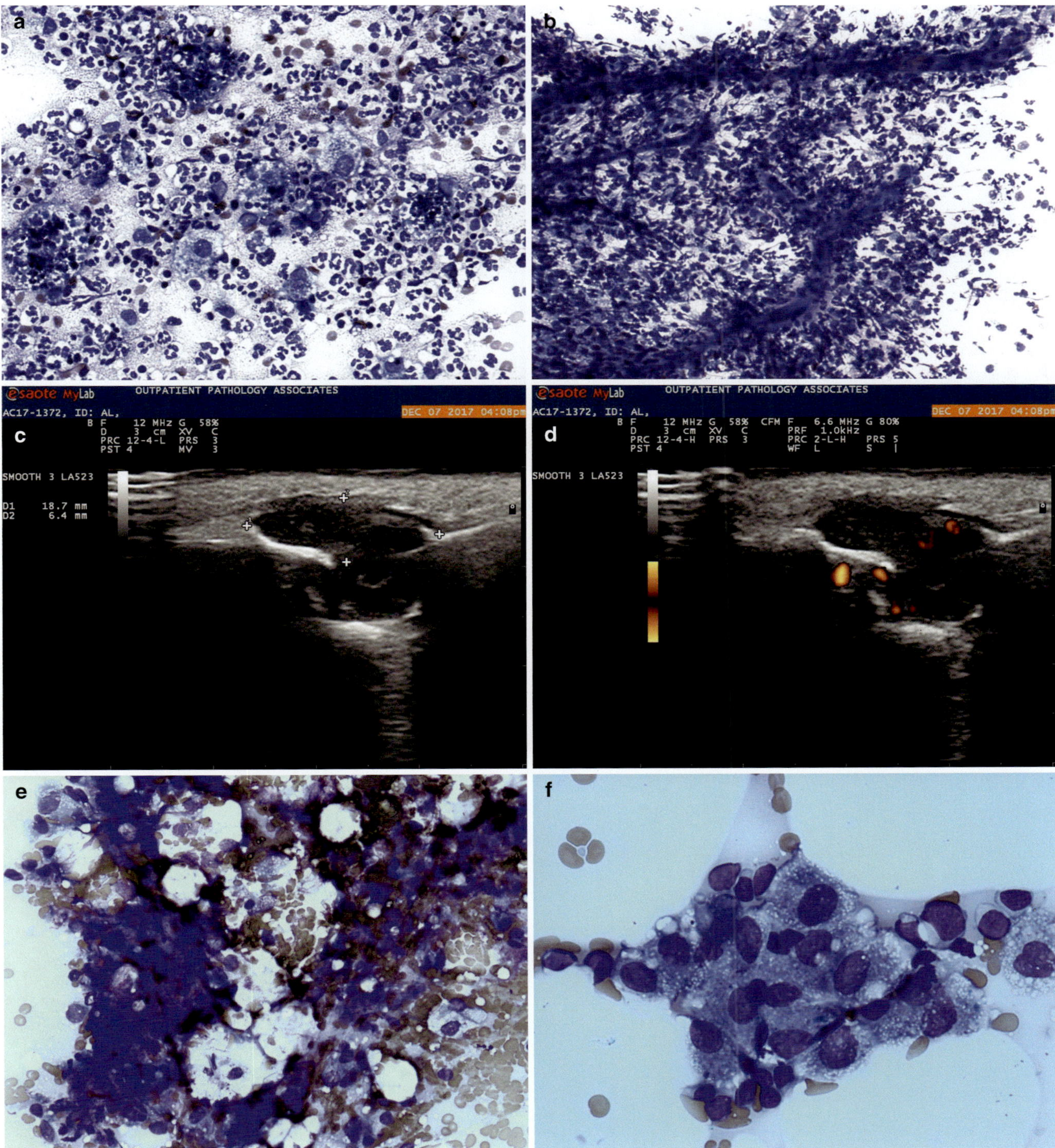

Fig. 6.34 (**a–m**) Infectious and inflammatory skin lesions. An abscess with acute inflammation and granulation tissue is present (**a**, **b**). US shows a hypoechoic, heterogeneous, and well-circumscribed mass with minimal vascular blood flow extending deep into the soft tissue of the nasolabial fold (**c**, **d**). Panniculitis with fat necrosis is present in the USG-FNA smears prepared from a the chest subcutaneous tissue mass of a patient with a history of recent external radiation for breast carcinoma (**e**, **f**); US shows multifocal diffuse and nodular hyperechoic areas with fuzzy borders and incipient cobblestoning that corresponded to areas of fat necrosis (**g**, **h**). A foreign-body giant-cell reaction is present in the smears harvested from nodular areas of the face of this 52-year-old woman who had a history of local injections of hyaluronic acid for cosmetic purposes (**i**, **j**); US shows an ill-defined heterogeneous hypoechoic mass in the dermis of the parotid region (**k**). Polarizable hydroxyapatite crystals were present in a patient with a history of a cosmetic procedure in her face (**l**, **m**). Smears made from a white granular material drained from the skin of a patient's neck level IV with clinical diagnosis of scleroderma and calcinosis show crystals and granular matter with no inflammation or foreign-body giant-cell reaction (**n**, **o**); US shows isoechoic, well-defined nodules with punctate echogenic foci corresponding to calcium deposits (**p**). (**a**, **b**, **e**, **f**, **i**, **l**, **n**, MGG stain, high magnification; **j**, **o**, Papanicolaou stain, high magnification; **m**, polarization microscopy, high magnification; **c**, **d**, **g**, **h**, **k**, **p**, US high frequency, transverse view)

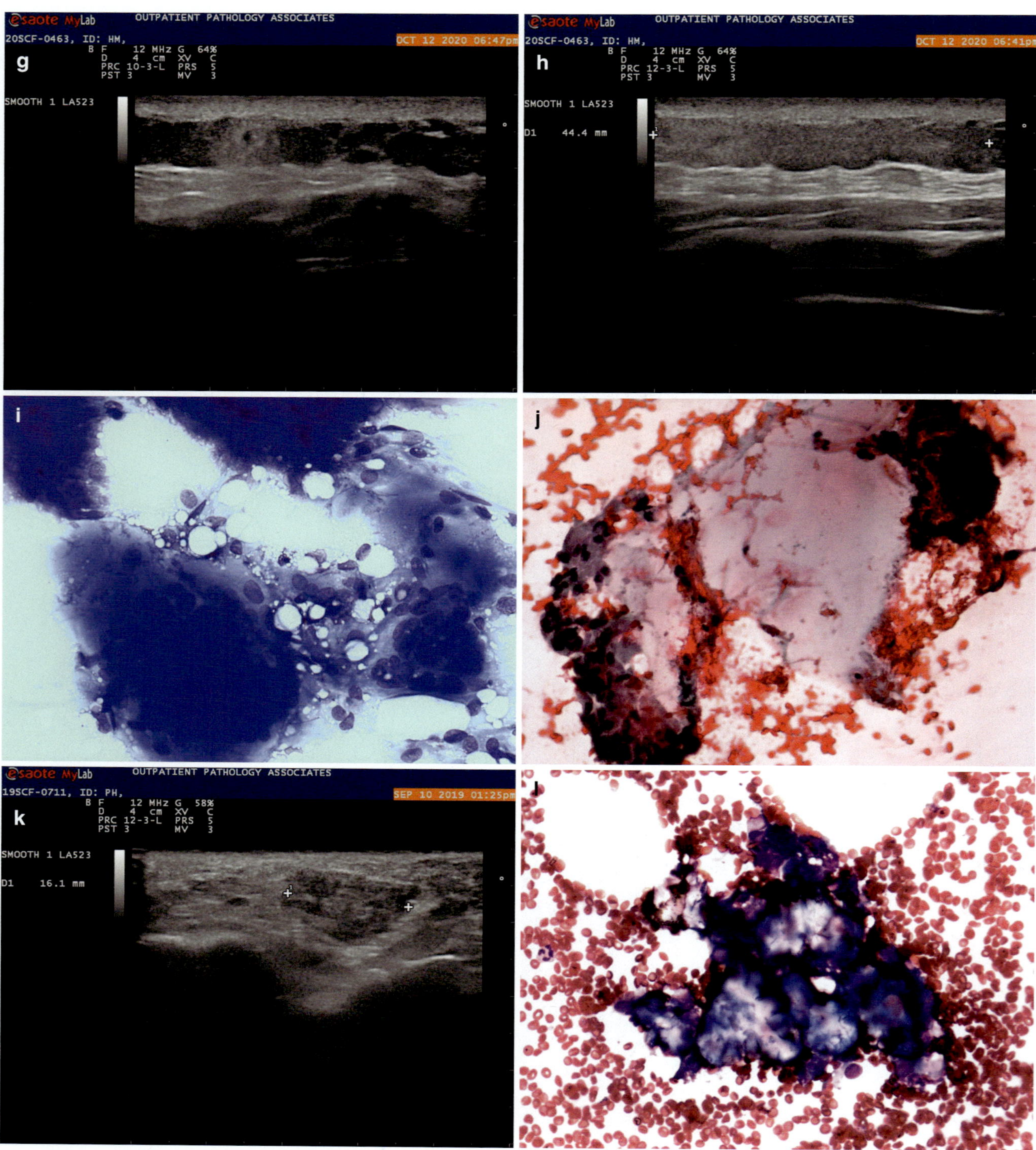

Fig. 6.34 (continued)

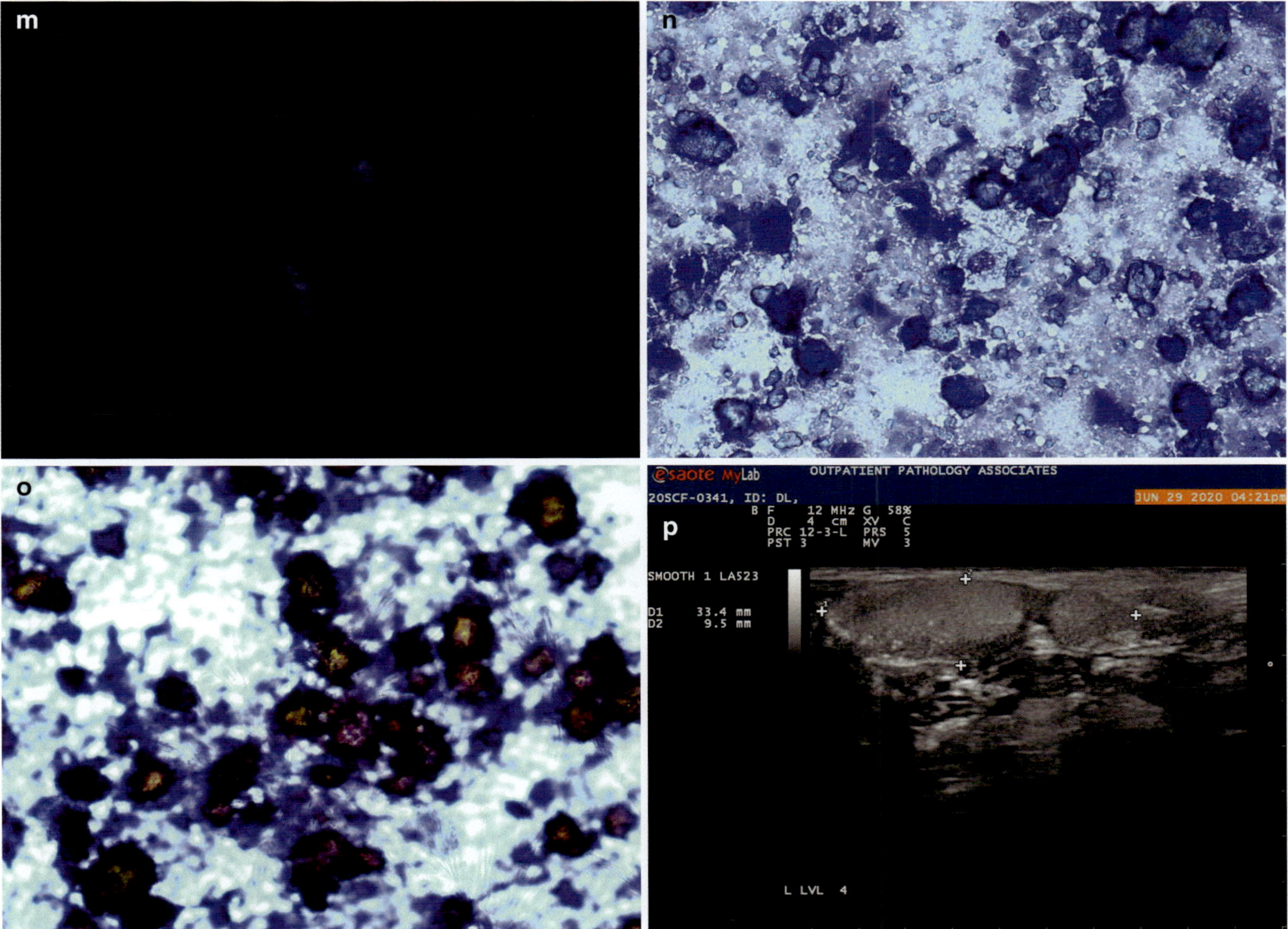

Fig. 6.34 (continued)

Adipocytic Tumors: Lipoma and Variants

Clinical Findings Lipomas are the most common benign soft-tissue tumors in adults and are usually non-tender, with exception of angiolipomas that may be tender on touch. They are superficial, usually palpable as a solitary doughy mass, but they may be multiple, develop in the subcutaneous tissue or rarely intramuscularly, and are seen most frequently in women and in obese individuals. Large, deeply seated lipomatous tumors are usually liposarcomas. Pleomorphic lipoma/spindle cell lipoma often occurs in the posterior neck and shoulders.

Atypical lipomatous tumor/well-differentiated liposarcoma of the deep soft tissue is a locally aggressive tumor that is commonly present in the proximal extremities. Both tumors show identical histopathology and genetic abnormalities (amplification of *MDM2* and/or *CDK4* is almost always present). Currently, the WHO renames both tumors to "atypical lipomatous tumor/well-differentiated liposarcoma."

Histopathology Conventional lipomas are composed of mature adipose tissue. Variants of lipoma include angiolipoma, myolipoma of soft tissue, spindle cell / pleomorphic lipoma, chondroid lipoma, and hibernoma.

FNA Findings Oily material with tissue fragments is usually harvested under suction. However, a cytologic interpretation is difficult because most material dissolves during preparation, resulting in smears of limited cellularity. Therefore, smears should be placed in a fixative solution for a few hours before processing. Smears show fragments of mature adipose tissue supported by a thin, almost invisible stroma. Adipocytes have vacuolated lipid-laden cytoplasm and peripheral regular oval and uniform nuclei. Atypical lipoblasts and a conspicuous vascular pattern are absent (Fig. 6.36a). Myxolipoma, except for the presence of adipocytes, resembles myxoma on FNA. Angiolipoma shows mature adipocytes, red blood cells, and capillaries (Fig. 6.36c). Smears from intramuscular lipoma show small fragments of mature adipocytes

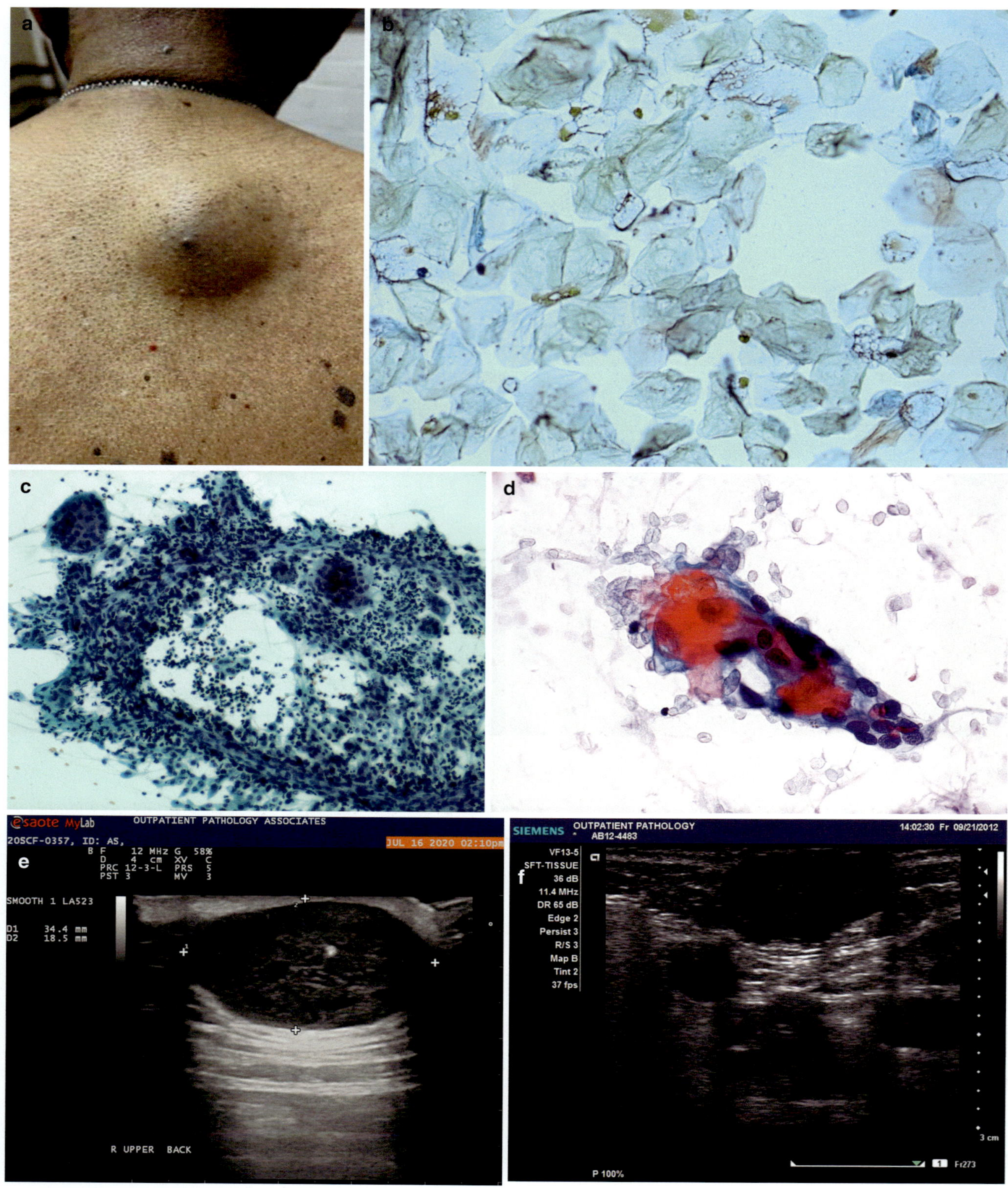

Fig. 6.35 (**a–f**) Epidermal inclusion cyst. A prominent "punctum" is visible in this large epidermal inclusion cyst (**a**). Smears show single and clustered anucleated squamous cells (**b**). Reactive squamous changes, multinucleated foreign-body-type giant cells, granulation tissue, and inflammation are present in a ruptured cyst (**c, d**). US in non-ruptured cysts shows a thin and uniform capsule (**e**). In the presence of rupture, the cyst wall is ill-defined, thick, and fuzzy (**f**). Note the posterior acoustic enhancement in both examples and the heterogeneous echotexture, which is more prominent in (**F**). (**b, c** MGG stain, high magnification; **d**, Papanicolaou stain, high magnification; **e, f**, US, high frequency, transverse views)

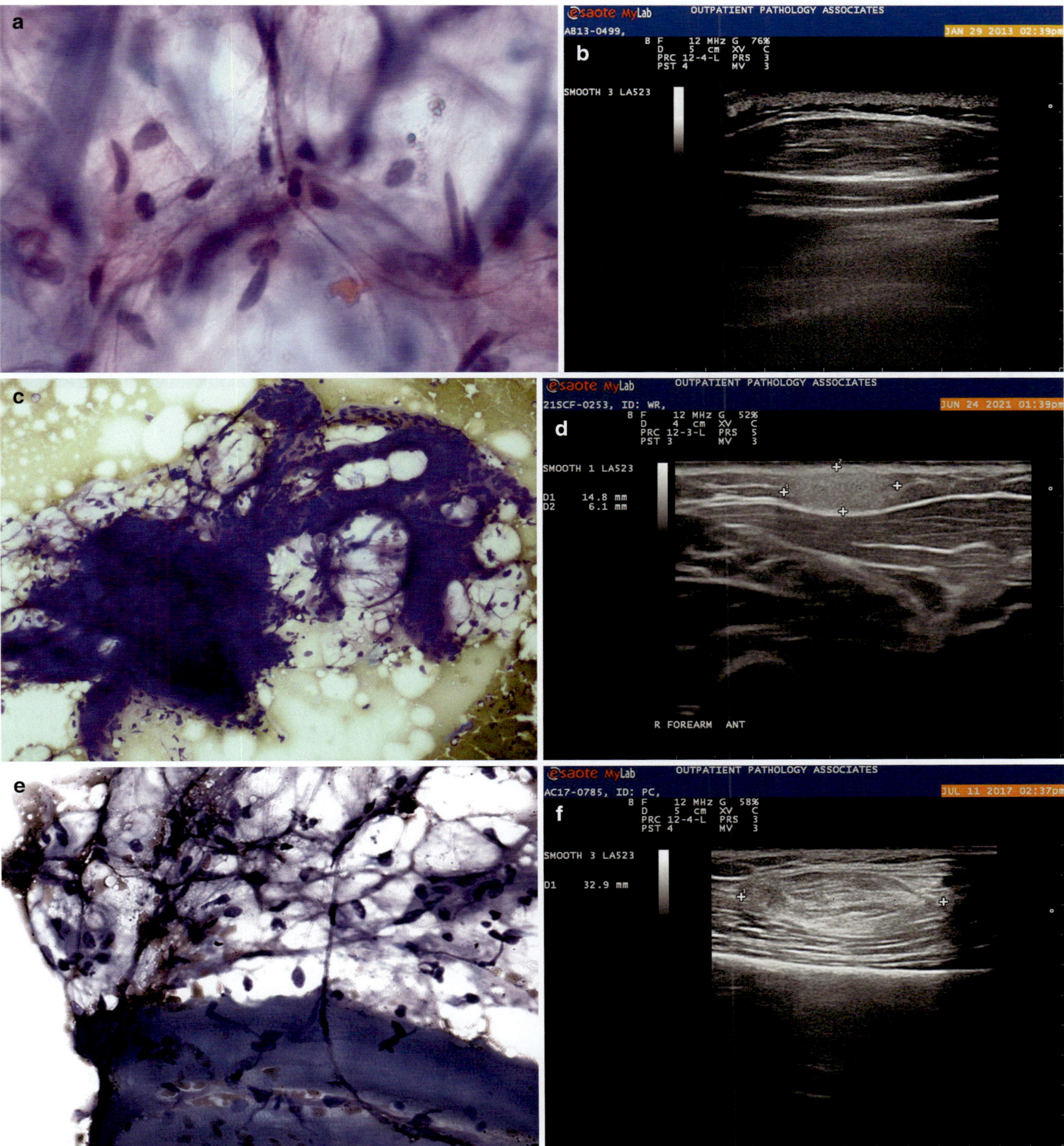

Fig. 6.36 (**a–d**) Lipoma and variants. Adipose tissue without atypia or pleomorphism is present (**a**). Mature adipocytes admixed with capillaries, skeletal muscle fibers, and fragments of spindle cells are seen in angiolipomas, intramuscular lipomas, and spindle-cell lipomas, respectively (**c, e, g**). US of lipomas shows a characteristic "feathering" (**b**). Hyperechogenicity and lack of "feathering" are seen in these examples of angiolipoma and spindle-cell lipoma (**d, h**). Lipoma within the skeletal-muscle substance is seen in intramuscular lipoma (**f**). (**a**, Papanicolaou stain, high magnification; **c, e, g**, MGG stain, medium magnification; **b, d, f, h**, ultrasound, high frequency, transverse views)

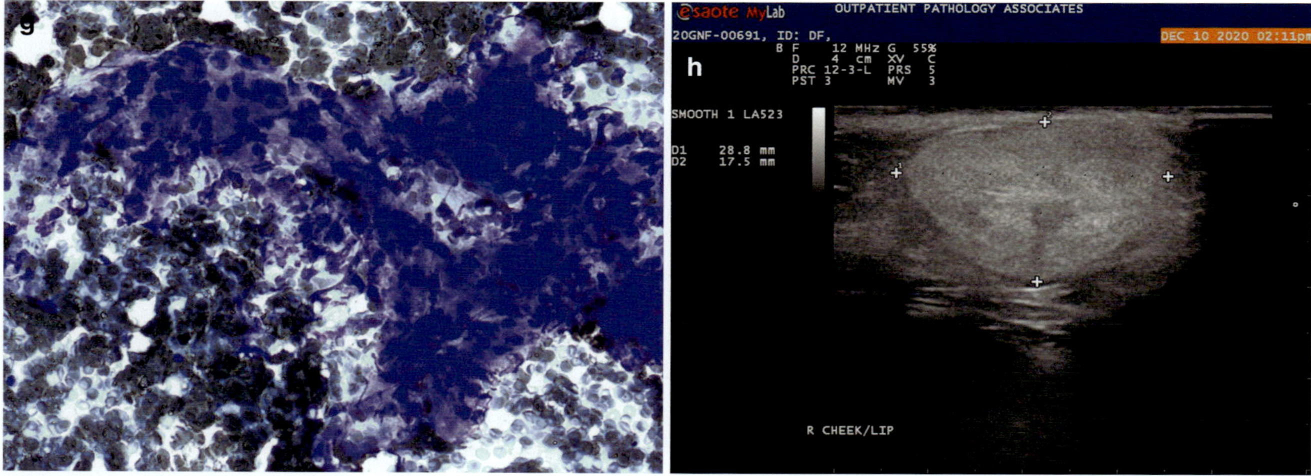

Fig. 6.36 (continued)

surrounding skeletal muscle fibers (Fig. 6.36e). Spindle cell/pleomorphic lipoma smear displays mature adipocytes, spindle cells, collagen fibers, and variable amounts of a myxoid background. Pleomorphic lipoma shows pleomorphic, bizarre, multinucleated giant cells (Fig. 6.36g). Smears of atypical lipomatous tumor/well-differentiated liposarcoma contain small fragments of fatty tissue similar to those of lipomas; however, numerous capillaries, occasional nuclear atypia, and lipoblasts are present.

Smears of atypical lipomatous tumor/well-differentiated liposarcoma show mature and rare, atypical adipocytes with anisocytosis and pleomorphic hyperchromatic nuclei. Involvement of adjacent muscle may be seen on imaging studies including US. FNA in these cases may show fragments of skeletal muscle, and intramuscular lipoma must be considered in the differential diagnosis.

The FNA diagnosis requires clinical correlation. One must make sure that the sampling needle is inside the mass to yield an adequate specimen and prevent an inconclusive or non-diagnostic interpretation.

US Features Typical lipomas are oval, well-circumscribed, homogeneous, and usually isoechoic and solid when compared with the subcutaneous tissue. They are surrounded by an echogenic capsule. The lipoma has fine linear striations ("feathering") that characteristically remain unchanged while the operator moves the US probe over the mass (Fig. 6.36b). Intramuscular lipomas show a distinct lipomatous mass within the skeletal muscle substance (Fig. 6.36f). Angiolipomas, spindle cell lipomas, and pleomorphic lipomas may appear hyperechogenic with a variable heterogeneous echotexture (Fig. 6.36d, h).

Hemangioma

Clinical Findings Hemangioma is a common soft tissue tumor that affects young individuals, with a slight preference for women. Superficial hemangiomas develop in the skin and subcutis, particularly in the head and neck area.

Histopathology There is a proliferation of small capillaries (capillary hemangioma) or large dilated vessels (cavernous hemangioma). Synovial, intramuscular (painful and most common in the thigh), arteriovenous, and venous are variants of hemangioma. Anastomosing and epithelioid (also known as angiolymphoid hyperplasia with eosinophilia) are rare variants.

FNA Findings Smears are bloody and variably cellular; but in general, they are poorly cellular. Rare small aggregates of spindle cells with blunt and pointy ends embedded in a variably dense fibrillary magenta stroma may be seen in good samples. Rare single endothelial cells may be present in sparsely cellular smears. Nuclei are bland-appearing with smooth contours, occasional longitudinal grooves, and no visible nucleoli (Fig. 6.37a, b).

US Features An iso- to hypoechoic mass without well-defined borders and with heterogeneous echotexture is commonly seen. Color Doppler examination shows varying vascularity in the "anechoic" spaces in most cases (Fig. 6.37c, d).

Nodular Fasciitis

This lesion is included in the WHO Classification of Soft Tissue and Bone Tumors, 5th edition under "Fibroblastic/myofibroblastic tumors."

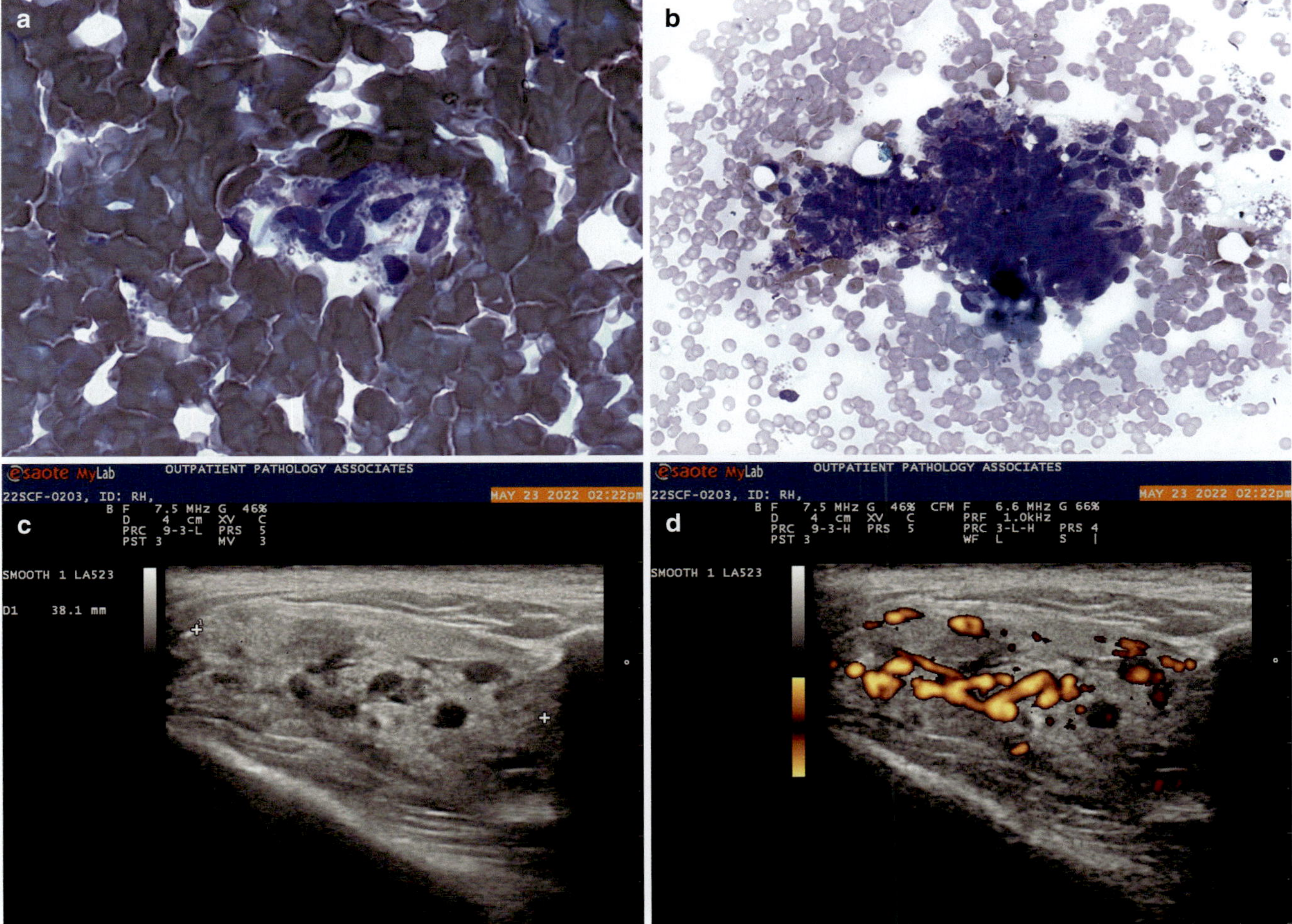

Fig. 6.37 (**a–d**) Hemangioma. FNA of a temple hemangioma shows rare single and small aggregates of spindle and endothelial cells in a background of abundant blood (**a**, **b**). Ultrasound with corresponding Doppler examination showing an isoechoic, poorly marginated mass with vascular lakes (**c**, **d**). (**a**, **b**, MGG stain, high magnification; **c**, **d**, ultrasound, high frequency, transverse view)

Clinical Findings This reactive lesion is commonly seen in the upper extremities, trunk, and neck of young adults. The usually palpable, rapidly growing mass (less than a month) is tender and usually less than 2 cm in size. The clinical evolution of the lesion should be monitored carefully because it will regress in a period of 8– 10 weeks.

Histopathology This lesion is directly associated with the fascia and extending into the subcutaneous tissue and muscle. It is usually well-circumscribed and shows a haphazard proliferation of fibroblasts and myofibroblasts in a loose myxoid stroma. Cells have reactive features, mitotic activity is variable, and there is mixed inflammation. This lesion is considered neoplastic, does not recur if resected, and has *MYH9-USP6* translocations.

FNA Findings Spindle and plump fibroblastic and myofibroblastic cells are present singly and in small interwoven clusters in a loose myxoid stroma and admixed with various

numbers of mixed acute and chronic inflammatory cells. Large myofibroblasts ranging in shape from elongated to polygonal with stellate appearance and dense cytoplasm, eccentric nuclei, and prominent nucleoli are also seen. Capillaries and typical mitotic figures are frequently encountered (Fig. 6.38a, b).

The differential diagnosis includes fibromatosis, inflammatory myofibroblastic tumor, and low-grade sarcomas with a myxoid component. Diagnostic keys are the clinical picture, adequate sampling, lack of anaplasia, and the presence of reactive nuclei. Immunostaining that is positive for smooth muscle antigen and negative for ß-catenin distinguishes nodular fasciitis from fibromatosis that stains positive for both.

US Features This is a solid, homogeneous, round to oval, isoechoic to hypoechoic, well-defined nodule of deep subcutaneous tissue adjacent to or extending into the fascia

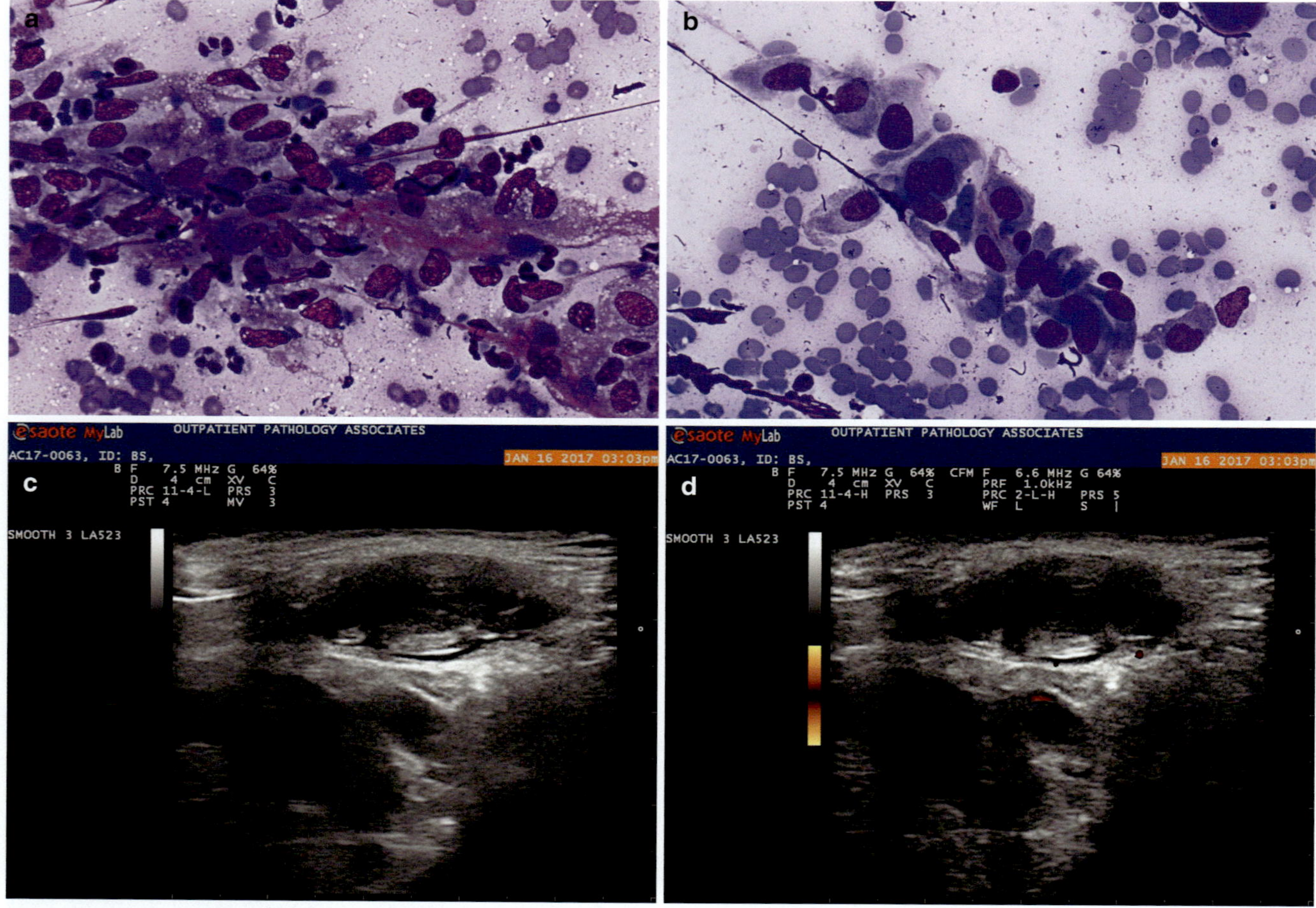

Fig. 6.38 (**a–d**) Nodular fasciitis. Spindle plump fibroblastic cells (**a**) and myofibroblasts (**b**) are present along with myxoid stroma and inflammatory cells. Ultrasound shows a deep soft-tissue, well-marginated hypoechoic heterogeneous mass with nodular echo-genic foci and variable vascular blood flow by Doppler examination. The lesion resolved spontaneously in less than 3 months. (**a**, **b**, DiffQuik stain, high magnification; **c**, **d**, US, high frequency, transverse view)

and the underlying skeletal muscle. It has echogenic foci or peripheral hyperechoic nodules. Variable vascular blood flow is present (Fig. 6.38c, d).

Fibromatosis

Desmoid-type and plantar/palmar fibromatosis are included in the WHO Classification of Soft Tissue and Bone Tumors, 5th edition, under "Fibroblastic/myofibroblastic tumors."

Clinical Findings This locally aggressive tumor is more common in women than in men, is seen particularly in the first five decades of life, and it can affect any part of the body; however, the head and neck are involved in approximately 20% of cases of extra-abdominal fibromatosis. The tumor has slow growth, is rubbery, non-tender, and recurs after local resection. It does not metastasize, but locally invades vital organs particularly in the head and neck.

Histopathology Interlacing bundles of fibroblasts with mild cytologic atypia are seen. Cellularity is variable, usually low to moderate, with predominance of collagen bundles. The margins of the tumor are infiltrative, frequently involving skeletal muscle. Mitotic activity is low. This tumor is seen as part of the Gardner syndrome, a variant of familial adenomatous polyposis (multiple osteomas, fibromas, and epidermal cysts), which has a cytogenetic abnormality involving the long arm of chromosome 5.

FNA Findings Smears show scant cellularity. Single bland-appearing spindle and oval cells are present, and in some areas, they are embedded in a fibrillary stroma. Nuclei are elongated with smooth nuclear contours and inconspicuous nucleoli. Inflammatory cells are absent (Fig. 6.39a–c). USG-FNA with the use of 25- or 23-G needles under suction for harvesting of material for a cell block and for performing immunohistochemical stains is strongly recommended.

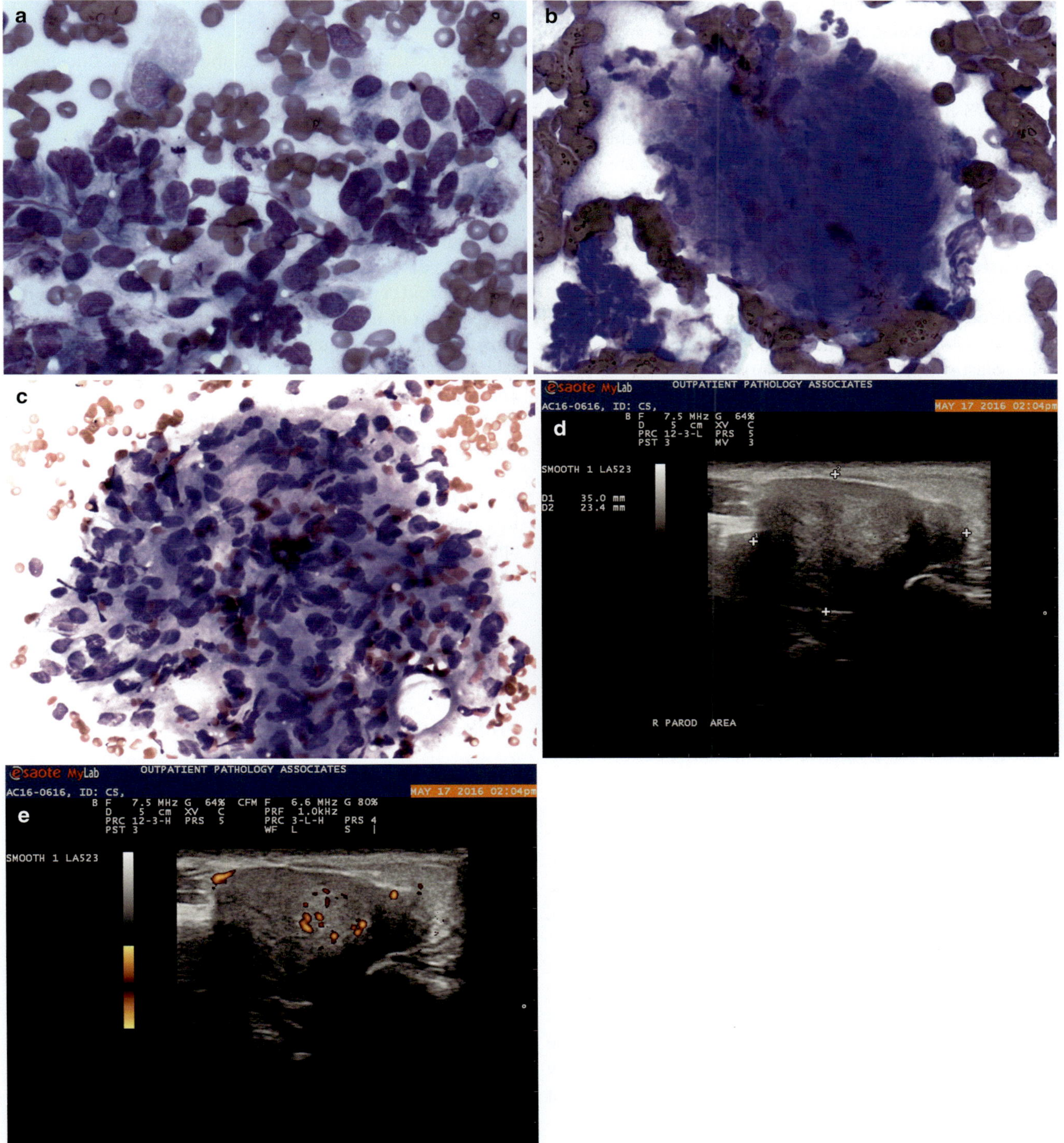

Fig. 6.39 (**a–e**) Desmoid fibromatosis. Parotid-area mass in a patient with known history of fibromatosis. Smears show aggregates of spindle cells in a fibrillary stroma. Rare myofibroblasts are present. The spindle-cell fragments may be conspicuous and resemble the cell fragments of Schwannoma (**a–c**). Ultrasound shows a well-circumscribed, vascular, hypoechoic heterogeneous mass (**d**, **e**). (**a–c**, MGG stain, high magnification; **d**, **e**, US, high frequency, transverse view)

US Features Tumors are hypoechoic, well-circumscribed, and variably vascular. Scattered echogenic foci may be present and may be correlated with areas of collagenization (Fig. 6.39d–e).

The US findings are non-specific; however, clinical features, cytologic findings, and positive immunostainings for vimentin, smooth muscle antigen, and ß-catenin are helpful for making the diagnosis.

Palisade Myofibroblastoma

Myofibroblastomas are included in the WHO Classification of Soft Tissue and Bone Tumors, 5th edition, under "Fibroblastic/myofibroblastic tumors."

Clinical Findings This rare, benign, slow-growing, solitary, and painless tumor of myofibroblastic origin is commonly found in the inguinal area but can be seen in the mediastinum and neck, clinically resembling lymphadenopathy, Schwannoma, and soft-tissue tumors. Resection is curative with rare recurrences, but with no malignant transformation or metastases.

Histopathology This is a well-circumscribed tumor, and a residual rim of lymphoid tissue may be present. A proliferation of bland-appearing spindle cells with scant eosinophilic cytoplasm and fusiform nuclei forming interlacing bundles is admixed with eosinophilic aggregates of "amianthoid" collagen fibers that have variable calcification. Foci of hemorrhage and hemosiderin deposition may be noted (Fig. 6.40c).

Immunohistochemistry is positive for smooth muscle actin and vimentin stains in the spindle cells and for trichrome and elastic stains in the "amianthoid" fibers/deposits. Desmin stain is negative. Epithelial, neurogenic, melanoma, and neuroendocrine markers also are negative.

FNA Findings Smears show dissociated and small aggregates of spindle cells with bland cytologic features. Nuclei are oval and fusiform with blunt ends surrounded by a fine fibrillary stroma. Small fragments of variably dense fibrillary eosinophilic matrix, hemosiderin-laden macrophages, mast cells, and red blood cells may be present. Acute inflammatory cells are absent (Fig. 6.40a, b).

US Features A well-circumscribed hypoechoic solid tumor with smooth borders, echogenic capsule, homogeneous echotexture, and posterior acoustic enhancement is seen. Small areas of heterogeneity may be identified when prominent and coalescing "amianthoid" deposits are present. No calcifications are identified. A non-chaotic vascular blood flow is present (Fig. 6.40d, e).

Myositis Ossificans

Myositis ossificans is included in the WHO Classification of Soft Tissue and Bone Tumors, 5th edition, under "Fibroblastic/myofibroblastic tumors."

Clinical Findings Myositis ossificans is a localized, heterotopic ossification of skeletal muscle and commonly follows trauma of the lower extremities in young individuals and in paraplegics. This localized lesion can also occur in the trunk and head and neck, is usually post-traumatic, and affects the sternocleidomastoid or masseter muscles. The progressive not trauma-related form of myositis ossificans affects the muscles of the face and neck and progresses to the thoracic musculature.

Histopathology The findings are similar to those of nodular fasciitis. Osteoid is usually absent; the presence of abundant osteoid favors the diagnosis of osteosarcoma.

FNA Findings In addition to findings seen in nodular fasciitis, osteoblasts, osteoclasts, and fibroblasts with reactive-appearing large nuclei are commonly seen. Lack of nuclear anaplasia or atypical mitoses distinguishes this process from sarcomas.

Clinical and imaging studies are helpful for distinguishing between myositis ossificans and osteosarcoma.

Proliferative Myositis

Proliferative myositis is included in the WHO Classification of Soft Tissue and Bone Tumors, 5th edition, under "Fibroblastic/myofibroblastic tumors."

Clinical Findings This is a painless and rapidly growing reactive solid tumor of unknown etiology. It may be associated with trauma, usually affecting the shoulders, upper trunk, and sternocleidomastoid muscles. A checkerboard appearance felt on physical examination reflects the mixture of affected and non-affected muscle tissue. Tumor growth is self-limited and local resection is curative.

FNA Findings The findings are like those of nodular fasciitis, including the presence of plump myofibroblasts, myxoid stroma, and inflammatory cells. In addition, fragments of skeletal muscle fibers, degenerated multinucleated muscle cells, large polygonal cells with prominent nucleoli, and reactive fibroblasts are present (Fig. 6.41a–c). The differentiation from sarcoma is based on a lack of nuclear anaplasia.

The cytology of proliferative myositis is like that of proliferative fasciitis that commonly occurs in the subcutaneous tissue of the lower extremities.

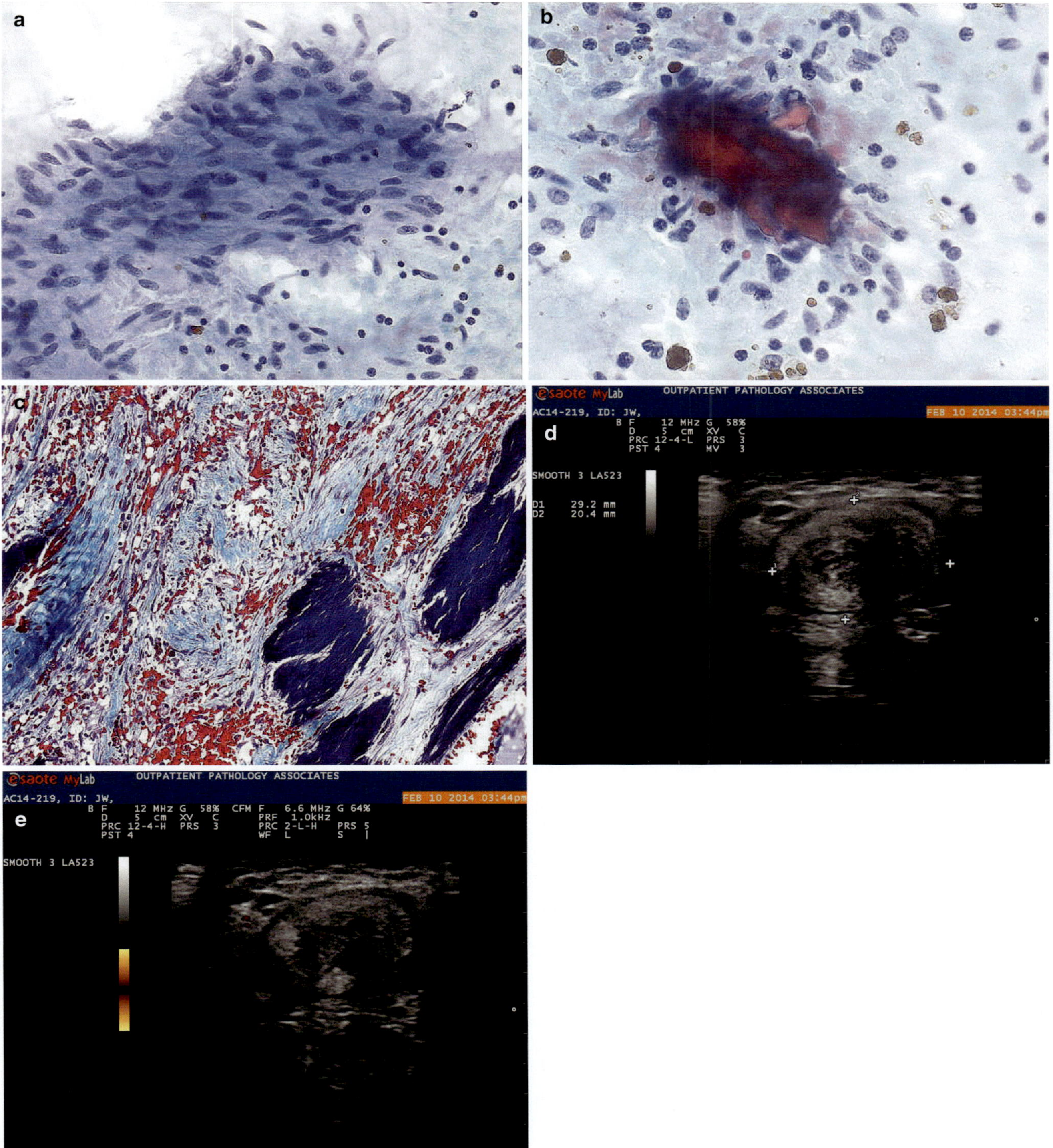

Fig. 6.40 (**a–e**) Palisade myofibroblastoma. Inguinal lymphadenopathy was the presumptive clinical impression in this case. Fragments of and single bland-appearing spindle cells with both blunt and pointy ends are present along with small lymphocytes, hemosiderin deposits, and eosinophilic aggregates of collagen fibers (**a**, **b**). Histopathology shows bundles of spindle cells, basophilic calcific aggregates, and blood (**c**). US shows a soft-tissue well-circumscribed, hypoechoic, heterogeneous mass with punctate echogenic foci, as well as mild vascular blood flow by Doppler examination, (**d**, **e**). (**a**, **b**, H&E stain, high magnification; **c**, H&E, low magnification; **d**, **e**, ultrasound, high frequency, transverse view) **a–c**, courtesy Dr. Javier Saenz de Santamaria, Badajoz Hospital, Spain

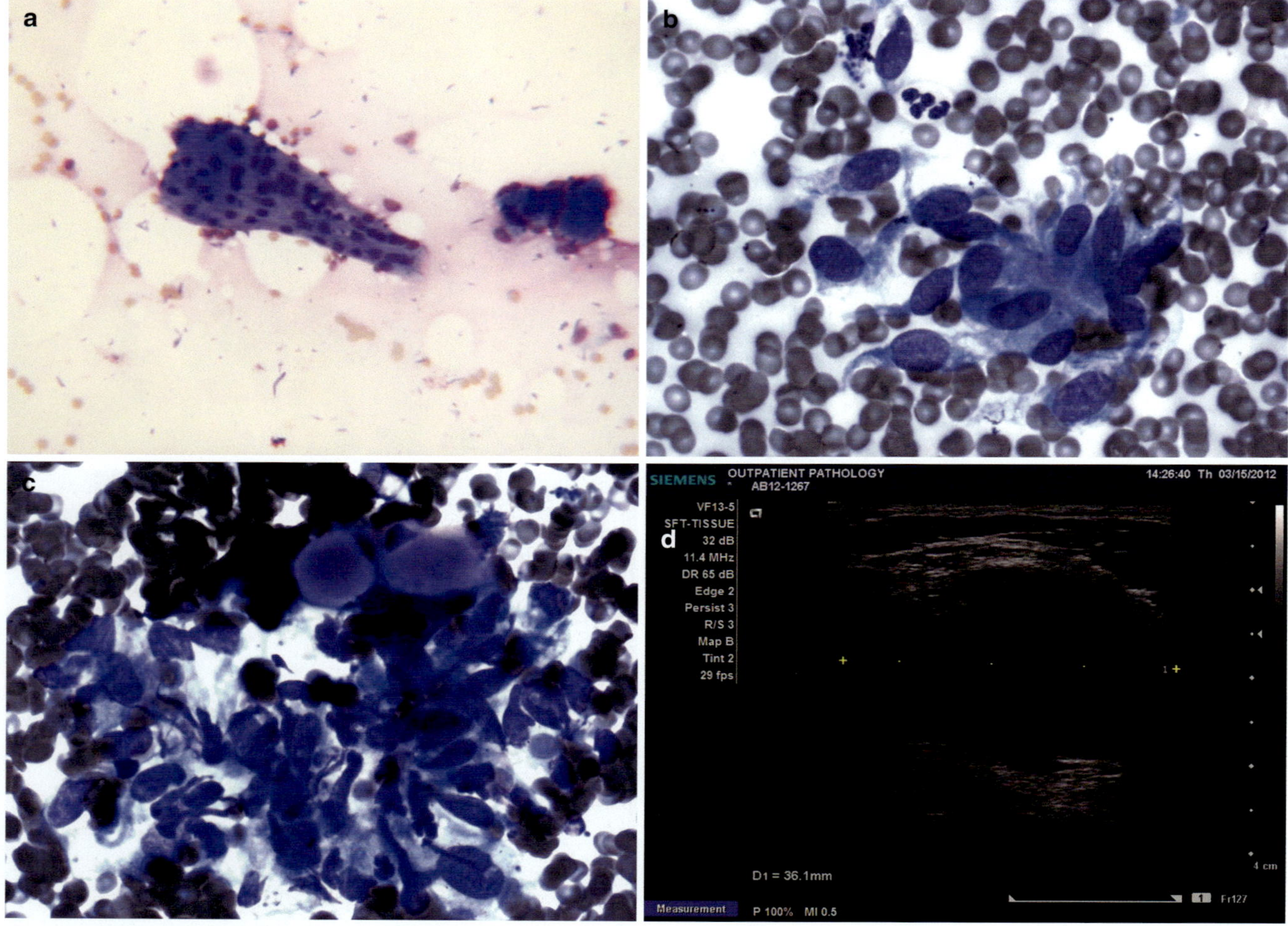

Fig. 6.41 (**a–e**) Proliferative myositis. Fragments of skeletal muscle fibers, plump spindle cells, and myofibroblasts with scattered acute inflammatory cells are present (**a–c**). US shows an intramuscular hypoechogenic and heterogenous mass with poorly defined borders (**d**). (**a–c**, MGG stain, high magnification; **d**, **e**, ultrasound, high frequency, transverse view)

US Features The mass is hypoechoic, heterogeneous, poorly marginated, and has variable vascular blood flow (Fig. 6.41d).

Dermatofibrosarcoma Protuberans (DFSP)

Dermatofibrosarcoma protuberans is included in the WHO Classification of Soft Tissue and Bone Tumors, 5th edition under "Fibroblastic/myofibroblastic tumors."

Clinical Findings DFSP exhibits a spectrum of spindle-cell tumors with fibroblastic differentiation that typically involves both the dermis and subcutis of the trunk, proximal extremities, and occasionally the scalp of patients in the third to sixth decades of life. It is a firm, nodular, protuberant cutaneous mass growing over a period of months to years and can be large, in cases larger than 20 cm in diameter (Fig. 6.42a). DFSP is a locally aggressive tumor with a high rate of local recurrence and with metastatic potential. Wide local resec-tion is the treatment of choice for localized tumors. Imatinib and radiation therapy can be used in cases of advanced disease.

Histopathology The dermis is the center of origin for this tumor that infiltrates adipose tissue, but spares adnexal struc-tures. Bundles of spindle cells forming a storiform and whorled pattern are present in a collagenous, myxoid, or microcystic background stroma. Oval to elongated nuclei are uniform. The mitotic index is variable (Fig. 6.42d). Almost all tumors have fusion genes, *COL1A1::PDGFB* being the most common fusion product. The clinical findings, histopa-thology, and a diffuse positive stain for CD34 and vimentin are paramount for making the diagnosis. Smooth muscle and melanoma markers are negative.

FNA Findings Aspirates are of variable cellularity and are frequently bloody. Useful cytologic features are the presence of storiform stromal fragments, entrapped adipose tissue, and fibrohistiocytic spindle cells. The fat entrapped within

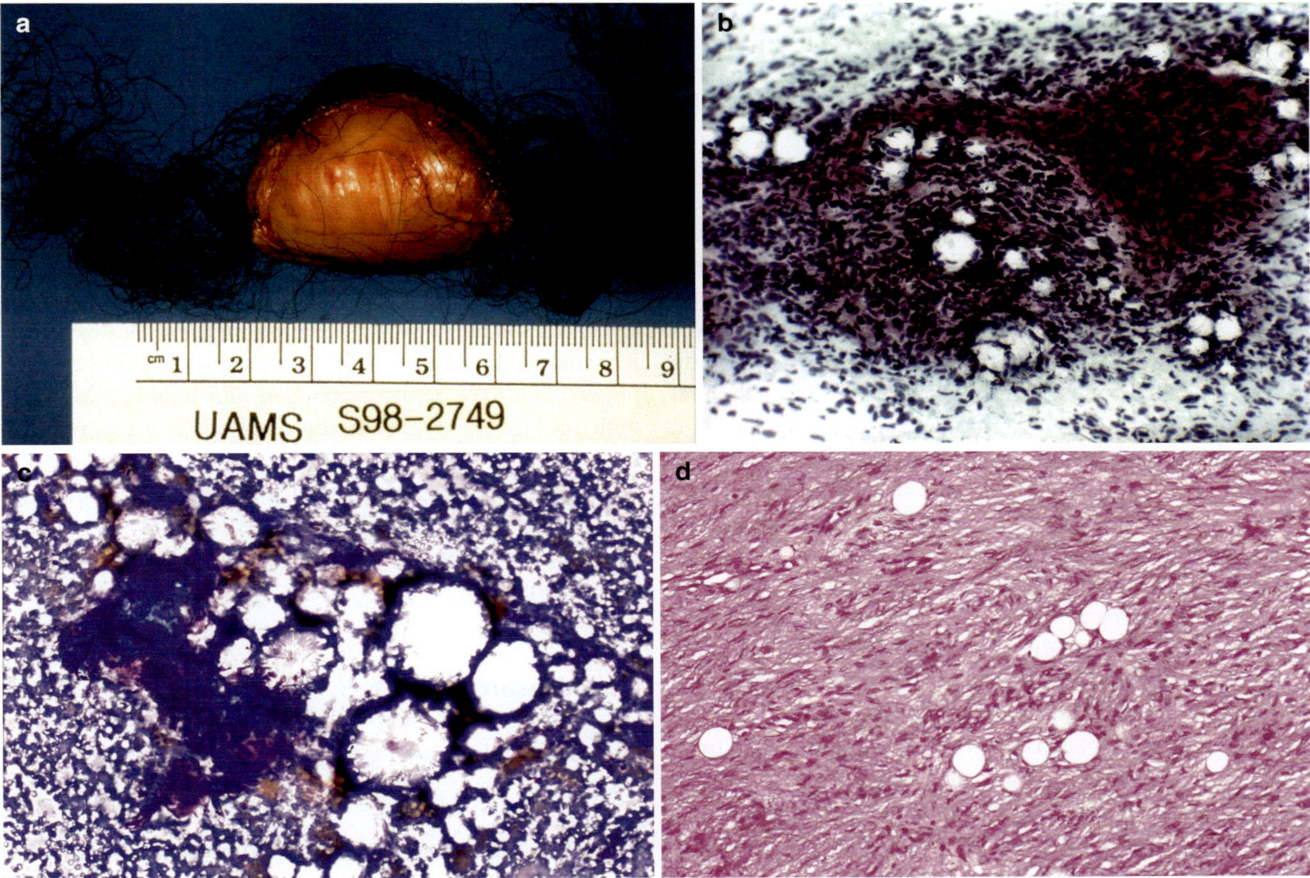

Fig. 6.42 (**a–d**) Dermatofibrosarcoma protuberans, an excised large nodular mass (**a**). Cellular smear shows fascicles of bland-appearing spindle cells admixed with adipose tissue elements (**b, c**). The histopathology recapitulates the FNA pattern (**d**). (**b**, Papanicolaou stain, medium magnification; **c**, DiffQuik stain, medium magnification; **d**, H&E, low magnification)

the storiform fragments reflects the infiltrative growth pattern of DFSP. The stromal fragments (best seen with Romanowsky stains) are of variable cellularity, showing a finely fibrillar and metachromatic matrix. The spindle cells have abundant eosinophilic cytoplasm, ill-defined cytoplasmic borders, and bland nuclear features. Occasional mitotic figures and pleomorphic spindle cells may be found. The absence of inflammatory cells is a prominent feature (Fig. 6.42b, c).

The differential diagnosis includes both benign and low-grade malignant spindle-cell lesions. Nodular fasciitis shows more angular fibroblasts with prominent nucleoli mixed with inflammatory cells. Fibrous histiocytoma shows multinucleate giant cells with hemosiderin deposition, as well as inflammatory cells. Kaposi's sarcoma contains delicate spindle cells and abundant blood. Spindle-cell melanoma displays pleomorphic nuclei. Clinicopathologic correlation is necessary, and occasionally a specific diagnosis may not be possible.

US Features Tumors are oval, heterogeneously hypoechoic, with posterior acoustic enhancement or with mixed echogenicity and with hyperchoic streaks that reflect the presence of adipose tissue and of collagenized stroma. They have well-defined and focally lobulated margins, and a thin hypoechoic rim that may be disrupted by tumor protrusions.

Synovial Sarcoma

Synovial sarcoma is included in the WHO Classification of Soft Tissue and Bone Tumors, 5th edition, under "Tumors of uncertain differentiation."

Clinical Findings Synovial sarcoma frequently occurs in the lower extremities, but occasionally occurs in the head and neck, in particular the mouth and larynx, most frequently in young adults. Metastases mainly occur to lungs and lymph nodes and may be biphasic or monophasic. The average 5-year survival rate is 50%.

Histopathology Multiple morphologies have been described, but the biphasic pattern with fibrous and epithelioid components is usually seen in typical lesions. There is a characteristic chromosomal translocation t(X;18)(p11;q11) involving genes *SS18* and *SSX1, SSX2,* or *SSX4*. The diagnosis is confirmed by molecular or cytogenetic testing for *SS18-SSX* fusion.

FNA Findings Aspirates of tumors with biphasic pattern have both epithelial and spindle cell components. Smears are highly cellular, showing tightly packed, monomorphic, bipolar spindle cells with oval nuclei, and faintly staining cytoplasm. A background of numerous small free-lying, monotonous, oval or spindle nuclei with a bland chromatin pattern and small nucleoli is usually present. The epithelioid cells are larger and cuboidal, columnar, or polygonal with round vesicular nuclei and rounded and distinct cell borders, and they occur in clusters of different sizes. Mast cells, cystic change, and calcific deposits are often seen. Only the spindle or epithelioid component is present in aspirates of monophasic synovial sarcoma. The presence of calcific deposits and mast cells suggests the diagnosis (Fig. 6.43a–c). Immunohistochemistry is positive for EMA and cytokeratins. Positive immunoreactivity for bcl-2 and CD99 (membranous) is seen in most cases. Positive stain for TLE1 is seen in 90% of synovial sarcomas and is helpful for distinguishing it from its mimics. Melanoma markers including SOX10 and S100 are negative. Large clusters of epithelioid cells may suggest a diagnosis of adenocarcinoma; however, the presence of a spindle-cell component is very unusual in such cases.

US Features Small tumors are homogeneous, hypoechoic, solid, and oval, or slightly lobulated with well-defined borders. The echogenicity is usually like that of skeletal muscle. Larger tumors show lobulated and irregular borders, a heterogeneous echotexture with areas of cystic change/necrosis (anechoic), and fibrosis and calcification (hyperechogenic foci). Synovial sarcoma from the abdominal wall may show a "honeycomb" pattern of echotexture (Fig. 6.43d, e).

Chordoma

Clinical Findings This neoplasm arises from remnants of the notochord, develops along the spinal axis, involves the sacrocoxygeal area, and may be found in the spheno-occipital region extending into the nasal cavity, sinuses, and nasopharynx. Chordomas are essentially intraosseous tumors; however, in rare cases they are soft tissue-based. They are more common in men than in women and can occur at any age; however, they are more common in the 4th to 8th decades of life. Tumors of the head and neck region occur more frequently in children and young adults. The tumor has an infiltrative growth pattern and may involve the base of the skull, causing neuro-ophthalmologic and otologic symptoms.

Histopathology Globules of mucoid material, neoplastic cells with vacuolated cytoplasm, and fibrous bands are present. Cellular atypia and mitotic activity are variable but are usually mild. Neoplastic cells are positive for EMA, S100, brachyury, cytokeratins, and vimentin; this is helpful for distinguishing chordoma from epithelial malignancies such as metastatic mucin-producing adenocarcinomas, as well as mesenchymal neoplasms such as chondrosarcomas (Fig. 6.44a).

FNA Findings Aspirates show an abundant thin mucoid-myxoid fibrillary substance of magenta color (with Romanowsky stains). Two cell types can be identified: The larger cells have multi-vacuolated and bubbly cytoplasm with round, bland nuclei; the smaller cells exhibit oval nuclei and are usually present in lesser numbers. The larger cells, arranged in nests and clusters, correspond to the physaliphorous cells seen in tissue sections of this tumor. Binucleation and multinucleation are occasionally observed (Fig. 6.44b, c).

Chondrosarcoma

This rare neoplasm affects the jaw, nasal septum, larynx, and trachea.

FNA Findings Aspirates show extracellular matrix and cells in various proportions. The extracellular matrix is magenta colored with Romanowsky stains. Cellularity depends on the grade of the sarcoma. The neoplastic chondrocytes are single, can be located in lacunae, and range from being oval to round. The cells have a well-demarcated, vacuolated cytoplasm encasing bubble-like peripheral vacuoles. No mitotic figures are seen, except in a de-differentiated form of chondrosarcoma. A fibroblast-like cell component may be present. Intermediate- to high-grade chondrosarcomas have characteristic cytologic features, but low-grade cases require tissue confirmation. Clinical and radiographic correlation is necessary.

Osteogenic Sarcoma

Head and neck osteosarcomas are rare and comprise 6% of all osteogenic sarcomas. Sites of involvement include the mandible, maxilla, paranasal sinuses, and skull. Depending on which component predominates, osteosarcomas are divided into osteoblastic, chondroblastic, and fibroblastic types.

FNA Findings The stromal cells are spindled to polygonal with hyperchromatic nuclei, with or without nucleoli, and exhibit variable anaplasia. Necrosis and mitoses are com-

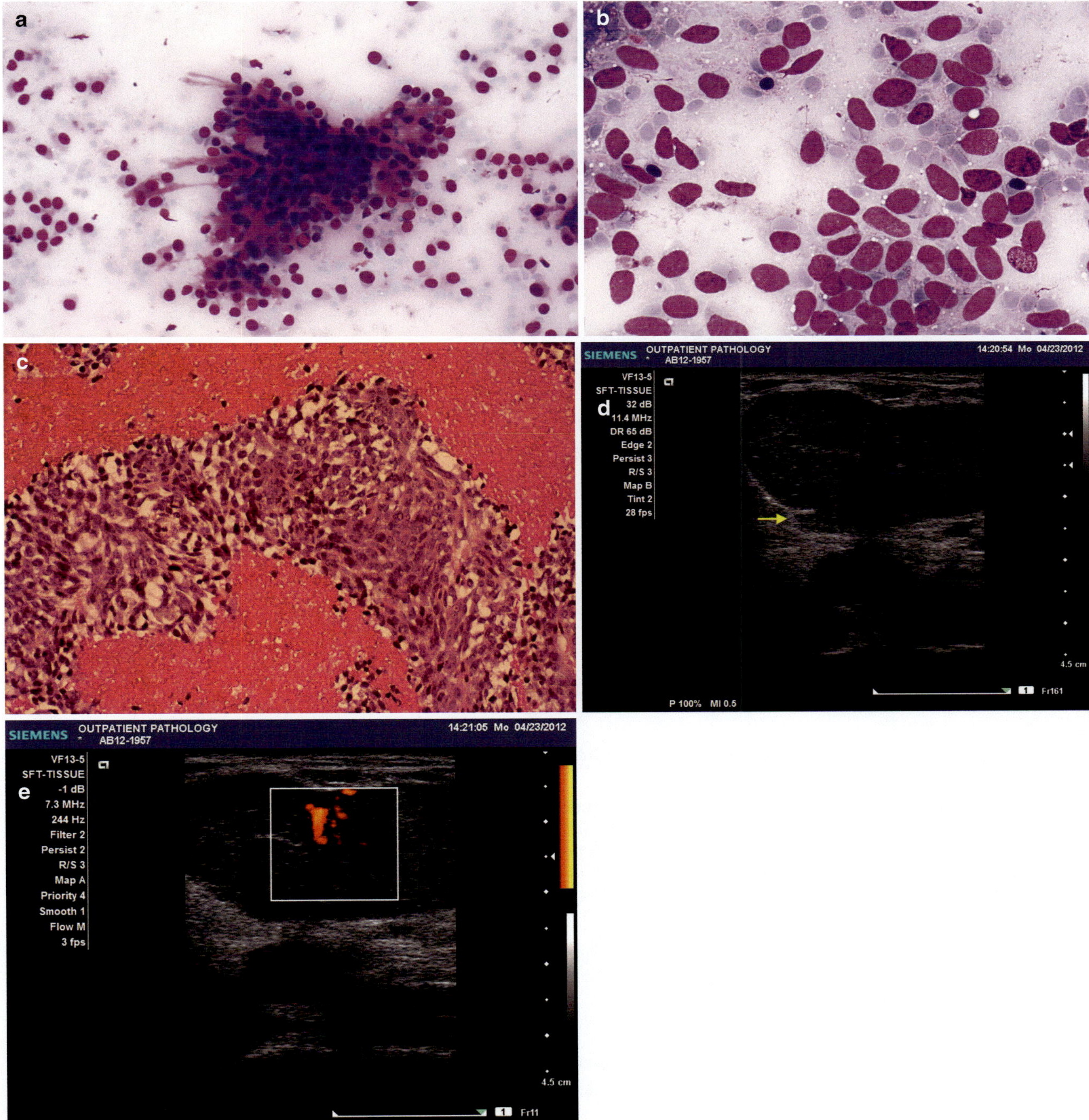

Fig. 6.43 (**a–e**) Synovial sarcoma. Both epithelioid (**a**) and spindle (**b**) cell components are seen. The cell block preparation shows the spindle-cell component (**c**). US shows a large hypoechoic mass with homogeneous echotexture, well-defined and smooth borders, and an area of stromal invasion (**d**, arrow). Vascular flow is moderate by Power Doppler (**e**). (**a**, DiffQuik stain medium magnification; **b**, DiffQuik stain, high magnification; **c**, H&E stain, low magnification)

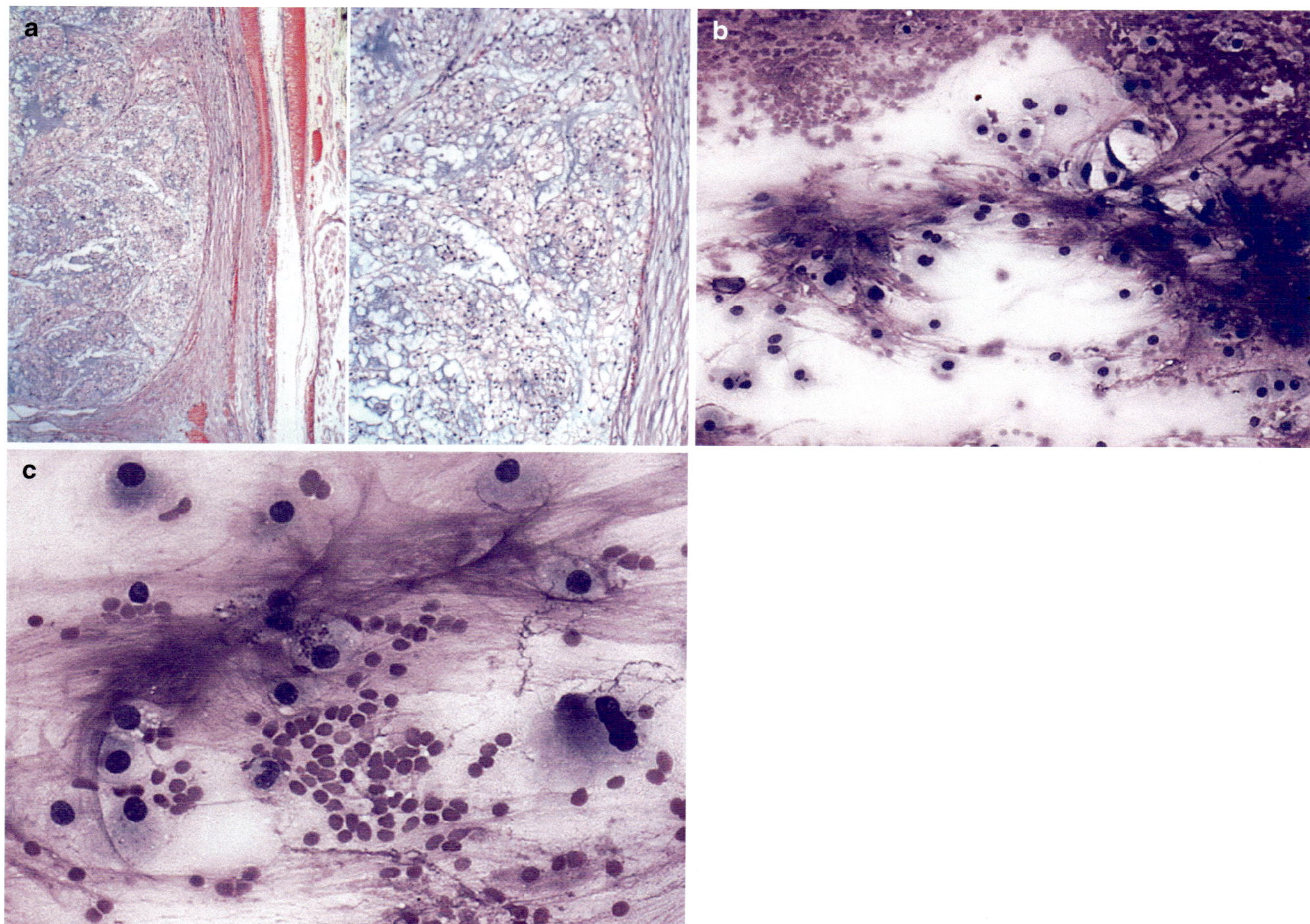

Fig. 6.44 (**a, b**) Chordoma. Globules of mucoid material, neoplastic cells with vacuolated cytoplasm, and fibrous bands are present (**a**). Smears show abundant thin fibrillary myxoid matrix that appears metachromatic on Romanowsky stain. Large cells with vacuolated cytoplasm and bland appearing, eccentrically placed nuclei are present admixed with the matrix. Some cells exhibit binucleation and multinucleation (**b, c**). (**a**, H&E stain, intermediate magnification; **b, c**, DiffQuik stain, medium magnification). **a**, Courtesy Dra. Vilma Perez-Valle, Managua, Nicaragua; **b, c**, Courtesy Dr. Javier Saenz de Santamaria, Badajoz Hospital, Spain

monly seen. Fragments of pink osteoid and chondroid and multinucleated osteoclast-type tumor giant cells are frequently found (Fig. 6.45a–c).

Differential Diagnosis When the osteoclast-type tumor giant cells predominate, differential-diagnostic consider-ations are given to giant-cell tumors, giant-cell reparative granulomas, and brown tumors of hyperparathyroidism. Anaplastic stromal cells are a key diagnostic feature for osteosarcoma. Recognition of the osteoid matrix distinguishes osteosarcomas from other sarcomas. Radiographic correlation is crucial.

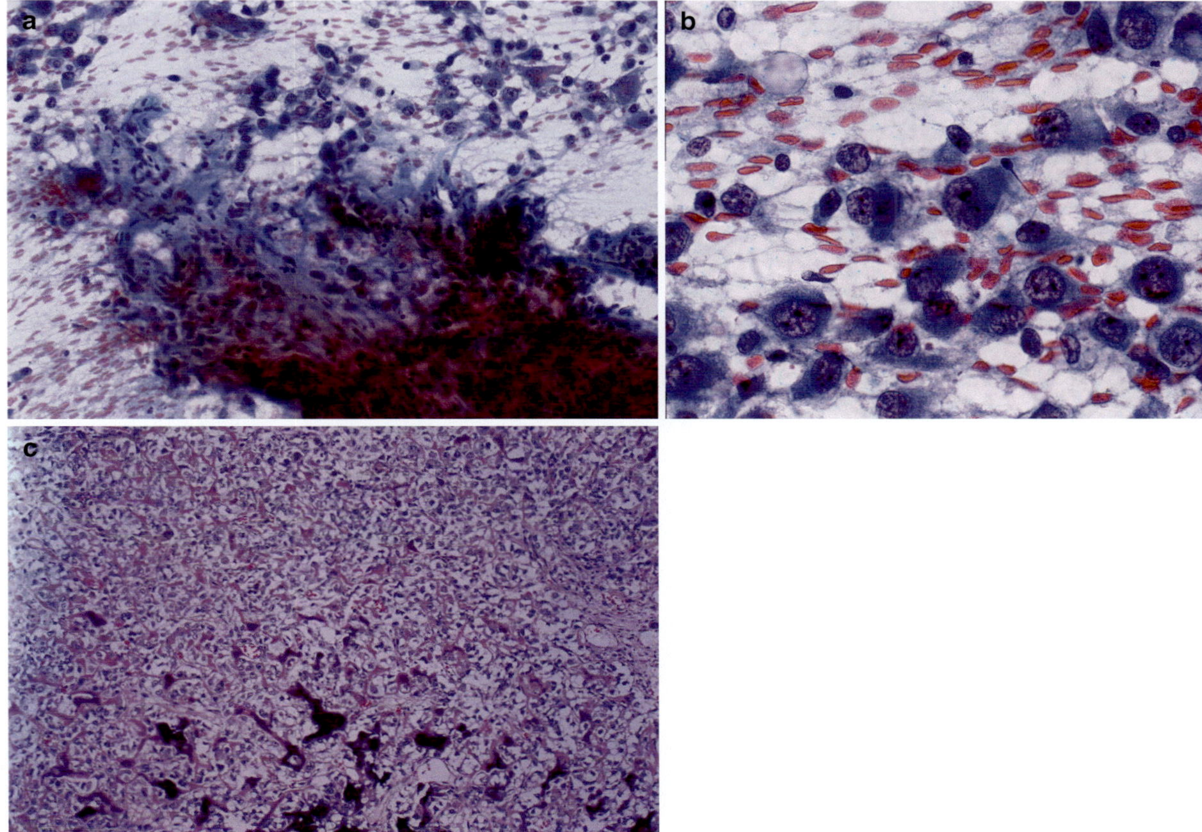

Fig. 6.45 (a–c) Osteosarcoma of the maxillary bone. Smears are cellular (a) and show spindle cells and pleomorphic epithelioid cells with anaplasia (b). The osteoid is evident in the tissue section (c). (a, b, Papanicolaou stain, medium and high magnification; c, H&E stain, low magnification)

Further Reading

Ahuja A, Evans R. Lumps and bumps in the head and neck. In: Practical head and neck ultrasound. London: Greenwich Medical Media; 2000. p. 87–104.

Bardales R. The invasive cytopathologist. In: Ultrasound guided fine-needle aspiration of superficial masses. New York: Springer; 2014.

Barnes L, Tse LLY, et al. Carotid body paraganglioma. In: Barnes L, Eveson JW, Reichart P, Sidransky D, editors. Pathology and genetics of head and neck tumors. Lyon: IARC Press; 2005. p. 364–5.

El-Naggar AK. Cellular and molecular pathology of head and neck tumors. In: Bernier J, editor. Head and neck cancer: multimodality management. New York: Springer; 2011. p. 57–79.

Fletcher CD. Distinctive soft tissue tumors of the head and neck. Mod Pathol. 2002;15(3):324–30.

Hamilton BE, Nesbit GM, et al. Characteristic imaging findings in lymphoceles of the head and neck. AJR Am J Roentgenol. 2011;197(6):1431–5.

Klijanienko J, Caillaud JM, et al. Cytohistologic correlations of 24 malignant peripheral nerve sheath tumor (MPNST) in 17 patients: the Institut Curie experience. Diagn Cytopathol. 2002;27(2):103–8.

Layfield LJ. Cytopathology of bone and soft tissue tumors. New York: Oxford University Press; 2002.

Lee YYP, Wong KT, et al. Ultrasound investigations in head and neck cancer patients. In: Bernier J, editor. Head and neck cancer: multimodality management. New York: Springer; 2011. p. 221–33.

Leonardo E, Bardales R. Practical immunocytochemistry in diagnostic cytology. Cham: Springer; 2020.

Leyfield L. Cysts and neoplasms of the neck. In: Cytopathology of the head and neck. Chicago: ASCP Press; 1997. p. 141–58.

Rhys R. Ultrasound of the neck. In: Allan PL, Baxter GM, Weston MJ, editors. Clinical ultrasound, vol. 2. London: Churchill Livingstone; 2011. p. 890–919.

Shin YR, Kim JY, et al. Sonographic findings of dermatofibrosarcoma protuberans with pathologic correlation. J Ultrasound Med. 2008;27(2):269–74.

Stanley MW, Skoog L, et al. Nodular fasciitis: spontaneous resolution following diagnosis by fine-needle aspiration. Diagn Cytopathol. 1993;9(3):322–4.

WHO Classification of Tumours Editorial Board. Soft tissue and bone tumours. Lyon: International Agency for Research on Cancer; 2020. https://publications.iarc.fr.

Yuan WH, Hsu HC, et al. Differences in sonographic features of ruptured and unruptured epidermal cysts. J Ultrasound Med. 2012;31(2):265–72.

Ricardo H. Bardales

Clinical Considerations

Lymph nodes are "absent" by palpation in newborns. They are more numerous in children than in adults and are soft and oval. Anterior cervical, axillary, and inguinal lymph nodes may be found in healthy children and measure <1 cm. The only palpable lymph nodes in adults may be found in the inguinal region and measure <1.5 cm.

Localized or regional lymphadenopathy is defined as lymph node enlargement in contiguous anatomic regions. *Generalized lymphadenopathy* is defined as the involvement of more than two noncontiguous lymph node regions.

Lymphadenopathy may be the result of a local or systemic etiologic process, i.e., metastases, lymphoma, infection, or inflammation. The clinical differential diagnosis is based on the physical examination, location of the lymph node, and particularly the age of the patient. Although these factors are important, they should not overinfluence the interpretation. The history of immunosuppression contributes to the frequency of certain lymph-node-based reactive, malignant, or infectious processes. A non-neoplastic pathologic process is the most common cause of regional or generalized lymphadenopathy in children and adults.

In the pediatric age group, the most common causes of regional lymphadenopathy are viral, bacterial, and mycobacterial processes, depending on the geographic environment; the most frequent malignancies presenting as a cervical lymphadenopathy are small-blue cell tumors including, but not limited to, lymphomas and leukemias, followed by solid tumors such as neuroblastoma, rhabdomyosarcoma, and Wilms tumor. In the adolescent group, Hodgkin lymphoma (HL) and non-Hodgkin lymphoma (NHL), nasopharyngeal carcinoma, and metastatic germ cell tumors are the predominant malignancies present in a neck lymph node. Metastatic carcinoma, predominantly of the squamous type, from lung and head and neck organs becomes the most common diagnostic consideration in or above the fourth decade of life.

In general, a round, firm, well-defined lymph node present for >6 weeks or a lymph node that is fixed to surrounding tissues including skin, deep anatomic planes, or other lymph nodes should be considered for FNA regardless of clinical findings. Likewise, a regional or generalized lymphadenopathy associated with localized (i.e., sore throat, dysphonia, dysphagia if the node is in the neck) or constitutional (i.e., weight loss, night sweats, anorexia, asthenia, fever) symptoms should be considered for FNA. Also, neck lateral-superior lymph nodes (level II) >3 cm and those >2 cm in other neck regions should be closely monitored for a short period of time and if there is growth, a FNA must be strongly considered.

Lymph Node Anatomy, Histology, Cytology, and Immunophenotype

The normal lymph node has a bean shape, measures <1 cm, has a cortex and medulla, and is surrounded by a capsule. The afferent lymphatic vessels penetrate the convex surface of the lymph node, and the efferent vessels exits at the level of the hilum, which is indented, contains the vein and artery, and is contiguous with the medulla.

Histology The cortex contains the lymphoid follicles, which have germinal centers. The medulla contains the sinuses, stroma, and vessels. The sinuses converge in the hilum. The afferent lymphatic vessels drain into the subcapsular sinus, a remarkably important structure because it is the first site of entry for any benign or metastatic process.

Supplementary InformationThe online version contains supplementary material available at https://doi.org/10.1007/978-3-031-73702-2_7.

R. H. Bardales (✉)
Precision Pathology, Outpatient Pathology Associates,
Sacramento, CA, USA

Cytomorphology Papanicolaou and Romanowsky are complementary stains used for the cytology evaluation of lymphoid cells. A normal lymph node exhibits a heterogeneous population of lymphoid cells: (1) small lymphocytes with scant cytoplasm, round nucleous, and coarse chromatin; (2) centrocytes (follicular center cells of medium size) with slightly irregular nuclei, and inconspicuous nucleoli; (3) centroblasts (follicular center cells of large size) with scant basophilic cytoplasm, round vesicular nuclei, 1–3 peripheral nucleoli placed close to the nuclear membrane; (4) immunoblasts with large size, moderate or abundant clear or basophilic cytoplasm, round nuclei with fine chromatin, and one central prominent nucleolus; (5) macrophages with tingible bodies, ample cytoplasm with debris, round/oval nuclei with fine chromatin, and an inconspicuous nucleoli; (6) interdigitating dendritic cells with spindle shape, abundant cytoplasm, and oval nuclei that may be indented; (7) dendritic follicular cells with ovoid/spindle shape and tend to aggregate forming bundles or storiform structures.

Positive Immunostains The small lymphocytes are partly B (CD19, CD20, and PAX5) and partly T (CD2, CD3, CD4, CD8, CD5, and CD7) cells. Follicular center cells are CD10, CD19, CD20, PAX-5, and bcl-6. Macrophages are CD68 and lysozyme. Follicular dendritic cells are vimentin, clusterin, desmoplakin, fascin, EGF-R, and HLA-DR and occasionally express CD21, CD23, CD35, CAN-42, and KiM4p.

Ultrasound (US) Features US is the preferred modality for the initial evaluation of lymphadenopathy and complements a careful physical examination that in many cases may not be fully revealing and reliable. The US findings reflect the histology. The cortex is densely cellular with little stroma and appears hypoechogenic and essentially avascular on Doppler examination. In contrast, the medulla has more stroma, converging sinuses, and vessels and appears hyperechogenic and vascular. Also, since the antigenic stimulus triggers lymph node enlargement, vascular increment, and follicular response, the cortex becomes variably vascular (Fig. 7.1a, b).

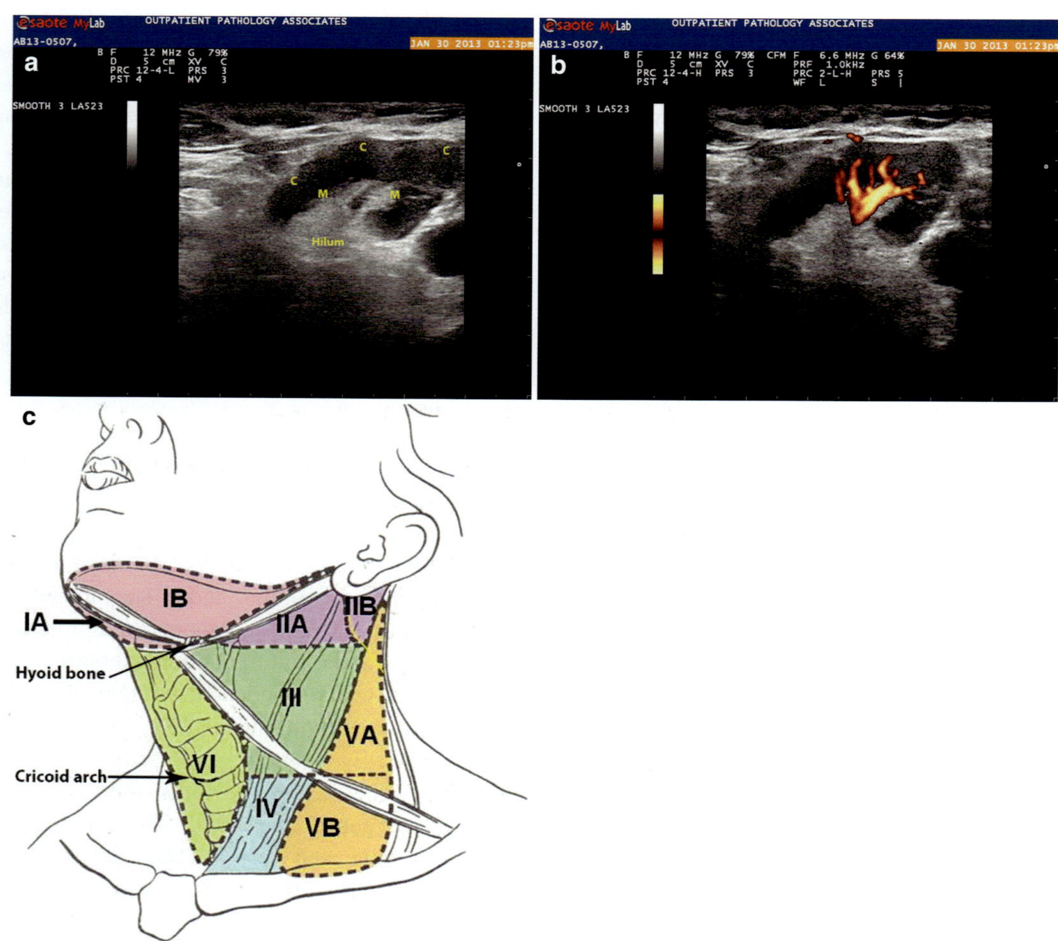

Fig. 7.1 Ultrasound anatomy of a reactive lymph node showing cortex (C), medulla (M), and hilum with a prominent vascular pole by Doppler examination (**a**, **b**). Anatomic levels of the neck are seen in (**c**)

The Neck Levels, US Examination, and Lymphatic Drainage

There are more than 300 lymph nodes in the head and neck region and range from 3 mm to 3.0 cm in size. The neck has been divided in topographic compartments / levels to facilitate the localization of a particular lymph node. Neck levels have clinical significance since different lymph node pathologic processes may prefferentially affect lymph nodes of certain neck levels based on the lymphatic drainage pattern. They were first described to map metastases from head and neck squamous cell carcinomas to cervical lymph nodes. The six levels of the neck are: (1) submental and submandibular, (2) upper lateral, (3) mid-lateral, (4) lower lateral, (5) posterior, (6) antero-lateral, and (7) suprasternal/superior mediastinum (Fig. 7.1c).

Level I Submental (Ia) and submandibular (Ib) area lymph nodes. Level I lymph nodes are the main lymphatic drainage for non-thyroid head and neck carcinomas, particularly those located in the oral cavity.

US Examination For *submental nodes*, elevate the chin, place the probe transverse to the chin, and scan from the chin down to the hyoid bone. The nodes are superficial in the midline between the anterior bellies of both digastric muscles; they drain the anterior tongue, floor of the mouth, lips, chin, and cheeks (Fig. 7.2a–d). For *submandibular nodes*, turn the head to the opposite side, place the probe transverse to the neck parallel to the mandible, and scan from the chin back to the angle of the mandible and identify the submandibular gland. The nodes are grouped superior and anterior to the submandibular gland and lateral to the anterior belly of the digastric muscle; they drain the anterior face, anterior oral cavity, and floor of the mouth (Fig. 7.3). Of note, there are no lymph nodes within the submandibular gland.

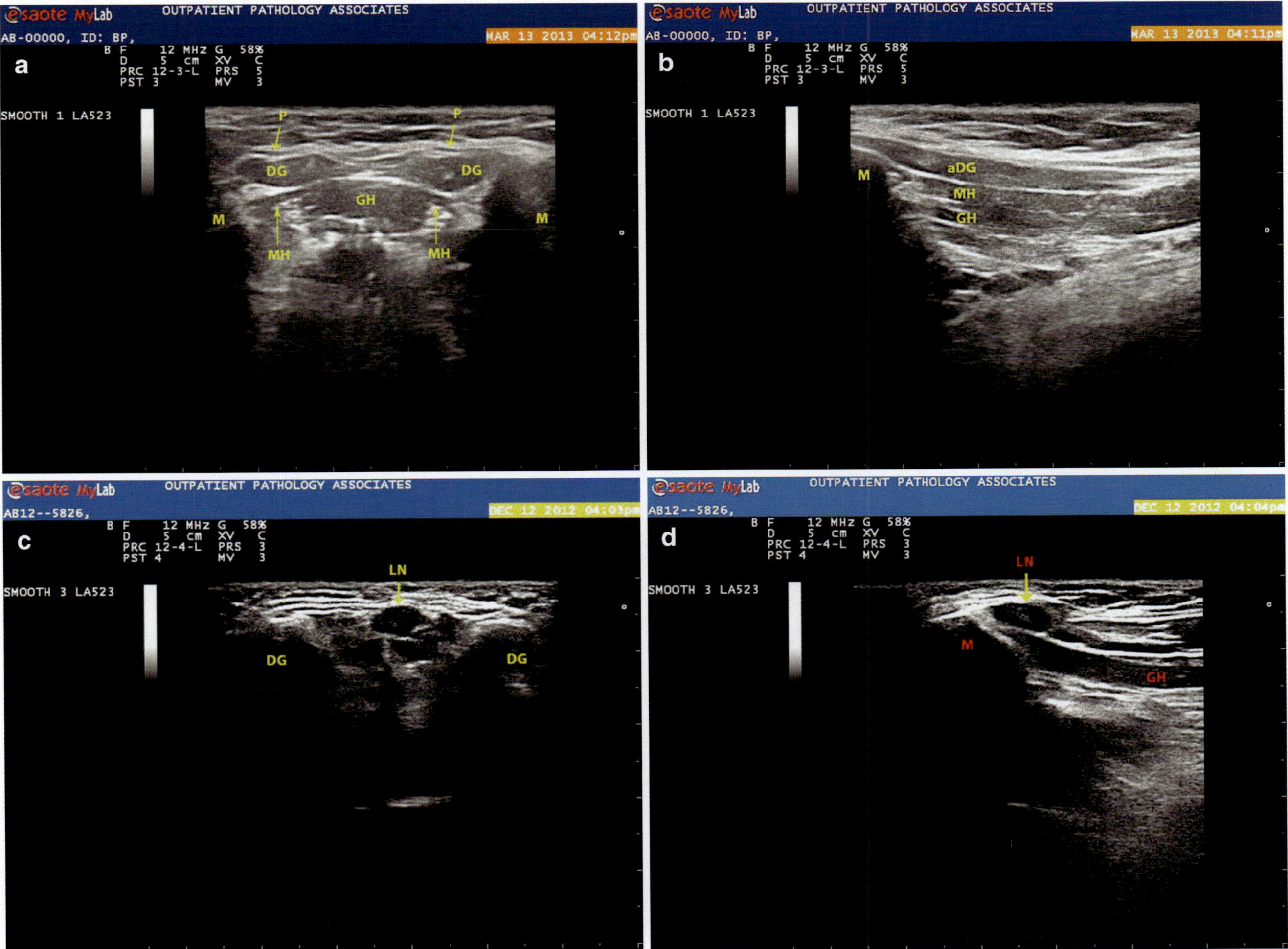

Fig. 7.2 Submental (level Ia) region. The normal anatomy is shown in (**a**) (transverse view) and (**b**) (longitudinal view along the midline). A small reactive lymph node between the digastric muscles is shown in (**c**) (transverse view) and (**d**) (longitudinal view). *P* platysma, *aDG* digastric muscle, anterior belly, *M* mandible, *GH* geniohyoid muscle, *MH* mylohyoid muscle, *LN* lymph node

Levels II, III, and IV These levels correspond to lymph nodes deep to the cervical/internal jugular chain that follows the course of the internal jugular vein extending from the angle of the mandible to the mid-clavicular region along the posterior border of the sternocleidomastoid muscle. They conform the anterior triangle of the neck and are the main lymphatic drainage for lesions located in the head and neck, draining the submental, submandibular, parotid, and retropharyngeal nodes. The jugulodigastric node is the most superior and prominent node in the chain, lies behind the submandibular gland, and is virtually visible by US examination in all individuals, measuring up to 4 cm in length in healthy young teenagers.

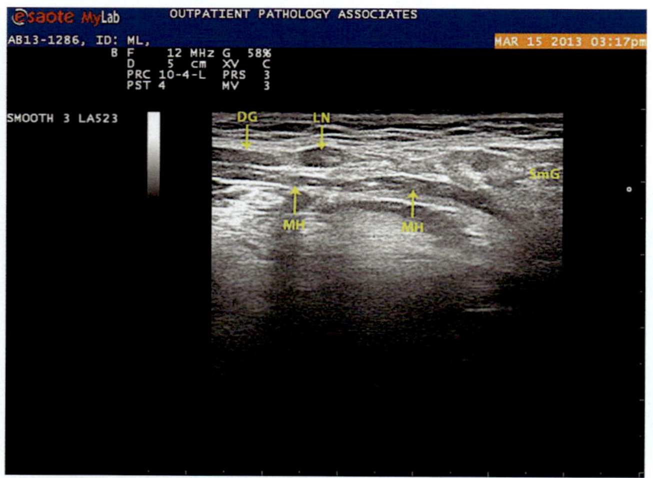

Fig. 7.3 Left submandibular region (level Ib). The transducer is placed parallel to the mandible. There is a small reactive lymph node posterior to the anterior belly of the digastric muscle. *LN* lymph node, *DG* digastric muscle, anterior belly, *MH* mylohyoid muscle, *SmG* submandibular gland

US Examination Identify the jugulodigastric node with the transducer transversally placed below the angle of the mandible and smoothly sweep down the chain keeping the internal jugular vein in the center of the field while evaluating all levels. In the mid-cervical region, the omohyoid muscle that divides levels III and IV lies deep to the sternocleidomastoid muscle and crosses the vessels mimicking a lymph node; the issue is solved by placement of the transducer in a longitudinal position.

Level II Lymph nodes located from the skull base to the level of the hyoid bone along the submandibular gland anteriorly and the posterior border of the sternocleidomastoid muscle (Fig. 7.4a, b, Video 7.1). Level II is further subdivided into level *IIa* (lymph nodes anterior to the internal jugular vein) and level *IIb* (posterior to the internal jugular vein).

Level III Lymph nodes located between the levels of the hyoid bone superiorly and the cricoid cartilage inferiorly between the omohyoid muscle anteriorly and the posterior border of the sternocleidomastoid muscle (Fig. 7.5, Video 7.2).

Level IV Lymph nodes located below the levels of the cricoid cartilage and the clavicle, from the the anterior border of the sternocleidomastoid mucle to the lateral edge of the anterior scalene muscle (Fig. 7.6a, b, Video 7.3).

Level V This level, also termed the posterior triangle of the neck corresponds to lymph nodes located in the supraclavicular fossa posterior to the sternocleidomastoid muscle and superior to the subclavian vein. The boundaries of the triangle are the sternocleidomastoid muscle anteriorly, the

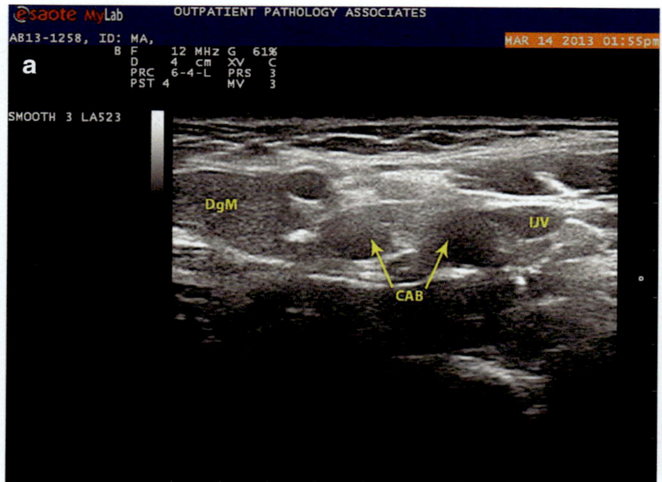
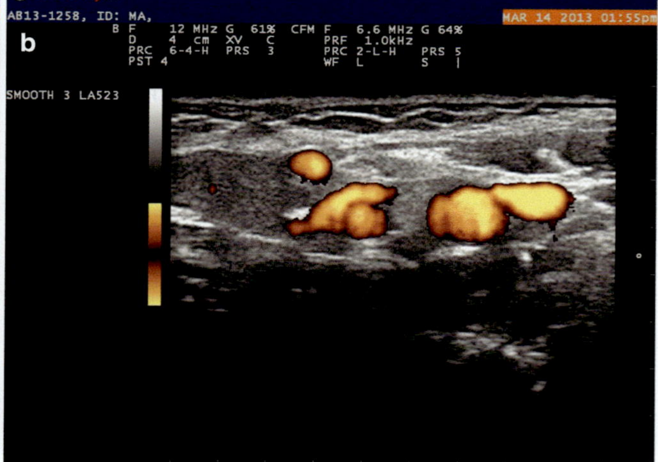

Fig. 7.4 Left neck level II. The transducer is placed slightly superior to the carotid bulb and both carotid branches are visualized in (**a**). The corresponding findings by Doppler examination are seen in (**b**). *DgM* digastric muscle, posterior belly, *CAB* carotid artery bifurcation, *IJV* internal jugular vein (Video 7.1)

clavicle inferiorly, and the trapezius muscle posteriorly (Fig. 7.7). The lymph nodes are located *superficially* within this triangle filled with adipose tissue. Enlargement of the left supraclavicular lymph node (Virchow's node) often indicates a primary malignancy located below the diaphragm. The posterior-triangle lymph nodes drain the skin of the occipital and mastoid regions, posterior scalp, lateral neck, and the postnasal space.

US Examination Scan transversally along the superior border of the mid clavicle to the lateral end of the clavicle to evaluate the supraclavicular fossa. The posterior triangle is scanned with the transducer transverse to the mastoid process, moving inferiorly along the posterior border of the sternocleidomastoid muscle toward the acromioclavicular joint and the anterior border of the trapezius.

Level VI These lymph nodes are located in the anterior central neck compartment. The prelaryngeal and pretracheal lymph nodes are superficial and the paratracheal are lateral to the trachea, medial to the carotid artery, and deeper in the tracheo-esophageal groove. The prelaryngeal and pretracheal nodes drain the skin and muscles of the anterior neck and the thyroid gland. The prelaryngeal lymph node drains

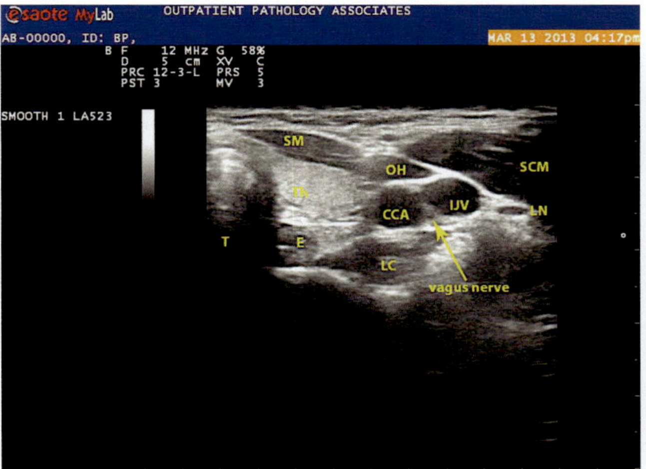

Fig. 7.5 Left neck level III. Normal US anatomy showing the trachea (T), esophagus (E), left thyroid lobe (Th), strap muscles (SM), omohyoid muscle (OH), common carotid artery (CCA), internal jugular vein (IJV), sternocleidomastoid muscle (SCM), and longus colli (LC). A small lymph node with hilum (LN) and the vagus nerve are also seen (Video 7.2)

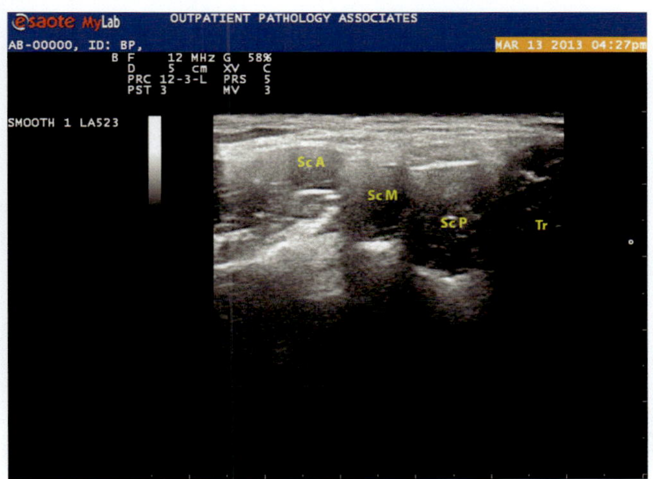

Fig. 7.7 Left neck level V, supraclavicular area. Normal anatomy is seen in this image and include the trapezius muscle (Tr), and anterior, medial, and posterior scalene muscles (ScA, ScM, ScP)

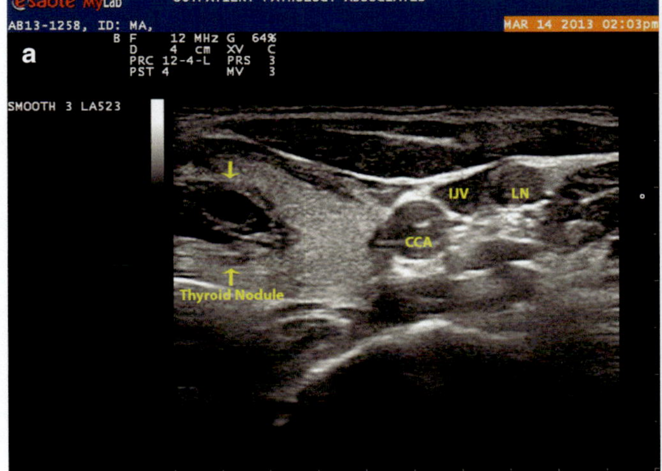

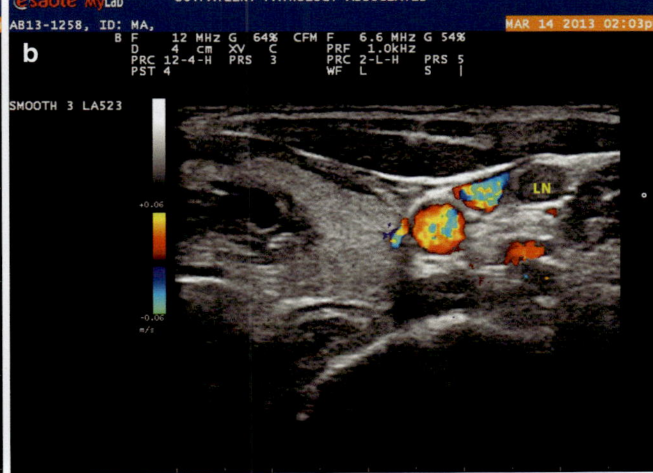

Fig. 7.6 Left neck level IV. US images show a predominantly cystic complex left thyroid nodule, the common carotid artery (CCA), internal jugular vein (IJV), and a round-shaped lymph node (LN) posterior to the IJV. US-guided FNA of both the thyroid nodule and lymph node showed papillary thyroid carcinoma (Video 7.3)

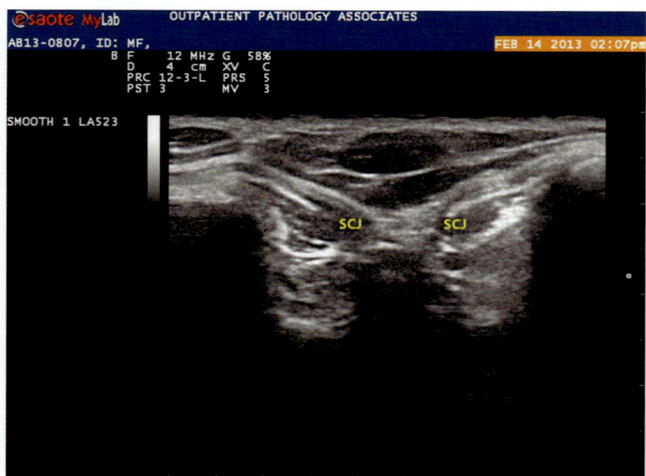

Fig. 7.8 Neck level VII. The transducer is placed above the sternal notch and is used for evaluation of suprasternal/superior mediastinum lymph nodes. *SCJ* sternoclavicular joint (Video 7.4)

the subglottic area of the larynx. The paratracheal lymph nodes are difficult to visualize by US because they lie posterior to the thyroid gland; they drain the larynx, the pyriform fossae, the thyroid gland, and the esophagus.

US Examination Scan moving the probe in the transverse plane with the probe in a longitudinal position from the level of the hyoid bone down to the sternal notch.

Level VII These lymph nodes are located in the suprasternal/superior mediastinum. Best evaluated using a small-footprint curvilinear probe placed above the sternal notch (Fig. 7.8, Video 7.4).

The *parotid-area lymph nodes* have no numbered level. They drain the skin of the lateral forehead, temple, external auditory meatus, posterior cheek, gums, and buccal mucosa. Likewise, the *buccal-region lymph nodes* are not numbered, lie anterior to masseter muscle adjacent to the facial artery in the buccal fat space, and drain the facial skin from the upper eyelid to the upper lip.

The retroauricular and occipital lymph nodes drain corresponding areas of the scalp and should be examined in cases of scalp malignancy.

There are more than 300 lymph nodes in the normal neck, and US can typically identify between 6 and 20 neck lymph nodes. Most enlarged lymph nodes are reactive secondary to inflammatory or infectious processes located in the head and neck area. Levels Ia and Ib, anterior triangle (levels II, III, IV), and posterior triangle (level V) lymph nodes are easier to detect and amenable to USG-FNA. Levels VI and VII lymph nodes are more difficult to detect by US and be sampled using US guidance.

US Features in Lymph Node Evaluation

The US features to be evaluated in a lymph node include, size, shape, border, confluence, echogenicity, hilum, calcification, necrosis, parenchymal reticulation, intranodal vascular pattern, and surrounding edema. Because no abnormality of these features by itself is diagnostic of malignancy, a combination of the ultrasound findings helps in predicting malignancy. The lymph-node number in a given lymph-node chain is a consideration for abnormality when >3 US-abnormal lymph nodes are present.

1. Size. Lymph node size is an important consideration; however, it may be of limited value in differentiating benign from malignant nodes (Fig. 7.9a, b). The most important factor is the variation in the lymph node size over a period of time. Most benign lymph nodes measure <5 mm. If a head and neck malignancy is known, a lymph node >6 mm is considered suspicious for a metastatic deposit. Nodal size is important for TNM staging: N1 <3 cm, N2 3–6 cm, and N3 >6 cm. The lymph node size should be measured transversally and not longitudinally.

2. Shape. A normal node has a flat bean shape. An irregular or round shape is seen in metastasis instead of the oval shape often seen in benign and reactive lymph nodes. An irregular lymph-node cortex is suggestive of a subcapsular metastatic deposit. It has been found that 85% of benign lymph nodes have a ratio of long (L) axis/short (S) axis >2, and 85% of malignant nodes have an L/S axis ratio <2 (Fig. 7.10a, b). Of note, level Ia and Ib benign lymph nodes may not follow that rule.

3. Border. The border of a normal lymph node is well-defined, smooth, and slightly indistinct from the surrounding tissue. A sharp lymph-node border is seen in metastasis and lymphoma instead of a less defined border seen in a reactive lymph node. Extracapsular nodal involvement of malignancy and response to radiotherapy also cause ill-defined borders. Ill-defined and spiculated/irregular margins in a metastatic node indicate extranodal metastatic spread (Fig. 7.11a, b).

4. Confluence. Matted lymph nodes can be seen in tuberculosis, post- radiation, chemotherapy, metastasis, and lymphoma as a result of perinodal inflammation and fibrosis (Fig. 7.12).

5. Echogenicity. Hypoechogenicity is seen in metastatic malignancies; however, metastatic oncocytic, medullary, and occasionally papillary thyroid carcinoma may be hyperechogenic when compared with adjacent muscle. A "pseudo cystic" pattern (marked hypoechogenicity with posterior acoustic enhancement) is seen in lymphoma when evaluated at conventional US resolution (Fig. 7.13a, b).

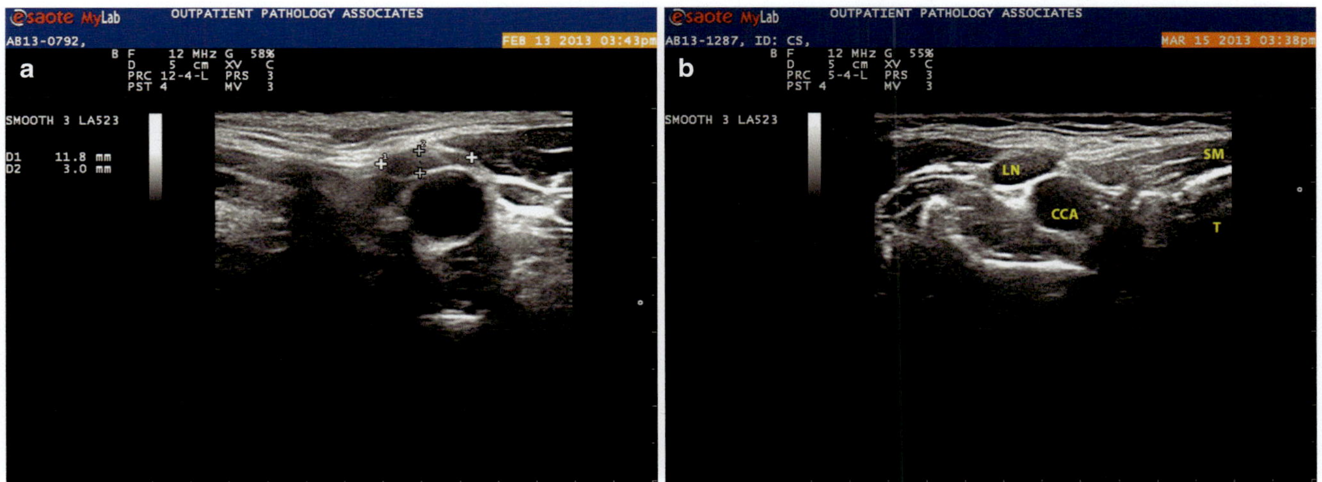

Fig. 7.9 Lymph node size. Small oval level III left (**a**) and right (**b**) neck lymph nodes. Metastatic papillary thyroid carcinoma (calipers, **a**) and reactive follicular hyperplasia (**b**) were the US-guided FNA diag- noses. *LN* lymph node, *CCA* common carotid artery, *SM* strap muscles, *T* trachea

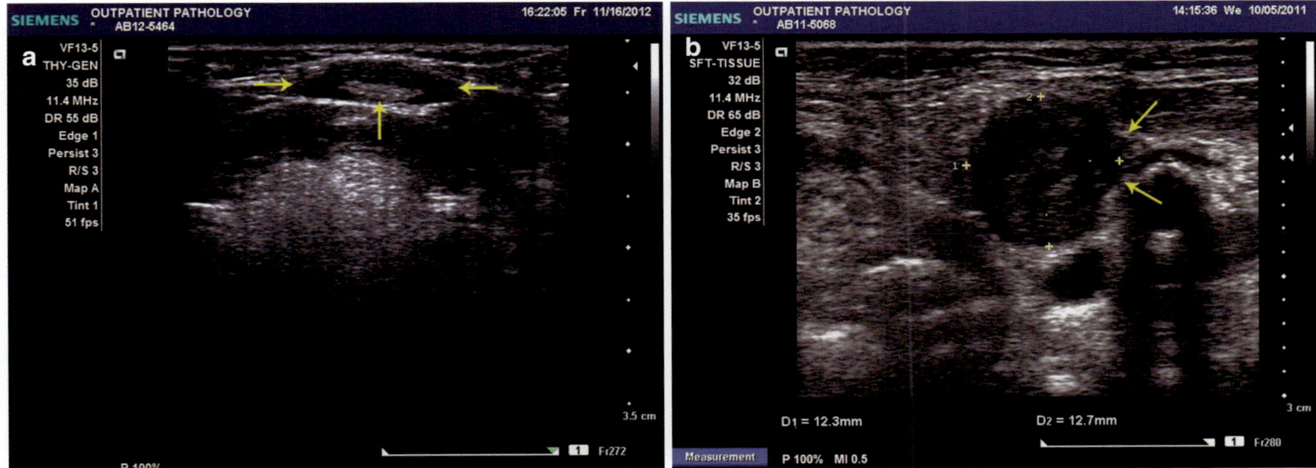

Fig. 7.10 Lymph node shape. Oval level Ia lymph node (horizontal arrows) with regular borders and prominent hilum (vertical arrow) (**a**, US-guided FNA diagnosis was reactive follicular hyperplasia). Left neck lymph node with heterogeneous echotexture, irregular borders (arrows), and taller than wide in the transverse view (**b**, US-guided FNA diagnosis was poorly differentiated metastatic squamous cell carcinoma)

(a) Hilum. A vascular hilum is usually seen in 90% of lymph nodes >5 mm. An enlarged lymph node with a prominent echogenic vascular hilum is probably benign (Figs. 7.1a, b and 7.14a, b). Metastatic lymph nodes usually lack a hilum; however, a hilum can be seen in metastasis, particularly in early metastatic nodal involvement. Thus, hilum absence in an enlarged lymph node is highly suspicious for malig- nancy. Of note, tuberculous lymph nodes usually lack a hilum.

6. Calcification. Metastasis from papillary thyroid carci- noma, medullary thyroid carcinoma, or in patients with a history of radiotherapy or chemotherapy may show foci of micro- or macrocalcifications. Macrocalcifications are also seen in tuberculous lymphadenitis (Fig. 7.15).

7. Necrosis. Cystic necrosis can be seen in metastases, i.e., squamous-cell carcinoma, papillary thyroid carcinoma, and benign processes such as tuberculosis (Fig. 7.16a, b). A cystic nodal metastasis >3 cm in squamous cell carci- noma appears anechoic and, if it involves the jugulo- digastric (level II) lymph node, should be differentiated from a branchial-cleft cyst, particularly in patients older than 30 years. Coagulative necrosis may appear hyper- echogenic and may be confused with hilum when located close to the nodal capsule; however, it is not continuous with the perinodal fat as the hilum is.

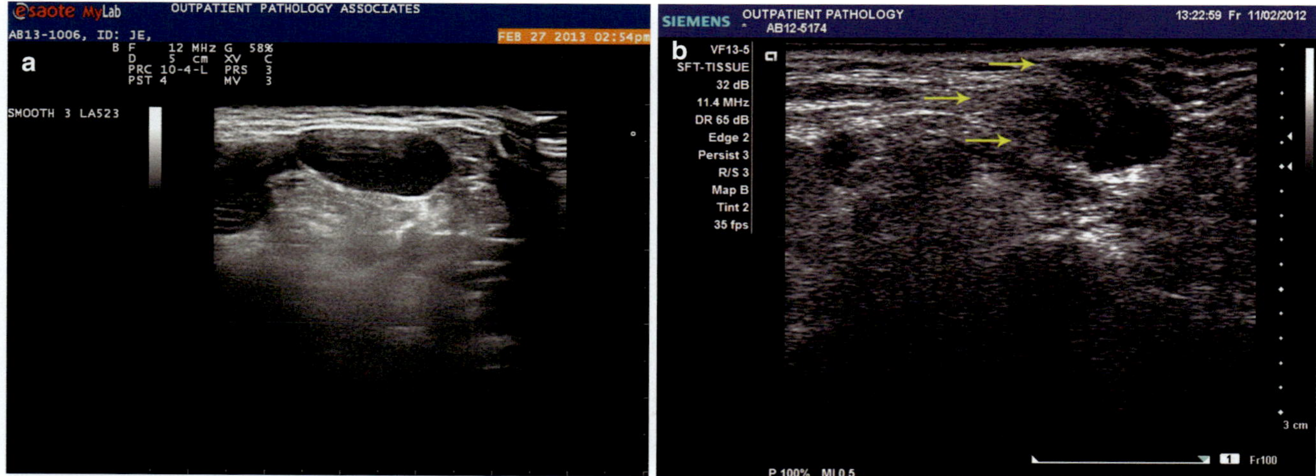

Fig. 7.11 Lymph node borders. Neck lymph node with oval, homogeneous, and slightly lobulated well-defined sharp borders (**a**, Hodgkin lymphoma was the US-guided FNA diagnosis). Neck level Vb lymph node with spiculated borders (arrows) and heterogeneous echotexture (**b**, metastatic breast carcinoma was the US-guided FNA diagnosis)

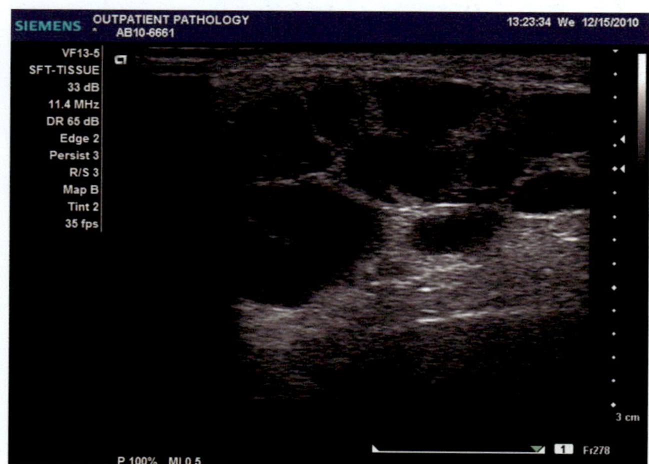

Fig. 7.12 Lymph node confluence. Matted hypoechoic homogeneous lymph nodes. Non-Hodgkin lymphoma was the US-guided FNA diagnosis

8. Intranodal reticulation. A micronodular reticulated pattern is seen in lymphoma when evaluated with high-resolution US. Under conventional resolution, lymph nodes have a "pseudo-cystic" appearance with marked hypoechogenicity and posterior acoustic enhancement (Fig. 7.13b).

9. Nodal vascular pattern. Normal or reactive lymph nodes usually have no vascularity when they measure <5 mm, or there may be symmetrical central radiating hilar vascularity only in larger nodes. Avascular lymph nodes are usually benign. Metastatic lymph nodes may have hilar and peripheral (mixed) or peripheral subcapsular flow and perfusion defects (Fig. 7.17a). Peripheral subcapsular flow is also seen in tuberculosis, which disrupts the nodal vascular architecture in a manner similar to malignancy. An exaggerated normal vascular appearance with a branching hilar vascular pattern is often seen in lymphoma (Fig. 7.17b).

Thus, the US characteristics, topographic distribution of lymph nodes (i.e, supraclavicular, epitrochlear, popliteal that are considered a significant finding), and the clinical scenario including age, symptoms, site, size, time of onset, remote and current medical history, pertinent laboratory test results, and physical examination, are paramount for the cytopathologist to provide a useful microscopic description and diagnostic interpretation using one of the five Sydney categories. In some instances, the diagnosis may not be specific, but only descriptive and the cytopathologist should include diagnostic possibilities and recommendations as clinically indicated.

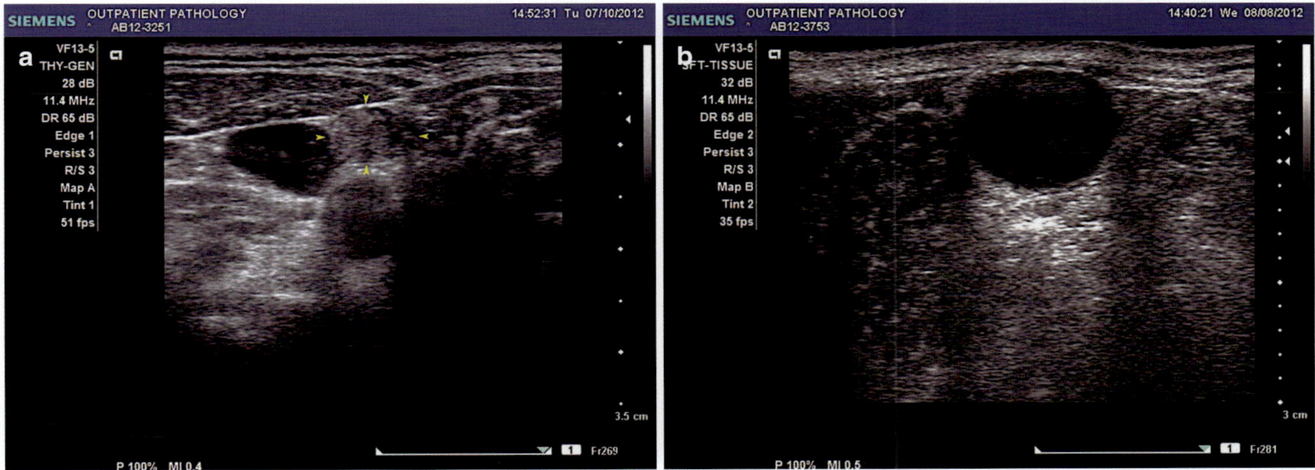

Fig. 7.13 Lymph node echogenicity. Iso- to hyperechogenic lymph node in a patient with metastatic oncocytic thyroid carcinoma (**a**). Lymph node with marked hypoechogenicity ("pseudocystic" pattern) and posterior acoustic enhancement in a patient with non-Hodgkin lymphoma (**b**)

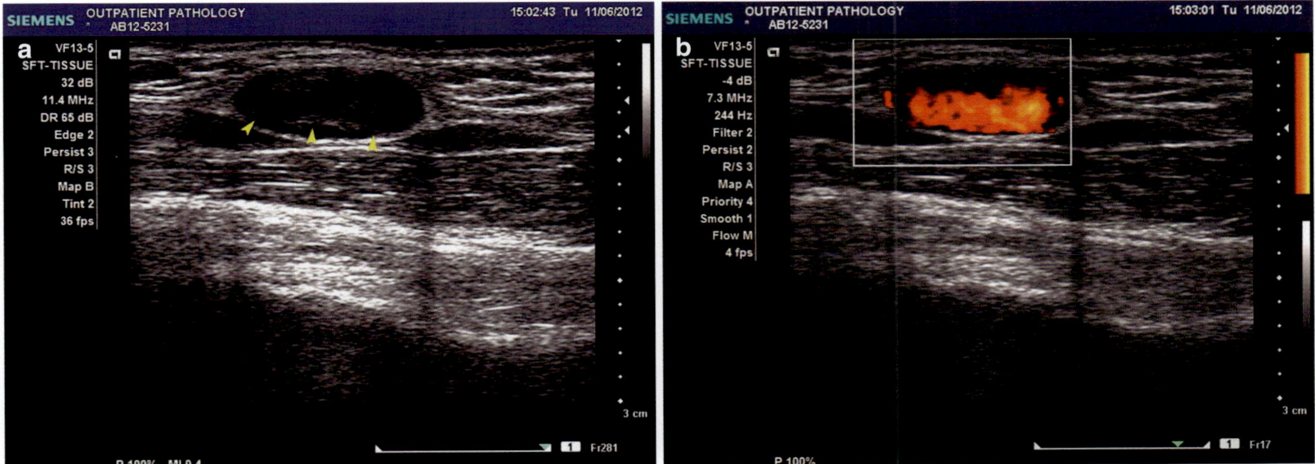

Fig. 7.14 Benign lymph node with a prominent hilum (**a**, arrow heads) highlighted by Doppler examination (**b**)

Fig. 7.15 Metastatic papillary thyroid carcinoma to a level V lymph node. Note microcalcifications/microreflectors in the upper part of this heterogeneous, hypoechogenic, taller than wide lymph node with fuzzy borders

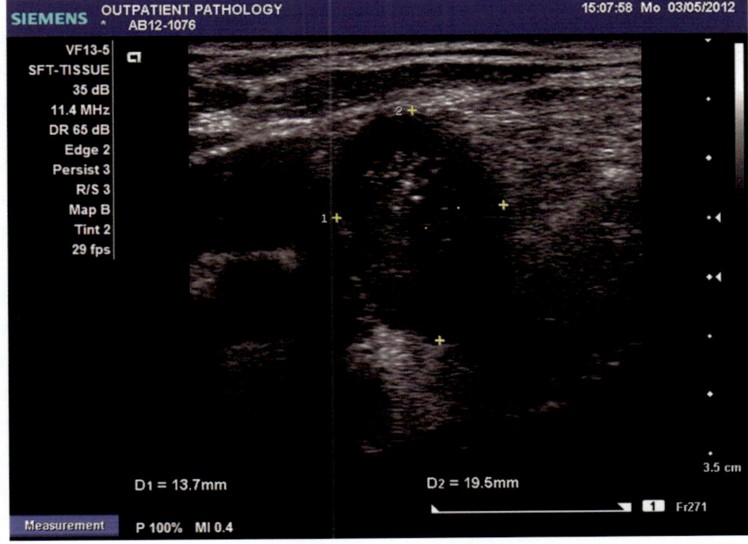

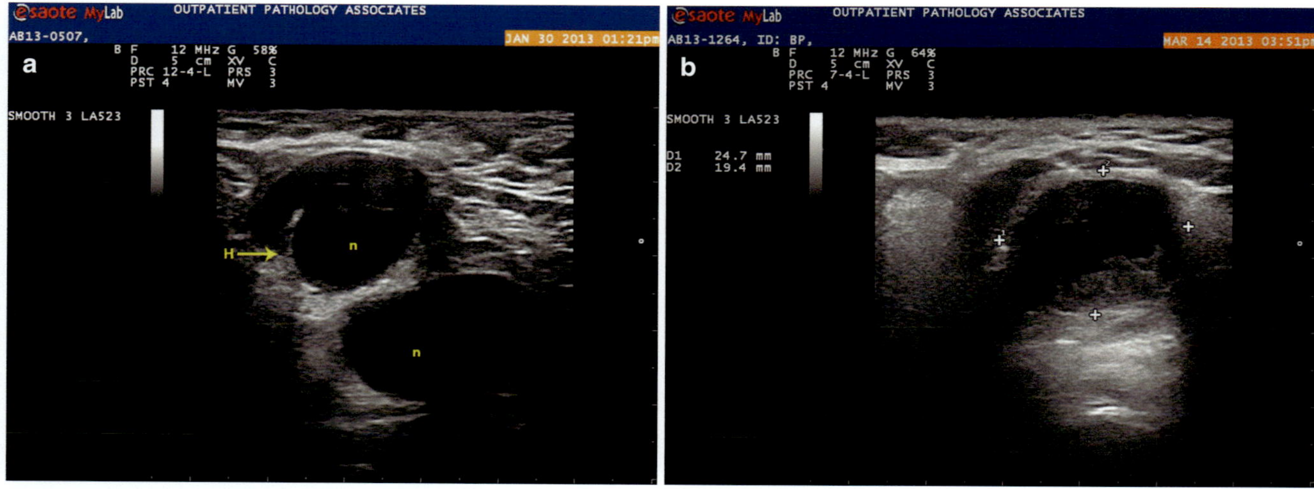

Fig. 7.16 Necrosis. Tuberculous lymphadenitis with focal necrosis (*n*) and preserved hilum (**a**, arrow). Level V cervical lymph node with metastatic squamous cell carcinoma with central necrosis. Note the hyperechogenic area towards the lower portion of the node that mimics a hilum (**b**)

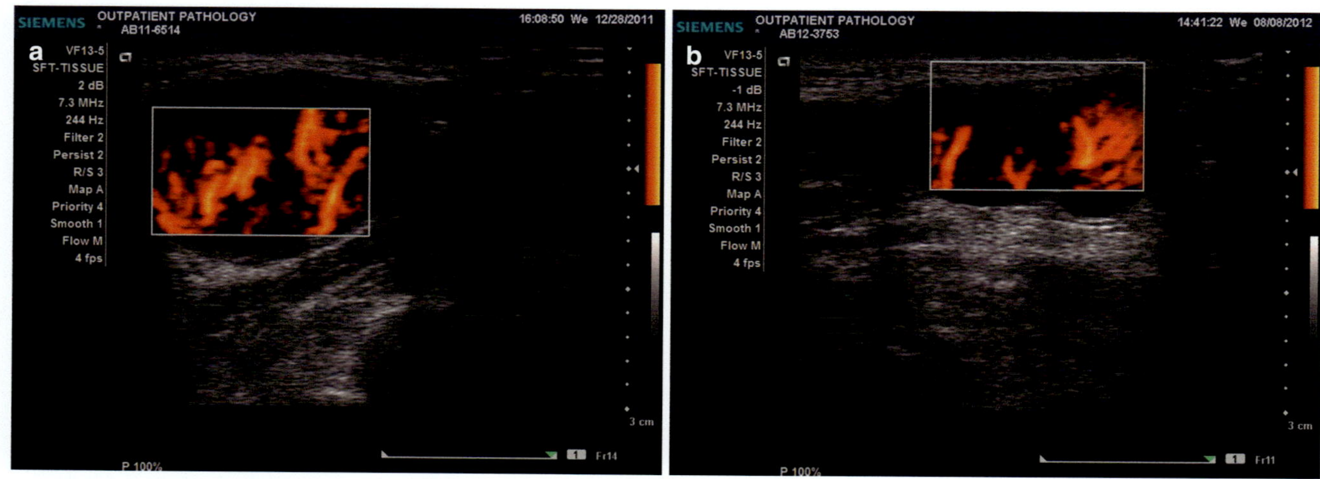

Fig. 7.17 Vascular pattern. Metastatic poorly differentiated carcinoma showing a chaotic vascular flow pattern (**a**). Non-Hodgkin lymphoma showing an exaggerated branching hilar vascular pattern (**b**)

Fine-Needle Aspiration of Lymph Nodes

FNA is the modality of choice for evaluating an abnormal lymph node and, in many instances, avoiding an unnecessary excisional biopsy. The use of US as an aid in locating and performing FNA of superficial and deep-seated lymph nodes is of paramount importance. Except for FNA of axillary lymph node that may be best sampled by palpation-guidance, ultrasound-guided (USG) FNA of lymph nodes is highly recommended and offers significant benefits, i.e., select the most significant or the most approachable lymph node in case of multiple enlarged lymph nodes, sampling of solid areas in cystic necrosis and reducing non-diagnostic samples, procurement of sample for cultures, obtain material for flow cytometry in lymphomas, measurement of thyroglobu-

lin, calcitonin, or parathyroid hormone (PTH) levels in needle rinses, cytogenetics and molecular estudies in lymphomas and some metastatic carcinomas, and immunostains in cellblocks and smears, among other ancillary tests that complement cytologic evaluation. USG-FNA has a sensitivity of >97% and a specificity of >93%. Of note, histological correlation is recommended for diagnosis of HL and NHL except for specific clinical situations (i.e., chronic lymphocytic leukemia/small lymphocytic lymphoma with supporting flow cytometry) or when surgery is contraindicated or not possible.

In my experience, the USG-FNA should be performed using 25-gauge needles with no suction (Zajdela technique). Two or three passes are sufficient. Rapid on-site interpretation is recommended in selected cases to triage the sample and harvest material for ancillary studies. The use of suction and 23- or 25-G needles is recommended to harvest material for a cellblock. USG-FNA procedure is detailed in Chap. 2 of this book.

A thorough cytologic evaluation answers questions which the cytopathologist should keep in mind when evaluating lymph node FNAs. The questions include: (1) is it really a lymph node?, (2) adequate?, (3) is it benign or malignant?, (4) if benign, is it infectious?, can we identify the infectious agent?, (5) if malignant, is it lymphoma?, metastasis?, (6) if lymphoma, NHL?, HL?, (7) if NHL, B- or T-cell type?, grade?, (8) if HL, sub-type?, (9) if metastasis, type?, source? Most answers can be based on morphologic evaluation, and others need the support of ancillary tests for reaching a definitive diagnosis.

The use of Romanowsky-type stains (DiffQuik®, Wright, May-Grunwald-Giemsa) performed on air-dried smears is fundamental for FNA cytologic interpretation, because they provide excellent evaluation of cell size, cytoplasmic detail, and background elements. Papanicolaou and hematoxylin-eosin stains performed on alcohol-fixed smears provide excellent visualization of nuclear morphology in both single cells and cell aggregates. Thus, both air-dried and alcohol-fixed stains are complementary. I caution against the use of liquid-based preparations for lymph node FNA because cells appear smaller, cell aggregates are fragmented, lymphocytes may become artificially aggregated, and background elements are difficult to evaluate.

Cell Patterns in Fine-Needle Aspiration of Lymph Nodes

To facilitate the cytologic interpretation, the FNA of lymph nodes can algorithmically be classified in the following smear cell patterns:

1. Polymorphous. Nonspecific reactive lymphoid hyperplasia, early HIV lymphadenitis, primary and secondary syphilis lymphadenitis, toxoplasma and leishmania lymphadenitis, rheumatoid arthritis, Castleman lymphadenopathy plasma cell variant, Kimura lymphadenopathy, Kikuchi-Fujimoto disease, autoimmune lymphoproliferative syndrome, early dermatopathic lymphadenopathy, Sézary syndrome, early cat-scratch lymphadenitis, follicular lymphoma (FL), marginal zone lymphoma (MZL).
2. Monotonous small size. Quiescent benign lymph node, Castleman disease hyaline vascular variant, B-cell chronic lymphocytic leukemia/small lymphocytic lymphoma (CLL/SLL), adult T-cell leukemia/lymphoma, B- and T-cell lymphoblastic leukemia/lymphoma, lymphoplasmacytic lymphoma (LPL), nodular lymphocyte predominant type (NLP) HL.
3. Monotonous intermediate size. FL, mantle cell lymphoma (MCL), MZL, Burkitt lymphoma (BL), precursors of B- and T-cell lymphomas, adult T-cell leukemia/lymphoma, Sézary syndrome, metastatic small-cell malignancies.
4. Monotonous large size. Diffuse large B-cell lymphoma (DLBCL) and its variants, grade 3 FL, Richter transformation of SLL, blastoid variant of MCL, peripheral T-cell lymphoma, NK/T cell lymphoma, granulocytic sarcoma, nodal Langerhans cell histiocytosis, dendritic cell neoplasms, and some metastases (carcinoma, melanoma, sarcoma, seminoma).
5. Pleomorphic. HL, anaplastic large-cell lymphoma (ALCL), Hodgkin-type Richter transformation of SLL, large B-cell lymphoma and variants, thymoma, metastatic melanoma, metastatic mesenchymal malignancies.

Clues for specific cytologic diagnoses and cytologic patterns are listed in Tables 7.1 and 7.2.

Table 7.1 Lymphadenitis/lymphadenopathy—clues for the cytologic diagnosis

Viral	
Infectious mononucleosis	Immunoblasts with marked atypia
Herpes simplex	Cowdry A inclusions, ground-glass nuclei, multinucleation
Cytomegalovirus	Large cells with large eosinophilic nuclear inclusion
Varicella-Zoster	Rare small intranuclear inclusions
Measles	Polykariocytes (not specific)
Human immunodeficiency virus	Polymorphous lymphoid cell pattern. Plasma cells in late stages
Bacterial	
Cat scratch	Granulomas, necrosis, acute inflammation
Lymphogranuloma venereum	Granulomas, necrosis, acute inflammation
Syphilis	Small granulomas and plasma cells
Tuberculosis	Granulomas and caseation necrosis
Mycobacterium avium-intracellulare complex	Histiocytes and background smear with numerous bacilli (Pseudo-Gaucher cells and negative images)
Leprosy, tuberculoid	Small non-caseating granulomas
Fungal	
Cryptococcus	Yeast with mucoid thick capsule. Mucous background. Narrow-based buds
Pneumocystis	Foamy exudates
Histoplasma	Intracytoplasmic yeasts. Granular calcific background
Coccidioides	Large spherules with yeast forms
Protozoal	
Toxoplasma	Crescent-shaped organisms (2–6 μm)
Leishmania	Amastigotes 1–3 μm with histiocytes (Donovan bodies) and multinucleated giant cells
Filaria	Fragments of dead calcified organisms

(continued)

Table 7.1 (continued)

Viral	
Non-infectious	
Kimura disease	Polymorphous lymphoid cell pattern with polykariocytes (not specific)
Kikuchi disease	Necrosis
Rosai-Dorfman disease	Histiocytes with emperipolesis (engulfment of lymphocytes, erythrocytes, plasma cells)
Sarcoidosis	Cell damage, non-necrotizing granulomas Schaumann and cytoplasmic asteroid bodies
Systemic lupus erythemathosus	Necrosis. Hematoxylin bodies
Rheumatoid arthritis	Polymorphous lymphoid cell pattern and plasma cells
Castleman disease, plasma cell variant Castleman disease, hyaline vascular	Plasma cells and dendritic cells Hyalinized capillaries and dendritic cells
IgG-4 related disease	Plasma cells, eosinophiles, dendritic cells
Dermatopathic	Lipid or pigment (melanin)-laden histiocytes
Amyloid	Amorphous "waxy" material, lymphocytes, multinucleated giant cells
Silicone	Histiocytes with clear cytoplasmic vacuoles, multinucleated giant cells
Lipid	Histiocytes with small cytoplasmic vacuoles, multinucleated giant cells (lipogranulomas)

Table 7.2 The various cytologic patterns as clues for the diagnosis

Necrosis	Granulomas with necrosis
Infectious mononucleosis (focal)	Cat-scratch disease
Herpes simplex (focal)	Mycobacterial infection
Kikuchi disease (marked)	Fungal infection
Systemic lupus erythematosus (marked)	Kikuchi disease
Pneumocystis (marked)	Lymphogranuloma venereum
Infarcted lymph node (marked)	Leishmania
Cat-scratch disease	Sarcoidosis (rare)
Neutrophils	**Granulomas without necrosis**
Bacterial infection (marked)	Toxoplasma
Anaplastic large cell lymphoma (scattered)	Sarcoidosis
Anaplastic carcinoma (scattered)	Syphilis
Hodgkin lymphoma (scattered)	Whipple disease
	Tuberculoid leprosy
	Filaria
	Tumor-associated lymphadenitis

The Sydney System for Performing and Reporting Lymph Node Fine-Needle Aspiration Cytopathology (TSS-RLN-FNAC)

In an effort for providing guidelines and a cytopathological diagnostic classification, a committee of cytopathologists developed the Sydney System of performance, classification, and reporting LN-FNAC in May 2019. The system integrates clinical data, imaging studies, and ancillary tests with cytopathological features that yields a standardized, reliable, and reproducible cytopathology report, which facilitates the communication among clinicians, surgeons, and cytopathologists.

The reporting system includes two diagnostic levels. The first level provides basic diagnostic information and includes five categories (inadequate, benign, atypical cells of udetermined sigificanace, suspicious, and malignant). The second level provides specific benign or malignant diagnostic entities with the use of ancillary tests.

The Sydney System diagnostic reporting categories, including cytologic patterns and recommendation are summarized in Table 7.3.

The LN-FNAC report should include clinical information including US features (recommended), description of the FNA procedure (suggested), one of the five diagnostic categories (recommended), microscopic description and ancillary tests if requested and done (suggested), and conclusions and recommendations for follow-up or management (suggested).

Some specific types of reactive lymphadenopathy, lymphadenitis, infection, NHL, HL, and metastases that are diagnosed by cytomorphology and ancillary tests are desbribed in the following sections of this chapter.

Table 7.3 The Sydney system for reporting lymph node fine-needle aspiration cytopathology (TSS-RLN-FNAC)[a]

LN-FNAC	Diagnostic categories (1–5)	Actions and recommendations
1st diagnostic level	(1) Inadequate/non-diagnostic (scant cellularity, necrosis, technical limitations)	Mandatory
	(2) Benign (reactive lymphoid hyperplasia, infectious)	Mandatory
	(3) AUS/ALUS (AUS, atypical small or large cells that may not be lymphoid; ALUS, suggestive of reactive lymphoid hyperplasia but follicular NHL can not be excluded)	Mandatory
	(4) Suspicious (…for NHL, HL, metastases)	Mandatory
	(5) Malignant (NHL, HL, metastases)	Mandatory
2nd diagnostic level (provide additional information)	Provide specific etiology in reactive processes	Recommended if available
	NHL subtyping and specific diagnosis[b]	Recommended if available
	HL[b]	Recommended if available
	Specific site of primary tumor in metastases and any possible prognostic or treatment markers (i.e., p16 or breast cancer makers)	Recommended if available
Management recommendations	(1) Inadequate/non-diagnostic	Repeat FNA, CNB, or excision
	(2) Benign	Clinical follow-up/specific treatment
	(3) AUS/ALUS	Repeat FNA for ancillary tests, CNB, or excision
	(4) Suspicious	Repeat FNA for ancillary tests, CNB, or excision
	(5) Malignant	Clinical correlation. LN histopathology correlation may not be necessary for NHL and HL relapses, CLL/SLL, or metastasis from known primary site

LN lymph node, *AUS/ALUS* atypia of undeterminaed significance/atypical lymphoid cells of udetermined significance, *NHL* non-Hodgkin lymphoma, *HL* Hodgkin lymphoma, *CNB* core needle biopsy, *CLL/SLL* chronic lymphocytic leukemia/small lymphocytic lymphoma
[a] Modified from Acta cytologica 2020;64:306-322
[b] Specific NHL and HL entities as listed in the 2022 WHO classification of hematolyphoid neoplasms

Select Examples of Non-malignant Lymphadenopathy

Reactive Lymphoid Hyperplasia

Reactive lymphoid hyperplasia is the prototype of a cytologic polymorphous lymphoid-cell pattern commonly associated with benign, reactive, and reversible, lymphadenopathy. The etiology remains unknown in most cases. Bacteria, viruses, chemicals, and iatrogenic drugs are identified in a minority of cases.

Clinical Findings The lymph nodes are small, oval, soft, and single or regional, often cervical in children and inguinal in all age groups. Location of the lymph node can suggest an underlying disease and additional ancillary tests are needed to confirm the diagnosis (i.e, cervical in infectious mononucleosis, posterior cervical in toxoplasmosis, parotid and epitrochlear in HIV infection, cervical and axillary in dermatopathic lymphadenopathy, and cat scratch disease, inguinal in sexually transmitted diseases).

FNA Findings The cytologic pattern reflects the expansion of a particular lymph node area (follicular, paracortical, medullary, sinusoidal), which depends on the antigenic stimulus. *Follicular hyperplasia* represents a B-cell response and includes the presence of small round lymphocytes, centroblasts, centrocytes, immunoblasts, plasmacytoid lymphocytes, plasma cells, and histiocytes/tingible-body macrophages in various numbers. *Paracortical hyperplasia* with predominance of B-immunoblasts admixed with a heterogeneous population of lymphoid cells admixed with fragments of germinal centers containing centrocytes, centroblasts, small lymphocytes, macrophages, and dendritic cells represents a T-cell response, which is often secondary to viral infections or drugs. An acute inflammatory pattern is frequently associated with bacteria and fungi. Occasionally, the differential diagnosis includes follicular lymphoma, and the use of ancillary tests on FNA material is needed. Prominent histiocytosis and plasmacytosis are also forms of lymphoid reactive processes.

After a single triggering factor, the smears show a polymorphous pattern lasting 3–4 weeks; progressively, the smear shows a predominance of small round lymphocytes and centrocytes for 3–4 weeks. The background shows histiocytes, scattered plasmacytoid cells, plasma cells, and lymphoglandular bodies (Fig. 7.18a, b). Of note, this pattern is seen as a smear background in HL and along with histiocytes in cases of draining lymph nodes in metastatic disease, regardless of the presence or absence of actual metastatic deposits.

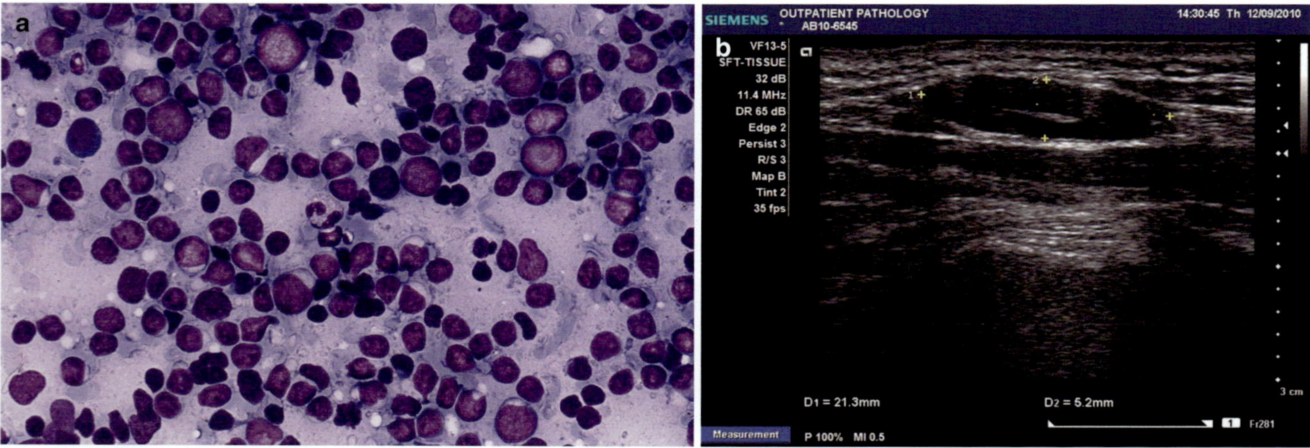

Fig. 7.18 Reactive lymph node. The smear shows a polymorphous population of lymphoid cells (**a**). The US evaluation shows an oval (AP/T <0.5 in the transverse view), hypoechoic, homogeneous, and well-defined lymph node with regular borders and a distinct hilum (**b**). (**a**, DiffQuik® stain, high magnification). *AP* anteroposterior axis (2), *T* transverse axis (1)

US Features A reactive lymphoid hyperplasia produces diffuse cortical widening; if the process continues, there is formation of germinal centers in the hilar area, causing widening of the hilum. Metastatic processes produce irregular cortical widening.

The immunophenotype is polytipic and B- and T-lymphocytes express normal markers with no immunoglobulin light-chain restriction or T-cell receptor rearrangement. PCR shows polyclonal immunoglobulin heavy chain gene rearrangement and no evidence of t(14;18)(q32;q21) or *IGL::BCL2* fusion, which is seen in classic FL.

Castleman Disease Lymphadenopathy

Clinical findings. Castleman desease (CD), also known as angiofollicular lymphoid hyperplasia, is a lymphoproliferative disorder that affects lymph nodes and/or extranodal sites of patients of all ages and genders. Patients with unicentric CD (UCD) are commonly younger (onset, 4th decade of life and commonly affects the mediastinum) than patients with multicentric (MCD) (onset, 6th decade of life and affects predominanly the neck). Patients with UCD are usually asymptomatic, in contrast to patients with MCD who have usually systemic symptoms including fever, weight loss, and organomegaly. MCD is prevalent in immunosuppressed patients and human herpes virus-8 (HHV-8) is commonly associated with this clinical presentation. MCD is particularly associated with malignancies such as Kaposi sarcoma, T-cell NHL, and HL.

Histopathology Three histopathologic CD types are described: hyaline vascular (HV-CD), plasma cell (PC-CD), and mixed type. LN excisional biopsy provides definitive diagnosis. HHV-8 can be highlighted by immunohistochemistry.

FNA Findings Presumptive diagnosis can be made by cytopathologic examination. The background is that of a nonspecific reactive follicular hyperplasia including small lymphocytes, centrocytes, centroblasts, and tigible body macrophages. Single and clustered dentritic cells with lymphocyte emperipolesis, increased number of plasma cells, and hyalinized capillaries in the appropriate clinical setting brings CD as a diagnostic possibility that should be confirmed by lymph node excision.

US Features Lymph nodes are variably enlarged, hypoechogenic, and well-circumscribed with identifiable hilum. HV-CD may show an increament of both peripheral and hilar vascular blood flow by Doppler exam.

Rosai-Dorfman Disease

Clinical Findings Rosai-Dorfman disease (RDD) is rare and can occur at any age with slight female predominance. Patients may have an underlying autoimmune disorder (collagen vascular disease) or a hematolymphoid malignancy. The lymph node involvement, also known as massive lymphadenopathy with sinus histiocytosis is often self-limited; however, RDD involving extranodal sites (central nervous system, retroperitoneum, sinus, orbit) is seen in 40% of cases and has an aggressive clinical course. Bilateral cervical lymphadenopathy is commonly found in young individuals with nodal RDD. Nodal and cutaneous involment are usually self-limited.

About 1/3 of cases harbor activated protein kinase pathways suggesting a pathogenesis like Langerhans cell histiocytosis.

Histopathology Lymph node sinuses are distended and contain histiocytes with engulfed intact lymphocytes or plasma cells (emperipolesis). A polymorphous population of lymphoid cells and plasma cells are in the background. Fibrosis and aggregates of neutrophis may be present.

FNA Findings Smears show a mixture of small lymphocytes, centrocytes, centroblasts, immunoblasts, and plasma cells. Emperipolesis (histiocytes with round to oval pale nuclei and abundant cytoplasm with vacuoles containing engulfed lymphocytes, red blood cells, and plasma cells) is the hallmark of the disease. Granulomas or necrosis are absent (Fig. 7.19).

The lymphocytes are immunoreactive with B- and T-cell markers with no light chain restriction. The histiocytes are immunopositive for S-100 protein, CD68, CD163, and cyclin D1. Langerin and CD1a are negative.

Langerhans Cell Histiocytosis

Clinical Findings This idiopathic proliferative disorder of abnormal Langerhans cells (antigen presenting cells) affects predominantly children in the first decade of life. Lymph nodes are involved isolated or as part of a multisystemic involvement in 25% of cases. Cervical lymph nodes are the most involved followed by inguinal, axillary, and mediastinal.

Histopathology There is a proliferation of Langerhans cells accompanied by a variable number of eosinophils, lymphocytes (T cells), and macrophages along with osteoclast-type multinucleated giant cells. Langerhanhs cell proliferation involves the lymph node interfollicular zones and sinuses.

FNA Findings Cytology shows a predominance of large, atypical cells along with lymphocytes, histiocytes, plasma cells, osteoclast-type giant cells, and numerous eosinophiles.

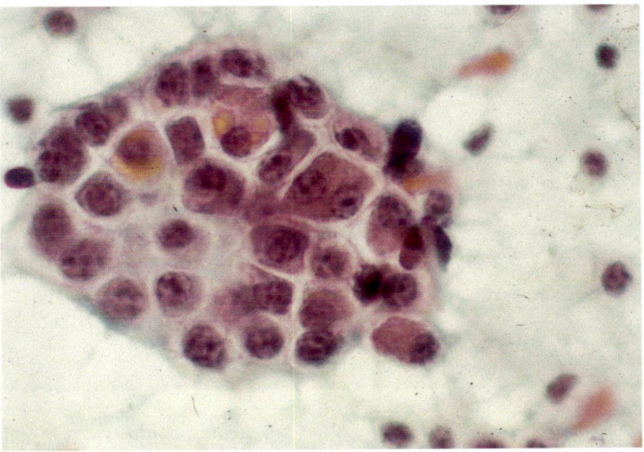

Fig. 7.19 Rosai-Dorfman disease. Emperipolesis of plasma cells is seen in this case (Hematoxylin and eosin stain, high magnification)

Langerhans cells are large (tree to five times the size of a small lymphocyte) and show a pale thin cytoplasm, an eccentrically placed reniform or contoured nuclei with deep grooves and folds, and indistinct nucleoli (Fig. 7.20a).

Immunophenotype Cells are positive for CD1a, S-100 protein, and langerin (CD207) that is a component of the Birbeck granules (hallmark of Langerhans cells by electron microscopy) and is more sensitive than CD1a for detecting Langerhans cells (Fig. 7.20b).

IgG4-Related Disease

Immunoglobulin (Ig) G4-related disease (RD) is a multisystemic chronic immune mediated fibroinflammatory disorder.

Clinical Findings IgG4-RD can affect people of any age and gender, predominantly middle age, and older men. Organ involvement can be synchronous or metachronous and include the pancreas, salivary glands, biliary system, retroperitoneum, lymph nodes, thyroid, lungs, and aorta, among others. Clinical manifestations vary by which organs are involved. Multiple organ involvement is seen in >50% of patients. Lymph node involvement commonly occurs in IgG4-RD; however, IgG4-lymphadenopathy must be associated with other organ involvement to be called as such, since IgG4-positive nodal lymphoplasmacytic infiltrate is not specific and can be associated with autoimmune disorders and primary or metastatic malignancies. Serum IgG4 levels are elevated with a cutoff level of >135 mg/dl to be a reliable marker predictive of IgG4-RD.

Histopathology Storiform fibrosis, obliterative flebitis, and IgG4-positive lymphoplasmacytic infiltrate are characteristic pathological findings of IgG4-RD; however, fibrosis and flebitis are rarely found in lymph nodes, and in contrast to IgG4-RD of other organs IgG4-positive lymphoplasmacytic infiltrate is more abundant in lymph nodes. IgG4-related lymphadenopathy has features that can overlap with Castleman disease, follicular dendritic cell tumors, and plasma cell-rich nodal proliferations. Thus, a comprehensive diagnosis includes (1) clinical and radiological features, (2) serological diagnosis, and (3) pathological diagnosis.

FNA Findings Smear findings are nonspecific and include sparse cellularity, lymphoplasmacytic infiltrate, few eosinophiles, and rare spindle cells, that must be correlated with clinical findings of other organ involvement by known IgG4-RD to suggest a probable lymph node involvement. IgG4-positive immunocytochemistry and high IgG4 serum levels support the presumptive diagnosis that must be proven histologically (Fig. 7.21a–c).

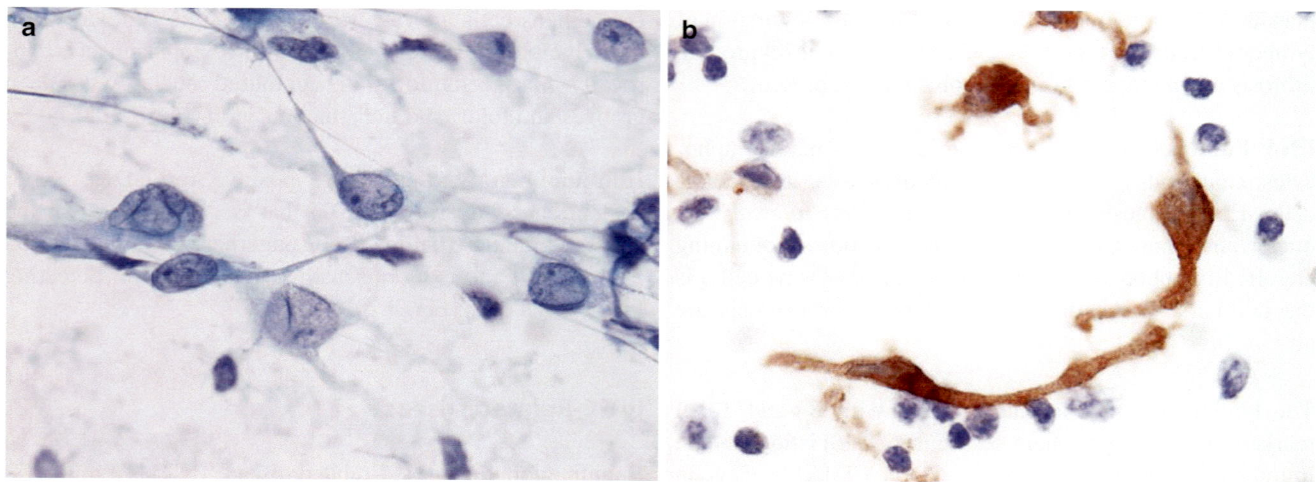

Fig. 7.20 Nodal Langerhans cell histiocytosis. The cells have bland cytologic features, nuclear grooves, slender cytoplasmic processes, and are CD1a-positive **a**, **b**). (**a**, Hematoxylin and eosin stain; **b**, immuno-cytochemistry, high magnification). Courtesy Dr. Javier Saenz de Santamaria, Pathologist, Department of Pathology, Complejo Universitario de Badajoz, Spain

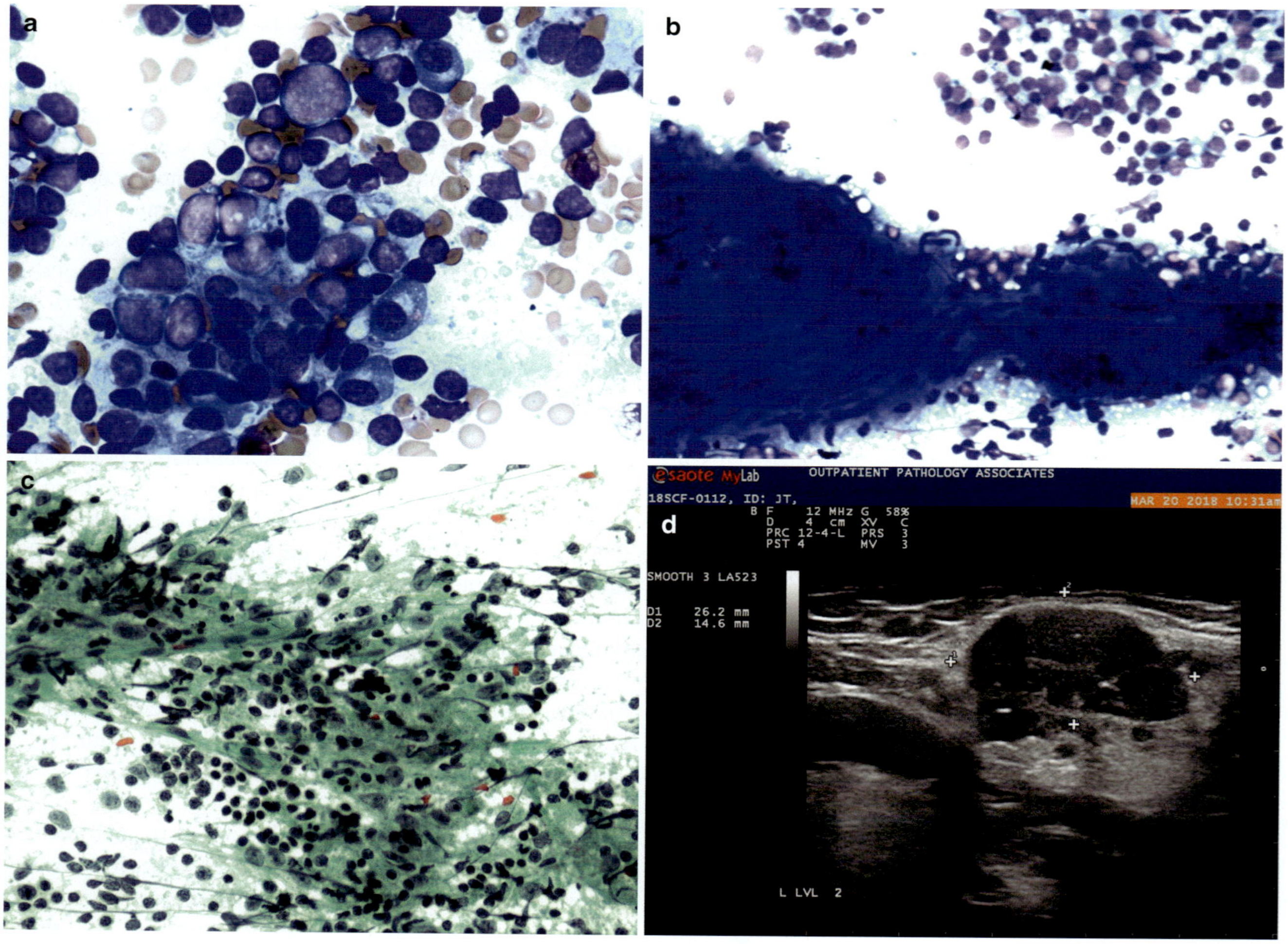

Fig. 7.21 IgG4-related disease. Reactive polymorphous lymphoid cells, numerous plasma cells, and few histiocytes are seen. Fibrous bands may be present (**a–c**). The US shows a hypoechoic, heteroge-neous lymph node with abnormal shape, distinct borders, and bright bands representing fibrosis. (**a**, **b**, MGG stain, high magnification; **c**, Papanicolaou stain, high magnification)

US Findings Single or multiple lymph nodes showing non-specific abnormal features are present. Lymph nodes are enlarged, hypoechoic, and heterogeneous with distinct borders, distorted hilum, and lobulated irregular cortex (Fig. 7.21d).

Dermatopathic Lymphadenopathy

This reactive lymphadenopathy is a T-cell immune response frequently associated with a dematologic lesion, either benign or malignant present in the area of lymphatic drainage. The eliciting agents include melanin or other skin antigens draining into the lymph node, commonly axillary and inguinal.

Histopathology There is paracortical hyperplasia and a proliferation of interdigitating dendritic cells (IDC), Langerhans cells, and histiocytes/macrophages.

FNA Findings Cytologic preparations show IDC, pigment-laden histiocytes with no cytoplasmic tingible bodies, plasma cells, eosinophiles, and lymphocytes. Histiocytes may contain lipid vacuoles or pigment, mostly melanin, in the cytoplasm (Fig. 7.22).

Immunophenotype Both IDC and Langerhans cells are positive for S100 protein and negative for CD68; however, IDC cells may sometimes express CD68. Histiocytes are positive for S100 protein and positive for CD68. In contrast to IDC, Langerhans cells are positive for CD1a.

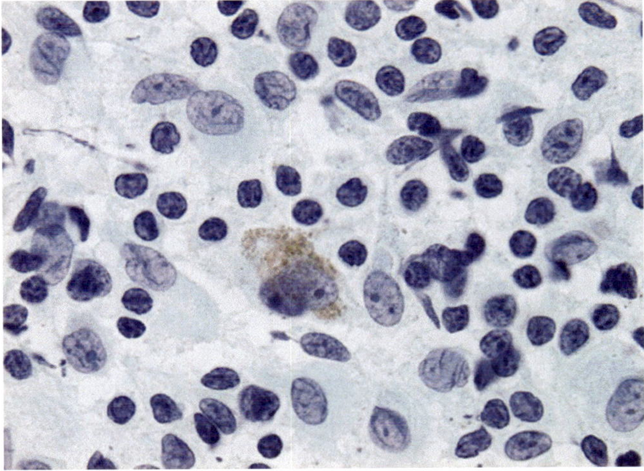

Fig. 7.22 Dermatopathic lymphadenopathy. A melanin-laden histiocyte is surrounded by Langerhans cells, and cerebriform lymphocytes corresponding to Sezary syndrome. (Papanicolaou stain, high magnification). Courtesy Dr. Javier Saenz de Santamaria, Pathologist, Department of Pathology, Complejo Universitario de Badajoz, Spain

Suppurative Bacterial Lymphadenitis

This process is often seen in the head and neck of children draining an area of bacterial infection. Patients have fever, the lymph node is enlarged and tender, and the overlying skin is usually hyperemic.

The smear pattern shows numerous intact and degenerated neutrophils; degenerated lymphoid cells and varying numbers of macrophages and plasma cells. Bacterial organisms may be seen best with Romanowsky-stained smears inside phagocytes and extracellularly (Fig. 7.23a, b). This pattern may be seen in systemic lupus erythematosus and rarely in HL.

Granulomatous Lymphadenitis

Etiologic agents for this smear pattern include infections (tuberculosis, fungi, virus, and protozoa), foreign-body reactions, and sarcoidosis.

In the US, *Mycobacterium tuberculosis* is prevalent in HIV-infected individuals and in foreign-born young immigrants. The most common form of extrapulmonary tuberculosis is lymphadenitis that commonly affects cervical (frequently posterior triangle) chains. The lymph nodes may be matted and markedly necrotic and fluctuant. The *M. tuberculosis* activates CD4+ T cells and produces tissue necrosis, and the macrophages transform into uni- or multinucleated epithelioid macrophages. Thus, the smears of tuberculous lymphadenitis usually show epithelioid granulomas, caseation necrosis, lymphocytes, and occasional Langhans-type giant cells with nuclei arranged peripherally in a horseshoe-shape rimming in the cytoplasm. Sometimes, smear shows acute inflammation, necrosis only, or less commonly granulomas without necrosis. The bacilli can be detected by special acid-fast staining and are detected predominantly in the background smear. The bacilli are bright red, slender, and beaded by the Ziehl-Neelsen acid-fast stain; however, only 20% of culture-positive cases have a positive stain. Culture in Lowenstein-Jensen medium can take up to 6 weeks for a definitive diagnosis, thus delaying treatment. Polymerase chain reaction (PCR) in fluids, smears, and tissue samples, including paraffin-embedded tissue, can detect the organism in less than 6 h.

Atypical mybobacteria are a cause of chronic granulomatous lymphadenitis in children. In adults, the infection occurs in the presence of immunosuppression. The organisms are widely spread in nature and include *M. marinum, M. fortuitum, M. scrofulaceum,* and *M. kansasii.* Commonly affected sites include cervical lymph nodes and may be associated with erythema of the overlying skin and with abscess formation. *Mycobacterium avium intracellulare* (MAI), found in the soil and in tap water, is highly pathogenetic in patients

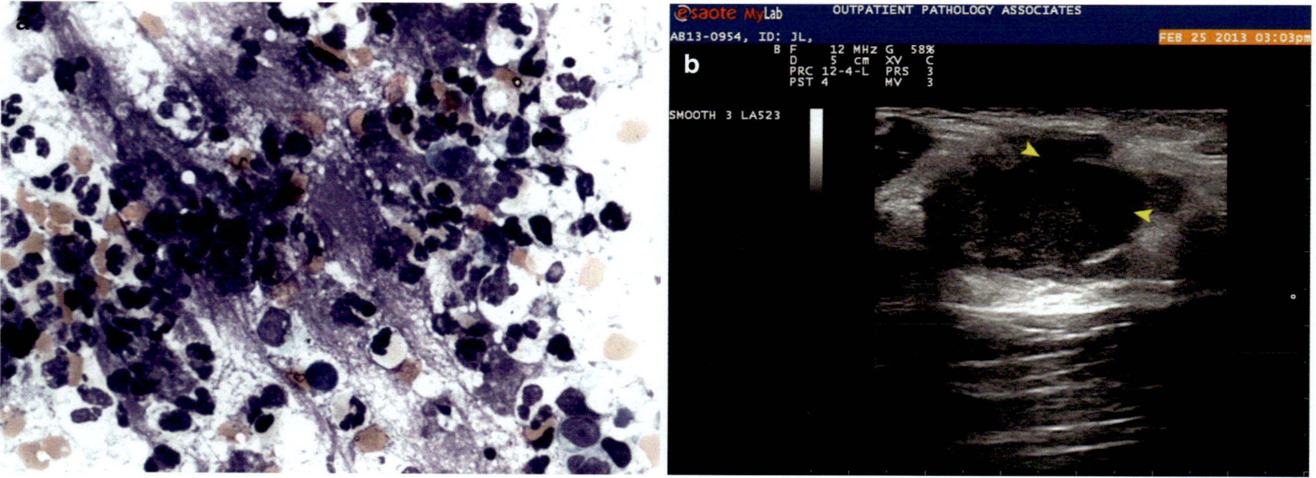

Fig. 7.23 Suppurative bacterial lymphadenitis. Smear shows a purulent smear pattern (**a**). The US exam shows a lymph node with ill-defined margins, heterogeneous echotexture, and a cystic component (**b**, arrow heads). (**a**, MGG stain, high magnification)

with AIDS and may produce regional or generalized lymphadenitis and systemic disease. The smears show necrosis, poorly formed granulomas, and numerous large histiocytes with foamy cytoplasm (pseudo-Gaucher cells) filled with bacilli. Occasionally, the histiocytes develop a spindle-cell phenotype (MAI spindle-cell pseudotumor). The characteristic negative images within the cytoplasm of macrophages and in the background are best seen in Romanowsky-stained smears. The definite diagnosis is made by cultures and PCR in cytological samples and formalin-fixed, paraffin-embedded tissue (Fig. 7.24a–f).

The differential diagnosis of granulomatous lymphadenitis includes tuberculosis, fungal infections, Kikuchi, and cat-scratch lymphadenitis, filaria, and sarcoidosis. Tightly packed histiocytes forming non-necrotizing granulomas and damaged lymphoid cells are seen in sarcoidosis; however, small foci of necrosis may be present; cultures are negative. Occasionally, Langhans type multinucleated giant cells showing the characteristic Schaumann (basophilic concentrically laminated) and asteroid bodies (red spider-like inclusions) are seen (Fig. 7.25a–d).

Fungal infections may involve the lymph nodes, particularly when immunocompetency is affected. The prevalence of these infections is influenced by the incidence of certain mycoses, i.e., histoplasmosis and coccidioidomycosis, in certain geographic areas. The identification of the organism in cytologic material by histochemical stains with periodic acid-Schiff (PAS), silver, and mucicarmine permits the application of early antifungal therapy before culture and serologic results are available (Fig. 7.26a–d). Protozoal lymphadenitis, i.e., toxoplasma and leishmania, are considerations when the smears show histiocytic aggregates and reactive lymphoid hyperplasia in the appropriate clinical setting (Fig. 7.26e, f). Occasionally, a malignant process (i.e., HL, metastases from keratinizing squamous carcinoma and seminoma) elicit a granulomatous reaction.

Cat-scratch Disease

Cat scratch disease is a common cause of chronic lymphadenitis in children and adolescents. In the US, 55% of cases occur in patients aged 18 years or younger, commonly in the months of September to January. The pathogenic organism is *Bartonella henselae*; a Gram-negative bacillus transmitted by fleas to kittens and then transmitted to humans by a cat bite or lick.

Clnical Findings The patients have enlarged, nodular, and matted regional lymphadenopathy that is fixed to surrounding tissues and commonly occurs in the upper extremities and face. The lymphadenopathy develops 1–3 weeks after the primary skin lesion and is usually accompanied by systemic symptoms. In immunocompetent individuals, the disease is self-limited and resolves in 6–12 weeks in the absence of treatment. Suppuration occurs in 10% of cases. A systemic life-threatening disease may occur in immunosuppressed patients.

FNA Findings The smears show a reactive lymphoid hyperplasia pattern with monocytoid cells and scattered tingible-body macrophages in the early stages of the disease. A suppurative granulomatous pattern with necrosis, neutrophils, epithelioid histiocytes, granulomas, and rare multinucleated Langhans-type giant cells is seen in more established processes. Numerous acute inflammatory cells may mask small granulomas (Fig. 7.27a–d).

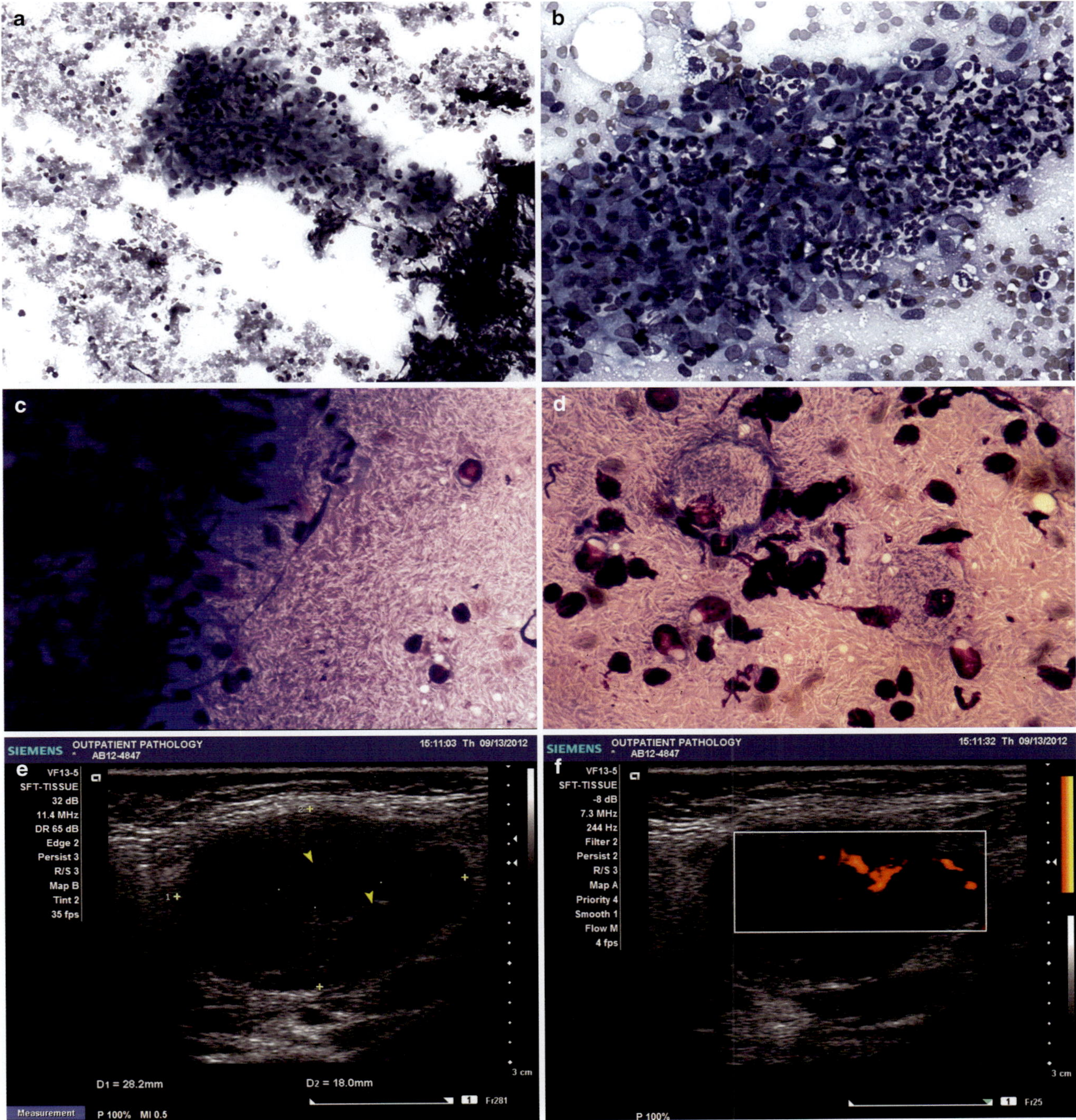

Fig. 7.24 Tuberculous lymphadenitis. Smears show necrosis, damaged inflammatory cells, histiocytes, multinucleated giant cells, and granulomas (**a**, **b** *Mycobacterium tuberculosis*). Atypical mycobacteria with numerous thick and long organisms that appear as "negative images" both in the background of the smear (**c**) and within histiocytes ("pseudo-Gaucher" cells) (**d**) (**c**, **d** *Mycobacterium avium intracellu-* *lare*). The US exam shows a large lymph node with hypoechogenicity, smooth distinct margins, foci of cystic degeneration (**e**, arrow heads), and mild central and peripheral vascular blood flow (**f**). (**a**, **b** MGG stain medium and high magnification, **c**, **d** DiffQuik® stain, medium and high magnification)

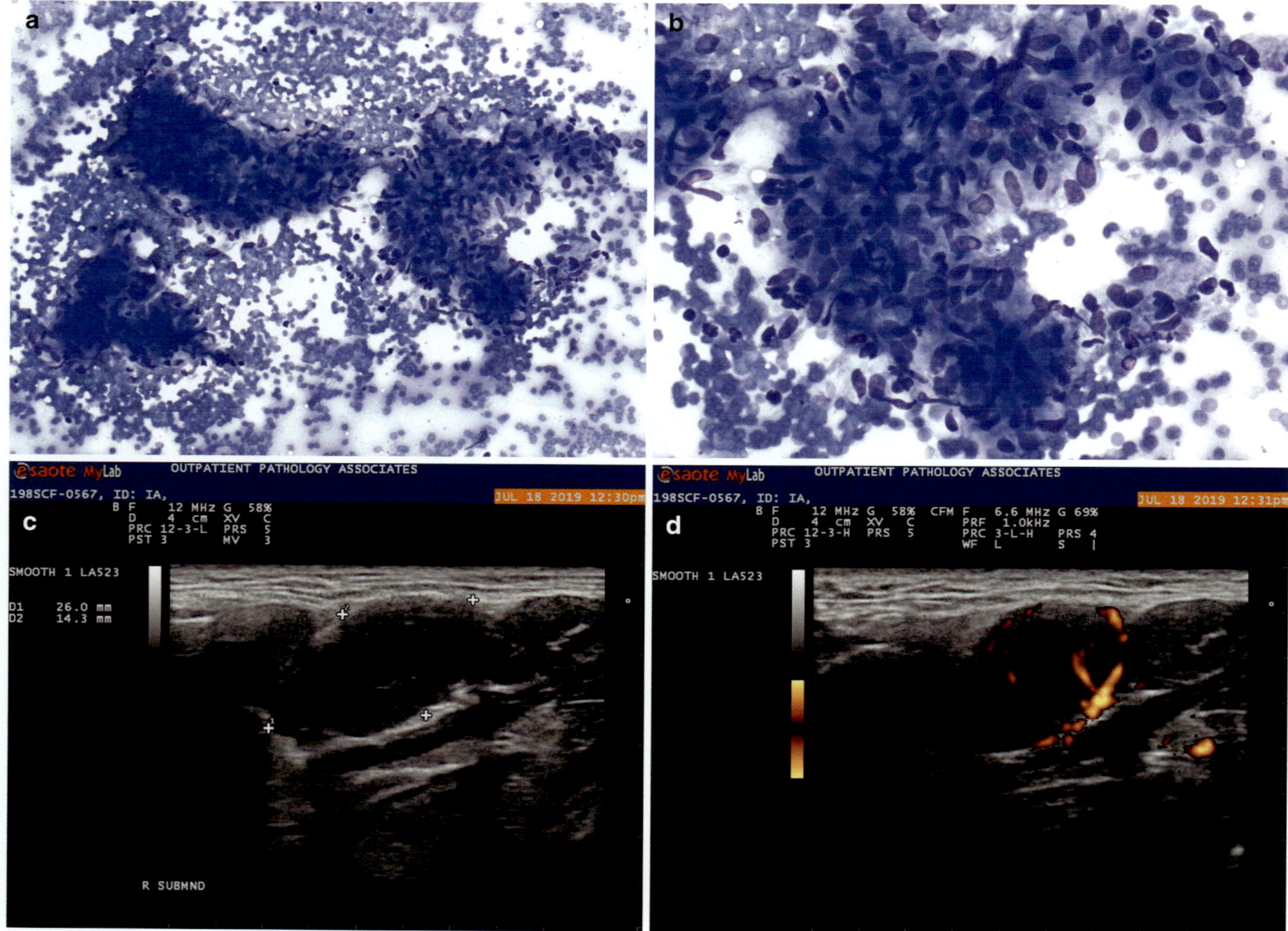

Fig. 7.25 Sarcoidosis. Tightly packed granulomas, few small lympho-cytes, blood, and absence of necrosis are seen (**a**, **b**). The US shows hypoechoic and coalescent submandibular lymph nodes with well-defined borders, heterogeneous echotexture, and hilar and focal subcapsular vascular blood flow (**c**, **d**). (MGG stain, medium and high magnification)

Microbiologic detection is difficult, and the diagnosis is supported by clinical history, serology, and histopathology. The organisms can be visualized by the Warthin-Starry silver stain, immunoperoxidase stain with anti-*B. henselae* antibod-ies in tissue sections, PCR, indirect immunofluorescence, and enzyme immunoassay. The diagnostic sensitivity of all tests is low. The silver stain is the most sensitive but is the least spe-cific. Lymphogranuloma venereum is cytologically identical, and immunofluorescence and serology are necessary for the diagnosis. The differential cytologic diagnosis also includes bacterial suppurative lymphadenitis, tularemia, and other granulomatous processes, including tuberculosis; special stains and cultures are needed to rule out these processes.

Infectious Mononucleosis

Infectious mononucleosis is an acute self-limited disease caused by the Epstein-Barr virus (EBV). The viral spread is via direct contact with oral secretions. The EBV infects both epithelial cells and B cells in the oropharynx; B cells can be infected via the CD3d complement receptor (CD21) causing an antibody response with cell proliferation during the first week of the disease.

Clinical Findings IM affects predominantly adolescents and young adults, who have fever, pharyngitis, and cervical or generalized lymphadenopathy. The lymph nodes are enlarged and soft, but not matted. Lymphocytosis with atypi-cal lymphocytes is commonly seen in the peripheral blood. The disease resolves in 3–4 weeks in most patients. A life-threatening disease is seen in immunosuppressed individuals.

FNA Findings The cytology preparations show numerous large reactive immunoblasts, variable numbers of small lym-phocytes, centroblasts, histiocytes, tingible-body macro-phages, and lymphoplasmacytes. Numerous mitoses and apoptotic nuclei are also present. The immunoblasts are large and show a basophilic cytoplasm, a large nucleus, and a sin-

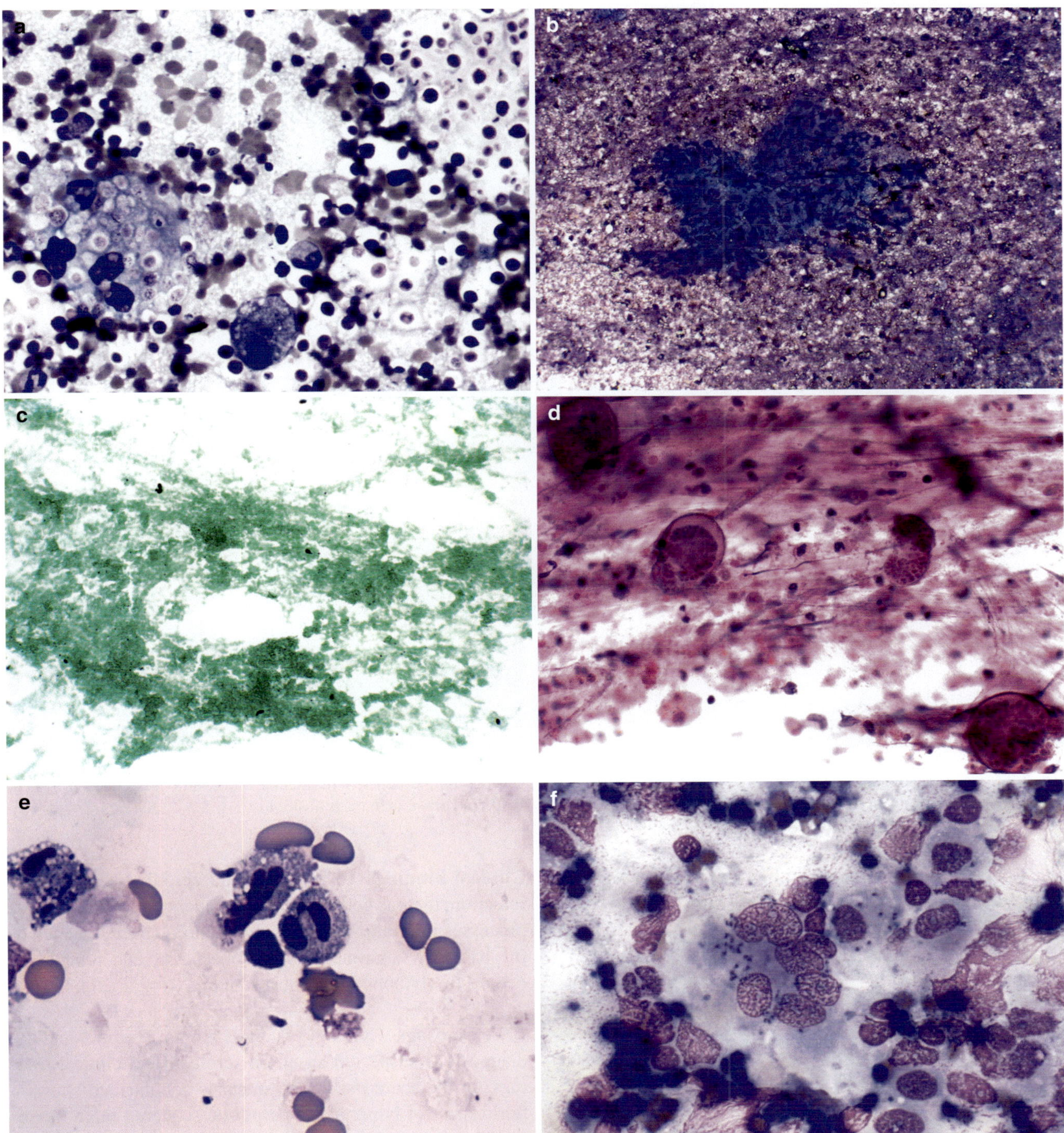

Fig. 7.26 Fungal and protozoal lymphadenitis. Cryptococcus with the characteristic clear "halo" around the yeast form are seen isolated in a "mucoid" background and inside a macrophage (**a**). A single granuloma is present in a granular background with crystals, which are hints for histoplasma lymphadenitis (**b**); the silver stain identifies the diagnostic narrow-budding yeasts (**c**). Numerous spherules packed with endo-spores are seen in coccidioidomycosis (**d**). Trophozoites are seen in toxoplasma lymphadenitis (**e**). Leishman-Donovan bodies within histiocytes are seen in leishmaniasis (**f**). (**a, b, e, f** DiffQuik® stain, medium and high magnification; **d**, Hematoxylin and eosin stain, high magnification) (**e, f** From Pambuccian and Bardales (2011). Reprinted with permission)

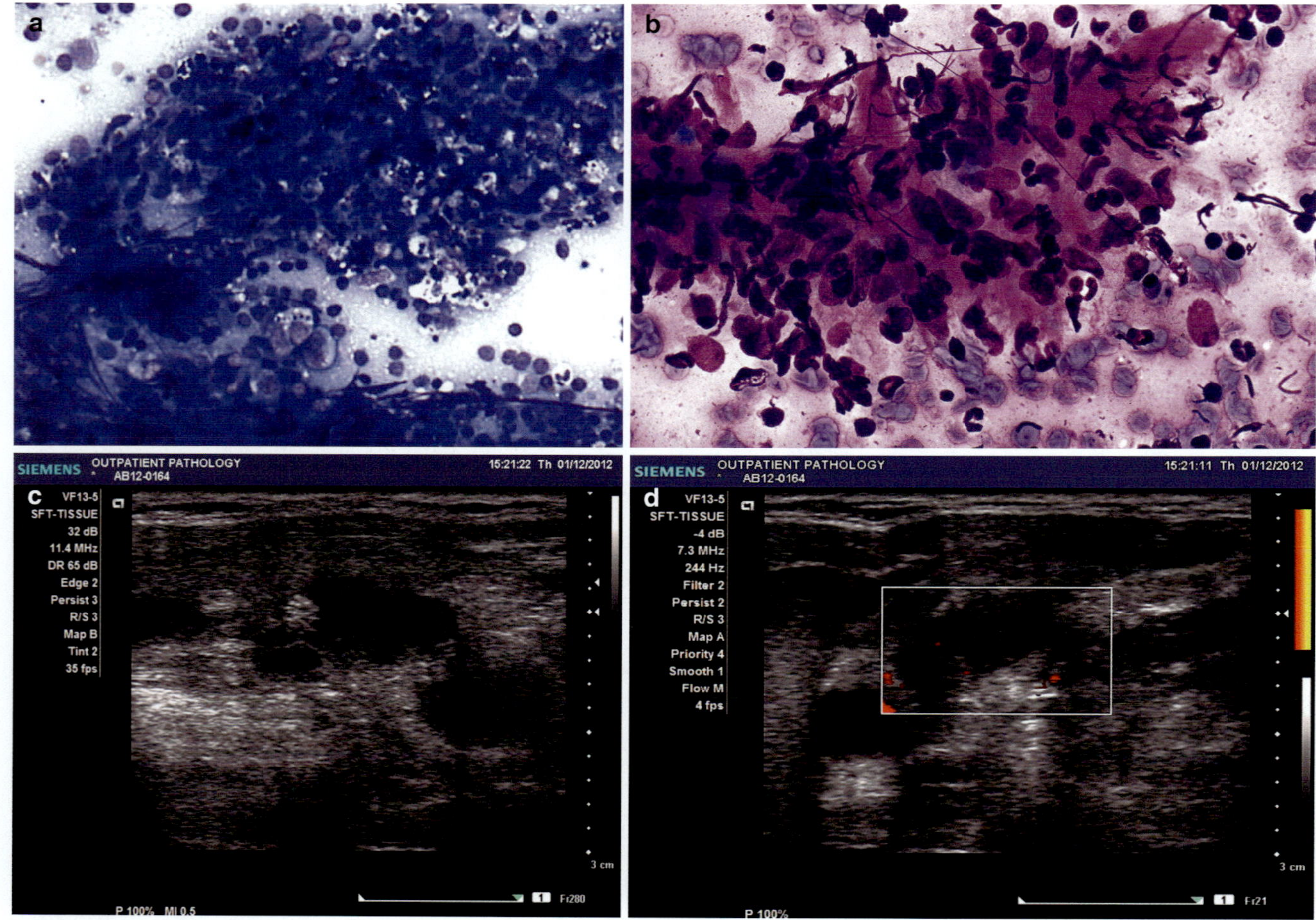

Fig. 7.27 Cat scratch disease. Smears show a purulent pattern with necrosis, acute inflammation, damaged lymphocytes, and granulomas (**a, b**). The US exam shows irregularly shaped, coalescent, and hetero-geneous lymph nodes. No vascular blood flow is seen (**c, d**). (**a, b**, DiffQuik® stain, high magnification)

gle central round or polyhedral nucleolus. Large Reed-Sternberg-like and Hodgkin-like cells may be observed. Necrosis may be present (Fig. 7.28a, b).

Polyclonality and no light-chain restriction are identified by FCM. EBV antigens and EBER positivity can be demonstrated by immunohistochemistry, in situ hybridization, and other molecular analysis. The differential diagnosis includes large-cell lymphoma, ALCL, NLPHL, and classical HL.

Human Immunodeficiency Virus

The human immunodeficiency virus 1 (HIV-1) is a lentivirus, a subfamily of retroviruses that infects CD4+ lymphocytes, macrophages, and dendritic cells; the first disseminates the virus, and the last two are the reservoirs. In the late stage, the CD4 lymphocytes and the dendritic cells are destroyed, the viremia resurges, and opportunistic infections and tumors develop in the immunosuppressed host. The main role of FNA in HIV patients is to rule out opportunistic infections and neoplasms such as lymphoma or Kaposi sarcoma.

Clinical Findings In the acute and chronic phase of HIV infection, there is generalized lymphadenopathy that harbors processes that may be reactive, infectious (bacterial including bacillary angiomatosis, mycobacterial, and fungal), or neoplastic (lymphoma, Kaposi sarcoma) (Fig. 7.29a, b).

FNA Findings Cytologic findings are not specific, and the diagnosis is suspected based on serology and clinical findings. In the acute phase, the smear is cellular and shows a florid reactive lymphoid hyperplasia, scattered large monocytoid cells with clear cytoplasm and round nuclei, neutrophils, multinucleated cells (polykaryocytes of Warthin-Finkeldey), and tingible-body macrophages. The smears are less cellular, and the presence plasma cells is notorious in the subacute phase of HIV lymphadenitis. Hypocellular smears with a paucity of lymphocytes and predominance of plasma cells are characteristic of the chronic burned-out phase of HIV infection.

Immunostains for p7, p9, p17, and p24 HIV protein recognizes the presence of the virus.

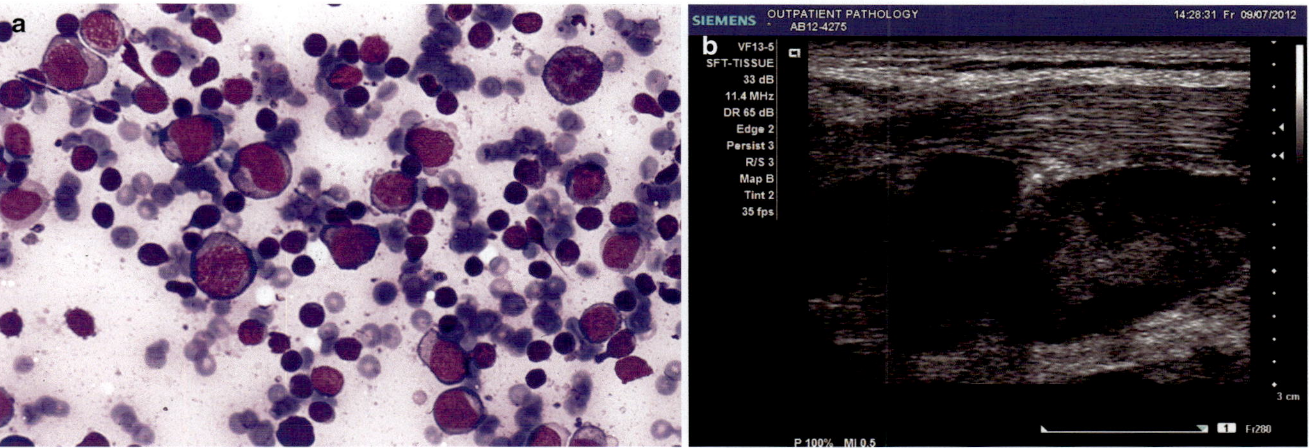

Fig. 7.28 Infectious mononucleosis. Smears show numerous reactive immunoblasts with bluish cytoplasm, large nuclei, prominent nucleoli, and scattered mitoses (**a**). The US exam shows large odd-shaped hypoechoic confluent lymph nodes that mimic a malignant process (**b**). (**a**, DiffQuik® stain, high magnification)

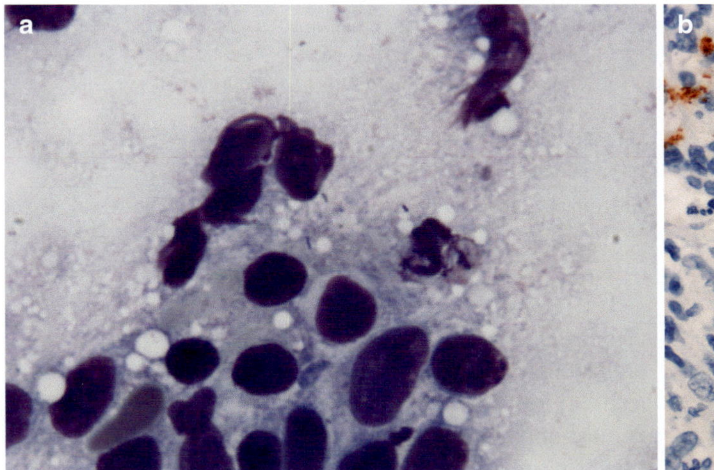

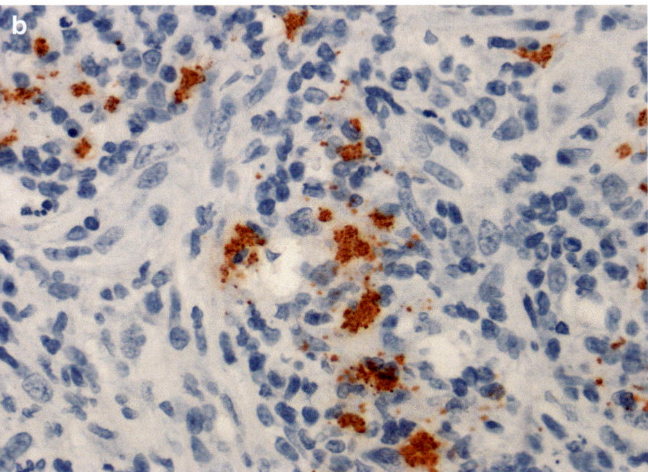

Fig. 7.29 Bacillary angiomatosis. Small aggregates of round, oval, and spindle cells and rare bacilli are seen in the smear (**a**). Immunohistochemistry confirms the presence of *Bartonella henselae* (**b**). (**a**, MGG stain high magnification). (Courtesy of Roberto Miranda, MD, Professor, Department of Pathology. MD Anderson Cancer Center)

Ultrasound Features of Reactive and Infectious Lymph Nodes

Reactive lymph nodes usually have the following characteristics: hypoechoic, slighty ill-defined margins, hilum present, hilar vascular pattern except lymph nodes <5 mm, lack of peripheral blood flow by Doppler examination, and flat or oval shape except lymph nodes involving neck level I, which may be round. Lymph nodes involved by granulomatous infectious processes including cat scratch disease and tuberculosis may have pronounced cystic necrosis and lymph node confluence in addition to the mentioned findings (Figs. 7.18b, 7.21d, 7.23b, 7.24e, f, 7.25c, d, 7.27c, d, 7.28b).

Select Examples Of Hematolymphoid Tumors

In the next section, I will discuss some lymphoid tumors following the 2022 WHO Classification of Hematolymphoid Tumors 5th edition: B- and T-cell proliferations and lymphomas, and stroma derived neoplasms of lymphoid tissues (Table 7.4).

Non-Hodgkin Lymphoma

The use of FNA cytology for diagnosing non-Hodgkin lymphoma (NHL) is well established. In fact, most ymphomas

Table 7.4 List of B-cell and T-cell lymphoid proliferations and lymphomas potentially encountered in FNA of palpable and/or US-visible superficial masses and lymph nodes[a]

Tumor-like lesions with B-cell predominance
Reactive B-cell-rich lymphoid proliferations that can mimic lymphoma
IgG4-related disease
Castleman disease
Tumor-like lesions with T-cell predominance
Kikuchi-Fujimoto disease
Precursor B- and T-cell neoplasms
B-cell lymphoblastic leukemia/lymphoma
T-lymphoblastic leukemia/lymphoma
Mature B-cell neoplasms
Pre-neoplastic and neoplastic small cell lymphocytic proliferations
Chronic lymphocytic leukemia/small lymphocytic lymphoma
Lymphoplasmacytic lymphoma
Lymphoplasmacytic lymphoma
Marginal zone lymphoma
Primary cutaneous marginal zone lymphoma
Nodal marginal zone lymphoma
Pediatric marginal zone lymphoma
Follicular lymphoma
Follicular lymphoma
Pediatric-type follicular lymphoma
Primary cutaneous follicle center lymphoma
Mantle cell lymphoma
Transformations of indolent B-cell lymphomas
Large B-cell lymphomas
Diffuse large B-cell lymphoma NOS (with *MYC* and *BCL6* but no *BCL2*)
T-cell/histiocyte-rich large B-cell lymphoma
Diffuse large B-cell lymphoma/high grade B-cell lymphoma with *MYC* and *BCL2* rearrangements
ALK-positive large B-cell lymphoma
Large B-cell lymphoma with *IRF4* rearrangement
High-grade B-cell llymphoma with 11q aberrations
EBV-positive diffuse large B-cell lymphoma
Diffuse large B-cell lymphoma associated with chronic inflammation
Plasmablastic lymphoma
Primary cutaneous diffuse large B-cell lymphoma leg type
High-grade B-cell lymphoma NOS
Burkitt lymphoma
KSHV/HHV8-positive large B-cell lymphoma
Lymphoid proliferations and lymphomas associated with immune deficiency and dysregulation
Polymorphous posttransplant lymphoproliferative disorders
Iatrogenic immunodeficiency-associated lymphoproliferative disorders, etc.
Lymphomas arising in immune deficiency/dysregulation
Monomorphic posttransplant lymphoproliferative disorders
Classic Hodgkin lymphoma posttransplant
Lymphomas associated with HIV infection, etc.
Mature T-cell and NK-cell neoplasms
Adult T-cell leukemia/lymphoma
Sezary syndrome

(continued)

Table 7.4 (continued)

Primary cutaneous T-cell lymphomas
Mycosis fungoides (10% has lymph node involvement)
Anaplastic large cell lymphoma
ALK-positive anaplastic large cell lymphoma
ALK-negative anaplastic large cell lymphoma
Breast implant-associated anaplastic large lymphoma
Nodal T-follicular helper (TFH) cell lymphoma
Nodal TFH cell lymphoma, angioimmunoblastic type
Nodal TFH cell lymphoma, follicular type
Nodal TFH cell lymphoma, NOS
Peripheral T-cell lymphomas, NOS
EBV-positive nodal T- and NK-cell lymphoma
Systemic EBV-positive T-cell lymphoma of childhood
Hodgkin lymphoma
Classic Hodgkin lymphoma
Nodular lymphocyte predominant Hodgkin lymphoma
Plasma cell neoplasms
Immunoglobulin-related (AL) amyloidosis
Plasma cell myeloma/plasmacytoma
Stroma-derived neoplasms of lymphoid tissues
Mesenchymal dendritic cell neoplasms
Follicular dendritic cell sarcoma
EBV-positive inflammatory follicular dendritic cell sarcoma
Fibroblastic reticular cell tumor
Myofibroblastic tumor
Intranodal palisaded myofibroblastoma

[a] Modified from Alaggio, R et al. The 5th edition of the World Health Organization Classification of Hematolymphoid Tumors: Lymphoid neoplasms. Leukemia 2022; 36:1720-1748

can be diagnosed and treated on the basis of cytomorphology and ancillary tests done on FNA material. Judicious use of ancillary tests including flow cytometry and molecular tests is most important in the detection of cell-surface markers to establish light-chain monoclonality and characterize the correct subtype of clonal proliferation. Normal mature B cells express CD19, CD20, CD22, and PAX5 and are good markers in B-cell lymphomas. Plasma cells lack such markers; instead, they express CD38 and CD138. CD10 is expressed by both early-B and T-cell progenitor cells and FL. The T-cell markers CD5 and CD43 may normally be expressed in a small percentage of B cells; CD5 is aberrantly coexpressed in some small-cell types of B-cell lymphomas. T-cell clonality is difficult to establish by flow cytometry.

The various types of NHL are defined by their morphology, immunophenotype, cytogenetics, and clinical features (Table 7.5).

In the following paragraphs, I will briefly review the characteristics of the common NHLs found in clinical practice.

Large B-cell Lymphoma

This is one of the most common neoplasms diagnosed by FNA, affects mainly adults in the 7th decade of life, and is aggressive. Young adults and children may be affected occa-

Table 7.5 CD5 and CD10 expression in most common nodal NHLs

CD5-positive, CD10-negative
Chronic lymphocytic leukemia/small lymphocytic lymphoma (CLL/SLL)
Mantle-cell lymphoma (MCL)[a]
Diffuse large B-cell lymphoma (DLBCL),[a] Richter transformation of CLL
CD5-negative, CD10-positive
Follicular lymphoma (FL)[a]
DLBCL
Burkitt lymphoma (BL)[b]
CD5-negative, CD10- negative
Marginal zone lymphoma (MZL)[c]
Lymphoplasmacytic lymphoma (LPL)

[a] FL, DLBCL, and MCL can be CD5$^+$/CD10$^+$ or CD5$^-$/CD10$^-$
[b] BL can be CD5$^+$/CD10$^+$
[c] MZL can be CD5$^+$

sionally. The primary presentation is usually nodal, but extranodal spread or presentation may be seen. One third of patients have systemic symptoms. B-cell is the most common phenotype, is usually diffuse (DLBCL), and does not meet the criteria for other WHO large B-cell lymphomas on tissue examination. Two molecular subtypes are described: activated B cell (ABC) and germinal center B cell (GCB).

The cytology shows monomorphous medium to large atypical lymphoid cells; however, the cytomorphology is variable, i.e., centroblasts, centroblasts and immunoblasts, and less frequently true immunoblasts may be seen. Variable anaplasia including large cells with abundant clear cytoplasm and irregular multilobed nuclei can also be seen in the anaplastic variant. This rare anaplastic B-cell lymphoma shows less pleomorphism than does the T-cell counterpart. The T-cell-rich B cell lymphoma shows rare large pleomorphic tumor cells and a background of numerous small lymphocytes and mimics HL, carcinoma, or melanoma (Fig. 7.30a–f).

DLBCL has a high proliferation index. Cells show light-chain monoclonality and positive B-cell markers CD19, CD20, CD79a, and PAX5. Neoplastic cells (centroblasts) of the GCB subtype are positive for CD10 and bcl-6, and negative for MUM-1. Cells are positive for CD30 in the anaplastic variant. The ALKoma variant expresses CD30, CD138, EMA, MUM-1/IRF, and ALK.

DLBCL with *MYC* and *BCL6* rearrangements (renamed as DLBCL-NOS) is biologically distinct from DLBCL with *MYC* and *BCL2* rearrangements, with or without *BCL6* (currently renamed as DLBCL with *MYC* and *BCL2* rearrangements); the latter being an aggressive lymphoma of GBC origin. Therefore, the diagnosis of large B-cell lymphoma requires immunophenotypic and cytogenetic studies.

Follicular Lymphoma

FL is a mature B-cell malignant neoplasm of the lymph node germinal center and is composed of centrocytes and centroblasts. It affects patients in the 6th to 7th decade of life, with slight female predominance who usually have an indolent generalized lymphadenopathy with a chronic and relapsing course. The clinical course depends on the stage and grade, and cure is rare. Large-cell malignant transformation occurs in 30% of patients and carries a poor prognosis.

Histopathology A follicular (nodular) pattern is present in variable proportions and most FLs show at least focal follicular architecture, and rarely are diffuse. If solely a diffuse pattern is present, the lymphoma is classified as DLBCL and needs further cytogenetic studies as described previously in the large B-cell lymphoma section. The lymphoma composition of centrocytes (small, cleaved cells) and centroblasts (larger cells) have more prognostic inplications for lymphoma grading (1, 2, 3A, 3B) than the histologic pattern (follicular vs diffuse). FL grading is as follows: grade 1, centrocytes and <6 centroblasts/high power field (HPF); grade 2, centrocytes and 6–15 centroblasts/HPF; grade 3A, few centrocytes and >15 centroblasts/HPF; grade 3B, >15 centroblasts/HPF and no centrocytes. Therefore, FLs need tissue confirmation for precise classification.

FNA Findings The cytology of the small-cell type shows a monotonous population of small lymphocytes (centrocytes) with irregular nuclear contours, i.e., indentations, notches, and clefts, which are best seen in Papanicolaou-stained smears; nucleoli are rarely identified. The mixed-cell type shows a variable mixture of centrocytes and medium-size atypical lymphocytes with a round nucleus and 1–3 peripheral nucleoli (centroblasts); macrophages are rare or absent; this pattern must be differentiated from that of reactive follicular hyperplasia. Small T lymphocytes are also present in the background. Cell aggregates may suggest a follicular pattern when smears are evaluated at low magnification (Fig. 7.31a–f).

Cells show light-chain monoclonality and CD19, CD20, CD79a, PAX-5, bcl-6, HGAL, LMO2, MEF2B, and CD10 positivity. CD5, cyclin D1, and CD43 are negative. Cells express bcl-2 in most cases. Almost all cases show a t(14;18) translocation.

Small Lymphocytic Lymphoma

This mainly B-cell neoplasm is the nodal counterpart of chronic lymphocytic leukemia.

Clinical Findings It affects middle-aged and older populations with male prepoderance, involves multiple lymph nodes, and is a low-grade malignancy. The clinical course is indolent; however, in rare instances it may undergo a high-grade large B-cell transformation (Richter syndrome or transformation). Hodgkin tranformation is a rare form of Richter transformation and requires the histology of classical HL.

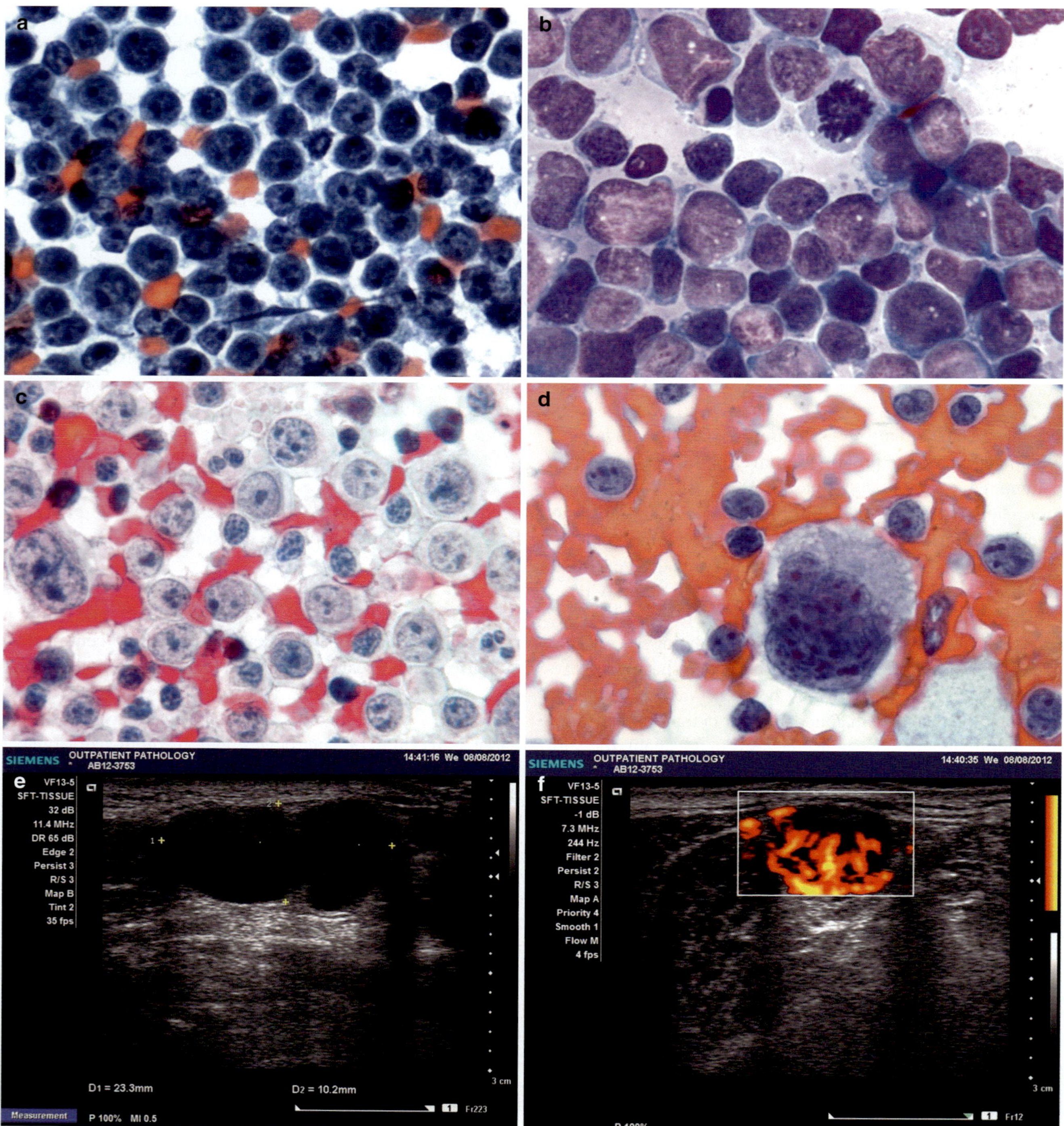

Fig. 7.30 Diffuse large B-cell lymphoma. Large monomorphous cells with dark blue cytoplasm, some plasmacytoid features, irregular nuclear contours, mitoses, and apoptotic bodies (**a**). Large cell with round nuclei, basophilic cytoplasm, and prominent nucleoli are characteristic of immunoblastic lymphoma (**b**). Large cells with centroblastic (**c**) and anaplastic (**d**) cytomorphology are seen in these two examples of DLBCL. The US exam shows dysmorphic coalescent lymph nodes with well-defined, margins, marked hypoechogenicity, and intense blood flow (**c**, **d**). (From Pambuccian and Bardales (2011). Reprinted with permission)

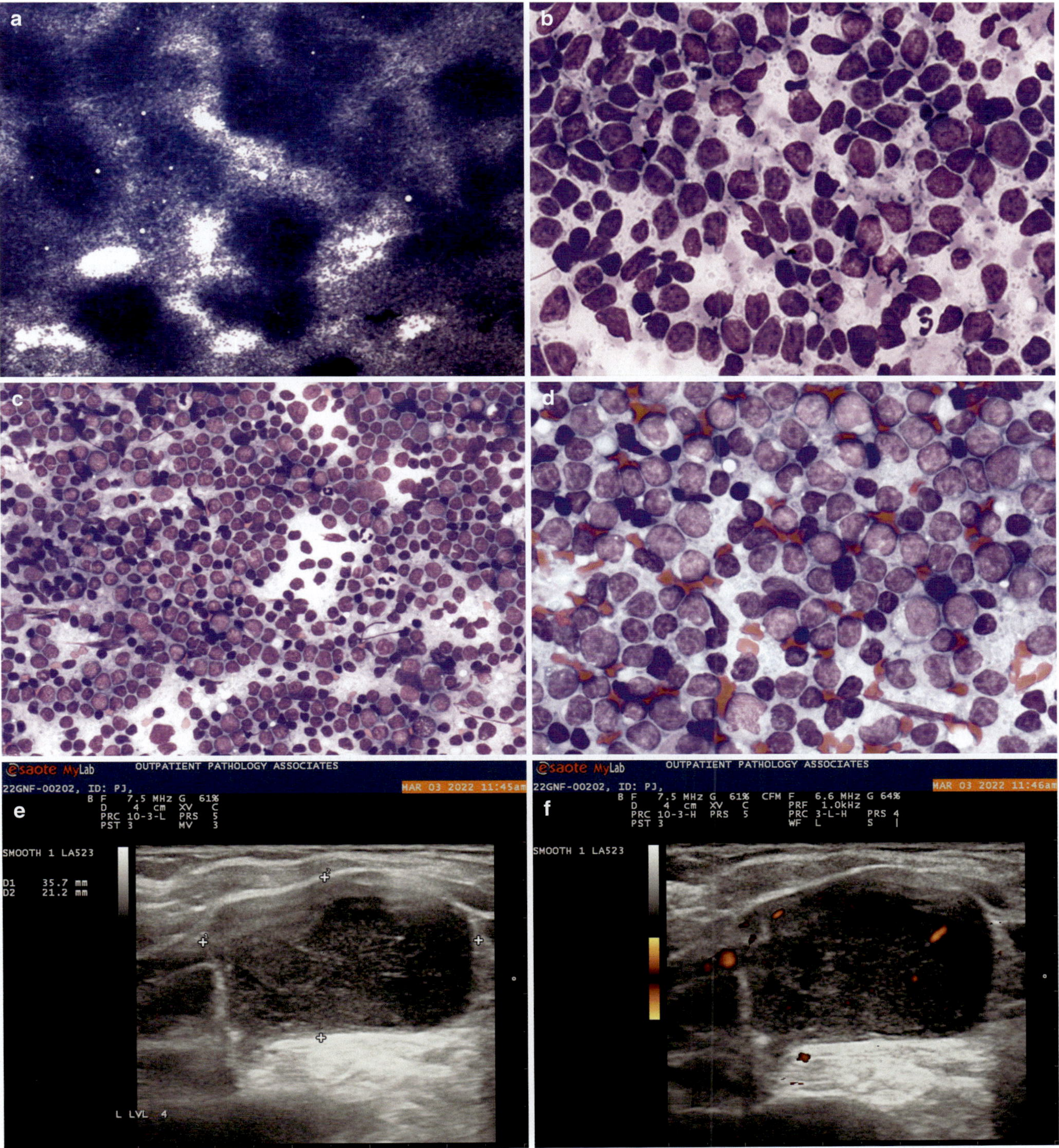

Fig. 7.31 Follicular lymphoma. Smear shows a follicular pattern at screening magnification (**a**). Cells are monomorphous of small to intermediate size and have irregular nuclear contours (**b**). A more conspicuous number of centroblasts is present in grades 2 and 3, as seen in these two examples (**c, d**). The US exam, in this case shows coalescent lymph nodes with absence of hilum, well-defined margins, hypoechogenicity, heterogeneous echotexture, and minimal peripheral vascular blood flow (**e, f**). (**a–d** MGG stain, low, medium, and high magnification)

FNA Findings The cytology shows a monotonous pattern of small lymphocytes with a scant cytoplasm, round nucleus, coarse chromatin, and inconspicuous nucleoli. Scattered paraimmunoblasts (large cells with large nucleus, dispersed chromatin, and enlarged nucleolus) and prolymphocytes (medium sized cells with round nucleus, coarse cromatin, and conspicuous central nucleolus) can be found. Distinction from other lymphomas of the small-cell type is based on flow cytometry and not on pure cytomorphology (Fig. 7.32a–f) (Table 7.6). Lymph node excision is not necessary unless to confirm the diagnosis of Richter transformation.

A dim light-chain immunoglobulin clonal restriction by FCM is characteristic. Cells show CD19, CD20, CD23, CD43, CD79a, bcl-2, and PAX-5 positivity. CD5 positivity is characteristic, and cells are negative for CD10 (positive in FL) and FMC7 (positive in MCL). CD38 and ZAP-70 are expressed in some cases and have been associated with adverse prognosis. Deletion (13q14) is present in 50% of the patients and is associated with a favorable prognosis. Trisomy 12, (13q14) deletion, and t(11;14) and t(14;19) translocations have been described.

Mantle Cell Lymphoma

MCL is a clinically aggressive mature B-cell NHL.

Clinical Findings It occurs in middle-aged to older individuals, with male predominance. Most patients can not be cured and have generalized lymphadenopathy, hepatosplenomegaly, and GI and bone marrow and peripheral-blood involvement. Progression to blastoid or pleomorphic variants in seen in approximately 20% of cases.

FNA Findings Cytologic preparations show monotonous lymphoid cells of small to intermediate size with irregular nuclear contours resembling centrocytes with dispersed chromatin and inconspicuous nucleoli; the larger cells may have single small, distinct nucleoli. Rare plasmacytoid lymphocytes may be seen. Scattered epithelioid histiocytes and plasma cells are commonly present. Cytologically, the blastoid variant resembles lymphoblastic lymphoma and the pleomorphic variant resembles DLBCL (Fig. 7.33a–f).

Cell show CD5+, FMC7+, PAX5+, CD43+, BCL2+, BCL6−, LEF-1−, and CD10− (Table 7.6). All cases express bcl-2, SOX-11, and cyclin D1. Neoplastic cells show t(11;14) (q13;q32) with *IGH/CCND1* translocation in almost all cases.

Nodal Marginal-Zone Lymphoma

Nodal MZL is a postgerminal center B-cell lymphoma that overlaps morphologically and immunophenotypically with extranodal MZL (mucosa-associated lymphoid tissue or MALT lymphoma and splenic MZL).

Clinical Findings The nodal type comprises <2% of all NHL, is a primary lymph node B-cell neoplasm without splenic or extranodal involvement and affects mostly adults and older individuals with no gender predominance. It is clinically indolent, and most patients have asymptomatic regional, often cervical or generalized lymphadenopathy and survive longer than 5 years. Some patients may have serologic evidence of hepatitis C infection or autoimmune disorders.

Histopathology The neoplastic proliferation is commonly nodular and rarely diffuse involving interfollicular and perifollicular areas with variably preserved germinal centers.

FNA Findings The cytology shows monocytoid cells, or medium-sized cells with irregular nuclear contours (centrocyte-like cells), or cells resembling small/intermediate-size round lymphocytes, or a combination of the three in various proportions. Plasma-cell differentiation may be prominent in some cases, and scattered eosinophils may be present (Fig. 7.34a–d).

As seen in Table 7.6, CD5, CD10, BCL6, SOX11, LEF-1, HGAL, LMO-2, and cyclin D1 are negative. CD19, CD20, BCL-2, PAX-5, BCL2, IRTA-1, MNDA, and CD43 are positive. CD23 may be faintly positive. Ki67 is low. Trisomy 3 (60%) or t(11;18) may be seen.

Lymphoplasmacytic Lymphoma

LPL is a mature B-cell neoplasm that originates in the post-germinal center memory B cell and composed of small lymphocytes, plasmacytoid lymphocytes, and plasma cells.

Clinical Findings It occurs in older individuals with slight male predominance, and usually involves bone marrow and sometimes the spleen. The incidence is higher is patients with hepatitis C and autoimmune disorders. The clinical course is indolent but incurable. Serum and urine electrophoresis show a monoclonal IgM paraprotein.

Histopathology Two main architectural patterns of nodal involvement can be seen: (1) classic with subtotal effacement of the architecture by a monomorphous cell population, and (2) total effacement by a nodular or a diffuse polymorphous cell proliferation.

FNA Findings The cytology shows small lymphocytes, plasmacytoid lymphocytes, plasma cells, epitheloid histiocytes, and variable numbers of large, transformed cells. Transformation to a DLBCL with immunoblasts or Reed-Sternberg-like cells is seen in approximately 10% of cases (Fig. 7.35a, b).

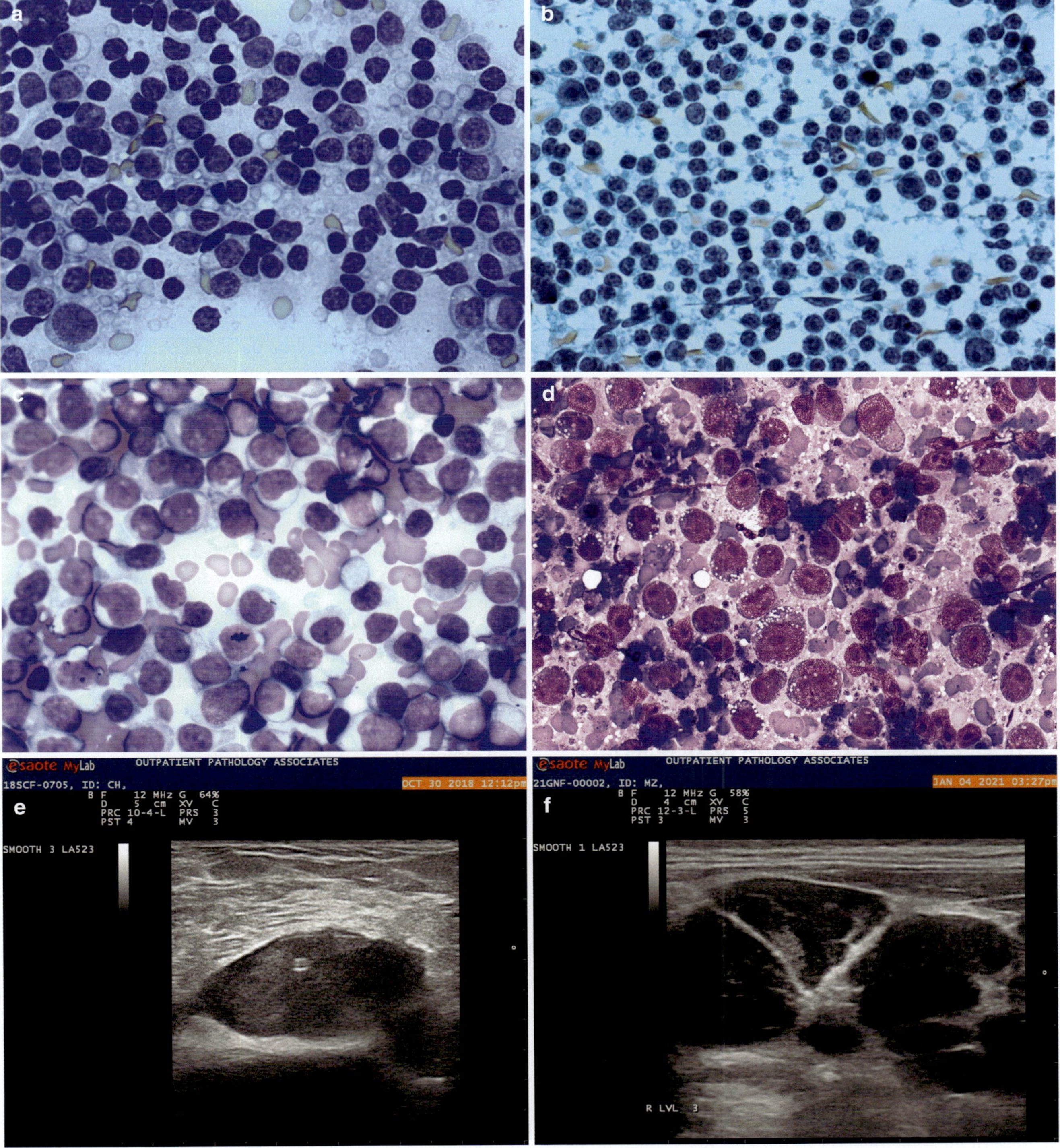

Fig. 7.32 Small cell lymphocytic lymphoma. The smear shows a monotonous population of small round lymphoid cells (**a**, **b**). The precise diagnosis is made based on flow cytometric analysis. Large cell lymphoma (Richter transformation) (**c**) may occur, and the vacuolated cytoplasm is often the result of prior chemotherapy (**d**). The US evaluation showed enlarged, irregularly shaped, coalescent, hypoechoic, and heterogeneous cervical lymph nodes (**e**, **f**). (**a**, **c**, **d** DiffQuik® stain, high magnification; **b**, Papanicolaou stain, high magnification)

Table 7.6 Immunophenotypic profile of small- and intermediate-sized-cell lymphomas

	B-CLL/SLL	MCL	MZL	FL-1	LPL
Surface κ/λ	+ dim	+ strong	+ strong	+ strong	+ strong
CD5	+	+	+ dim 10%	–	–
CD10	–	–	–	+	–
PAX5	+	+	+	+	+
CD20	+ dim	+	+	+	+
CD23	+ 90%	+ dim 10%	+ 10%	–	+dim/–
FMC7	–	+	+	+	+
BCL-1	–	+	–	–	–
BCL-2	+	+	+ most cases	+	+
BCL-6	–	–	–	+	–
Cyclin D1	–	+	–	–	–
SOX-11	–	+	–		–
LEF-1	+	–	–		–

B-CLL/SLL B-chronic lymphocytic leukemia/small lymphocytic lymphoma, *MCL* mantle cell lymphoma, *MZL* marginal zone lymphoma, *FL-1* follicular lymphoma, grade 1, *LPL* lymphoplasmacytic lymphoma, *LEF-1* lymphocyte enhancer-binding factor 1

Cells are positive for CD19, CD20, CD22, CD79a, PAX5, FMC7 and are negative for CD5, CD10, CD23, with variable CD38 stain. Cytoplasmic immunoglobulin, CD43, and CD138 are positive in plasma cells. *MYD88* mutation is found in >90% of cases.

Small Non-cleaved Cell (Burkitt) Lymphoma (BL)

BL is an aggesive mature B-cell neoplasm. Historically, three variants, endemic, sporadic, and immunodeficiency-associated, have been described and differ clinically, morphologically, and biologically. Evidence suggests that a dual mechanism, viral/EBV-positive and mutational/EBV-negative drives the pathogenesis of BL. The Epstein-Barr virus (EBV) genome is present in the neoplastic cells in all cases of endemic BL, and in approximately 30% of sporadic and immunodeficiency-associated BL. Currently, the WHO recommends subtyping of BL according to the EBV status instead of the epidemiological context.

Clinical Findings Endemic BL occurs in equatorial Africa in areas of endemic malaria and affects predominantly children. Sporadic BL is seen throughout the world, represents <2% of all non-Hodgkin lymphomas in the US, and affects predominantly children and young adults. Immunodeficiency-associated BL is often associated with HIV infection. Patients have bulky disease and signs and symptoms of a few weeks' duration due to the short doubling time of the tumor. Endemic and sporadic BL may be cured with intensive chemotherapy regimens.

FNA Findings The cytology shows tumor cells of medium size with round nuclei and evenly distributed chromatin with multiple nucleoli. The amount of cytoplasm is moderate, deeply basophilic, and usually contains clear-lipid-containing vacuoles. Numerous mitoses are present as well as numerous macrophages with ingested apoptotic tumor cells. The spectrum of BL is wide, and some cases may show tumor cells with plasmacytoid features or nuclear pleomorphism with prominent nucleoli (Fig. 7.36a–f).

Tumor cells have a germinal center-B-cell phenotype CD10, bcl-6, CD19, and CD20, CD22, and PAX5 positive. bcl-2 is negative or weak. Ki67 index is >95%. MYC protein is expressed in most cells. Most cases have an t(8;14) (q24;q32), t(2;8)(p12;q24), or t(8;22)(q24;q11) translocations.

Precursor B- and T-cell Lymphomas

These are two highly aggressive neoplasms of precursor lymphoid cells with blastic cytomorphology. The term lymphoblastic lymphoma (LBL) is used when the process is confined to a mass lesion with minimal or no peripheral blood and bone marrow involvement. Whereas the B-cell lineage predominates in lymphoblastic leukemia, only 10% of LBLs have a B-cell phenotype.

Clinical Findings In general, LBLs are seen often in children and adolescents. The most frequent sites of involvement in B-LBL are skin, soft tissue, bone, and lymph nodes. Mediastinal (thymic) involvement is often present in T-LBL and infrequent in B-LBL. Lymphadenopathy, hepatomegaly, and splenomegaly are frequent in B- and T-LBL.

FNA Findings The cytology shows cells of small or intermediate size. The small cells are uniform and have scant cytoplasm, round nuclei with occasional clefting and indentations, homogeneous, fine, and delicate chromatin, and multiple variably prominent nucleoli. When intermediate-size cells predominate, the pattern shows more anisocytosis, moderate cytoplasm, fine and delicate chromatin, often irregular, clefted, and indented nuclear contours, and two to three small nucleoli. Mitotic figures are often numerous (Fig. 7.37a, b).

Tumor cells are positive for the enzyme terminal deoxynucleotidyl transferase (TdT) in most cases of B- and T-LBL. The lymphoblasts in B-LBL are almost always positive for the B-cell markers CD10, CD19, and PAX5. CD20, CD22, CD24, CD79a are usually expressed in the cytoplasm. The lymphoblasts in T-LBL are positive for the T-cell markers CD3 and CD7, and depending on the grade of "maturation," the neoplastic cells may be positive for CD1a, CD2, CD4, CD5, CD8, CD10, CD34, and CD38. Almost all cases of B-LBL have cytogenetic abnormalities. T-cell receptor gene rearrangements, commonly of α and δ loci are usually present in T-LBL.

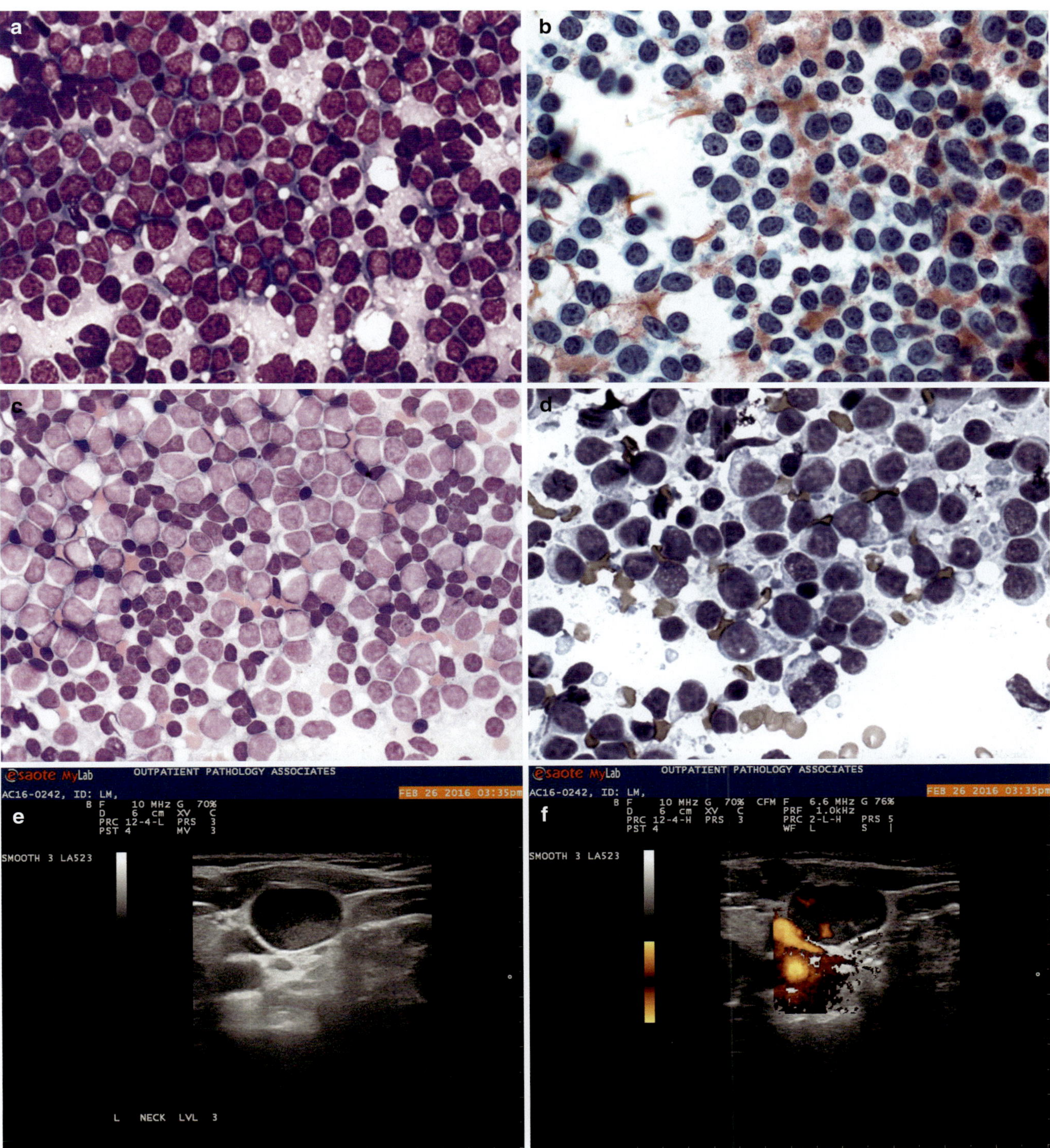

Fig. 7.33 Mantle cell lymphoma. The smear shows a monotonous population of small slightly irregular lymphoid cells (**a, b**). The blastoid variant and cells with plasmacytoid features are seen in these two cases (**c, d**). The diagnosis needs flow cytometry evaluation in material obtained by FNA. The US exam shows a lymph node with well-defined margins, hypoechogenicity, homogeneous echotexture, and internal vascular blood flow (**e, f**). (**a, c**, DiffQuik® stain, high magnification; **b**, Papanicolaou stain, high magnification; **d**, MGG stain, high magnification)

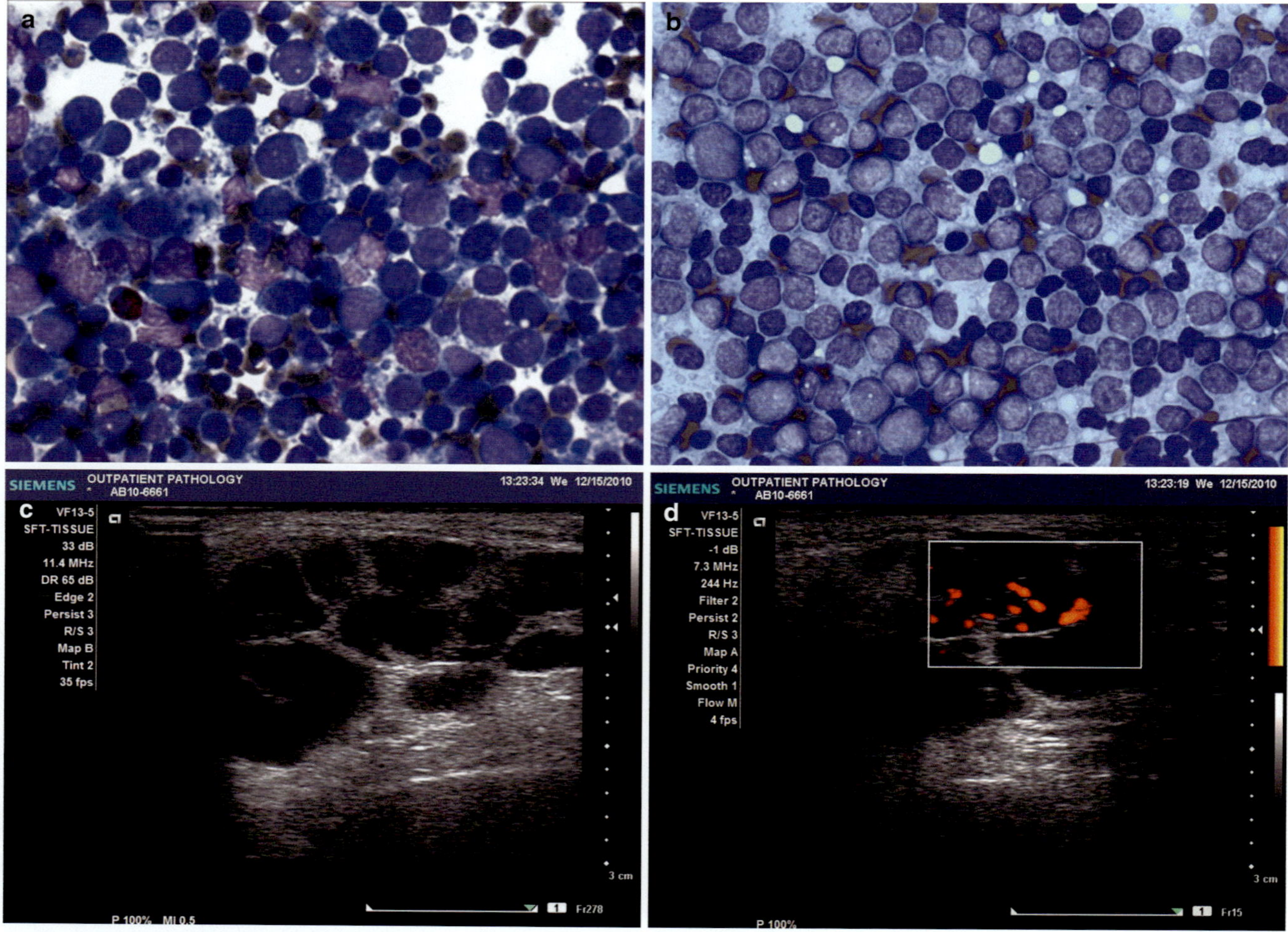

Fig. 7.34 Marginal zone lymphoma. A monotonous population of intermediate size centrocyte-like lymphoid cells with slightly irregular nuclei is seen (**a, b**). The diagnosis is made by flow cytometry on FNA material. Ultrasound shows coalescent lymph nodes with hypoechogenicity, well-defined margins, and chaotic vascular flow (**c, d**). (**a**, DiffQuik® stain, high magnification; **b**, MGG stain, high magnification)

Adult T-cell Leukemia/Lymphoma

ATLL is a rare and aggressive peripheral T-cell neoplasm associated with the human T-cell leukemia virus type-I (HTLV-I) that is endemic in southwestern Japan, the Caribbean basin, and Central Africa. HTLV-1 is transmitted from mother to child through breastfeeding, blood transfusion, or sexual interaction.

Clinical Findings ATLL is clinically sclassified into four subgroups: acute, chronic, lymphomatous, and smouldering. Most patients have generalized disease with lymphnode and peripheral-blood involvement. Generalized lymphadenopathy, skin rash, leukocytosis, eosinophilia, and hypercalcemia are common in acute ATLL. Generalized lymphadenopathy without peripheral-blood involvement is seen in the lymphomatous variant of ATLL. Due to severe immunosuppression, all ATLL patients are at increased risk of infections and infestations, particularly strongyloidiasis.

FNA Findings The cytology shows neoplasic lymphocytes of intermediate to large size with marked nuclear irregularities, coarse chromatin, and distinct nucleoli. Giant cells with convoluted nuclei may be present (Fig. 7.38a, b).

The tumor cells express T-cell-associated antigens (CD2, CD3, CD5, CD25, CD29, CD30, CD38, CD71, CCR4, FOXP3, and HLA-DR) and lack CD7. Most cases show CD4 positive cells; CD8 positive cells are present in rare cases. The large cells may be CD30[+] but are negative for ALK. Multiple chromosomal abnormalities are described, particularly in the aggressive forms: trisomy 3, trisomy 7, and monosomy X, and defects in chromosomes 6 and 14. Neoplastic cells have a clonal rearrangement of T-cell-receptor genes and monoclonal integration of HTLV-I.

Peripheral T-cell Lymphoma

Peripheral T-cell lymphoma (PTCL) originates in the activated mature CD4 memory T cell.

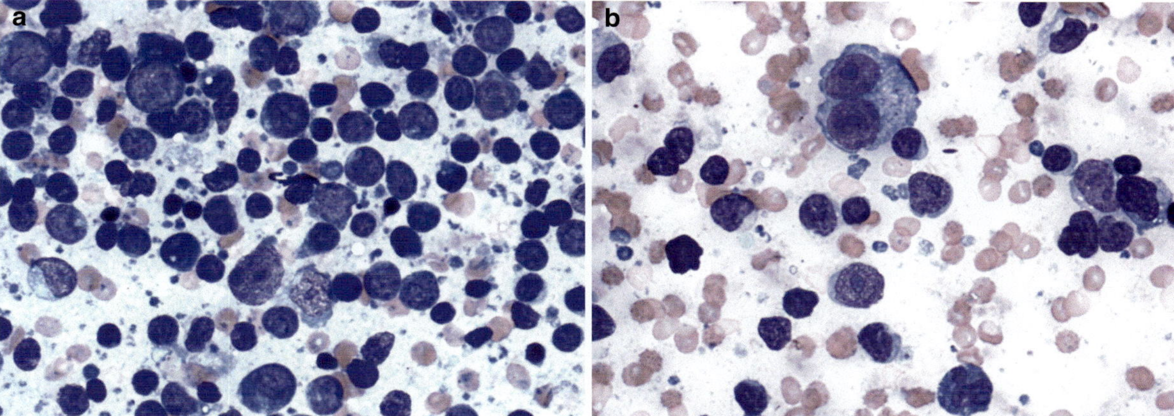

Fig. 7.35 Lymphoplasmacytic lymphoma. Distinct plasmacytoid features and a Reed-Sternberg-like cell are seen. (**a**, **b**, MGG stain, high magnification)

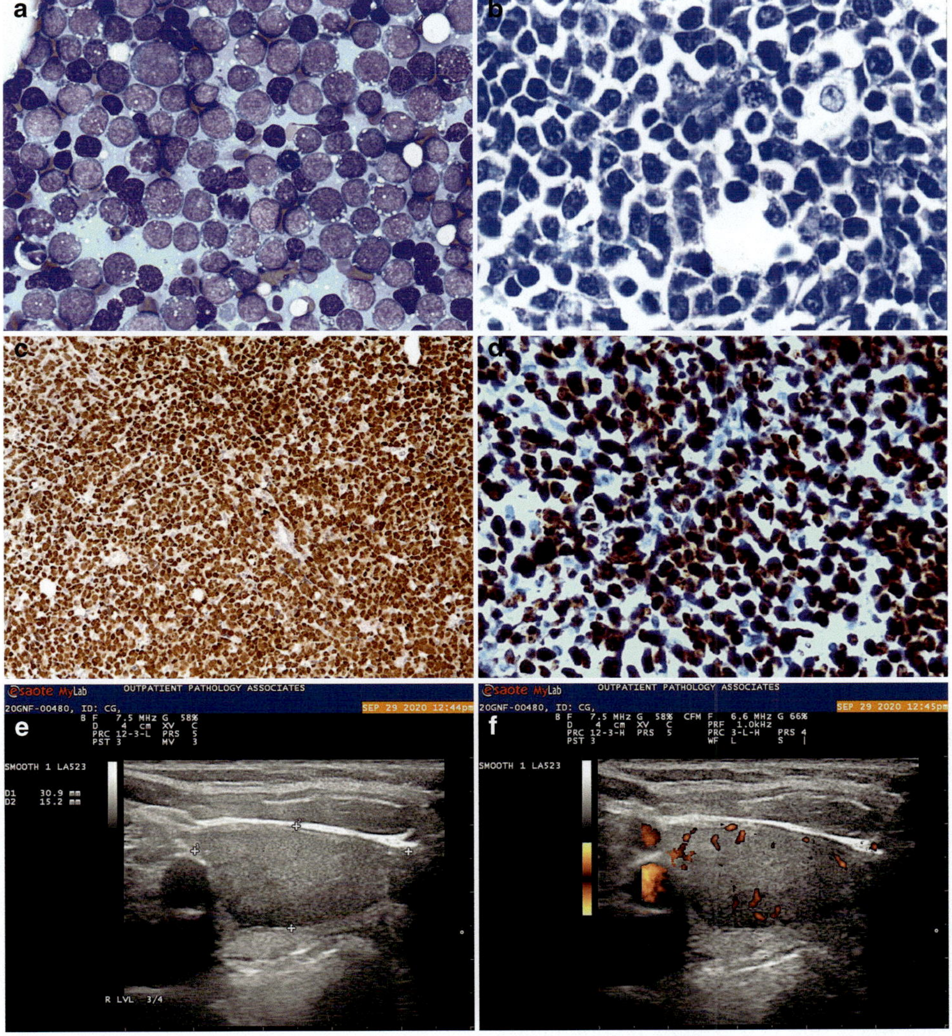

Fig. 7.36 Burkitt's lymphoma. The smear shows a population of intermediate-size cells with multiple nucleoli and distinct minute cytoplasmic vacuoles (**a–f**). Positive immunostaining for c-myc (**c**) and for EBER in situ hybridization (**d**) are seen. The US shows an irregularly shaped and isoechoic lymph node with distinct borders and internal vascular blood flow (**e**, **f**). (**a**, MGG stain, high magnification; **b**, DiffQuik® stain, high magnification) (**c**, **d** From Leonardo and Bardales (2020). Reprinted with permission)

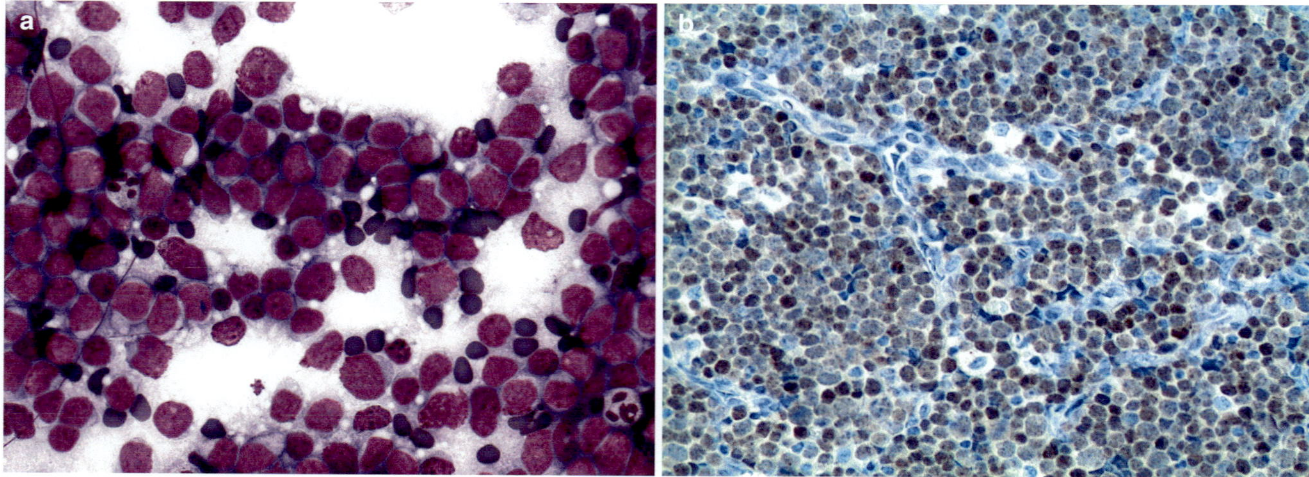

Fig. 7.37 Lymphoblastic lymphoma. The smear shows a monotonous population of intermediate-size lymphoid cells some with scant cytoplasm and slight nuclear irregularities (**a**). Positive TdT immunostain (**b**). (**a**, MGG stain, high magnification) (**b** From Leonardo and Bardales (2020). Reprinted with permission)

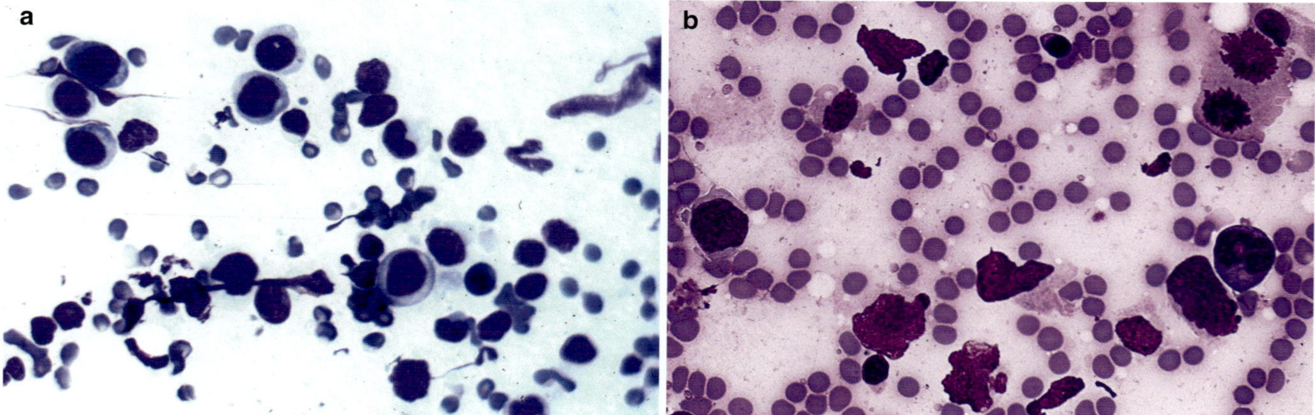

Fig. 7.38 Adult T-cell leukemia/lymphoma. Large neoplastic cells with marked anisonucleosis, nuclear irregularities, and mitoses. (**a**, **b**, MGG stain, high magnification)

Clinical findings. PTCL is rare, usually has aggressive behavior, and is especially common in African American males in the 6th decade of life or older. Patients commonly present with lymphadenopathy, and have extranodal (skin, GI tract, liver, spleen, bone marrow) involvement, and systemic symptoms. Pruritus, eosinophilia, and hemophagocytic syndrome may be present, but leukemia is uncommon.

Histopathology There is paracortical or diffuse effacement of the nodal architecture.

The cytology shows small, intermediate, and large cells in various combinations resulting in a polymorphous pattern or may be monotonous when one cell pattern predominates. The small-cell pattern is the least common. Cells exhibit clear cytoplasm, irregular nuclei, prominent nucleoli, and numerous mitoses. Clear cells and Reed-Sternberg-like cells

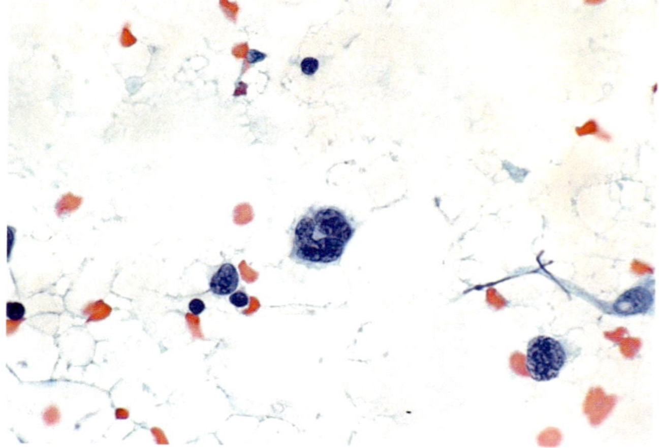

Fig. 7.39 Peripheral T-cell lymphoma. Large cell with multilobated nuclei and coarse chromatin. (Papanicolaou stain, high magnification)

may be seen (Fig. 7.39). In addition, small lymphocytes, histiocytes, eosinophils, and plasma cells are present. Tight sarcoid-like granulomas can be present.

The neoplastic cells express pan-T-cell and T-cell-associated antigens including CD2, CD43, and CD45RO. Most are CD4 and CD30 positive, and express TCR αβ. T-cell-receptor genes are clonally rearranged in most cases. ALK, EMA, and TdT are negative. Most markers of T-cell helper are negative. Rare cases lack CD4 and express CD8.

Sézary Syndrome

This type of primary cutaneous T-cell lymphoma is rare.

Clinical findings. It occurs in adults, usually older than 60 years, and has a male predominance. It is an aggressive disease with an overall survival of 20% at 5 years. Patients have erythroderma and generalized lymphadenopathy. Palmar and plantar hyperkeratosis and onychodystrophy may be present. The cell of origin is the skin resident CD45RO⁺ memory T cell.

FNA Findings The neoplastic T cells are of small to intermediate size, have irregular "cerebriform" nuclei (Sézary cells), and are found in the skin, lymph nodes, and peripheral blood. The cells have moderate amounts of cytoplasm, and the nucleus may have a monocytoid appearance with one to three nucleoli. The smear background may show melanin-laden histiocytes as a manifestation of dermatopathic lymphadenopathy (Figs. 7.22 and 7.40).

Tumor cells are immunoreactive with CD2, CD3, TCRβ⁺, CD5, cutaneous lymphocyte antigen (CLA), and the skin-homing receptor CCR4. Most cases are CD4 positive and

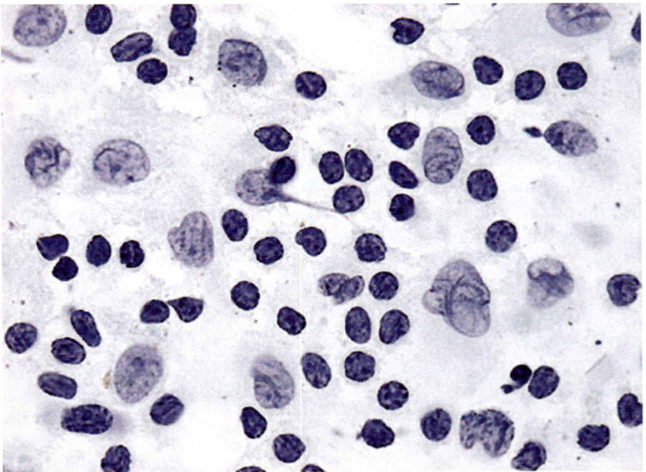

Fig. 7.40 Sezary syndrome. Monotonous population of intermediate-size lymphocytes with prominent nuclear irregularities. Dermatopathic lymphadenopathy was seen in other areas of the smear (see Fig. 7.22). (Papanicolaou stain, high magnification) Courtesy Dr. Javier Saenz de Santamaria, Pathologist, Department of Pathology, Complejo Universitario de Badajoz, Spain

rare cases are CD8 postive. T- cell-receptor gene rearrangement is present.

Anaplastic Large-Cell Lymphoma

Anaplastic large cell lymphoma (ALCL) is a mature T-cell lymphoma that accounts for approximately 20% of all T-cell lymphomas. According to the presence or absence of ALK protein expression, it can be divided into the morphologically indistinguishable but clinically distinct ALK-positive ALCL (50–80% of cases) and ALK-negative ALCL.

Clinical Findings It occurs in young adults but may occur in children. ALK-positive ALCL involves both lymph nodes and extranodal sites (skin, musculoskeletal system, lungs, liver) of young, predominantly male patients, whereas ALK-negative ALCL tends to affect elderly patients. Based on its distinct pathogenesis, the response to treatment and the prognosis of patients with ALK-positive ALCL are better than that for ALK-negative ALCL and other peripheral T-cell lymphomas.

Of note, **breast implant-associated ALCL** is an entity distinct from ALK-negative ALCL, is usually non-invasive, arises in association with surface breast implants, and the outcome is excellent.

Histopathology ALCL has a few morphologic variants or patterns, the *common* (or *classic*) (75%), the *lymphohistiocytic* (10%), and the *small cell* (5–10%). The small cell variant is composed of neoplastic cells that are neither large nor anaplastic and may enter the differential diagnosis of small blue cell tumors and of lymphomas composed of intermediate-sized neoplastic cells.

FNA Findings Common to all morphologic variants of ALCL is the presence of "hallmark" cells, large or very large cells, with horseshoe-shaped or kidney-shaped nuclei, abundant clear cytoplasm and prominent perinuclear clear hofs, corresponding to the Golgi regions. Nucleoli are round or angular and prominent. The cytoplasm may show peripheral blebs and small vacuoles. A continuum of sizes of the abnormal cells can usually be seen. Other characteristic neoplastic cells include "half-doughnut cells", "doughnut cells", multinucleated giant "wreath cells", "embryo cells," "tennis racket" or "hand mirror" cells, and cells with polylobed nuclei and Reed–Sternberg-like cells. Frequent mitoses and apoptotic cells are present. Erythrophagocytosis or cell cannibalism, reactive lymphocytes, neutrophils, histiocytes, or eosinophils can occasionally be seen (Fig. 7.41a–f).

Immunohistochemistry is useful in the differentiation of ALCL from HL and metastatic malignancies (Table 7.7). The large, pleomorphic neoplastic cells of ALCL are positive for CD30 in a membranous and Golgi pattern. Most cases

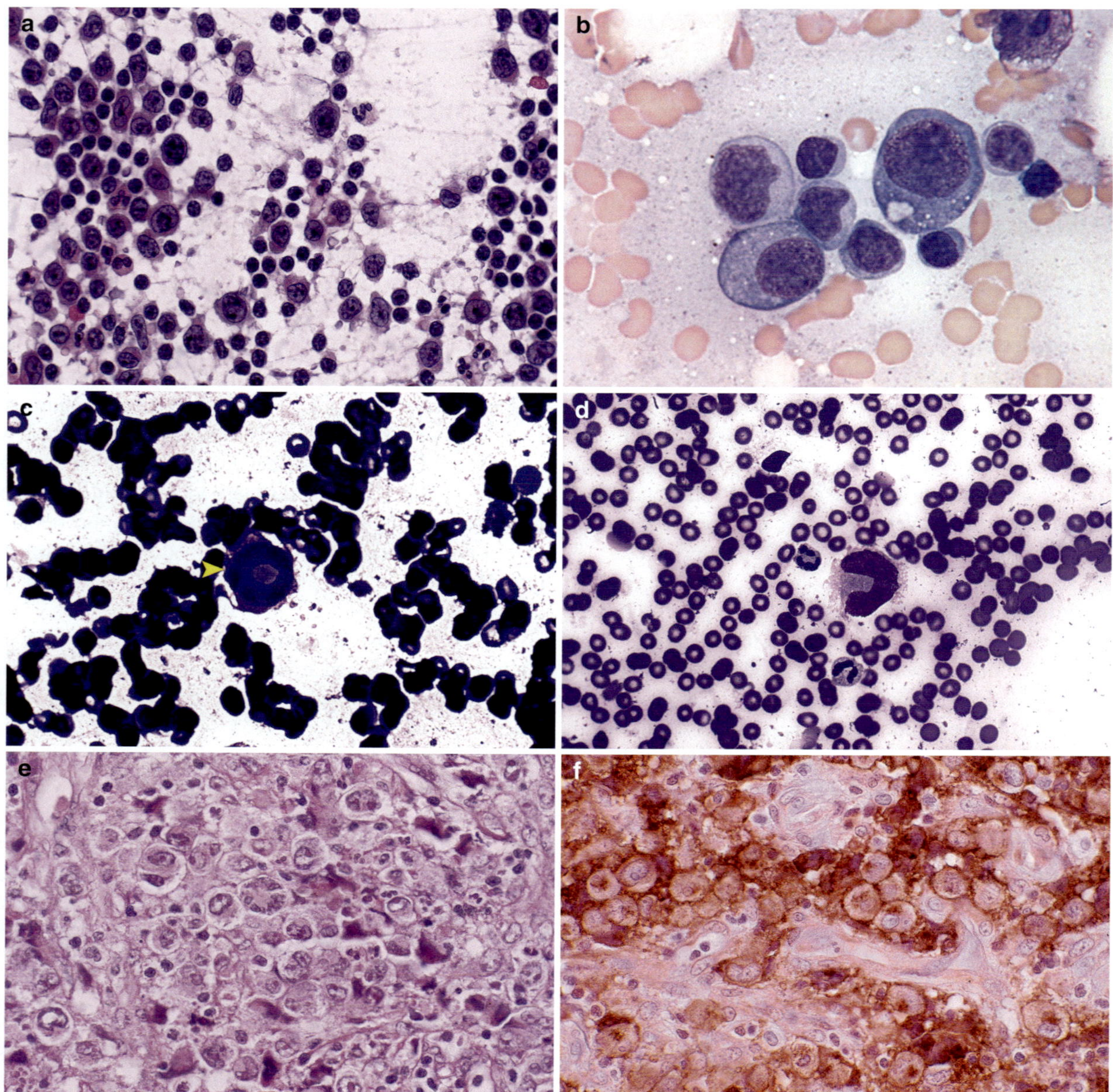

Fig. 7.41 Anaplastic large cell lymphoma. A pleomorphic population of large cells with anisocytosis and anaplasia is characteristic of this lymphoma (**a**, **b**). "Doughnut" (**c**, arrowhead) and "half-doughnut" (**d**) cells also are some of the pleomorphic cells seen. Histopathology shows prominent cell anaplasia including a wreath cell (center of frame) (**e**). Positive immunostain for CD30 in the tissue section (**f**). (**a**, MGG stain, medium magnification; **b–d**, DiffQuik® stain, high magnification; **e**, hematoxylin and eosin, high magnification; **f**, immunoperoxidase stain, high magnification)

Table 7.7 Immunohistochemistry in Hodgkin lymphoma and its mimics

	CD15	CD30	CD45	CD3, CD5, CD7	CD20	PAX5	EMA
cHL	+	+	−	−	−80%	+	−
NLPHL	−	−	+	−	+	+	+/−
TC/HRLBCL	−	−	+	−	+	+	−/+
ALCL	−	+	+	+/−	−	−	+
pTCL	−	−	+	+/−	−	−	−
PMBL	−	+ weak	+	−	+	+	−

cLH classical Hodgkin lymphoma, *NLPHL* nodular lymphocyte-predominant Hodgkin lymphoma, *TC/HRLBCL* T-cell/histiocyte-rich large B-cell lymphoma, *ALCL* anaplastic large-cell lymphoma, *pTCL* peripheral T-cell lymphoma, *PMBL* primary mediastinal B-cell lymphoma

express one or more T-cell markers (CD2, CD4, CD5), but CD3 is frequently lost. The neoplastic cells are consistently positive for CD45 and EMA. The t(2;5) or t(1;2) translocation is present in 90% of systemic cases.

Hodgkin Lymphoma

Hodgkin lymphoma (HL) is a B-cell derived lymphoma that accounts for 30% of lymphomas, has a bimodal age distribution, adolescents and young adults and 6th and 7th decade of life, and initially involves cervical and mediastinal lymph nodes. Lymph nodes are enlarged and usually non-tender, and patients are often asymptomatic at diagnosis. HL tends to spread to contiguous lymph node regions. Constitutional symptoms including fever, night sweats, and weight loss usually occur with widespread disease. Treatment with radiation and chemotherapy results in a >85% cure rate.

The current 2022 WHO classification of HL includes:

1. Nodular lymphocyte predominant HL (NLPHL)—5% of all HL cases.

    Of note, NLPHL has been renamed under The International Concensus Classification of Lymphomas as nodular lymphocyte predominant B cell lymphoma (NLPBL). The term NLPBL is pending to be adopted by the WHO.
2. Classical Hodgkin lymphoma (cHL)—95% of all HL cases
    (a) Nodular sclerosis cHL—65–70% of all HL cases
    (b) Mixed-cellularity cHL—20% of all HL cases
    (c) Lymphocyte-rich cHL—5% of all HL cases
    (d) Lymphocyte-depleted cHL—1% of all HL cases

The mononuclear Hodgkin (H) and bi- and multi-nucleate Reed-Sternberg (R-S) cells of cHL are collectively called HRS cells. The lymphocytic and/or histiocytic (L&H) cells of NLPHL are also named LP or popcorn cells; by polymerase chain reaction, it has been demonstrated that HRS cells have immunoglobulin gene rearrangements with somatic mutations that indicate their clonal origin in the germinal center. Likewise, the LP cells of NLPHL have cell rearrangements and mutations similar to those of HRS. However, the B-cell differentiation program is downregulated in HRS cells and fully active in LP cells. Thus, neoplastic cells have lost most B-cell markers in cHL and are preserved in NLPHL. The neoplastic cells of cHL are variably positive for EBV; however, no EBV positivity is found in NLPHL.

FNA Findings Smears show a background of reactive polymorphous lymphoid cells with predominance of small mature lymphocytes. The cellularity is variable, and neoplastic cells are found scattered in the background. The cellularity is the lowest due to fibrosis in nodular-sclerosis HL, the most common form of HL. The background also shows variable numbers of eosinophils, plasma cells, and even epithelioid cells and granulomas to the point that such findings in a lymph-node aspirate should trigger the diligent search for neoplastic cells of HL. These findings may also be present in lymphadenopathies secondary to allergic reactions and parasitic infestations. Occasionally, the background shows numerous neutrophils and simulates bacterial lymphadenitis. Of note, the syncytial variant of nodular sclerosis HL, particularly when present in the mediastinal lymph nodes, must be distinguished from metastatic carcinoma and primary mediastinal large B-cell lymphoma. Large-cell T- and B-cell lymphomas, metastatic malignancies, especially melanoma and carcinoma or viral-driven lymphadenitis, should be included in the differential diagnosis.

The FNA diagnosis requires finding the neoplastic cells. Classic R-S cells usually have a moderate amount of pale cytoplasm with two or more eccentrically placed large, complex, or lobulated nuclei exhibiting irregular borders, coarse chromatin, and prominent irregular inclusion-like nucleoli. The mononuclear variants show similar nuclear features. Immunoblasts, commonly mistaken for the mononuclear variant are smaller, and show basophilic cytoplasm, round nucleus, and a prominent but smooth round nucleolus (Figs. 7.42a–d, 7.43a–d, 7.44a–f, 7.45a–d).

Immuno-Profile Table 7.7 summarizes the markers that are useful in the differential diagnosis of HL.

Ultrasound Features of Lymph Nodes Involved by Lymphomas

Lymphomas commonly involve the levels I and V of the neck, in addition to other neck levels. Lymph nodes are usually round or oval, very hypoechoic reticulated/micronodular, rarely necrotic, have sharp margins, and the hilum may be absent or present, usually with an exaggerated vascular pattern (Figs. 7.30e, f, 7.31e, f, 7.32e, f, 7.33e, f, 7.34c, d, 7.42c, d, 7.43d, 7.44e, f).

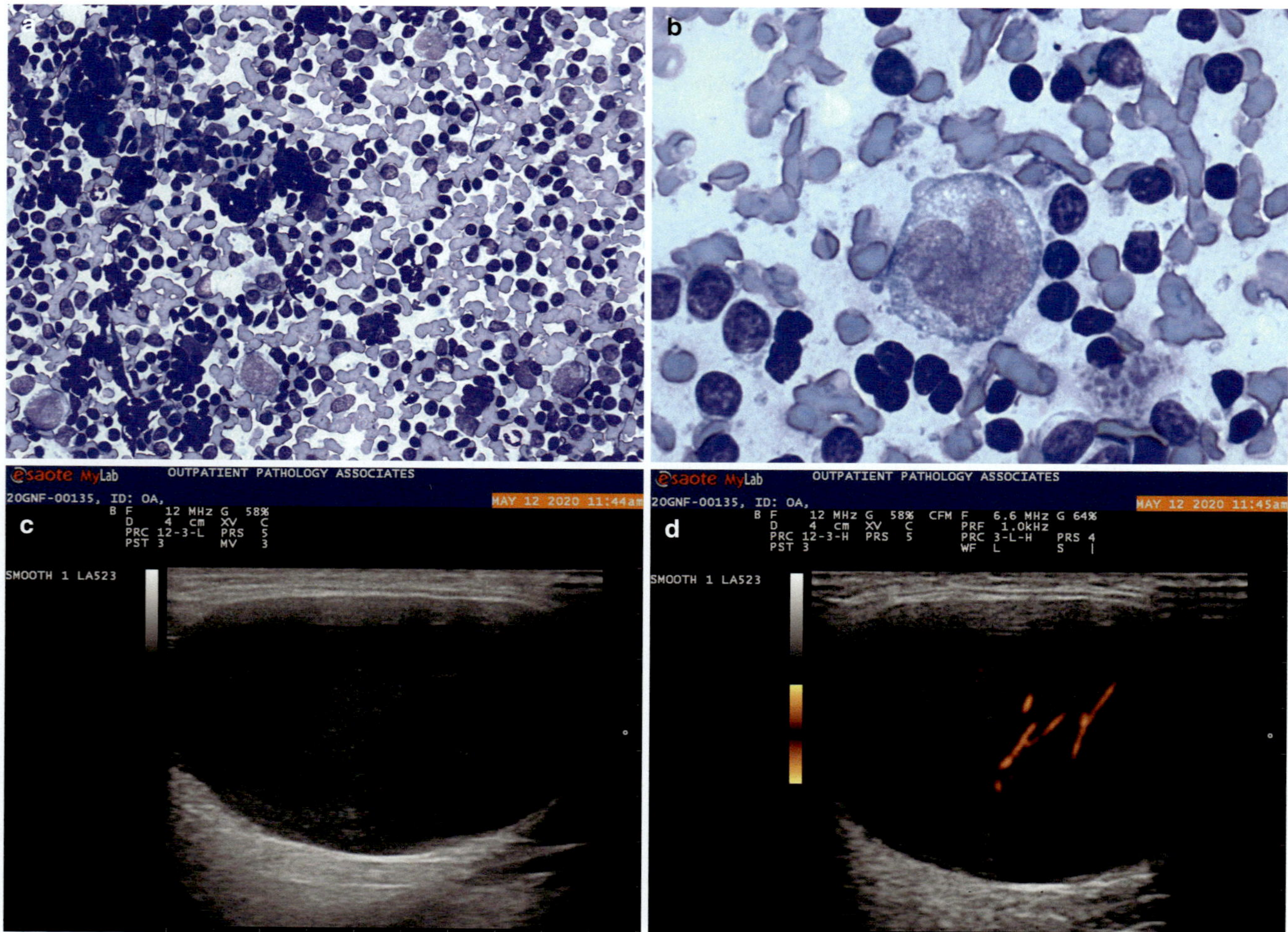

Fig. 7.42 Hodgkin lymphoma, nodular lymphocyte predominant. Large cells with pleomorphic nuclei are seen, mainly in the lower portion of frame along with numerous reactive lymphoid cells (**a**). A large pleomorphic cell with a "popcorn-like" convoluted nuclei and finely vacuolated cytoplasm (**b**). The US shows a large deeply hypoechoic lymph node with sharp borders, posterior acoustic enhancement, and internal vascular blood flow (**c**, **d**). (**a**, **b**, MGG stain, medium and high magnification)

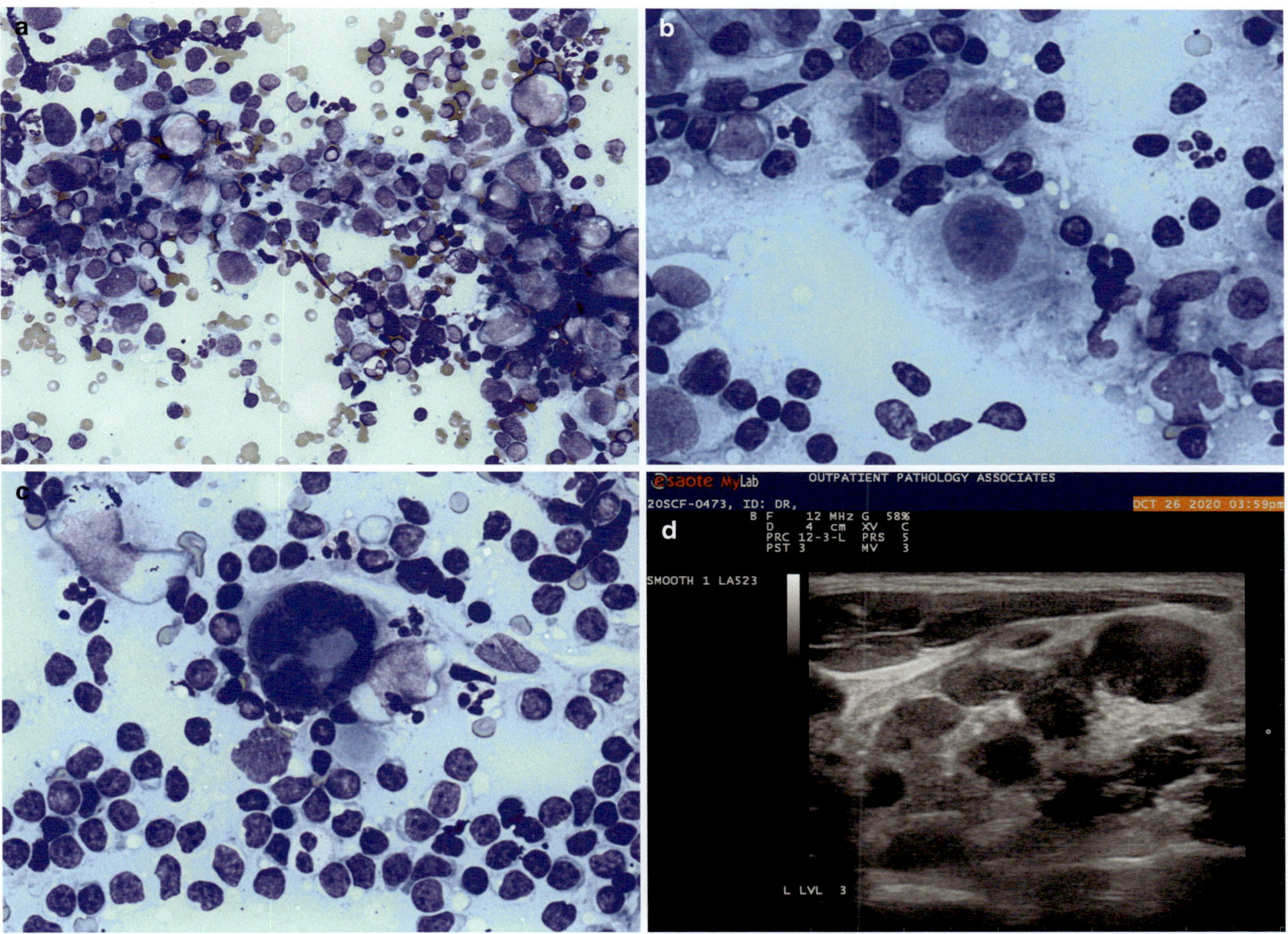

Fig. 7.43 Hodgkin lymphoma, nodular sclerosis. Numerous large pleomorphic cells (**a**), a Hodgkin mononuclear cell with large nucleolus (**b**) surrounded by pleomorphic cells, and a "wreath-like" cell (**c**) are seen. The US shows confluent lymph nodes of varying sizes and abnormal shapes surrounded by dense stroma (**d**). (**a–c**, MGG stain, medium and high magnification)

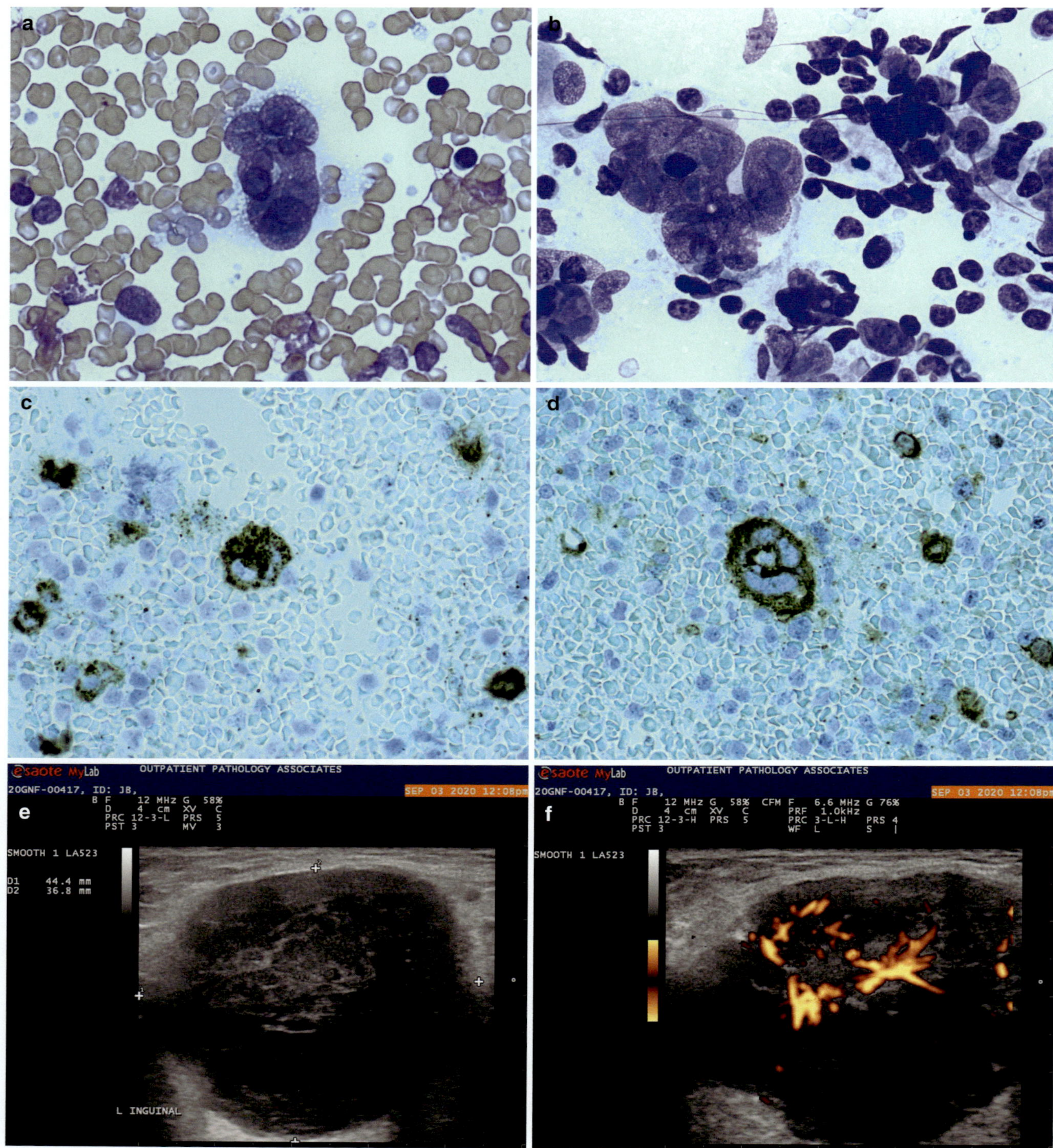

Fig. 7.44 Hodgkin lymphoma, mixed cellularity. A single "popcorn-like" cell (**a**) and a multinucleated Reed-Sternberg cell (**b**) were present in this case. Immunostains for CD15 (**c**) and CD30 (**d**) are positive. The US shows a large hypoechogenic inguinal lymph node with heterogeneous echotexture, fuzzy borders, lobulated contours, and chaotic internal vascular blood flow (**c**, **d**). (**a**, **b**, MGG stain, high magnification; **c**, **d**, immunoperoxidase stain, high magnification)

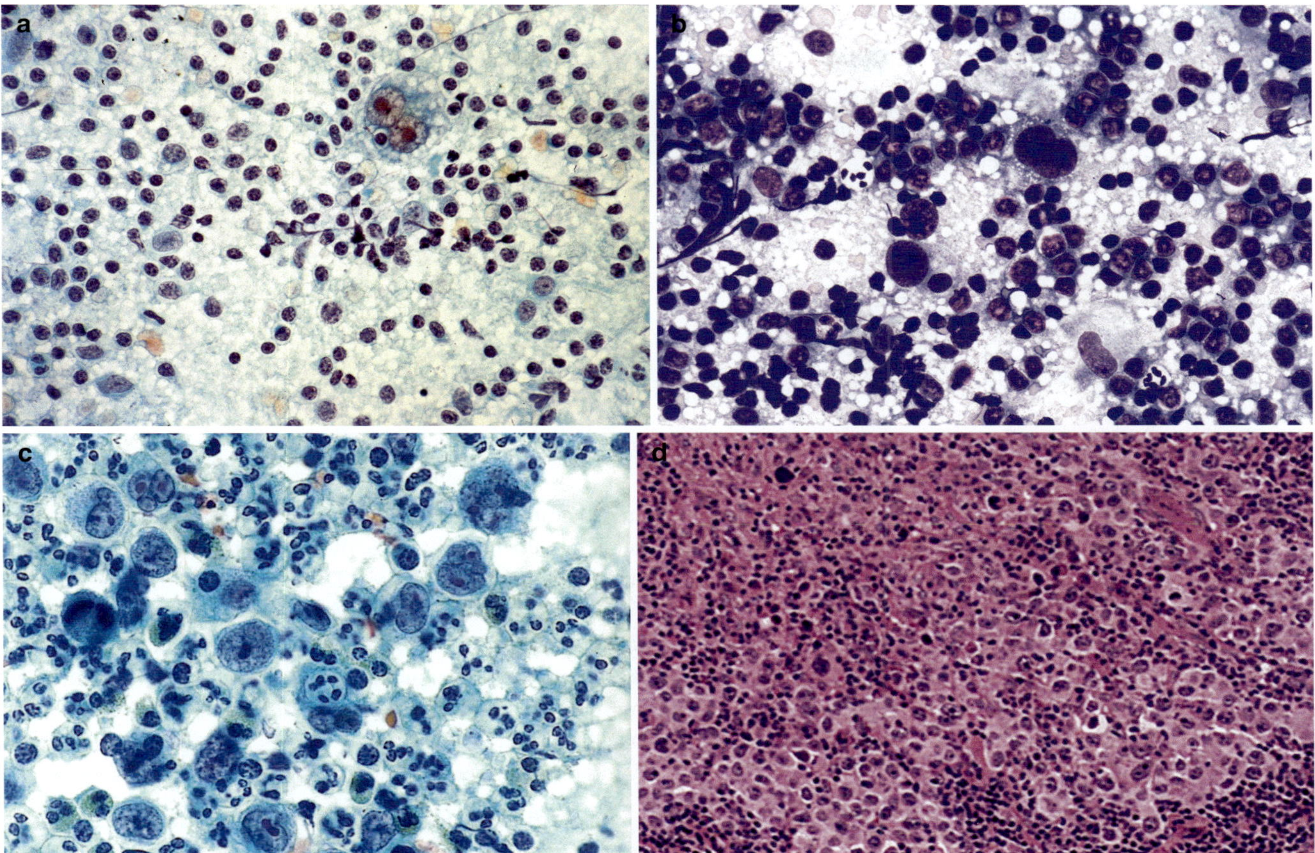

Fig. 7.45 Hodgkin lymphoma. The smear shows polymorphous reactive lymphoid cells, rare eosinophils, and plasma cells. Present in this background are Reed-Sternberg cells, mononuclear variants, and multinucleated cells (**a**, **b**). The suppurative type shows Hodgkin–Reed-Sternberg cells in a background of neutrophils (**c**). The syncytial type of Hodgkin lymphoma shows sheets of large cells in a background of lymphoid cells that mimic a metastatic malignancy (**d**). (**a**, Papanicolaou stain, high magnification; **b**, MGG stain, high magnification; **c**, DiffQuik® stain, high magnification; **d**, hematoxylin and eosin stain, medium magnification)

Select Examples of Lymph Node Metastases

Lymph nodes are the most common sites of metastasis, and metastatic malignancies outnumber primary lymphoid malignancies in most lymph-node locations. The topography of lymph-node chains and their territories of lymphatic drainage covered early in this chapter and Chap. 6 are helpful clues for determining the primary site of malignancy. Common metastases to lymph nodes by regions are summarized in the next paragraphs.

Axilla Metastases from breast carcinoma, melanoma, and squamous cell carcinoma in decreasing order of frequency.

Neck Supraclavicular Supraclavicular lymphadenopathy should be considered pathologic in any age group. In children, it often reflects associated mediastinal pathology including HL and neuroblastoma arising from the high thoracic or cervical sympathetic ganglia. In adults, less than 1% of carcinomas of the thorax and abdomen lead to malignant supraclavicular lymphadenopathy. Abdominal and pelvic malignancies are more likely to metastasize to the left supraclavicular lymph nodes (Virchow's node). Occasionally a left supraclavicular lymphadenopathy may be the first manifestation of an unknown malignancy, as seen in aggressive prostatic adenocarcinoma. Lung, breast, and head and neck malignancies show no differences in metastatic patterns to the left and right supraclavicular lymph nodes and the metastasis is usually ipsilateral to the primary tumor. Most patients have a strong suspicion or a known primary malignancy.

Inguinal Unilateral lymphadenopathy from malignancies of the skin of the lower extremities, cervix, vulva, skin of the trunk, anus/rectum, ovary, and penis are seen in decreasing order. Of note, bilateral lymphadenopathy may occur in lymphoma.

When possible, the cytomorphology of the primary malignancy and metastasis should be compared. In the absence of a known primary malignancy, a metastatic deposit can be correctly classified only by the cytomorphology in many

Table 7.8 Panel of immunostains helpful in classifying lymph node metastasis

General markers	Malignancy
CD45RB (leukocyte common antigen)	Hematolymphoid
Cytokeratin cocktail (AE1/ AE3 and 8/18)	Epithelial
EMA (epithelial membrane antigen)	Epithelial
S100 protein	Melanocytic
Vimentin	Mesenchymal and others
Specific markers	Organ-specific malignancy
Thyroglobulin	Thyroid
Calcitonin	Thyroid (medullary carcinoma)
HepPar1	Liver
Renal cell carcinoma antigen	Kidney
Uroplakin	Urothelium
TTF1 (thyroid transcription factor 1)	Thyroid, lung
CDX2, pS2 protein, CK20	GI tract, neoplasms with intestinal differentiation
CK7 and CK20	Lung, GI tract, urothelium
GATA-3, mammaglobin, ER, PR, GCFDP15	Breast
CK7, WT1, PAX8, CA125, EMA, B72.3	Ovarian serous papillary carcinoma

Table 7.9 Lymph node metastasis by cell patterns

Monotonous intermediate cell	• Neuroendocrine tumors: carcinoid, atypical carcinoid, small-cell carcinoma, Merkel cell carcinoma • Basal cell carcinoma • Melanoma • Small blue cell tumors: metastatic neuroblastoma, Ewing sarcoma/peripheral neuroectodermal tumor, rhabdomyosarcoma • Nasopharyngeal carcinoma
Monotonous large cell	• Carcinoma • Melanoma • Sarcoma • Seminoma
Pleomorphic cell	• Carcinoma • Melanoma • Sarcoma

cases. However, poorly differentiated, or undifferentiated malignancies, particularly of the small cell type (blue cell tumors), may be difficult to distinguish from each other and from lymphomas. Immunostains for the diagnosis of carcinoma, lymphoma, melanoma, or other malignancies can be done in cell block and smear preparations (Table 7.8). In summary, the clinical data and cytomorphology suggest the nature and origin of tbe metastatic deposit, and immunostains, molecular tests, and genetic analysis may be used for refining and making the correct diagnosis.

Material from needle rinses may also be used for measurement of thyroglobulin and thyroglobulin antibody levels when differentiated thyroid carcinoma is suspected. Likewise, calcitonin levels in needle rinses are helpful when metastasis from medullary thyroid carcinoma is suspected.

The Table 7.9 summarizes metastatic malignancies by patterns, monotonous and pleomorphic, as an attempt to ease and narrow the differential diagnosis in lymph-node aspirates.

Metastatic Squamous Cell Carcinoma

This is the most common metastatic malignancy to the head and neck and frequently follows or presents with a primary tumor in the head and neck.

FNA Findings Well-differentiated squamous cell carcinoma shows high cellularity, with keratinized cells exhibit-

ing pyknotic, minimally irregular, and slightly enlarged nuclei, with no mitotic activity. Necrosis and cannibalism may be seen (Fig. 7.46a–d). The diagnosis is usually straightforward in these cases. Cystic squamous cell carcinoma shows scant cellularity, anucleated squamous cells, and scattered intermediate squamous cells with hyperchromatic and minimally irregular nuclei in a necrotic and variably inflamed background (Fig. 7.47a–d, Video 7.5). A granulomatous foreign-body-type reaction to the keratin may be seen.

The differential diagnosis of cystic squamous cell carcinomas includes inflamed branchial cleft cysts and abscesses. Malignant cells with anaplastic nuclei are important for diagnosis. Poorly differentiated squamous carcinomas may be difficult to differentiate from other high-grade neoplasms. Cell block material is useful to perform special stains such as p16, which is a subrogate for HPV-driven squamous carcinomas of the head and neck. Independent of cellular differentiation, immunostains are positive for CK5, desmocollin-3, p40, and sometimes p63 (Fig. 7.48a–f).

Metastatic Nasopharyngeal Carcinoma

This is particularly prevalent among the Asian ethnic group, is associated with Epstein-Barr virus infection, and has a bimodal age presentation with one peak between 15 and 25 years and the other between 60–70 years. Involvement of neck level II and III neck lymph nodes is frequent and is the first evidence of the tumor in 90% of cases. Histologic types include keratinizing, non-keratinizing, and undifferentiated.

FNA Findings The smears are cellular. The non-keratinizing type shows numerous tri-dimensional aggregates and single round or elongated cells with scant cytoplasm, large nuclei, and prominent nucleoli. The undifferentiated type shows single and aggregated basaloid cells and small lymphocytes within the cell aggregates and in the background. Mitosis

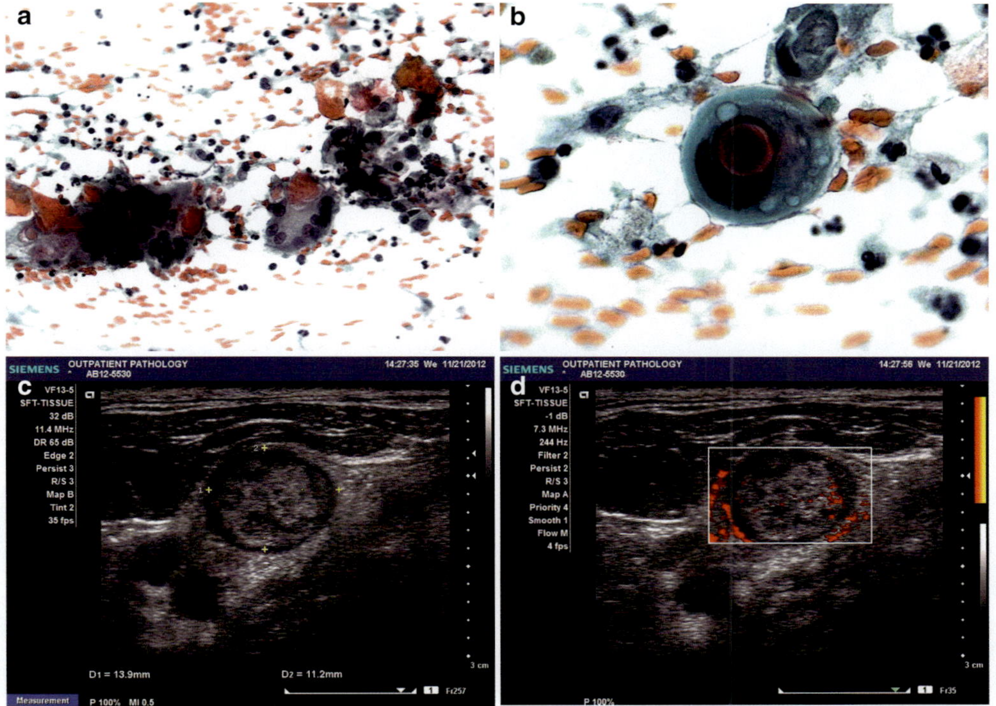

Fig. 7.46 Metastatic squamous carcinoma, well-differentiated. The smears show keratinization with anucleated squamous cells, foreign body type reaction with giant cells "engulfing" keratin flakes (**a**), and keratinized malignant cells showing cytophagocytosis with clearly malignant nuclear features (**b**). The US exam shows slightly hyperechoic round lymph node with lobulated borders and heterogeneous echotexture (**c**). Minimal peripheral and central vascularity are seen (**d**). (**a**, **b** Papanicolaou stain, high magnification)

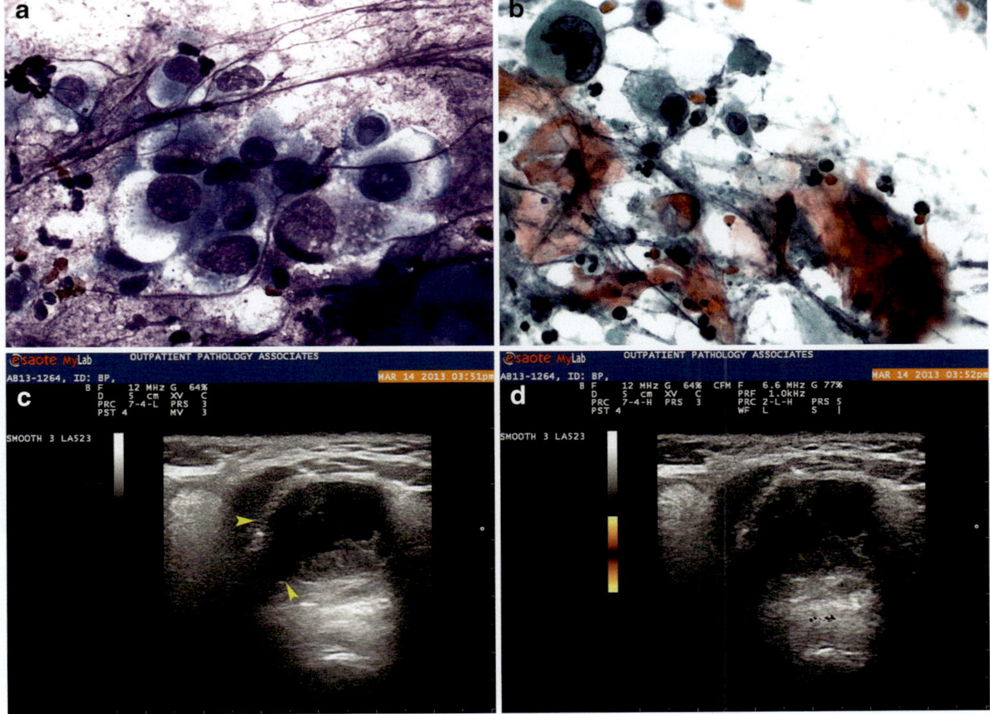

Fig. 7.47 Metastatic squamous carcinoma with cystic degeneration. Clearly malignant squamous cells with focal keratinization and a background of necrosis are seen (**a**, **b**). The US images show an irregular lymph node with cystic necrosis, ill-defined margins, focal extracapsular invasion (arrowheads), and no vascular blood flow (**c**, **d**). (**a**, MGG stain high magnification; **b**, Papanicolaou stain, high magnification) (Video 7.5)

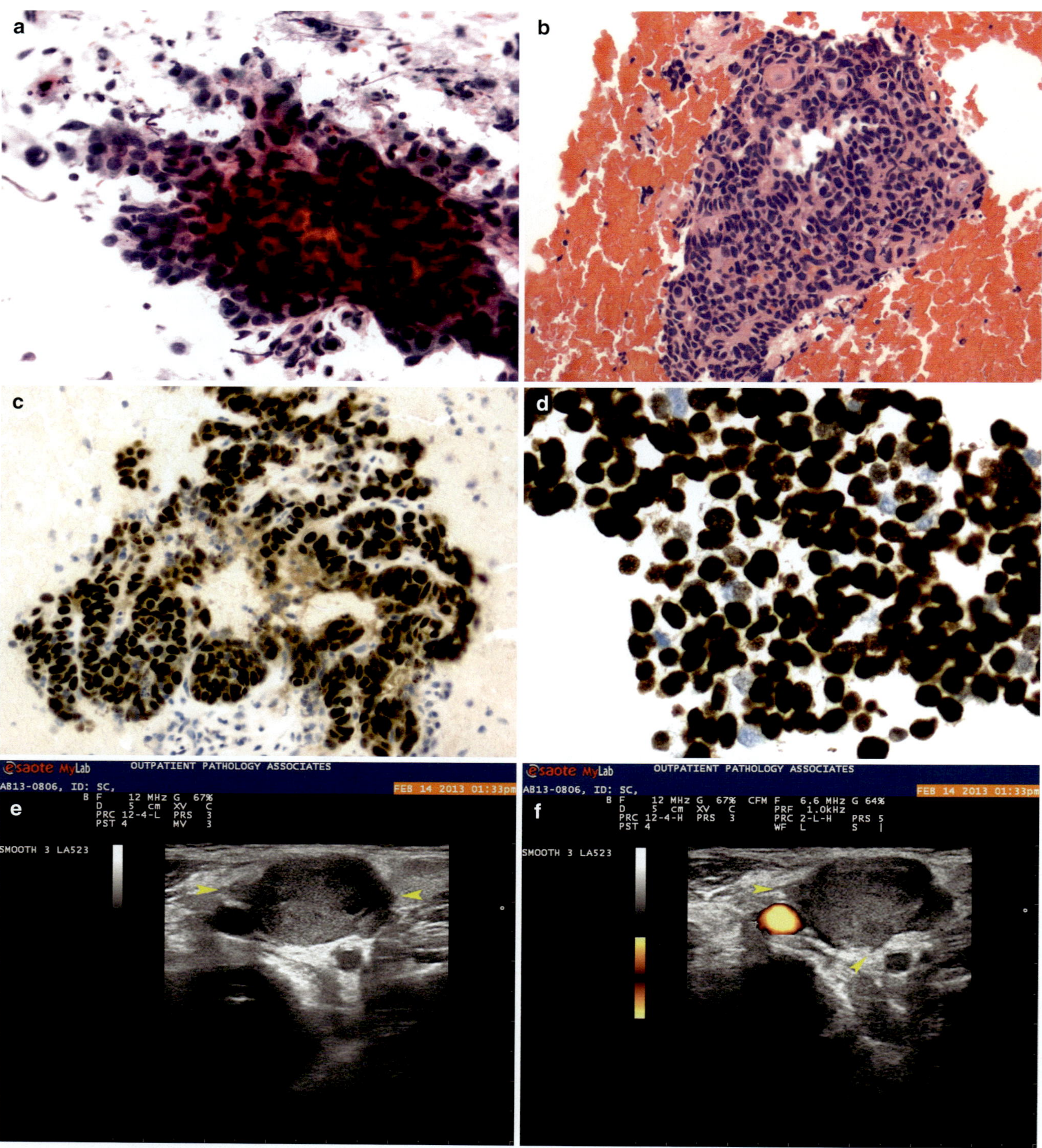

Fig. 7.48 Metastatic squamous carcinoma, poorly differentiated. The smear shows complex aggregates with spiculated ends and no evidence of keratinization (**a**). The cell block shows an aggregate of malignant squamous cells (**b**). Immunostains for p16 (**c**) and p40 (**d**) are positive. The US exam shows a hypoechoic lymph node with fuzzy margins, extracapsular invasion (arrowheads), and no vascularization (**d**, **e**). (**a**, Papanicolaou stain high magnification; **b**, H–E stain, medium magnification; **c**, **d**, immunoperoxidase stains, medium and high magnifications)

and necrosis are common (Fig. 7.49a–d). Tumors with similar histomorphology can arise in the palatine and lingual tonsils, thymus, and larynx.

Immunohistochemistry for CK5, CK14, and p40 and occasionally for p63, desmoplakin 1–2, and EMA is positive in the neoplastic cells. The neoplastic cells are positive for EBV-associated markers such as EBV-latent membrane protein type 1 and in situ hybridization for EBV small-encoded RNA (EBER). The differential diagnosis includes large-cell lymphoma, carcinomas, and germ-cell tumors and immunostains for leukocyte common antigen, alpha-fetoprotein, and β-chorionic gonadotropin are helpful for a correct diagnosis.

Metastatic Thyroid Carcinoma

US examination of neck lymph nodes is useful in the evaluation of patients with thyroid carcinoma. Of note, cystic changes are common in metastatic papillary carcinomas and the possibility of a metastatic papillary thyroid carcinoma must be strongly considered when a neck lymph node with cystic change (levels III, IV and less frequent in level II) is identified by US, at times as the first manifestation of the thyroid malignancy. US examinatioj must be followed by USG-FNA of the lymph node.

FNA Findings Solid lymph node metastases from papillary carcinoma show diagnostic features sufficient for a diagnosis (Fig. 7.50a–d, Video 7.6). Aspirates from cystic metastasis show small sheets of monolayered epithelium in a hemorrhagic cystic background; cytoplasmic septate vacuoles and macrophages are often seen, and other cytologic characteristics may be inconspicuous (Fig. 7.51a–d, Video 7.7). Metastatic follicular carcinoma consistently shows microfollicles with bland cytologic features. Metastasis of the oncocytic type may show a cytomorphology that is similar to medullary carcinoma in the absence of a pertinent clinical

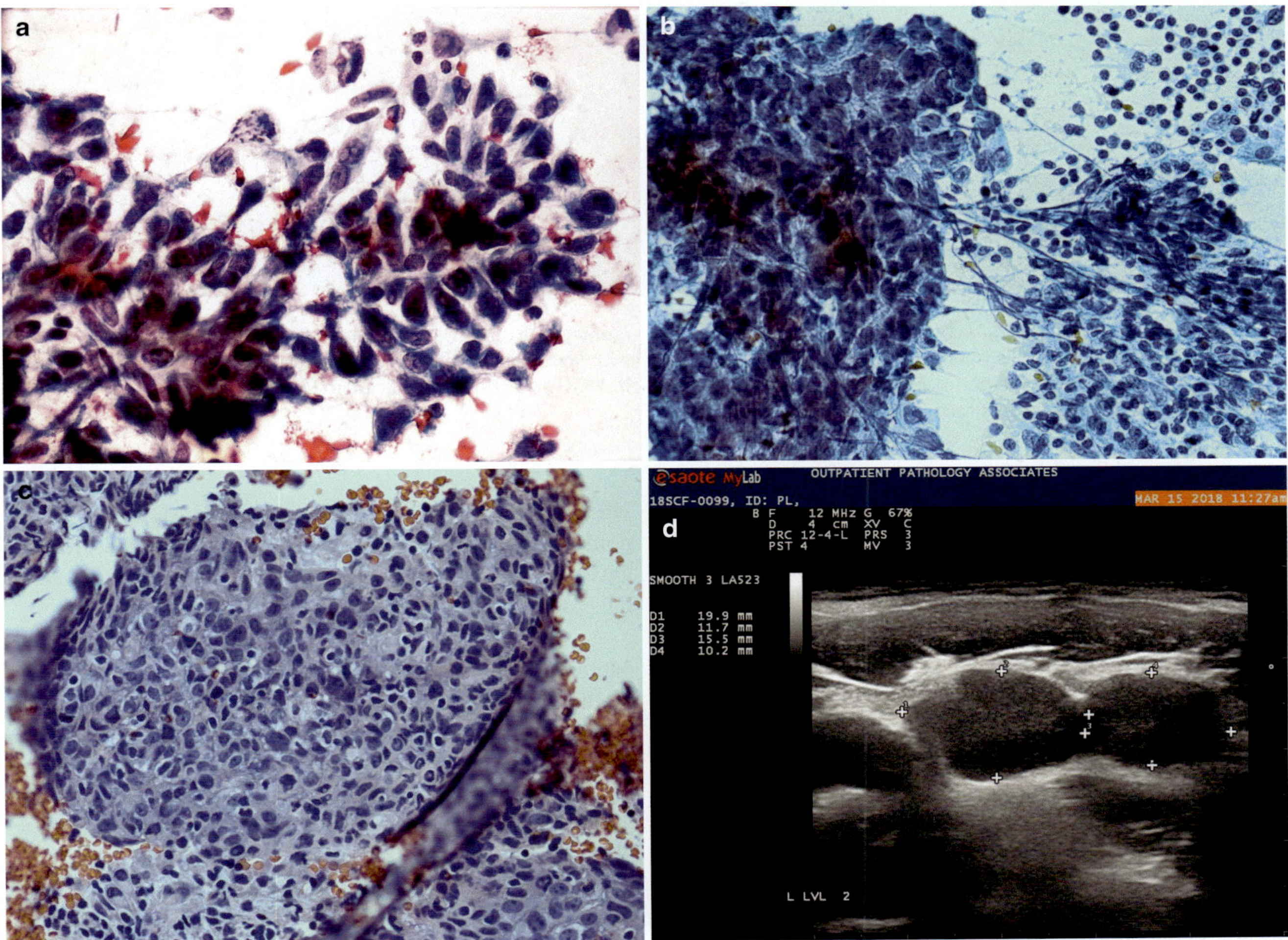

Fig. 7.49 Metastatic nasopharyngeal carcinoma. Undifferentiated carcinoma with spindle cell features (**a**) and non-keratinizing carcinoma (**b**) admixed with lymphocytes. Cell block (**c**) shows non-keratinizing carcinoma. The US features are not specific and include hypoechoic coalescent lymph nodes with lobulated sharp margins (**d**). (**a**, Papanicolaou stain, high magnification; **b**, **c**, MGG stain, high magnification)

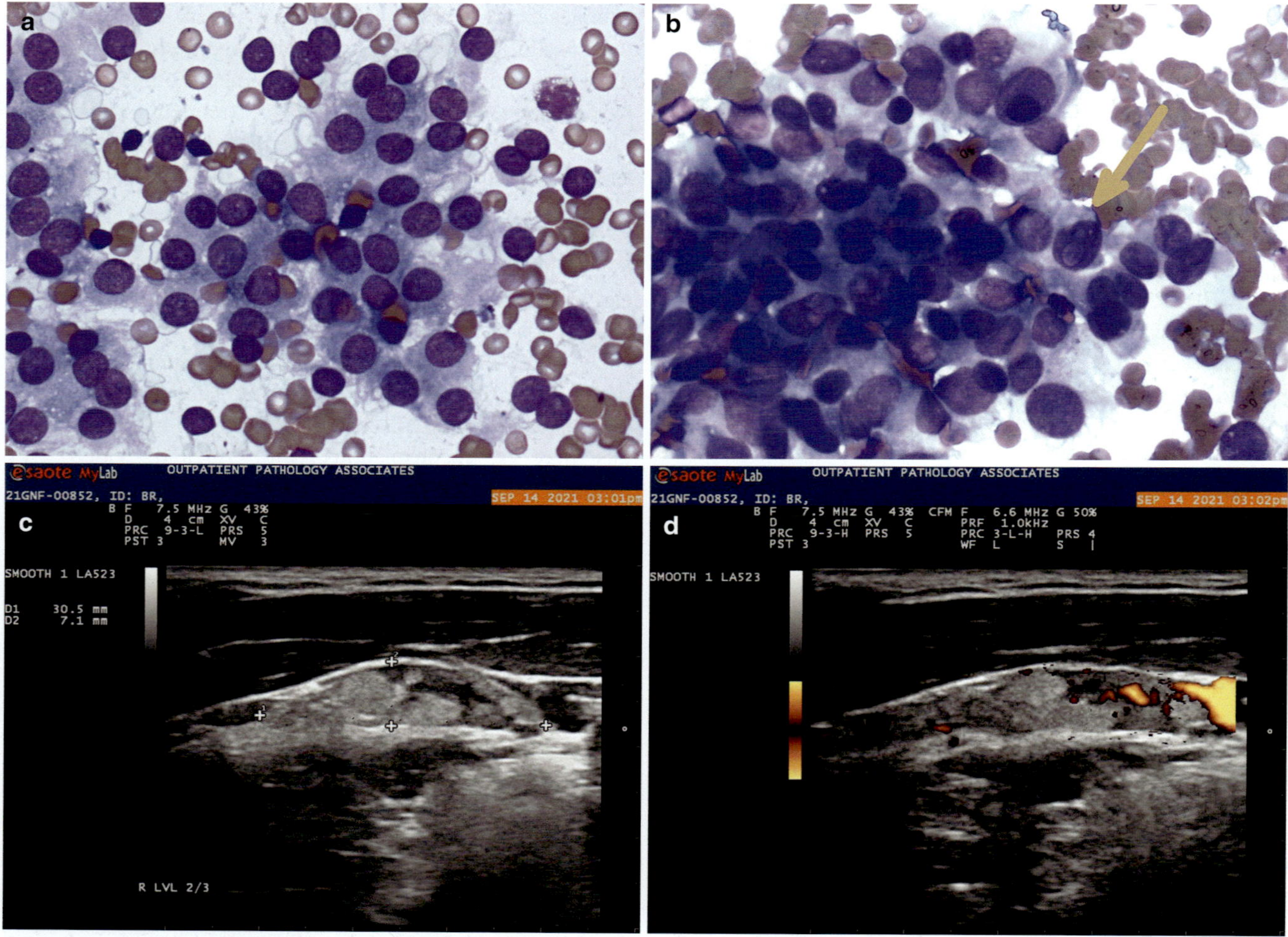

Fig. 7.50 Metastatic papillary thyroid carcinoma. This solid metastasis shows complex aggregates of follicular cells with hyperplastic features including ample finely vacuolated cytoplasm with lobulated and accentuated cytoplasmic borders and few intranuclear inclusions (arrow) (**a**, **b**). The US exam shows isoechoic, coalescent lymph nodes with nodular borders, and focal internal vascular blood flow (**c**, **d**). (**a**, **b**, MGG stain, high magnification) (Video 7.6)

information (Fig. 7.52a, b, Video 7.8). Medullary thyroid carcinoma shows dispersed small- to medium-sized cells with variable, usually ample cytoplasm, peripherally located round nuclei with fine chromatin, and small, inconspicuous nucleoli. Cells may be arranged in a pseudo-papillary pattern, and may show intranuclear inclusions and nuclear grooves, which may be erroneously interpreted as papillary carcinoma with oncocytic features. Furthermore, medullary thyroid carcinoma may show amyloid that resembles colloid, and macro- and microcalcifications by US, which are features that invite to render an erroneous diagnosis of papillary carcinoma (Fig. 7.53a–d). Measurement of thyroglobulin antibody levels for well-differentiated (papillary and follicular) carcinoma and calcitonin levels for medullary carcinoma, both in needle rinses complement the cytologic evaluation in these cases.

Papillary thyroid carcinoma cells can be highlighted by immunostainings with CK7, CK19, thyroglobulin, TTF1, HBME1, PAX8, COX2, and galectin 3. Medullary carcinoma cells are positive for low-molecular-weight CK (except CK7), calcitonin, chromogranin A, synaptophysin, NSE, CEA, CD56, and CD57.

Metastatic Breast Carcinoma The single most important predictor of clinical outcome is the sentinel lymph node, which is the ipsilateral axillary lymph node closest to the breast cancer tumor and likely to be the first to harbor a metastatic deposit. Intraoperative touch preparation cytology evaluation of a sentinel lymph node is the preferred technique. Alternatively, sampling by means of FNA can be done pre- or intraoperatively at the time of lumpectomy. If the sentinel lymph node is positive, the patient undergoes axillary lymph node dissection. Skip metastasis involving axillary lymph nodes other than the sentinel lymph node occurs in 5% of cases. Immunocytochemistry, independent of the subtype is positive for CK7 and GATA3, and variably positive

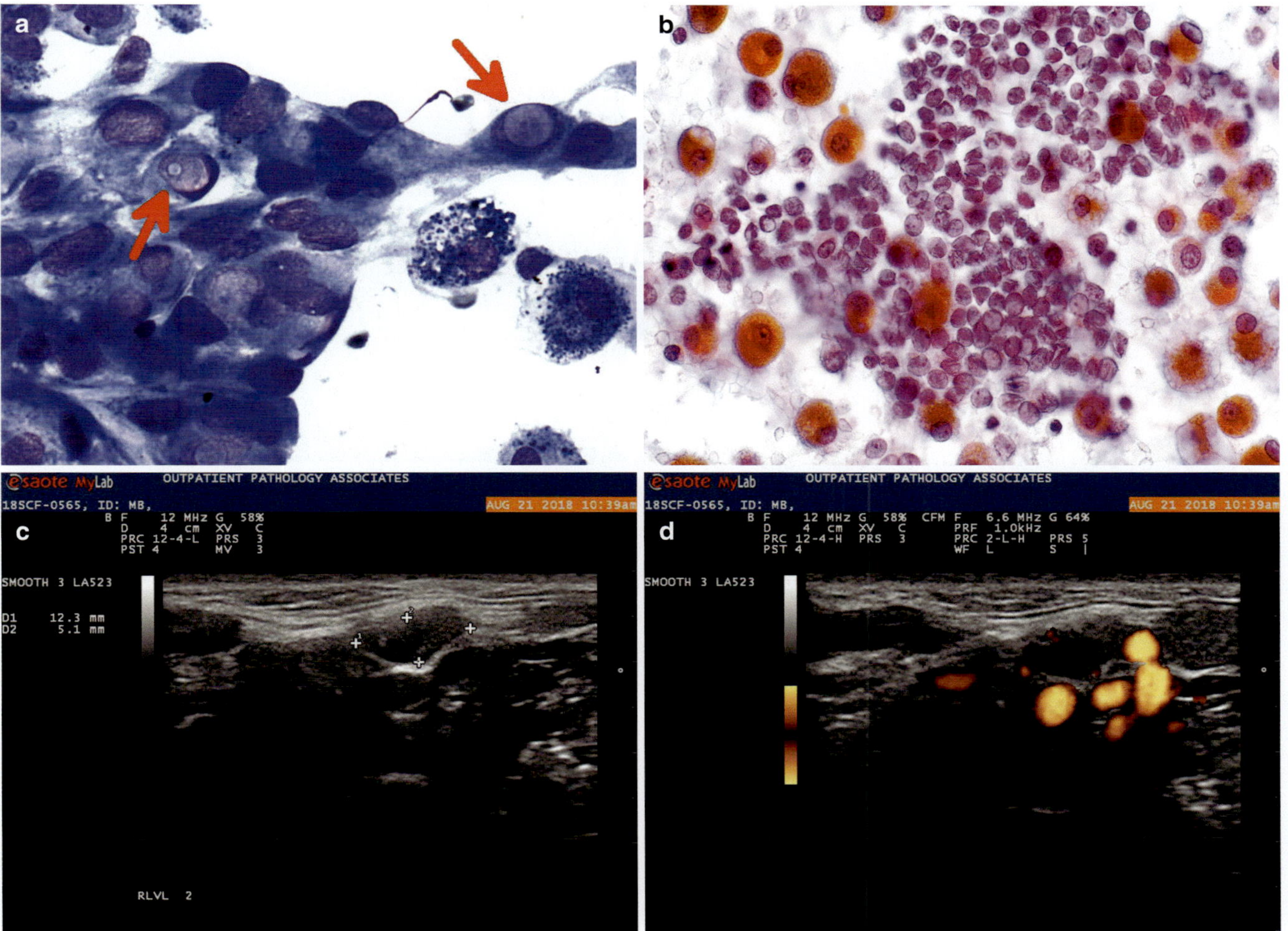

Fig. 7.51 Papillary thyroid carcinoma, cystic metastasis. Metaplastic cells with intranuclear cytoplasmic invaginations (arrows), numerous macrophages, and rare sheets of cells with pale chromatin, nuclear grooves, and intranuclear cytoplasmic invaginations (**a, b**). US exam shows an oddly shaped angulated lymph node with marked hypoechogenicity and no vascular blood flow by Doppler (**c, d**). (**a**, MGG stain, high magnification; **b**, Papanicolaou stain, high magnification) (Video 7.7)

for mammaglobin and GCFDP15. Positive ER, PR, and HER2 is seen in some cases (Fig. 7.54a–f).

Metastatic Melanoma

If the thickness of a cutaneous melanoma exceeds 0.76 mm, the risk of lymph node metastasis increases in parallel to the tumor thickness. The regional (sentinel) lymph nodes are involved before the melanoma spreads more distally. However, approximately 4% of melanomas show axillary, cervical, and inguinal lymph node metastases in the absence of a known primary site (spontaneous regression).

FNA Findings The diagnosis is facilitated by the clinical history and the demonstration of melanin pigment in tumor cells or histiocytes (melanophages), but melanin may be entirely absent, and a history of melanoma may not be available. Aspirates are usually cellular, containing round or oval, spindle-shaped, and pleomorphic cells in various proportions. This pleomorphic pattern is characteristic of metastatic melanoma; however, anaplastic nuclei, prominent nucleoli, intranuclear cytoplasmic invaginations, and melanin pigment may not be present in all cell types. In equivocal cases, stains for S100 protein, Melan A, HMB-45, and SOX10 are helpful. Of note, the S100 protein stain is also positive in the interdigitating reticulum cells of the lymph node (Fig. 7.55a–h). Melanoma may mimic the cytomorphology of any neoplasm, including large-cell lymphoma, although metastatic melanoma cells are usually larger and more pleomorphic. The rare amelanotic melanoma with lymphocyte-like or plasmacytoid-like cytomorphology may also resemble lymphoma or plasmacytoma; however, the smear background lacks lymphoglandular bodies. The spindle-cell type must be distinguished from spindle-cell neoplasms (Fig. 7.56a–d).

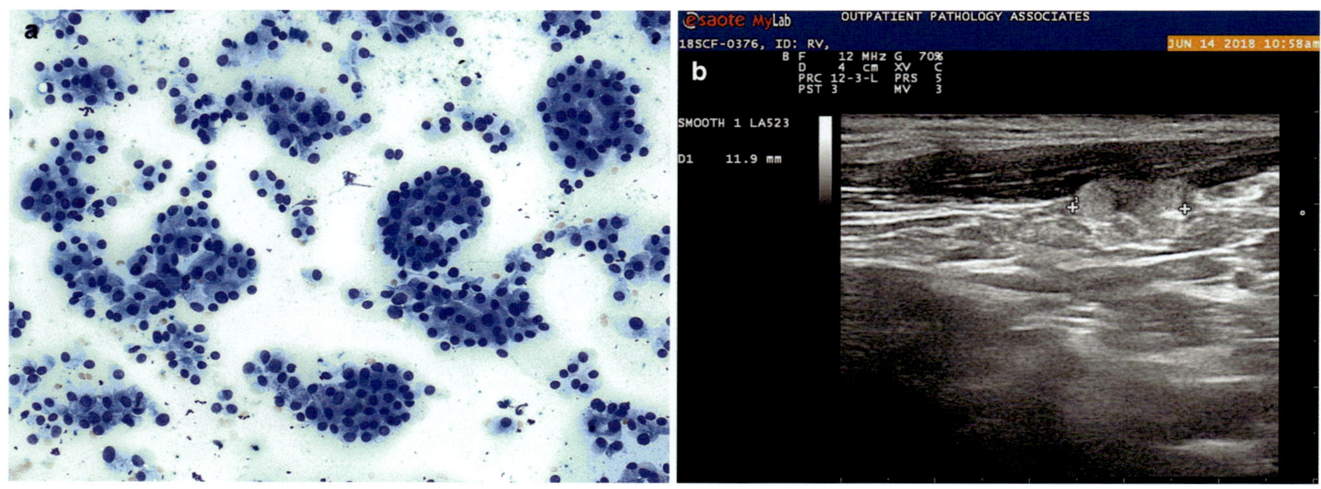

Fig. 7.52 Metastatic follicular thyroid carcinoma. A microfollicular pattern composed of bland-appearing follicular cells with oncocytic features (**a**). The US exam shows a small hyperechogenic metastatic lymph node encroaching upon the neck strap muscle (**b**). (**a**, MGG stain, medium magnification) (Video 7.8)

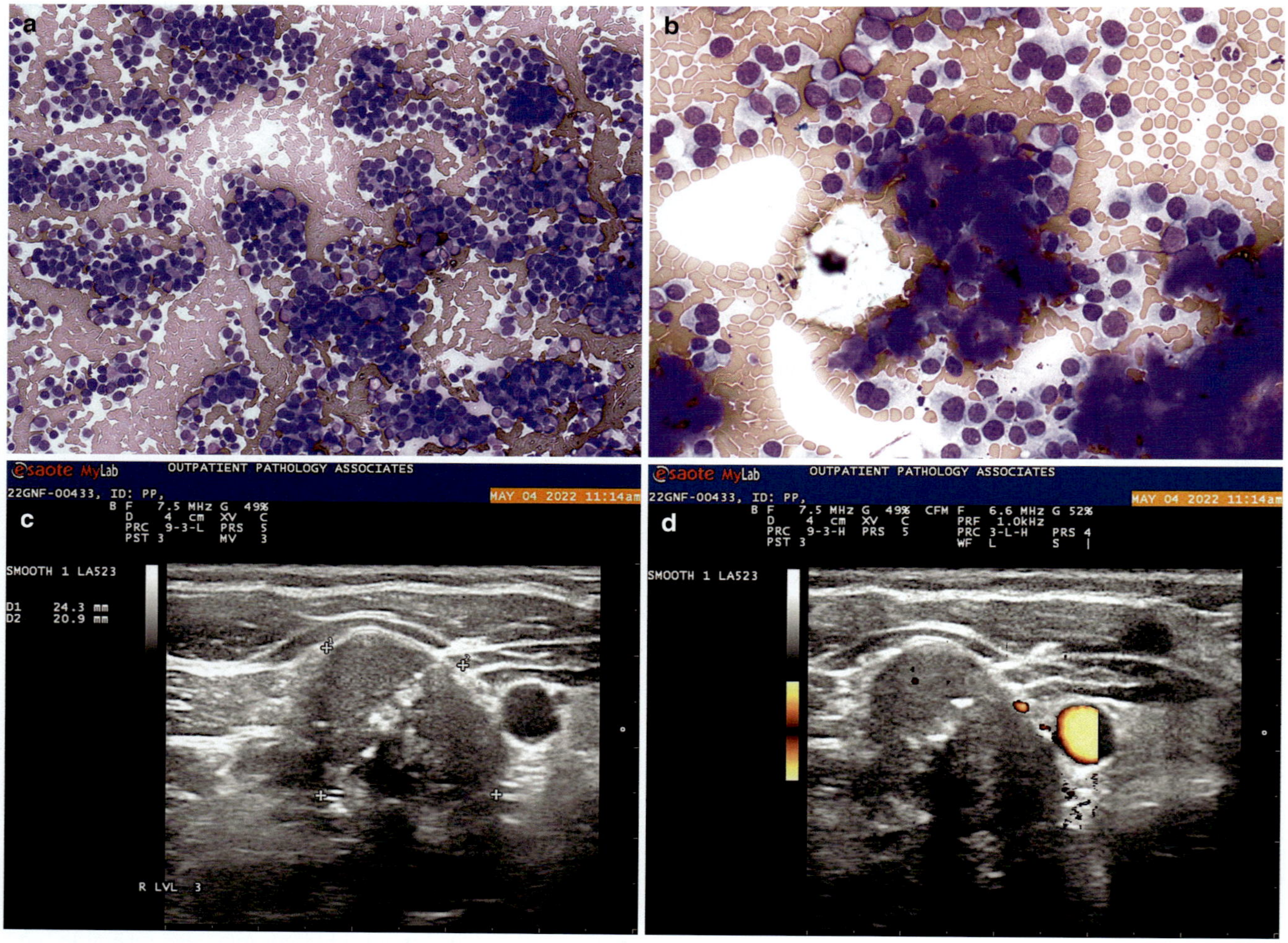

Fig. 7.53 Metastatic medullary thyroid carcinoma. Complex aggregates and microfollicles composed of medium size cells with slight anisonucleosis (**a**). Binucleation, peripheral nuclei, dense granular cytoplasm, inconspicuous nucleoli, and colloid-like amyloid (**b**). The US exam shows a hypoechogenic lymph node with abnormal shape, irregular ill-defined borders, macro- and microcalcifications, and no vascular blood flow (**a**, **b**, MGG stain, medium and high magnification)

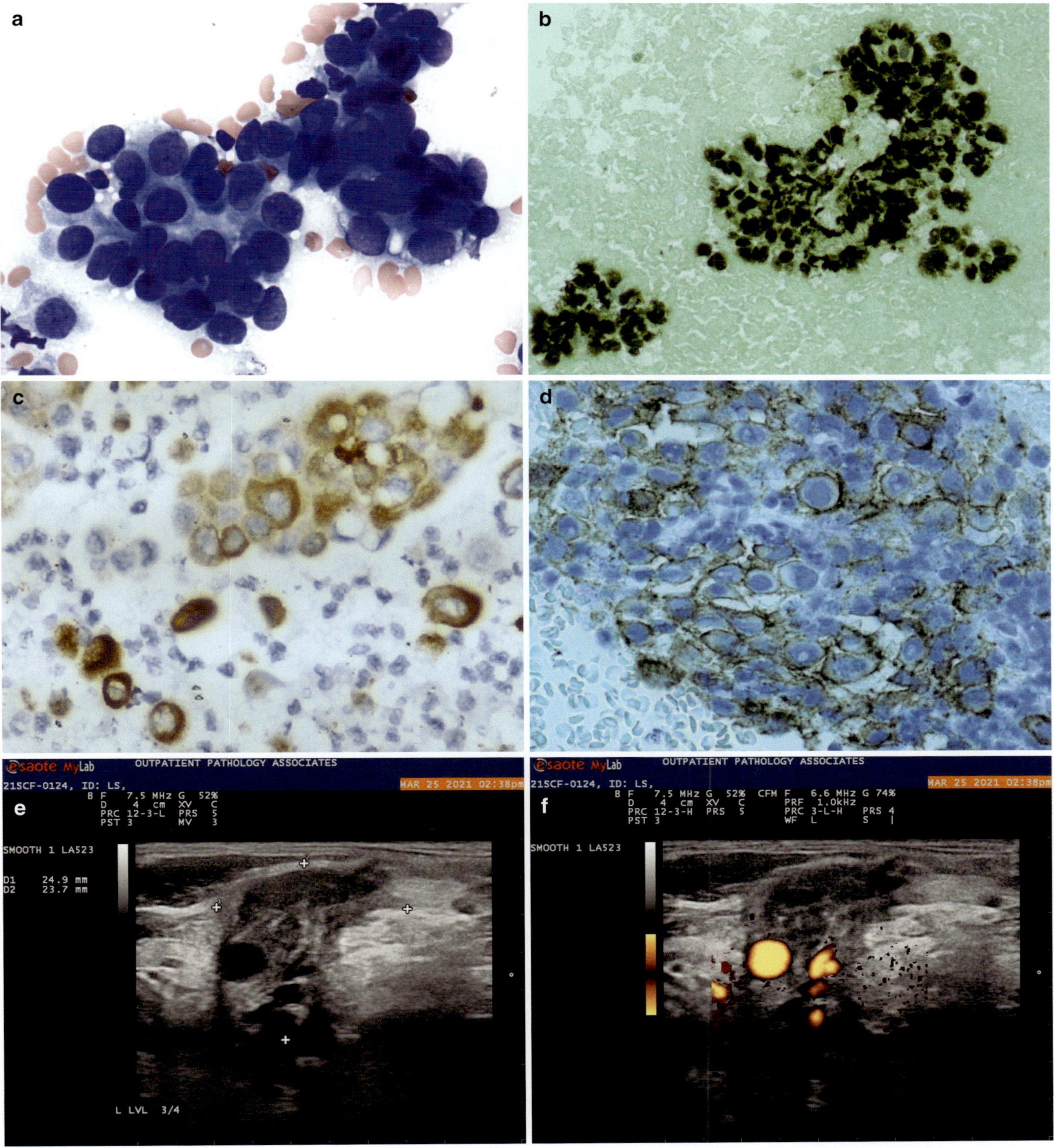

Fig. 7.54 Metastatic breast carcinoma. Neck level IV LN. Gland-forming aggregates of malignant cells with thin cytoplasm, ill-defined cytoplasmic borders, round nucleus, and inconspicuous nucleoli (**a**). Positive immunostains for GATA3, mammaglobin, and Her2 in the cell block (**b**–**d** respectively). The US exam shows a hypoechoic and hetero-geneous lymph node with ill-defined and spiculated borders, and poor vascular blood flow (**e**, **f**). (**a**, MGG stain high magnification; **b**–**d**, Immunoperoxidase stains, high magnification) (**c**, From Leonardo and Bardales (2020). Reprinted with permission)

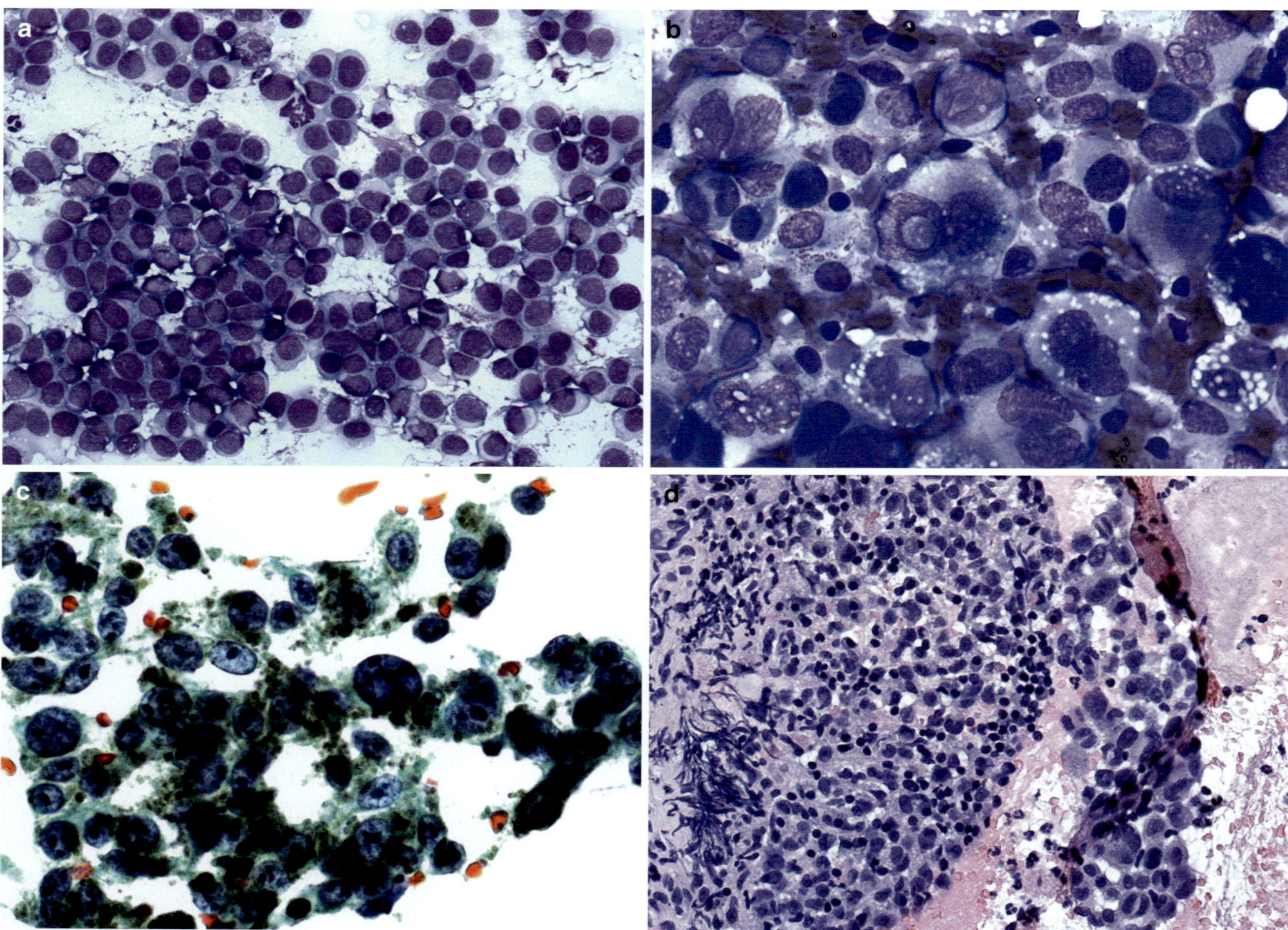

Fig. 7.55 Metastatic melanoma. Plasmacytoid cells, anisocytosis, an abnormal mitotic figure, finely vacuolated cytoplasm, and rare large cells with intranuclear cytoplasmic invaginations (**a**, **b**). Markedly pleomorphic cells with cytoplasmic brown melanin pigment, and prominent nucleoli (**c**). Corresponding cell block (**c**) with metastatic melanoma and positive immunostains for Melan A and SOX10 (**d**–**f**). The US evaluation shows a large hypoechogenic lymph node (inguinal) with abnormal shape, heterogeneous echotexture, lobulated borders, and internal abnormal vascular blood flow (**g**, **h**). (**a**, **b**, MGG stain, medium and high magnification; **c**, Papanicolaou stain, high magnification; **d**, hematoxylin and eosin, medium magnification; **e**, **f**, immunoperoxidase stains, high magnification)

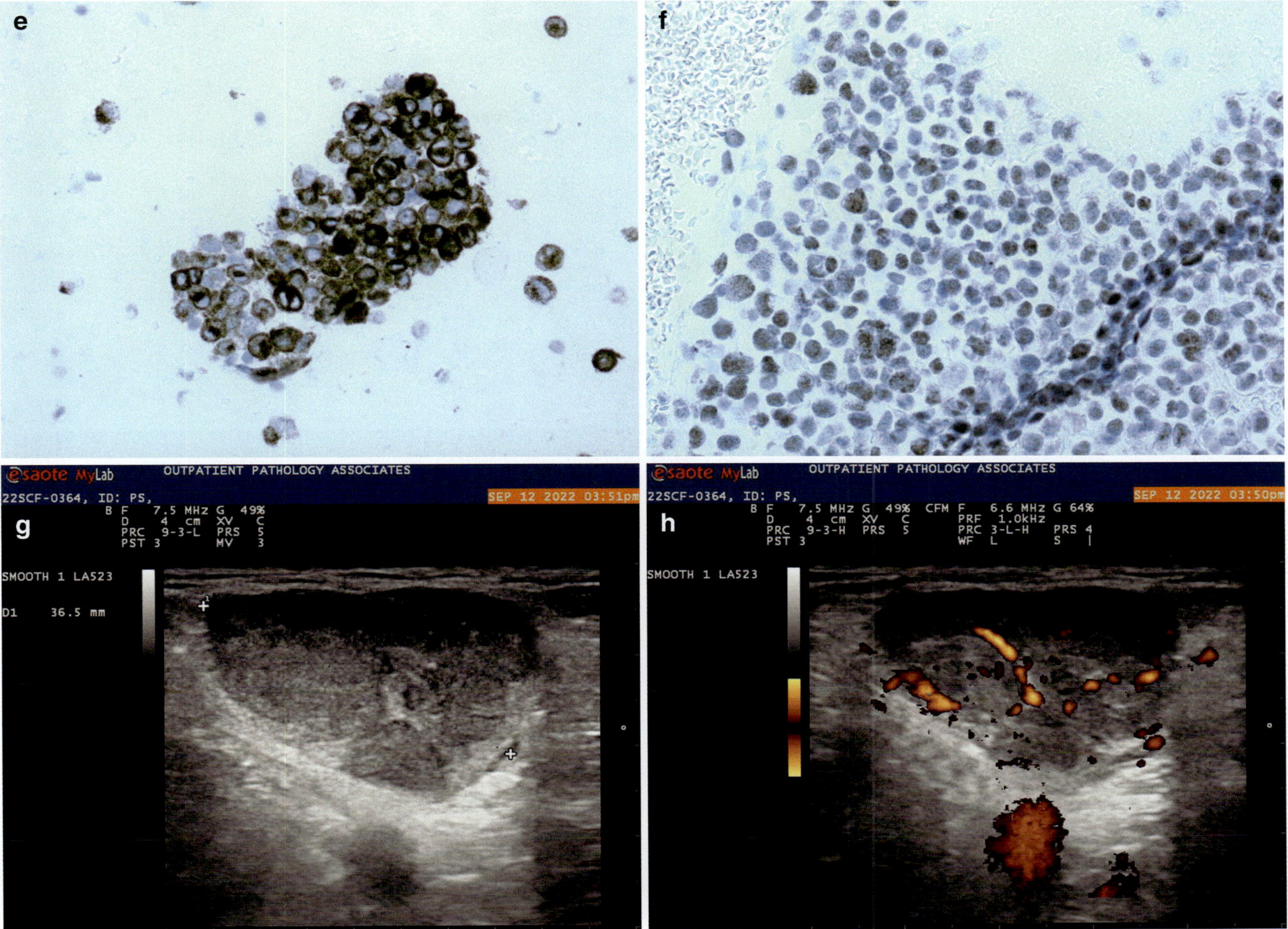

Fig. 7.55 (continued)

Metastatic Merkel Cell Carcinoma

Merkel cell carcinoma is a rare primary neuroendocrine tumor of the skin which occurs particularly in the head and upper extremities of elderly individuals. This tumor is aggressive and may produce multiple distant metastases, including lymph nodes.

FNA Findings Aspirates are cellular, composed of intermediate-sized cells with a variable degree of cohesiveness. Cells have uniform round or oval nuclei with fine chromatin, and small nucleoli. The cytoplasm is scant and fragile. Cell molding is not a feature. Scattered mitoses and apoptotic nuclei are present, and the background lacks lymphoglandular bodies. The most characteristic feature is the presence of an inconspicuous small spherical perinuclear cytoplasmic aggregate ("button") of intermediate filaments (keratin). The cells show a positive immunostain for CK8, CK18, CK19, CK20, chromogranin, synaptophysin, and NSE. The keratin stain highlights the cytoplasmic condensation (Fig. 7.57a–d).

The differential diagnosis includes small-cell carcinoma of salivary gland or lung origin, lymphoma, and solid adenoid cystic carcinoma. The presence of "buttons" and small perinuclear clear zones are important for diagnosing Merkel cell carcinoma. In some cases, the use of special stains is necessary. The demonstration of the Merkel cell polyomavirus is diagnostic.

Metastatic Mesenchymal Malignancies

Lymph node metastases from sarcomas are unusual; however, when they occur, they may mimic carcinomas or lymphomas of Hodgkin or non-Hodgkin type, including ALCL due to the presence of pleomorphic single cells or loose clusters in a lymphoid background. Of the metastatic mesenchymal neoplasms, the most likely to be confused with such entities are metastatic high-grade undifferentiated sarcomas (malignant fibrous histiocytomas), metastatic rhabdomyosarcomas, and metastatic neuroblastomas. Metastatic neuro-

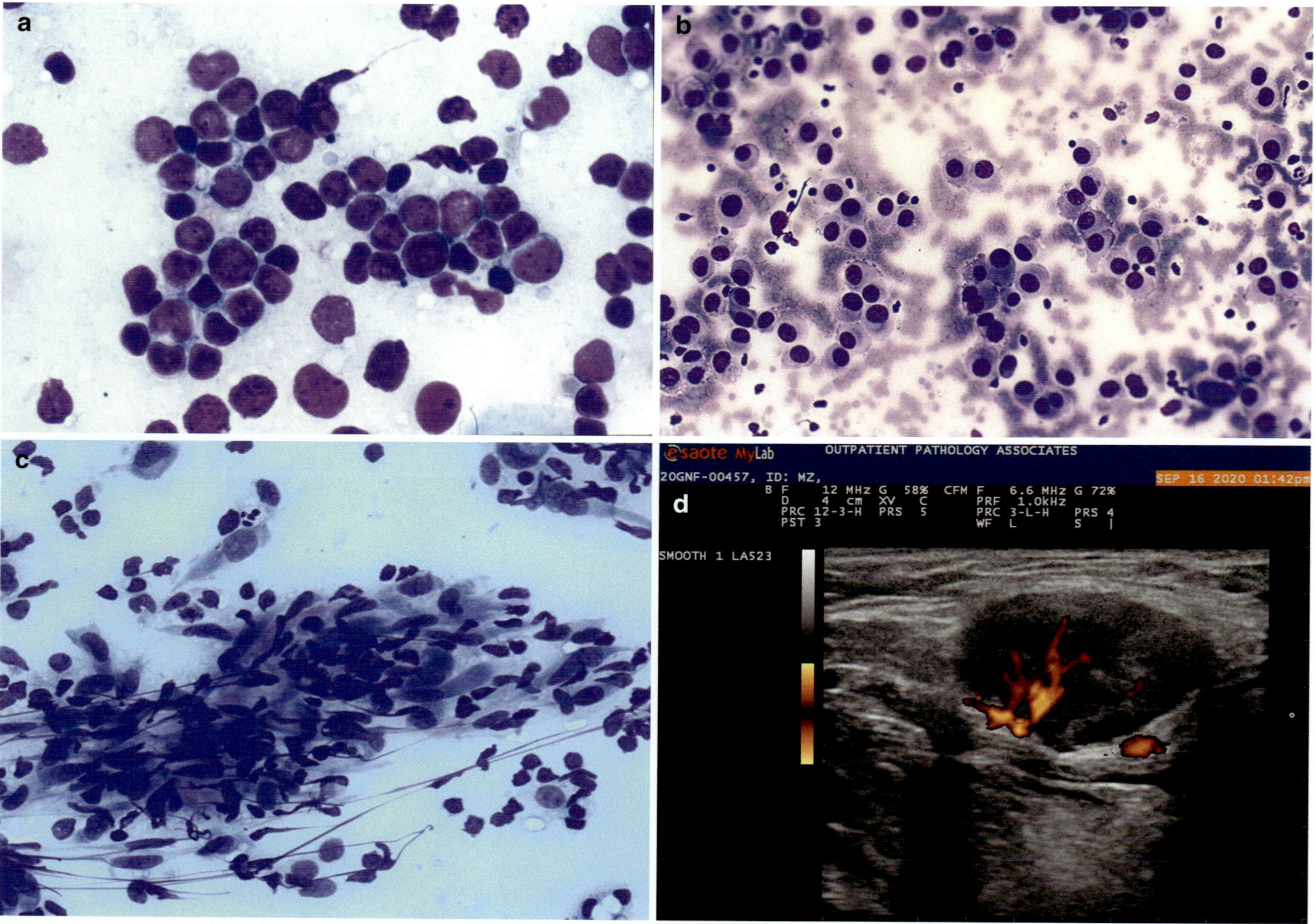

Fig. 7.56 Metastatic amelanotic melanoma of lymphoid, plasma, and spindle cell cytomorphology (**a–c**). US show hypoechoic lymph node with abnormal vascular blood flow (**d**). (**a–c** MGG stain, medium and high magnification)

blastoma may show a spectrum of neuroblastic to ganglion cell differentiation, with large, frequently multinucleated ganglion-like cells which may mimic Hogkin/Reed-Sternberg cells or ALCL cells. The identification of neuropil-like material in the background is diagnostically useful. The correct diagnosis is made by clinical correlation and immunostains (desmin and myogenin in rhabdomyosarcoma and NSE in neuroblastoma).

The Virchow's Lymph Node

The supraclavicular lymph nodes are the most likely site to harbor cancer. Left supraclavicular lymphadenopathy is usually an ominous sign of disseminated disease from a primary site in the lung (Fig. 7.58a–l), esophagus (Fig. 7.58m, n), breast, and below the diaphragm, including but not restricted to the stomach, ovary (Fig. 7.58o, p), colon (Fig. 7.58q–t), biliary tract, pancreas, uterus. It may be the first evidence of an aggressive disease in patients with prostatic adenocarcinoma (Fig. 7.58u, v).

Ultrasound Features of Lymph Nodes Involved by Metastases

Lymph nodes affected metastases are usually in the territory of lymphatic drainage of the primary tumor, unless is a widely metastatic process. In squamous cell and papillary thyroid carcinomas, the metastatic lymph node may be as small as 0.5 cm. Lymph nodes often have the following characteristics: taller than wide (>2×) or round, usually hypoechoic, confluent, absent hilum, eccentric cortical thickening, partial or total cystic necrosis, abnormal peripheral vascularization, and sharp margins. The lymph node margins are ill-defined or spiculated when there is lymph node extracapsular spread, or lobulated and irregular when there is subcapsular metastases. It may be hyperechoic with microcalcifcations in metastatic papillary thyroid carcinoma, metastatic medullary thyroid carcinoma, and ovarian serous papillary carcinoma (Figs. 7.46c, d, 7.47c, d, 7.48e, f, 7.49d, 7.50c, d, 7.51c, d, 7.52b, 7.53c, d, 7.54e, f, 7.55g, h, 7.56d, 7.57d, 7.58d, h, k, l, n, p, t, v).

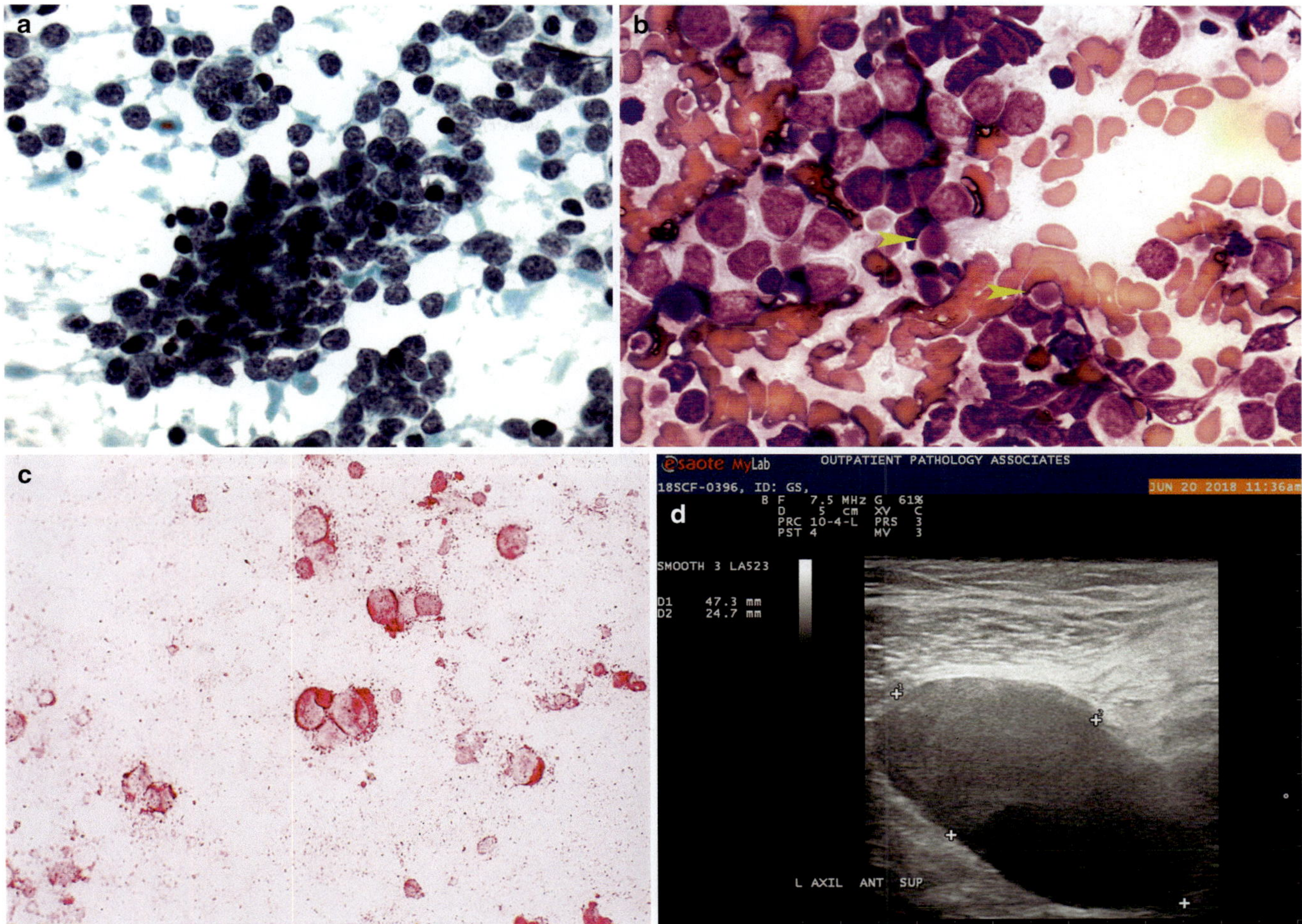

Fig. 7.57 Metastatic Merkel cell carcinoma. Complex aggregates of intermediate size cells with scant cytoplasm, granular coarse chromatin, and paranuclear dense cytoplasmic round aggregates of intermediate filaments or "buttons" (**a**, **b**, arrow heads) highlighted by the keratin immunostain (**c**). The US features are not specific and include oval, large, hypoechoic axillary lymph node with well-defined margins (**d**). (**a**, Papanicolaou stain high magnification; **b**, DiffQuik® stain high magnification; **c**, immunoperoxidase stain, high magnification)

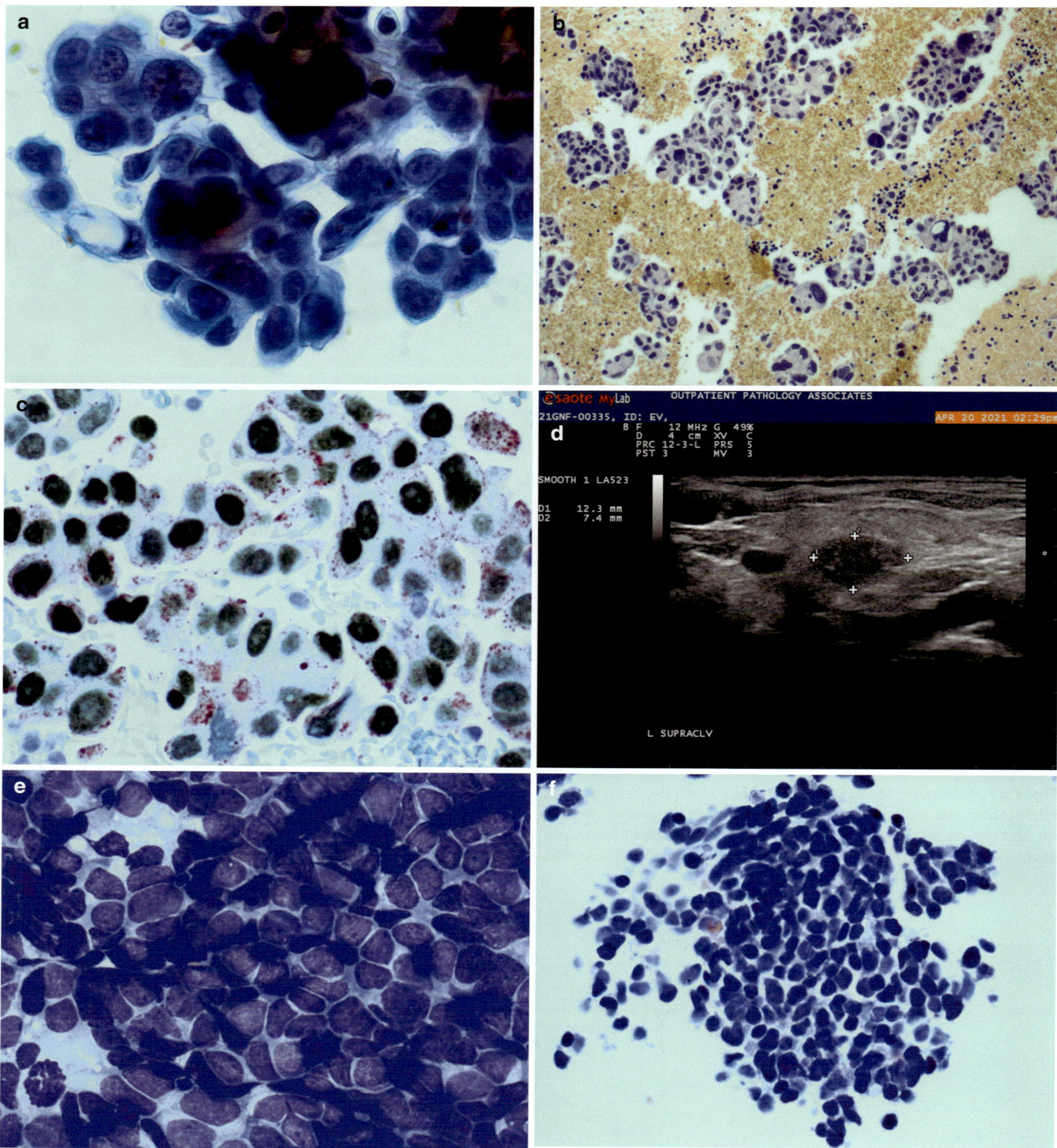

Fig. 7.58 The Virchows' lymph node metastases. Lung adenocarcinoma to a 12-mm lymph node with positive immunostain for TTF-1/Napsin A in the cell block (**a**–**d**). Lung small cell carcinoma to a left 18-mm lymph node with positive CD56 in the cell block (**e**–**h**) Lung anaplastic carcinoma to a 17-mm lymph node (**i**–**l**). Esophageal adenocarcinoma to a 24-mm lymph node (**m**, **n**). Ovarian serous carcinoma to a 16-mm lymph node (**o**, **p**). Colonic adenocarcinoma to matted lymph nodes with positive immunostains for CEA and CK20 (**q**–**t**). Prostate adenocarcinoma to an 18-mm lymph node (**u**, **v**). The US evaluation in these cases show hypoechogenic lymph nodes with heterogeneous echotexture, fuzzy, irregular, spiculated, or lobulated borders, and abnormal shape, some taller than wide with microcalcifications and abnormal vascular blood flow. (**a**, **m**, **o**, **q**, Papanicolaou stain, high magnification; **b**, **f**, cell block hematoxylin and eosin stain, medium magnification; **c**, **g**, **r**, **s**, immunoperoxidase stain, medium and high magnification; **e**, **i**, **j**, **u**, MGG stain, high magnification)

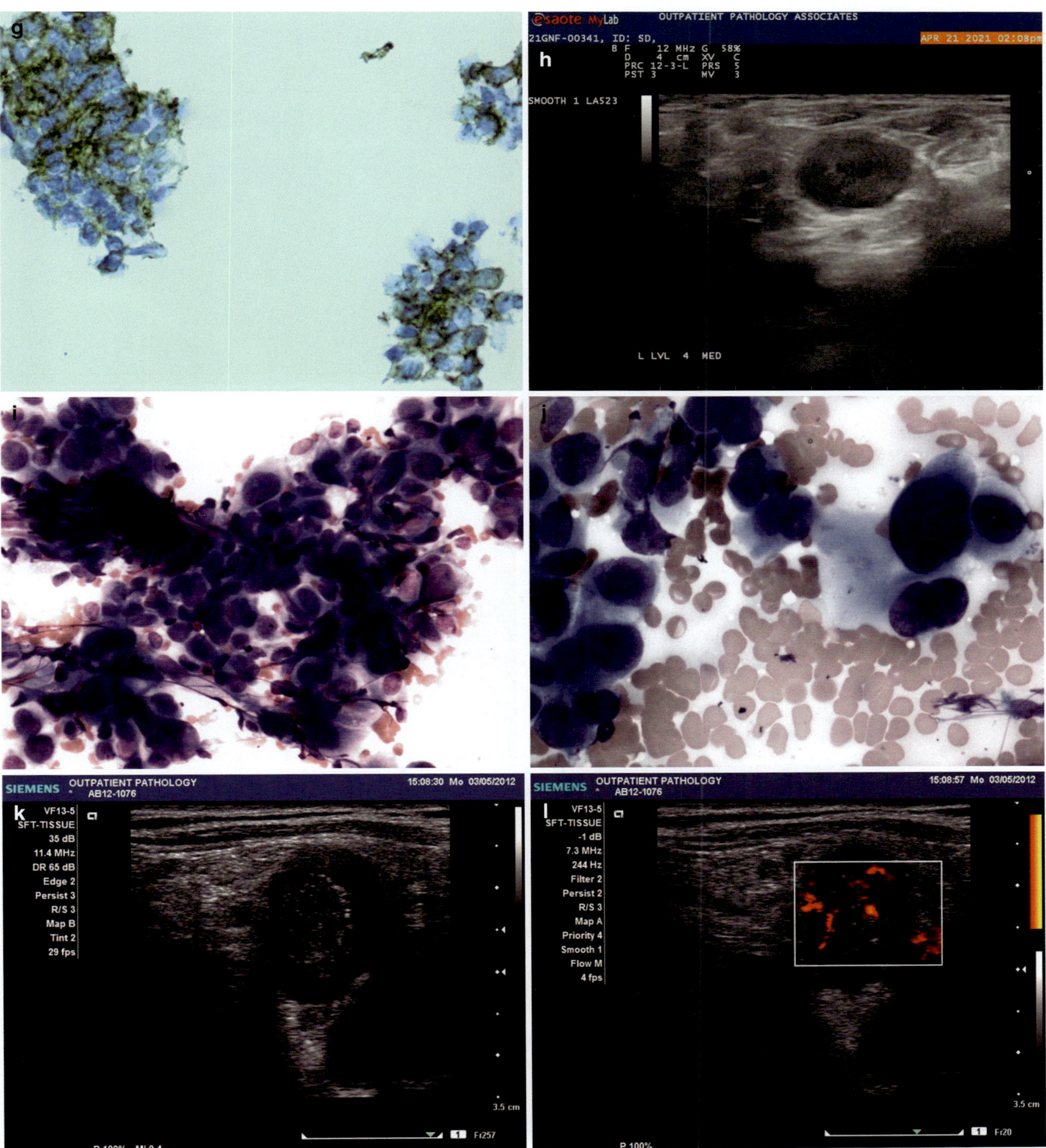

Fig. 7.58 (continued)

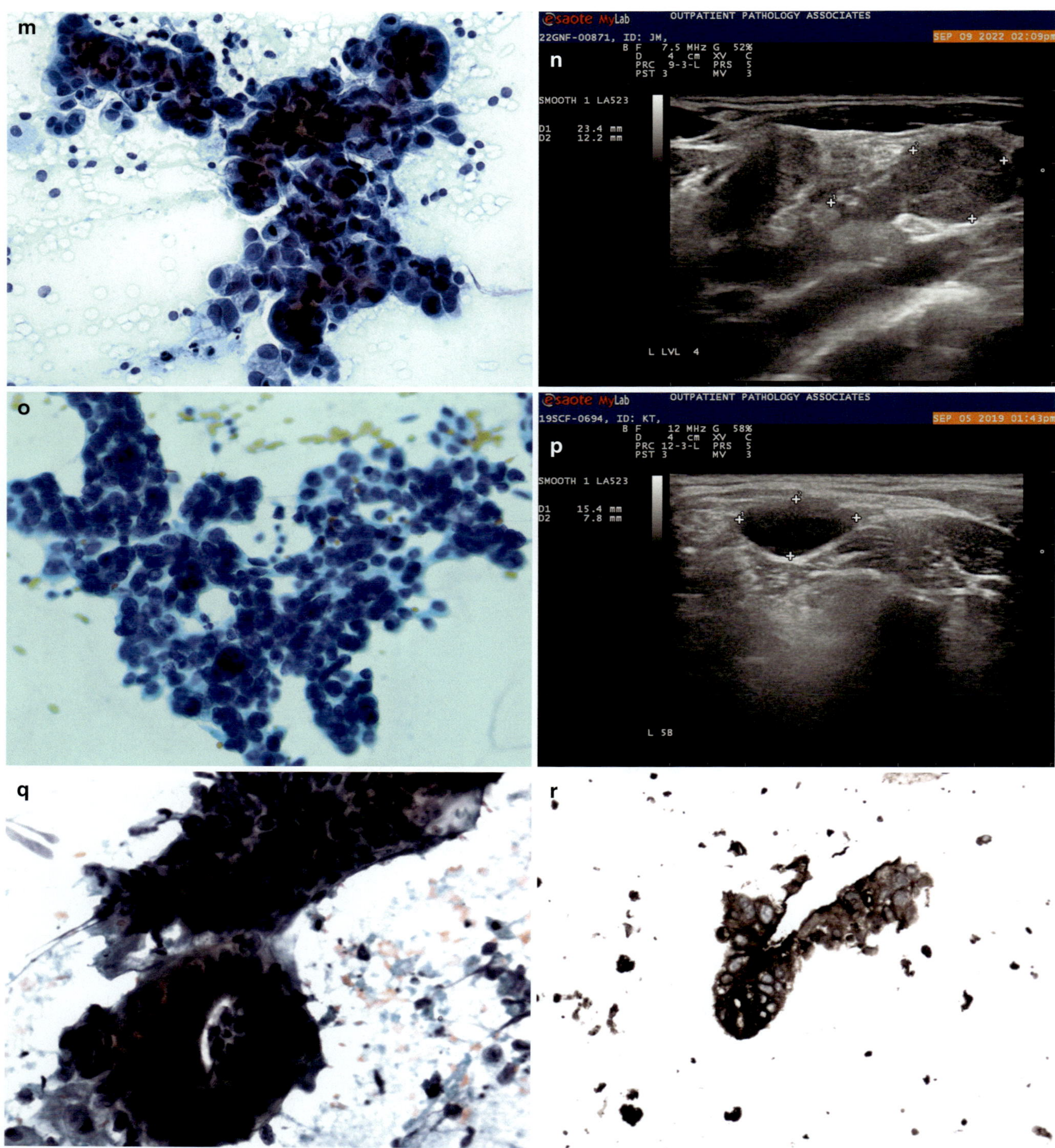

Fig. 7.58 (continued)

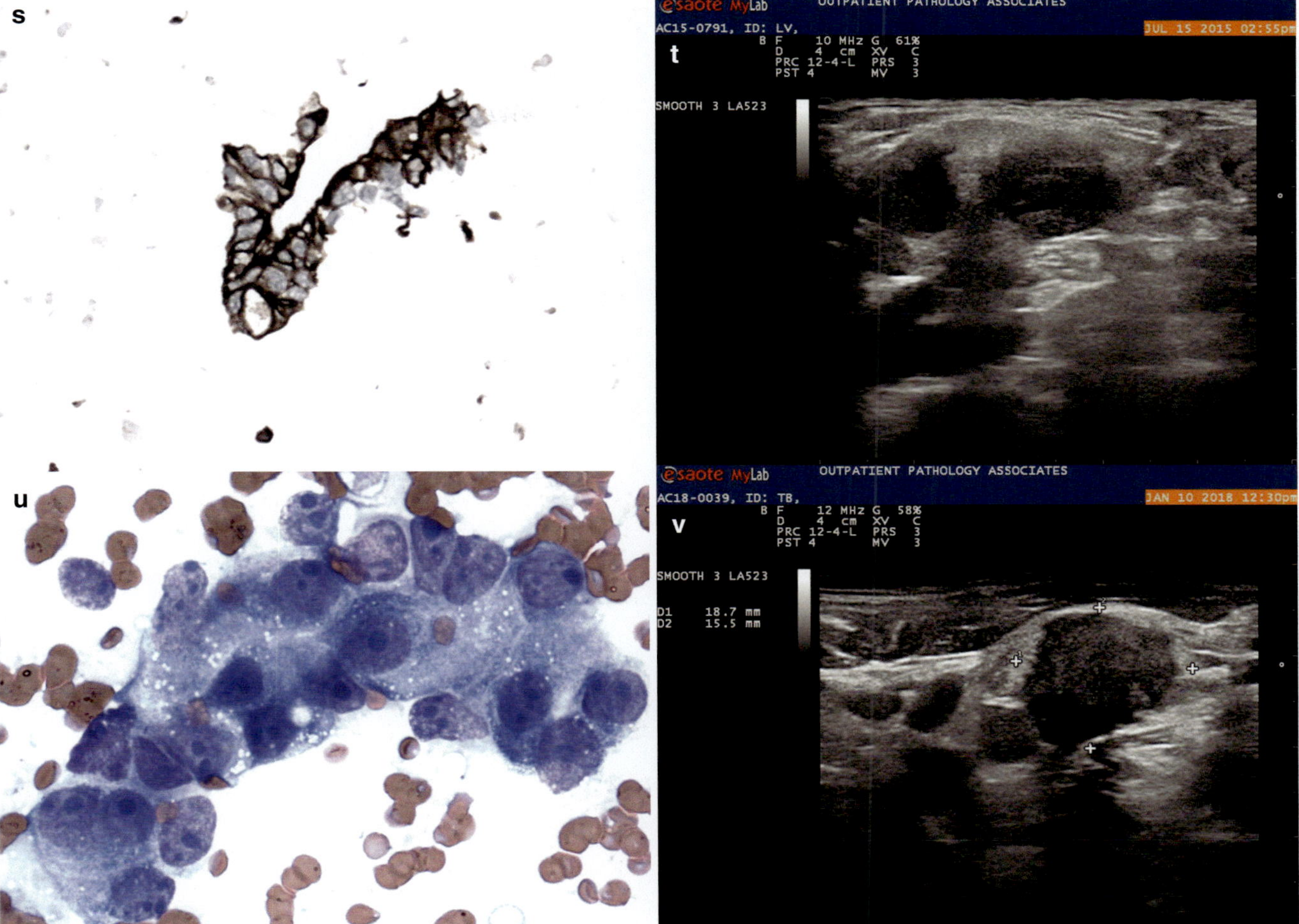

Fig. 7.58 (continued)

Further Reading

Al-Abbadi MA, Barroca H, Bode-Lesniewska B, Calaminici M, Caraway NP, Chhieng DF, et al. A proposal for the performance, classification, and reporting of lymph node fine-needle aspiration cytopathology: The Sydney system. Acta Cytol. 2020;64(4):306–22. https://doi.org/10.1159/000506497.

Alaggio R, et al. The 5th edition of the World Health Organization Classification of hematolymphoid tumors: lymphoid neoplasms. Leukemia. 2022;36:1720–48.

Bardales R. The invasive cytopathologist. Ultrasound guided fine-needle aspiration of superficial masses. New York: Springer; 2014.

Cook JR. Nodal and leukemic small B-cell neoplasms. Mod Pathol. 2013;26(Suppl 1):S15–28.

Ioachim HL, Medeiros LJ. Ioachim's lymph node pathology. Philadelphia: Lippincott Wlliams and Wilkins; 2009.

Leonardo E, Bardales RH. Practical immunocytochemistry is diagnostic cytology. Cham: Springer; 2020.

Nithagon P, Tsang P. WHO & ICC-B cell. 2022. PathologyOutlines. com website. https://www.pathologyoutlines.com/topic/lymphomaWHOHAEM5ICCBcell.html. Accessed 3 January 2024.

Pambuccian SE, Bardales RH. Lymph node cytopathology. Philadelphia: Springer; 2011.

Rhys R. Cervical lymph nodes. In: Allan PL, Baxter GM, Weston MJ, editors. Clinical ultrasound, vol. 2. London: Churchill Livingstone; 2011. p. 920–37.

Said JW. Aggressive B-cell lymphomas: how many categories do we need? Mod Pathol. 2013;26(Suppl 1):S42–56.

Skoog L, Tani E. FNA cytology in the diagnosis of lymphoma. Basel: Karger; 2009.

Swerdlow SH, Campo E, et al. WHO classification of tumors of haematopoietic and lymphoid tissues. Lyon: IARC; 2008.

Twist CJ, Link MP. Assessment of lymphadenopathy in children. Pediatr Clin N Am. 2002;49(5):1009–25.

Weiss LM, O'Malley D. Benign lymphadenopathies. Mod Pathol. 2013;26(Suppl 1):S88–96.

The Breast

Ricardo H. Bardales and Eugenio Leonardo

Background and General Concepts

Breast imaging has become the main tool in breast cancer screening and diagnosis and has a major impact on breast cancer staging. Interventional radiologists and cytopathologists may obtain adequate tissue samples for pathologic evaluation of palpable and non-palpable, but ultrasound (US)-visible lesions. However, the cytopathologist is more skilled in obtaining FNA cytology samples under US guidance (USG-FNA), a minimally invasive and cost-effective technique that avoids a more costly core needle biopsy (CNB) for a potentially benign condition. Microcalcifications without a palpable or US-visible lesion must be sampled under stereotactic guidance.

It is our experience that FNA sampling by capillarity without aspiration (Zajdela technique) with use of a 25-G needle may yield less cellular samples but provides sufficient material for diagnosis of most breast lesions. It has been suggested that adding aspiration lowers the yield of non-diagnostic specimens when benign breast lesions are studied. This is in part due to the fibro-fatty tissue composition of the normal breast tissue that yields sparsely cellular samples. For smaller or non-palpable lesions, USG-FNA samples are adequate and diagnostic.

In experienced hands, FNA of breast lesions can be highly accurate, with sensitivity between 80% and 100% and specificity of 99% when radiologic evaluation is provided and clinical evaluation and FNA are performed by the cytopathologist who also interprets the FNA. The so-called triple test (clinical, radiology, and FNA) results must be congruent for guiding an appropriate therapeutic management. If the cytopathologist did not perform the FNA, he or she must know the clinico-radiologic findings before the FNA interpretation is given. If one of the three is discrepant, CNB, open biopsy, or a frozen section may be required prior to definitive surgery.

Rapid on-site evaluation (ROSE) for evaluation of sample adequacy and often providing a preliminary diagnosis are important and will prompt the operator to obtain material to perform additional studies, i.e., hormonal receptor studies, cultures, flow cytometry. As mentioned in the technical section of this book, in our practice, the cytopathologist triages the material on site and, if necessary, obtains CNBs under US guidance. Alternatively, a cell block may be obtained for performing hormone receptor immunohistochemistry or other ancillary tests, including molecular studies (Fig. 8.1a, b, Videos 8.1 and 8.2).

In our laboratory, a specimen is considered adequate when at least six clusters or sheets of at least 15 epithelial cells each, or any number of well-smeared and stained (Romanowsky or Papanicolaou stain) epithelial cells each are present. Specimen adequacy is influenced by the clinical impression of the operator and by radiologic findings. Non-epithelial lesions such as an adipose tissue mammary prominence or lipoma do not have epithelial elements and should not be considered a non-diagnostic specimen.

FNA cytology cannot distinguish between in situ and invasive carcinoma and cannot further define all "atypias." For most benign conditions, cytology cannot give a specific diagnosis. However, when FNA diagnoses of "malignancy," "atypia," or "benign" are reached, CNB, open biopsy, or lumpectomy will follow in the first two instances and a conservative approach in the last, as outlined in the Yokohama System for Reporting Breast FNA Biopsy cytopathology covered in the next section of this chapter.

CNB and FNA are complementary tests for evaluating palpable and non-palpable US-visible breast masses and can

Supplementary Information The online version contains supplementary material available at https://doi.org/10.1007/978-3-031-73702-2_8.

R. H. Bardales
Precision Pathology, Outpatient Pathology Associates, Sacramento, CA, USA

E. Leonardo (✉)
Surgical Pathologist and Professor Emeritus, University Hospital of Trieste, Torino, Italy

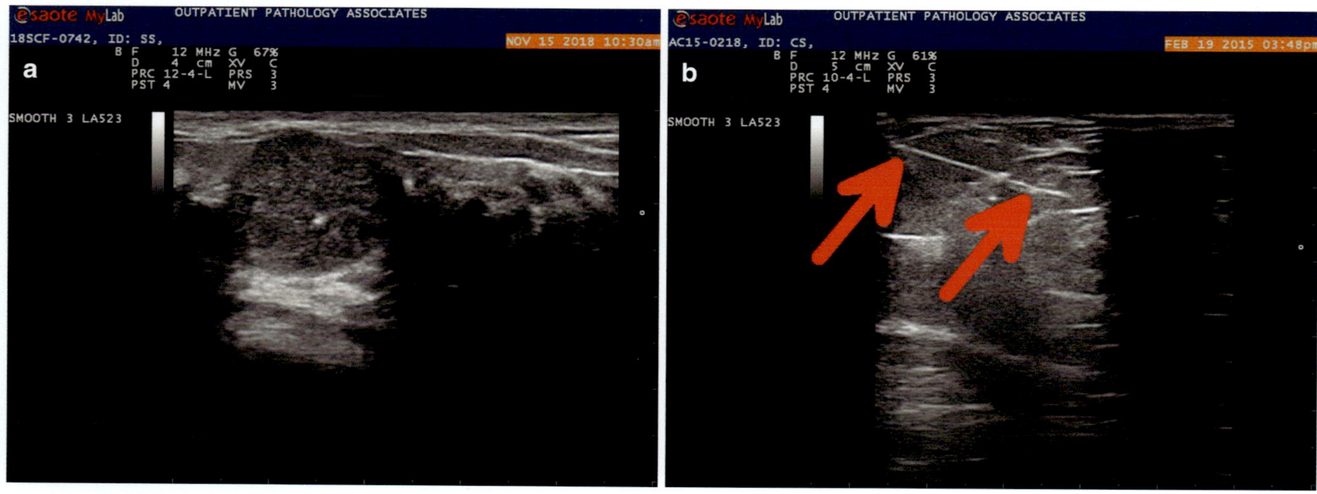

Fig. 8.1 US-guided fine-needle aspiration of fibroadenoma, perpendicular approach. Needle tip is visualized as a bright dot (**a**). US-guided core needle biopsy of an ill-defined adipose tissue prominence. Arrows point the visualized needle length (**b**)

modify decisions before surgery, may affect surgical outcome, or may avoid unnecessary surgery in benign conditions.

Complications of breast FNA are rare. Local pain and hematoma are the most common, and the latter can be minimized by applying firm pressure to the area of the FNA. Pneumothorax is a very rare complication. Needle track seeding of malignancy has been reported with large core needle biopsies, but is exceedingly rare with FNA. Histologic changes and epithelial displacement have been reported post FNA. The latter may be seen in breast carcinoma in situ and simulates invasive malignancy.

The FNA Report

The International Academy of Cytology (IAC) Yokohama System for Reporting Breast FNA Biopsy Cytopathology uses five categories, and each has a specific risk of malignancy. The FNA diagnostic categories are: "insufficient/ inadequate," "benign," "atypical," "suspicious for malignancy," and "positive for malignancy." The type of malignancy must be stated when a suspicious or malignant diagnosis is given.

The Yokohama System for Reporting Breast FNA Cytopathology

Category	ROM	Management	If imaging and/or CNB not available	Comment
Insufficient	2.6–4.8%	Review clinical and imaging findings. Repeat FNA if US findings are "benign" or proceed to CNB	Review clinical. Repeat FNA if necessary	At ROSE, if FNA still insufficient, perform US-guided FNA up to three times. If still insufficient proceed to CNB
Benign	1.4–2.3%	Review clinical and imaging findings. No further biopsy is required if both are benign ("triple test")	Review clinical and repeat FNA if incongruent. If repeat FNA atypical or worse consider excisional biopsy	At ROSE, correlate with "triple test." Follow-up and perform US-guided FNA up to three times. Proceed accordingly to CNB
Atypical	13–15.7%	Review clinical and repeat FNA or proceed to CNB	Review clinical and repeat FNA. If atypical, consider excisional biopsy	At ROSE, proceed to CNB
Suspicious	84.6–97.1%	Review clinical and imaging findings. CNB is mandatory	If no CNB available, perform excisional biopsy	At ROSE proceed to CNB
Malignant	99–100%	Review clinical and imaging findings. Proceed CNB if discrepant. If "triple test" is concordant and malignant proceed to definitive management	If no CNB available, perform excisional biopsy	At ROSE may proceed to CNB

ROM risk of malignancy, *CNB* core needle biopsy, *FNA* fine needle aspiration, *US* ultrasound, *ROSE* rapid on-site evaluation
Modified from: The International Academy of Cytology Yokohama System for Reporting Breast FNA Cytopathology. Field AS, Raymond WA, Schmitt F. Eds. 2020. Springer Switzerland Nature

In addition to the diagnostic category, the report also includes a brief clinical history and physical examination, microscopic description, and a note or assessment that correlates all findings. The note section is also used to address physician notification in case of a malignant diagnosis or other clinically relevant discussion. Although optional, our report includes photomicrographs and ultrasound images of the mass.

The Normal Breast

The normal female breast is a modified sweat gland showing ducts, ductules, and acini surrounded by stromal elements, mainly adipose tissue (Fig. 8.2). Aspiration cytology smears of a nonlactating breast show fibroadipose tissue stroma and few ductal and acinar elements. The ductal epithelial cells are arranged cohesively in monolayers with honeycomb architecture and have a cuboidal or columnar shape with oval nuclei, finely dispersed chromatin, and inconspicuous nucleoli (Fig. 8.3). The myoepithelial cells have indiscernible cytoplasm and appear as small dark, oval nuclei both admixed with the ductal cells (but in a different plane of focus) and in the smear background. Acinar cells are arranged in small aggregates and show a cuboidal shape and slightly granular cytoplasm; they are rarely seen in aspirates from normal breast (Fig. 8.4).

Immunohistochemistry

The wall of the terminal ducts and acini consists of secreting cells, cylindrical or cubic, resting on a *basal lamina* that can be highlighted by use of antibodies for vimentin, type IV col-lagen, and laminin. *Acinar cells* are usually positive for low-molecular-weight cytokeratins (CK7, CK8, CK18, and CK19). *Myoepithelial cells* in the interlobular and terminal ducts intensely express CK5, CK14, and CK17, and myoepithelial cells in the alveoli also show positivity for vimentin, α-SMA, smooth-muscle myosin heavy chain, and bone calponin. Myoepithelial cells are also positive for p63, maspin, and CD10. The terminal ducts have a mosaic of reactivity for cytokeratins, being positive for low-molecular-weight cytokeratins (except CK20) or CK5, CK14, and CK17. Some ductal cells are also positive with maspin and CD10. Cells positive for steroid receptors (ER and PR) are confined to the ducts and lobules. The lobule positive cells occupy a luminal position, or they are arranged in an intermediate zone between epithelial luminal cells and basal elements. In interlobular ducts, the positive cells are distributed predominantly in the basal level (Fig. 8.5, 8.6, and 8.7).

Ultrasound of the Normal Breast

Breast US is not a screening test; however, it can be used as an adjunct to mammography in palpable or not palpable breast masses. Breast US can also be used as an adjunct to mammogram in patients with dense breasts or breast cancer risk factors. In patients under the age of 35 years, US is the main tool for evaluating breast lesions. Of note, approximately 15% of US-visible lesions are not detected on mammography, particularly in young women with dense breasts or women with lobular carcinoma; on the contrary, US detects only few additional cancers in women with large breasts, increasing the screening cost and slightly lowering the speci-

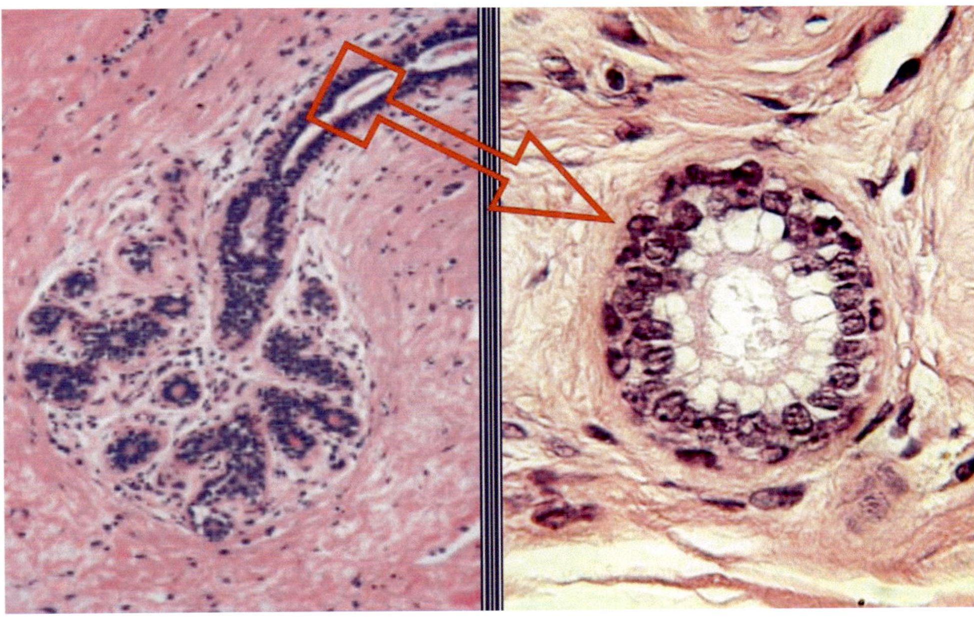

Fig. 8.2 Normal breast histology. Tubulo-lobular unit and cross section of the duct showing epithelial and myoepithelial cell layers. (H&E stain, medium and high magnification)

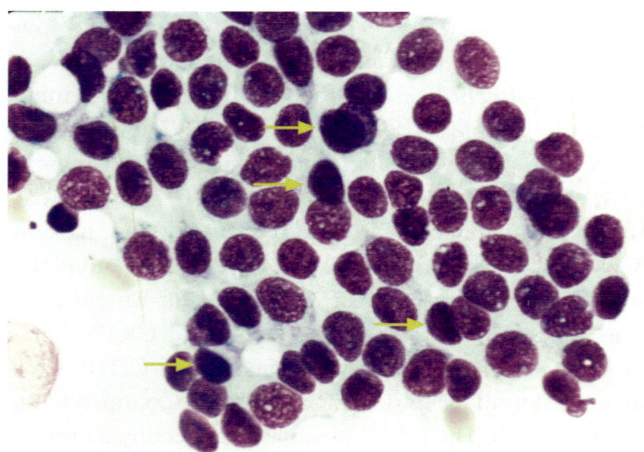

Fig. 8.3 Cytology benign ductal cells. Sheet of benign ductal epithelial cells and myoepithelial cell nuclei seen as small overlapping darker nuclei (arrows). (DiffQuik stain, high magnification)

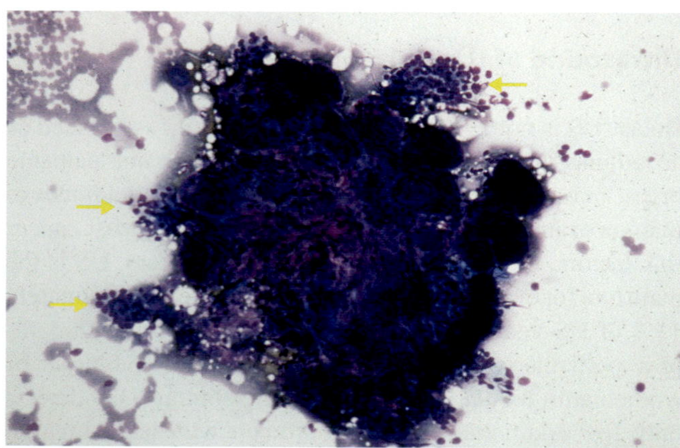

Fig. 8.4 Cytology benign breast lobule. Tightly packed lobular cells arranged as small nodular aggregates surrounded by stromal elements. Note a small sheet of terminal ductal epithelial cells in the periphery of the lobule (arrows). (DiffQuik stain, medium magnification)

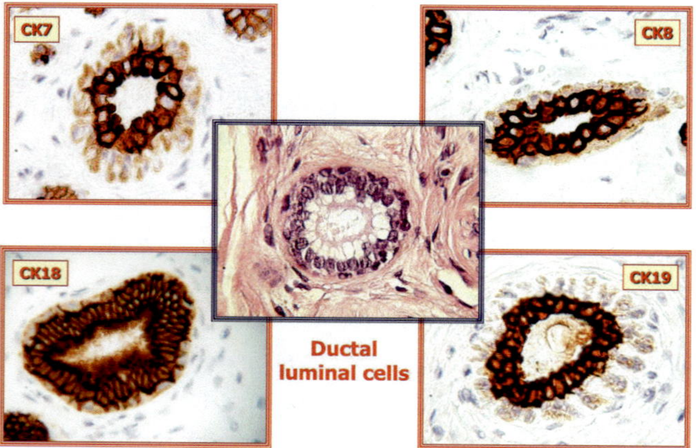

Fig. 8.5 Immunohistochemistry of normal ductal luminal cells. (Immunoperoxidase stain, high magnification)

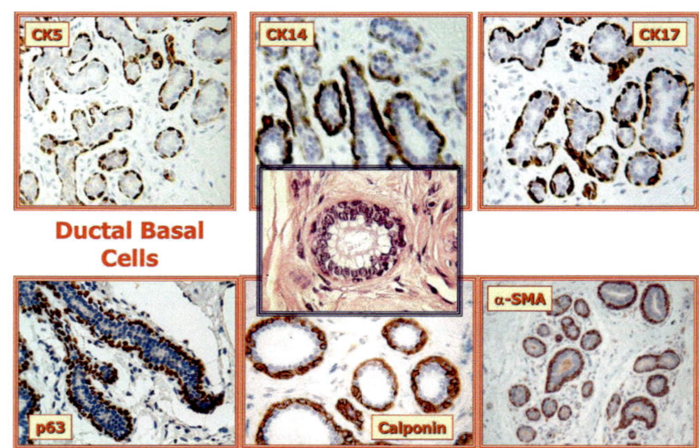

Fig. 8.6 Immunohistochemistry of normal ductal basal cells. (Immunoperoxidase stain, high magnification)

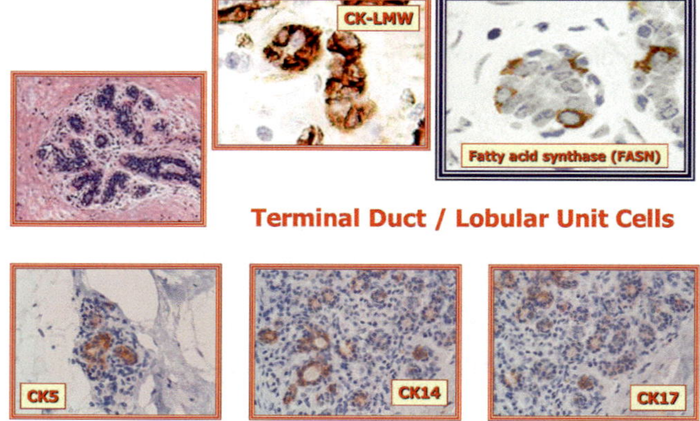

Fig. 8.7 Immunohistochemistry of the normal tubulo-lobular unit. (Immunoperoxidase stain, high magnification)

ficity. In women with a history of familial breast cancer, the preferred screening modality is MRI with a 91% detection rate in contrast to mammography (33%) and US (40%).

Fat in the breast is hypoechoic compared to glandular tissue, which is relatively hyperechoic. Thus, normal glandular breast tissue is isoechoic or slightly hyperechoic when compared with the pectoralis muscle. A dense fibroglandular tissue often shows round, oval, or elongated areas of hypoechogenicity in a more echogenic background. Breast tissues that can be distinguished by US include skin, fat, fibrous tissue stroma, Cooper's ligaments, fibroglandular tissue, and mammary ducts. The skin is 1–2 mm thick and has a hypoechoic band surrounded by a superficial and deep dermal echogenic lines. Bundles of fatty tissue are seen demarcated by echogenic lines coursing through tissue (Cooper's ligaments) (Fig. 8.8). The nipple can simulate a hypoechoic subareolar mass by US (Fig. 8.9); angling the transducer around the nipple helps to distinguish this artifactual shadowing also called hypoechoic nipple shadow. Ribs appear as

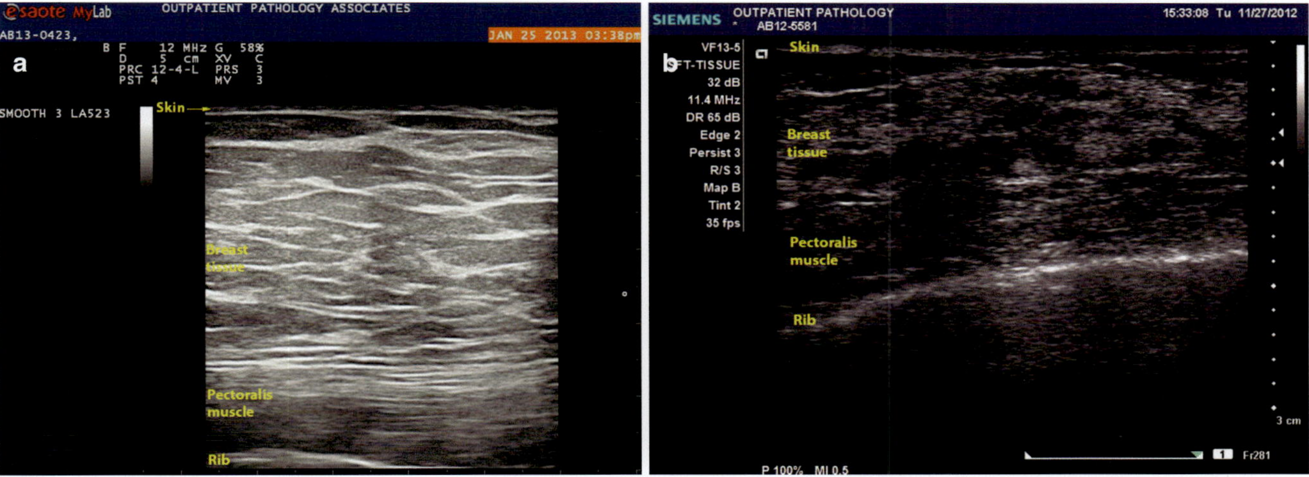

Fig. 8.8 Ultrasound features of normal breast in a young woman (**a**) and in a 65-year-old woman (**b**)

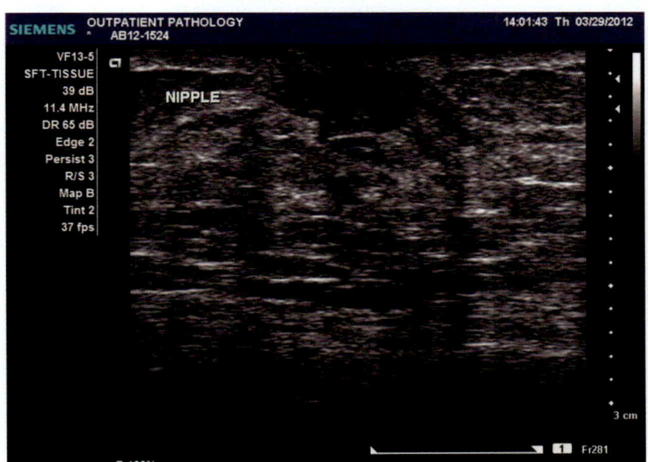

Fig. 8.9 Nipple. The nipple appears hypoechoic with irregular and poorly defined borders. These features may be confused with those of malignancy

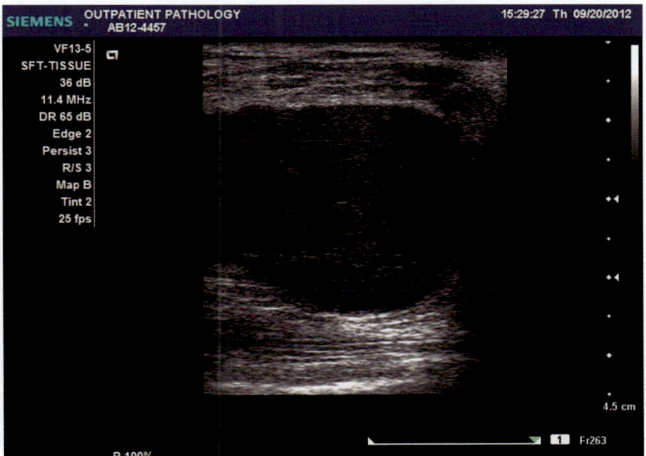

Fig. 8.10 Fibroadenoma. The mass is oval, hypoechoic, wider than tall, and shows circumscribed distinct margin, pushing borders, slight lobulation in the left upper portion, and posterior acoustic enhancement

oval hypoechoic masses and pleura as an echogenic line immediately below the rib. Pectoral muscle appears hypoechoic with parallel echogenic striations.

Ultrasound of Breast Masses

US features are not entirely specific or sensitive for predicting benign or malignant breast lesions. US features of benign conditions such as inflammation, fat necrosis, or radial scar can mimic a malignant lesion.

Benign solid lesions show hypoechogenicity compared with fat, and have an oval shape, well-circumscribed lobulated margins (macrolobulation), homogeneous internal echo pattern, posterior acoustic enhancement, parallel orientation (long axis of lesion parallels skin), compressibility, gentle bi- or tri-lobulation, and a thin echogenic pseudocapsule. For example, fibroadenomas are usually oval, well-circumscribed, smooth, and hypoechoic. These tumors have pushing borders and are oriented in a horizontal fashion and not vertically. They show posterior acoustic enhancement (Fig. 8.10). Intramammary lymph nodes are found more frequently in the upper outer quadrant of the breast, but they may be found in any quadrant.

However, not all well-circumscribed lesions are benign. Most circumscribed malignancies represent specific breast tumor types such as medullary carcinoma, colloid carcinoma, cystic papillary carcinoma, and high-grade infiltrating ductal carcinoma (Fig. 8.11). Some fast-growing malignant tumors are circumscribed by US due to a lack of tumor-induced desmoplastic stromal reaction. For the same reason, these tumors often show posterior acoustic enhancement that may be augmented by the presence of a host inflammatory response, as seen in medullary carcinoma.

Hyperchoic lesions are usually benign and include prominent and dense fibroglandular tissue, breast adipose tissue prominence, and lipomas (Fig. 8.12). Lesions that are anechoic are usually cystic and have posterior acoustic enhancement (Fig. 8.13). If a breast cyst has an echogenic vascular focus on Doppler examination, it is probably a papillary neoplasm, and USG-FNA (preferably using the Zajdela technique) must be directed to the solid component after cyst drainage. When the mass is heterogeneous, the sound waves do not pass through and an acoustic shadowing posterior to the mass is seen (Fig. 8.14).

Malignant breast lesions are typically hypoechoic and are easily identified in normal or dense breast tissue. These lesions appear white on screening mammogram. US findings suspicious for malignancy include: marked hypoechogenicity, spiculation, taller than wide or round, irregular angular ill-defined margins, posterior acoustic shadowing, microlobulated borders, intraductal extension, solid echotexture, inhomogeneous internal echotexture, ill-defined echogenic halo, no compressibility, and calcifications (Fig. 8.15). Some infiltrating breast cancers elicit a desmoplastic stromal reaction surrounding the malignant glandular component, which appears as slightly hyperechoic irregular rims (Fig. 8.16). Posterior acoustic enhancement may be seen in rapidly growing tumors such as poorly differentiated carci-

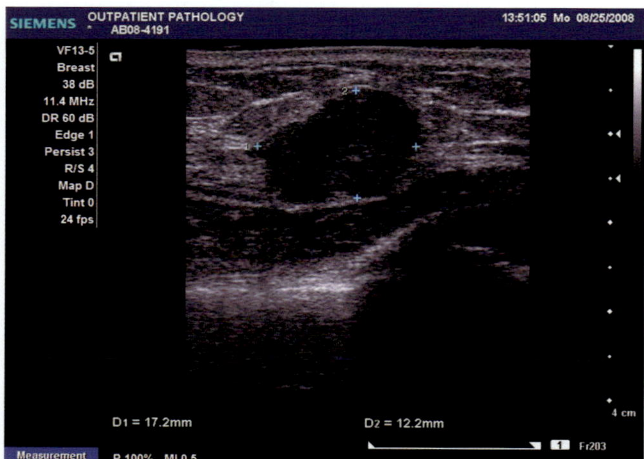

Fig. 8.11 Medullary carcinoma. The mass is oval, hypoechoic, wider than tall, and has a circumscribed slightly fuzzy margin, slight lobulation, slight spiculation at 5 o'clock, and disruption of surrounding breast parenchyma

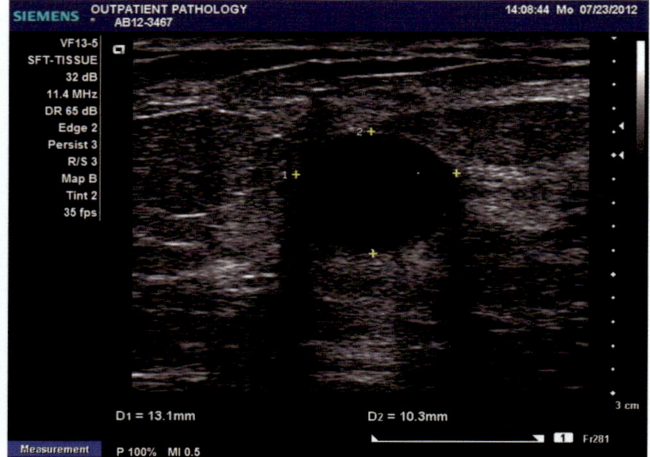

Fig. 8.13 Simple cyst. The mass is round, anechoic and has well-circumscribed distinct margin, with posterior acoustic enhancement, edge shadows (representing a thick cyst wall), and no lobulations or spiculations

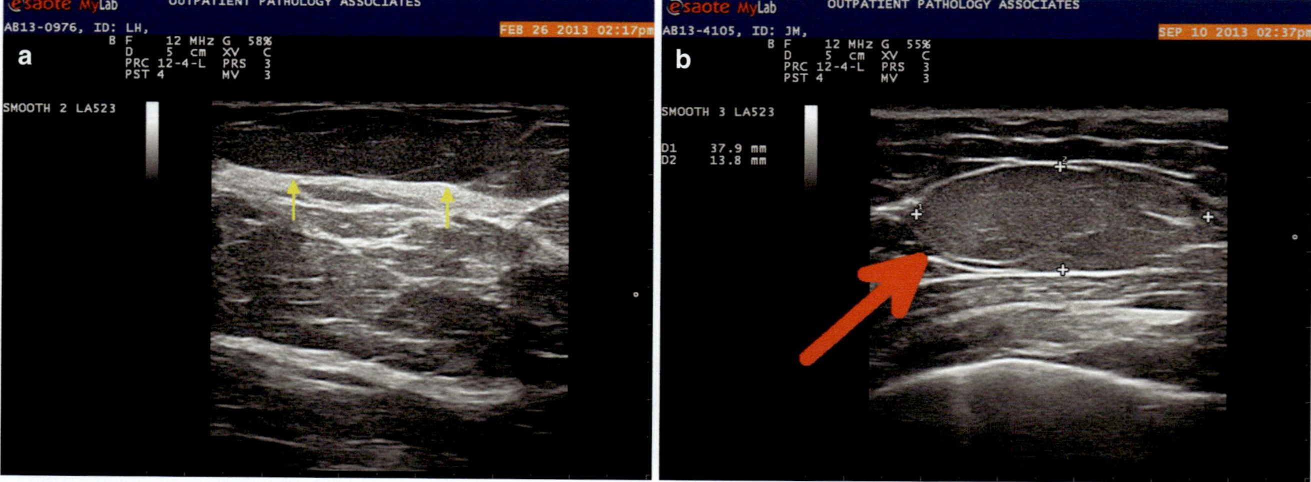

Fig. 8.12 Breast adipose tissue prominence (**a**) and lipoma (**b**). The mass (arrows) is oval, slightly hypoechoic, homogeneous, and has a circumscribed margin, with no lobulations, spiculations, or disruption of breast architecture. Lipoma has tapered ends and better defined margins

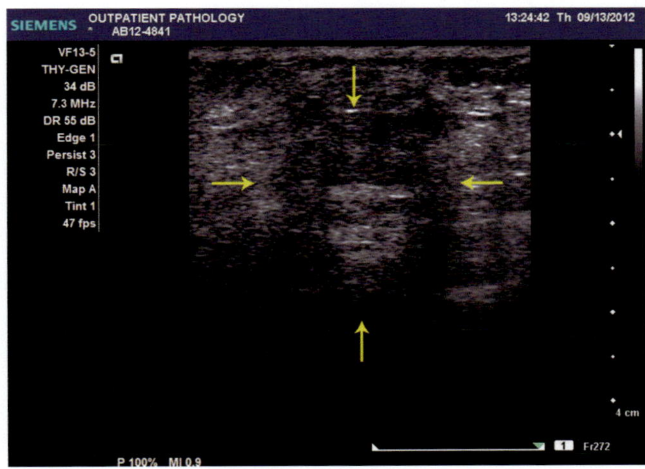

Fig. 8.14 Fat necrosis. The mass has an irregular shape, complex echotexture, poorly circumscribed and indistinct margins, and is taller than wide with disruption of breast architecture. The lesion mimics a malignant mass. The top arrow shows a hyperechoic linear area of dense fibrous tissue (also present in the center right and center low surrounded by a hyperechogenic area)

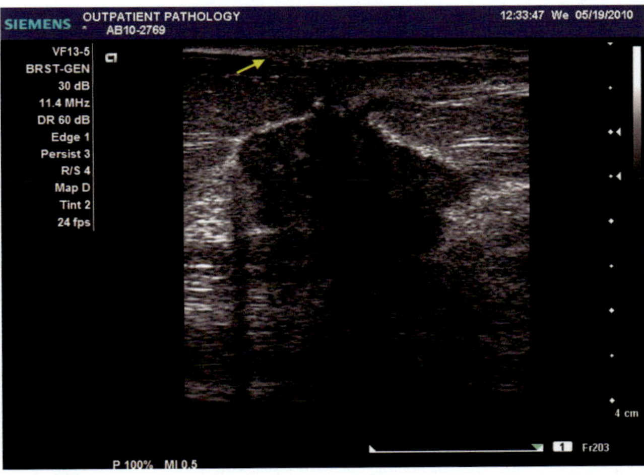

Fig. 8.15 Malignant lesion. The mass is wider than tall, and has an irregular shape, slight complex echotexture, poorly circumscribed and indistinct margins in the lower left part of the mass, and microlobulation. The mass seems to invade the superficial breast tissue causing slight retraction of the skin with disruption the deep subcutaneous tissue hyperechoic plate (arrow), superior and left from the area of spiculation

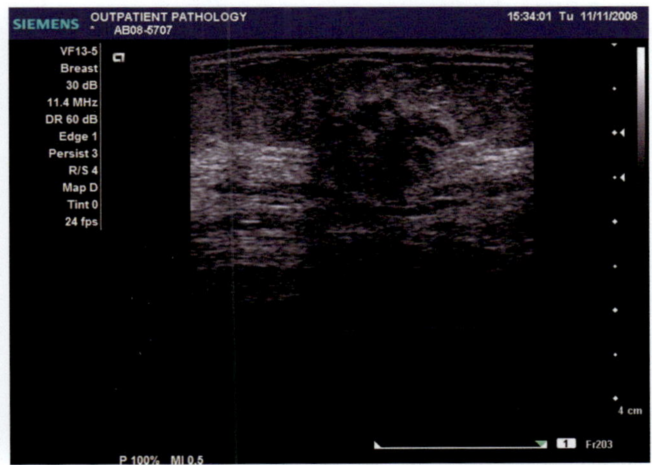

Fig. 8.16 Malignant lesion. Hyperechoic stromal reaction is seen in the right upper portion of the mass. The mass is slightly round with complex echotexture and ill-defined margins

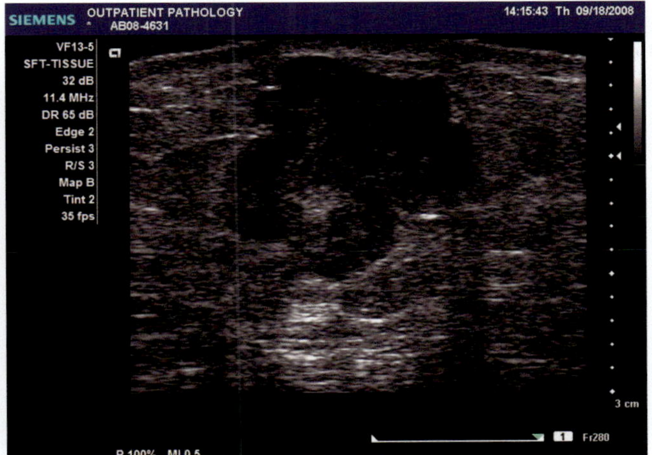

Fig. 8.17 Malignant lesion. The mass is irregular, hypoechoic, with slight heterogeneous echotexture, ondulations or macrolobulations, one spiculated border at 1 o'clock, and irregular posterior acoustic enhancement. Cooper's ligaments are disrupted

nomas and in colloid and intracystic papillary carcinoma (Fig. 8.17).

Spiculated lesions usually correlate with a slow tumor growth and the presence of tumor-induced desmoplastic stromal response formation as seen in low- and intermediate-grade ductal carcinoma, invasive tubular carcinoma, and lobular carcinoma. Also, these tumors show posterior acoustic shadowing by US (Fig. 8.18).

It must be remembered that not all smooth and well-circumscribed tumors are benign and spiculated ones malignant. The US error rate is 1–2%.

Useful US information essential for the cytopathologist to know in regard to a lesion include: (1) borders well-circumscribed or irregular, (2) echotexture solid, cystic, or solid and cystic, (3) size, (4) physical changes over time, (5) disappeared or collapsed after fluid drainage. Also important are the clinical findings, the patient's age, evidence of stability over a period of time, and mammographic findings, when evaluating the likelihood chance of malignancy of a solid mass.

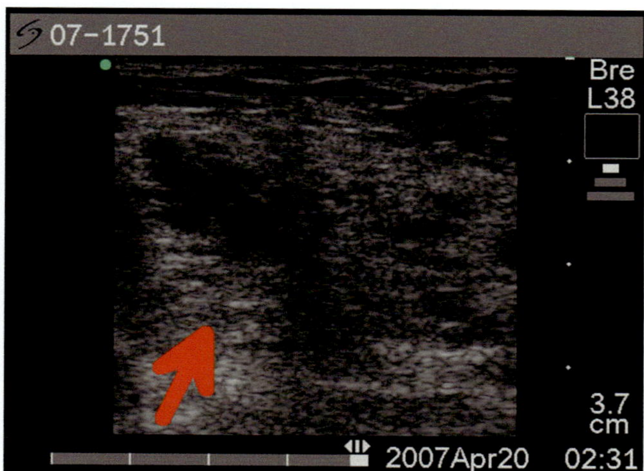

Fig. 8.18 Malignant lesion. The mass is large, irregular, and wider than tall, poorly circumscribed, heterogeneous, complex, and has irregular posterior acoustic enhancement. Breast architecture is disrupted

American College of Radiology Ultrasound: Summarized Bi-Rads[a] Terminology and Categories

- Mass
  - Shape: oval (may have slight undulations, macrolobulations), round, irregular
  - Orientation: long axis parallel to skin (wider than tall) or not parallel ("taller than wide")
  - Margin: circumscribed, not circumscribed (indistinct, angular, microlobulated or spiculated
  - Boundary: abrupt interface, echogenic halo
  - Echo pattern: (relative to fat) anechoic, hypoechoic, isoechoic, hyperechoic, complex
  - Posterior acoustic features: enhancement, shadowing, combined, none
  - Surrounding tissue changes: ducts, Cooper's ligament, edema, architectural distortion, skin thickening/retraction/irregularity
- Calcifications
  - Macrocalcifications (≥0.5 mm in size)
  - Microcalcifications out of the mass (<0.5 mm in size)
  - Microcalcifications in the mass
- Special cases
  - Clustered microcysts, complicated cysts, mass in or on skin, foreign body, lymph nodes (intramammary, axillary)
- Vascularity
  - Not present, present in lesion, present adjacent to lesion, diffuse in surrounding tissue
- Assessment categories
  - Category 0: incomplete, need additional imaging evaluation
  - Category 1: negative findings
  - Category 2: benign findings
  - Category 3: probably benign
  - Category 4: suspicious abnormality (consider biopsy)
  - Category 5: highly suggestive of malignancy
  - Category 6: known malignancy (biopsy proven)

[a] *BI-RADS* breast imaging-reporting and data system

Breast Masses

Palpable and US-visible breast masses can be neoplastic or non-neoplastic and can be sampled and interpreted by FNA under palpation or US guidance. Non-neoplastic masses include mastitis, breast abscesses, fibrocystic change, fat necrosis, cysts, lactation changes/adenoma, etc. An abridged current 2019 WHO classification of tumors of the breast is listed in Table 8.1. Modifications to the 2012 WHO classification of tumors of the breast and new entities incorporated in the current classification are listed in Table 8.2. Ductal carcinoma in situ (DCIS) may be palpable, and precursor and intraductal proliferative lesions may be visible by US and be targets for USG-FNA.

Table 8.1 Abridged 2019 WHO classification of tumors of the breast

Epithelial tumors	
Invasive breast carcinoma	Infiltrating duct carcinoma, NOS Invasive breast carcinoma of no special type (IBC-NST). Variants with … (medullary pattern, neuroendocrine differentiation, osteoclast-like stromal giant cells, pleomorphic pattern, choriocarcinomatous pattern, melanocytic pattern, oncocytic pattern, lipid-rich pattern, glycogen-rich clear cell pattern, sebaceous pattern) Lobular carcinoma, NOS Tubular carcinoma Cribriform carcinoma, NOS Mucinous adenocarcinoma Mucinous cystadenocarcinoma, NOS Invasive micropapillary carcinoma Carcinoma with apocrine differentiation Metaplastic carcinoma [adenosquamous carcinoma of low- and high-grade, fibromatosis-like carcinoma, spindle cell carcinoma, squamous cell carcinoma, metaplastic carcinoma with heterologous mesenchymal (e.g. chondroid, osseous, rhabdomyoid, neuroglial) differentiation, mixed metaplastic carcinomas]
Rare and salivary gland type tumors	Secretory carcinoma Acinic cell carcinoma Mucoepidermoid carcinoma Polymorphous adenocarcinoma Adenoid cystic carcinoma: classic, solid basaloid, and high-grade transformation Tall cell carcinoma with reversed polarity
Neuroendocrine neoplasms	Neuroendocrine tumor: grade 1, grade 2 Neuroendocrine carcinoma: small cell, large cell
Epithelial-myoepithelial tumors	Pleomorphic adenoma Adenomyoepithelioma Adenomyoepithelial carcinoma Epithelial myoepithelial carcinoma
Noninvasive lobular neoplasia	Atypical lobular hyperplasia Lobular carcinoma in situ: classic, florid, and pleomorphic

(continued)

Table 8.1 (continued)

Epithelial tumors	
Ductal carcinoma in situ (DCIS)	DCIS of low, intermediate, and high nuclear grade
Benign epithelial proliferations and precursors	Usual ductal hyperplasia Columnar cell lesions including flat epithelial atypia Atypical ductal hyperplasia
Adenosis and benign sclerosing lesions	Sclerosing adenosis Microglandular adenosis Radial scar/complex sclerosing lesion
Papillary neoplasms	Intraductal papilloma Ductal carcinoma in situ, papillary Solid papillary carcinoma: in situ and invasive Encapsulated papillary carcinoma
Adenomas	Tubular adenoma Apocrine adenoma Lactating adenoma Duct adenoma
Mesenchymal tumors	Benign and malignant
Fibroepithelial tumors	Fibroadenoma, NOS Phyllodes tumor NOS: benign, borderline, malignant Periductal stromal tumor Hamartoma
Tumors of the nipple	Nipple adenoma Syringoma Paget disease of the nipple[a]
Malignant lymphoma	B- and T-cell types
Metastatic tumors	
Tumors of the male breast	Gynecomastia Carcinoma: in situ and invasive

[a] Scraping of the lesion can provide cytologic material for diagnosis

Table 8.2 2019 WHO classification of tumors of the breast: Modifications to the WHO 2012 morphological subtypes

Entity	WHO 2012	WHO 2019
Carcinoma with medullary features	Separate entity	Classified as TIL-rich IBC-NST
Carcinomas: oncocytic, lipid-rich, glycogen-rich clear cell, sebaceous, pleomorphic, melanotic, choriocarcinomatous, with osteoclast-like giant cells	Separate entities	Classified as IBC-NST
Inflammatory, bilateral, and non-synchronous breast carcinomas	Separate entities	Recognized as clinical presentations rather than special subtypes
Lobular carcinoma in situ	Classic, pleomorphic types	Classic, pleomorphic, and florid types
Neuroendocrine neoplasms		Classified as NET, SCNEC, and LCNEC

(continued)

Table 8.2 (continued)

Entity	WHO 2012	WHO 2019
Neuroendocrine differentiation		Overridden by morphologic tumor type (NST, mucinous, solid, papillary)
Well-differentiated liposarcoma in phyllodes tumor	Histologic criterion of malignancy by itself	No longer a histological criterion of malignancy by itself
Mucinous cystadenocarcinoma		New entity
Breast tumor resembling the tall cell variant of papillary thyroid carcinoma; solid papillary carcinoma with reversed polarity		Grouped as tall cell carcinoma with reversed polarity
Periductal stromal tumor	Separate fibroepithelial tumor	Variant of phyllodes tumor

WHO World Health Organization, *TIL* tumor-infiltrating lymphocyte, *IBC-NST* invasive breast carcinoma no special type, *NET* neuroendocrine tumor, *SCNEC* small cell neuroendocrine carcinoma, *LCNEC* large cell neuroendocrine carcinoma
Modified from: Tan PH, Ellis I, et al. The 2019 World Health Organization classification of tumors of the breast. Commentary. Histopathology 2020; 77:181–185. https://doi.org/10.1111/his.14091

Non-neoplastic Breast Masses

Cysts

The most common lesions of the female breast are solitary or multiple cysts, particularly in the premenopausal age. The FNA is a diagnostic and therapeutic procedure and yields clear, opaque, or turbid fluid that may be yellow or red (bloody). Turbid and bloody fluids should be examined cytologically because they may harbor a papillary neoplasm, including papillary carcinoma. It is also important to re-examine the area manually and or by US after cyst drainage to search for a solid-phase component, which must be sampled by FNA, preferably under US guidance. The smears show macrophages in various numbers and epithelial cells, often of apocrine appearance (Fig. 8.19a, b).

The histiocyte/macrophage nature of foam cells can be confirmed by immunohistochemical staining for CD68, whereas the immunostaining for S-100 protein and CD1a is useful for distinguishing apocrine cells from a granular cell tumor (Schwannoma) or Langerhans cell histiocytosis. Immunostaining for androgen receptors identifies apocrine cells.

US Features Cysts have well-circumscribed margins, are anechoic, rounded or oval, and show thin edge shadows and a characteristic posterior acoustic enhancement due to the

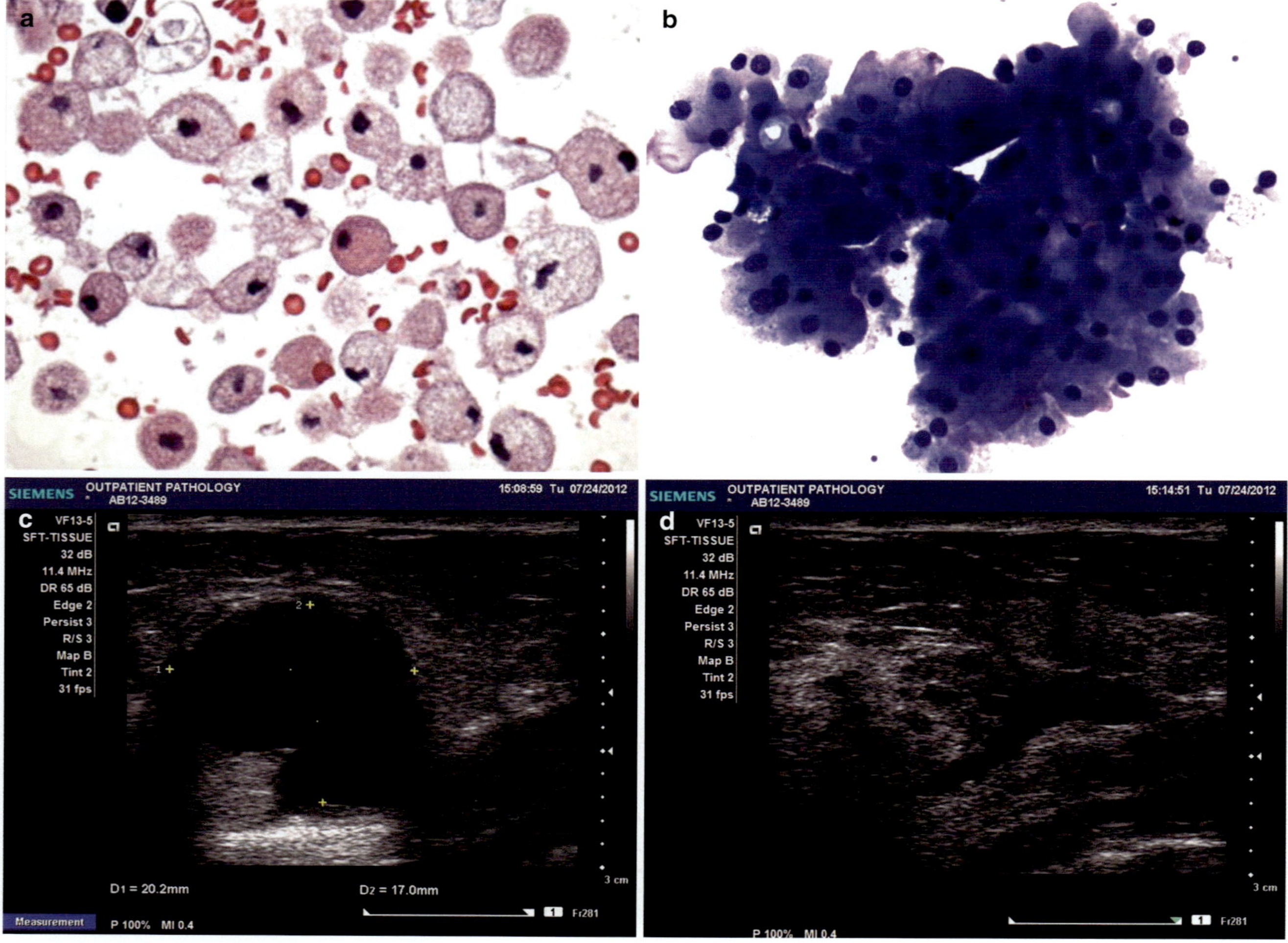

Fig. 8.19 Simple cyst. Macrophages (**a**) and apocrine metaplastic cells (**b**). The cyst is anechoic with no mural nodules (**c**) and collapsed after fluid drainage (**d**). (**a**, **b**, Papanicolaou stain, medium and high magnification)

presence of fluid (Fig. 8.19c). Posterior acoustic enhancement is not always seen in small cysts or in those located close to the chest wall. In some cysts, dot-like moving internal echogenic signals ("gurgling cyst") are seen upon cyst compression with the US transducer, confirming a fluid internal matrix. Occasionally, small echogenic septations may be seen, particularly when apocrine metaplasia is present. Again, a mural solid component present after fluid drainage must be sampled by USG-FNA (Fig. 8.19d, Video 8.3).

Mastitis

Bacterial, mycobacterial, fungal, parasitic, and viral among others are rare causes of mastitis. Less than 3% of lactating women develop acute suppurative mastitis, and staphylococci and streptococci are the most common agents. Localized acute mastitis may result in abscess formation. Inflammatory mastopathy may be associated with duct/cyst rupture and diabetes mellitus. Granulomatous mastitis may be due to sarcoidosis, infections, reaction to tumor, fat necrosis, foreign-body reaction (suture, ruptured squamous cyst, silicone implant leakage), and idiopathic granulomatous mastitis. These entities can clinically and radiologically mimic carcinoma. USG-FNA can be used as diagnostic and therapeutic tools, i.e., for abscess drainage associated with antibiotic therapy (Fig. 8.20a, b).

FNA Findings The inflammatory cells vary in type and number according to the type of mastitis; however, the epithelial cell morphology has variable reactive changes ranging from minimal to severe and can be confused with malignancy. The epithelial cells are arranged in cohesive sheets and have variable reactive inflammatory changes and reparative features (Fig. 8.20c, d). Polarity is maintained, and myoepithelial cells are present in the background. A purulent smear pattern including neutrophils, macrophages, and debris is found in *acute mastitis*. In *chronic mastitis*,

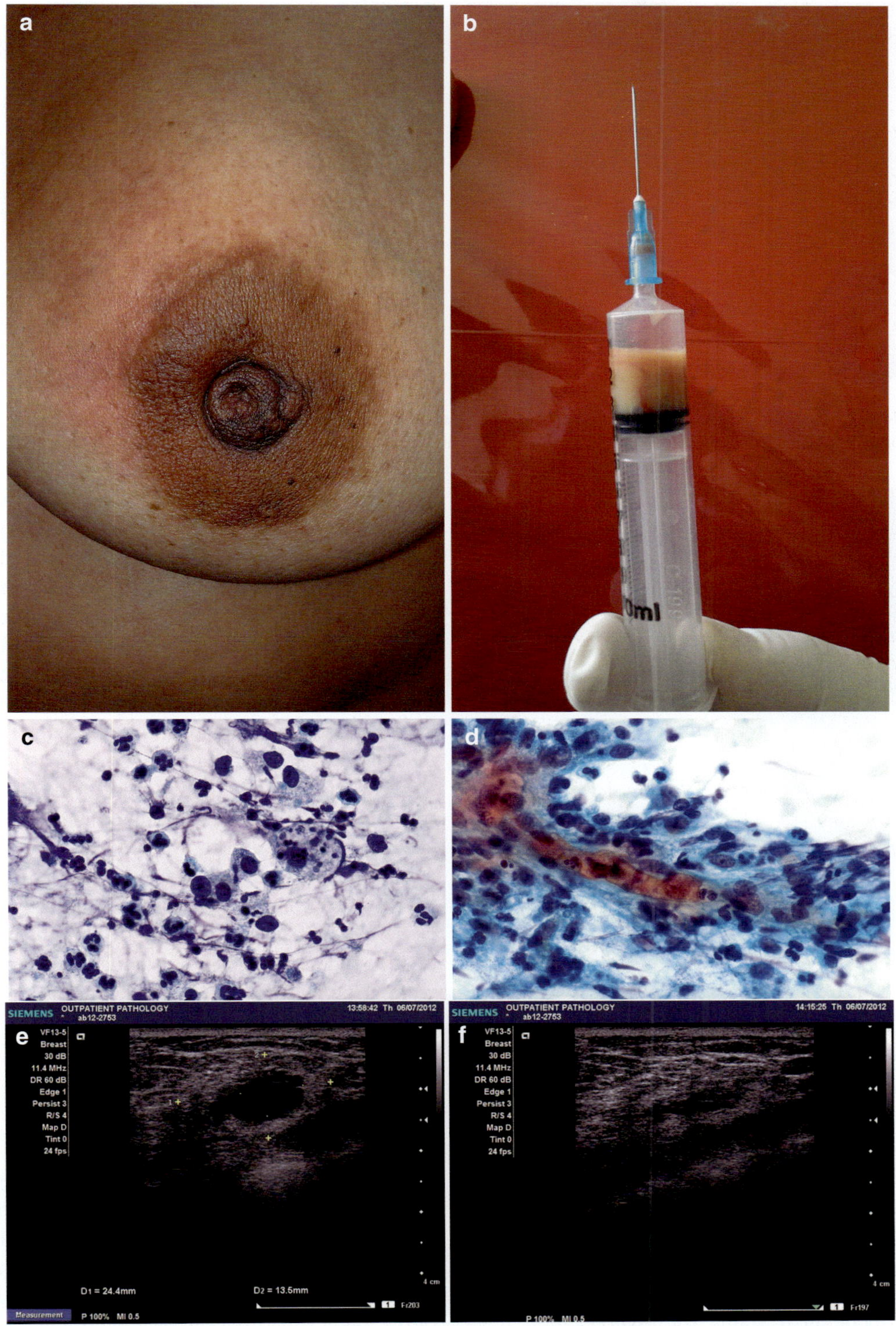

Fig. 8.20 Acute and chronic mastitis/abscess. Upper inner quadrant left breast visible mass (**a**). Abscess contents harvested using a 25-G needle (**b**). Acute inflammatory exudate, variable numbers of macrophages (**c**), and granulation tissue fragments (**d**) are seen. This US image shows an abscess with thick hyperechoic wall and anechoic center (**e**) that collapsed partially after drainage (**e**). (**c**, DiffQuik stain high magnification; **d**, Papanicolaou stain high magnification)

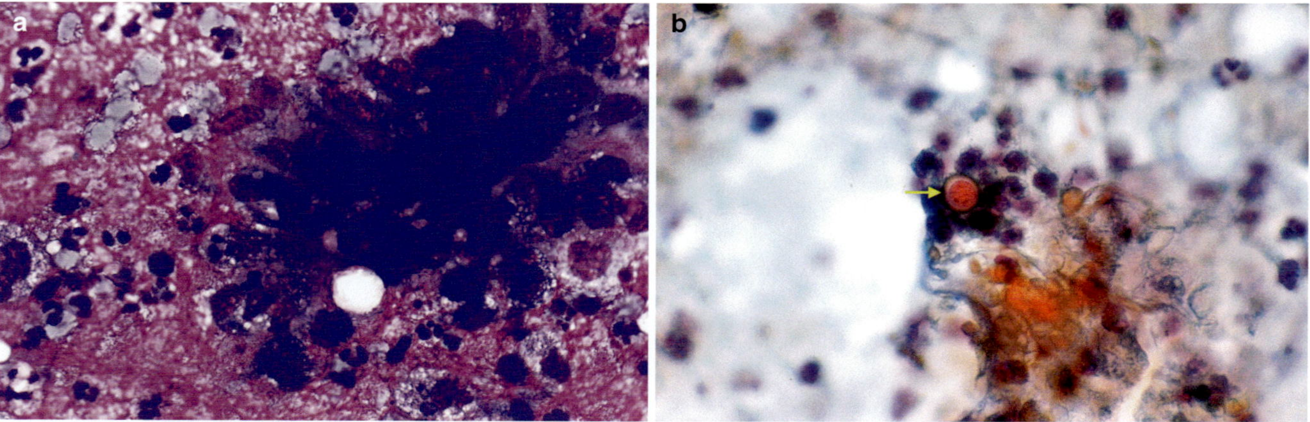

Fig. 8.21 Granulomatous mastitis. Blastomycosis. Necrosis, granulomas, markedly reactive stromal and epithelial elements resembling malignancy (**a**), and fungal organisms (**b**, arrow) are seen. (**a**, DiffQuik stain high magnification; **b**, Papanicolaou stain high magnification)

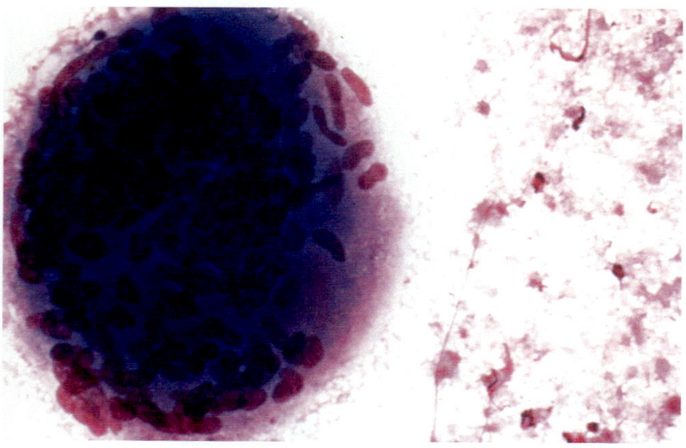

Fig. 8.22 Granulomatous mastitis. Tuberculosis. Multinucleated histiocytes and a background of necrosis. (DiffQuik stain, high magnification)

smears are less cellular due to underlying fibrosis and show plasma cells and lymphocytes. Multinucleated giant cells and macrophages may be present. Plasma cell mastitis is a common chronic inflammatory condition and is most probably caused by duct rupture. In *granulomatous mastitis*, smears show granulomas, a foreign-body type giant cell reaction, aggregates of epithelioid histiocytes, lymphocytes, and plasma cells, and variable necrosis (Figs. 8.21 and 8.22). Special stains for mycobacteria and fungus performed in smears or cell blocks are useful for rapid diagnosis and for initiation of therapy. However, histochemical and immunohistochemical stains for mycobacteria have poor diagnostic sensitivity. Of greater use, are molecular biology tests. Cultures are confirmatory and used to modify therapy according to sensitivity to specific drugs. *Silicone granulomas* can be suspected when histiocytes contain empty, round vacuoles and amorphous nonstaining material in Romanowsky stains; the clinical history is important (Fig. 8.23).

US Features Mastitis shows diffusely increased echogenic tissue with loss of normal tissue planes including Cooper's ligaments, reflecting the presence of tissue edema; increased vascularity may be seen on Doppler examination. Areas of increased echogenicity may be associated with areas of decreased echogenicity, resulting in a not well-circumscribed mass. An abscess is hypoechoic, well-defined, and may be uni- or multiloculated, showing interconnecting complex cystic masses that may extend to the skin. The abscess content has an echogenic signal that results in movement of particles when there is compression of the mass with the US transducer. The overlying skin and the surrounding soft tissue are thickened and show edema (Fig. 8.20e, f). A "snowstorm" appearance is characteristic of silicone granuloma; the same appearance can be seen in axillary lymph nodes in cases of extracapsular rupture of the implant and migration of the silicone to the lymph nodes. Immunocytochemistry with CD68 and/or CD163 can be performed to confirm histiocytic nature of epithelioid cells.

Subareolar Abscess

This process usually occurs in nonlactating premenopausal women who have recurrent abscess formation in the subareolar area and draining of a periareolar fistula. Squamous metaplasia of the distal lactiferous ducts with obstruction is considered to be the etiologic factor. The abscess is usually sterile, but a superimposed bacterial infection may occur.

FNA Findings Smears show a mixed acute and chronic inflammatory background, multinucleated giant cells of foreign-body type, and squamous cells (anucleated, parakeratotic). Variable numbers of foamy macrophages, cholesterol crystals, and reactive ductal epithelial cells and granulation tissue may be present (Fig. 8.24). Sebaceous cysts (aka., epider-

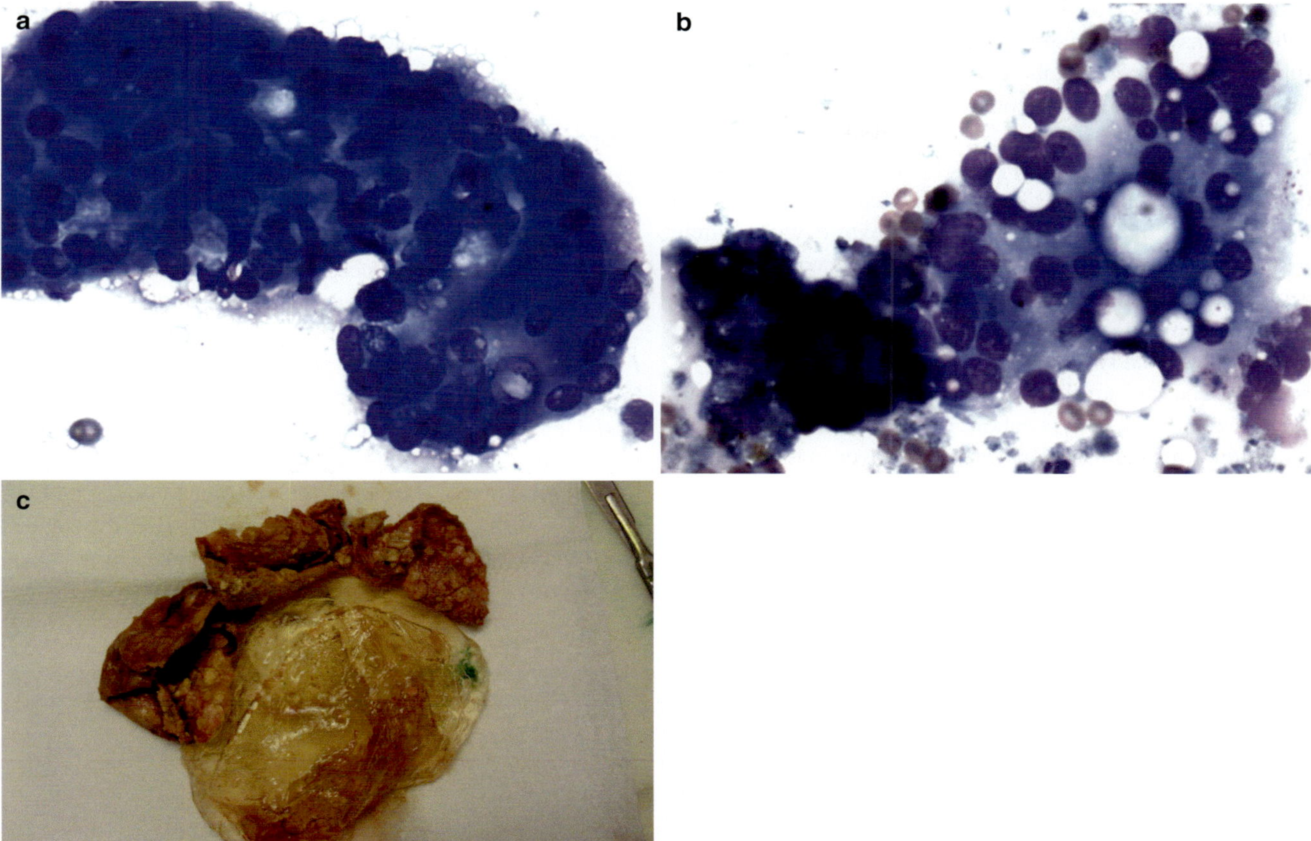

Fig. 8.23 Silicone mastitis. Granulomas and multinucleated giant cells containing round empty vacuoles (**a**, **b**). Ruptured breast implant containing silicone (**c**). (**a**, **b**, MGG stain, high magnification)

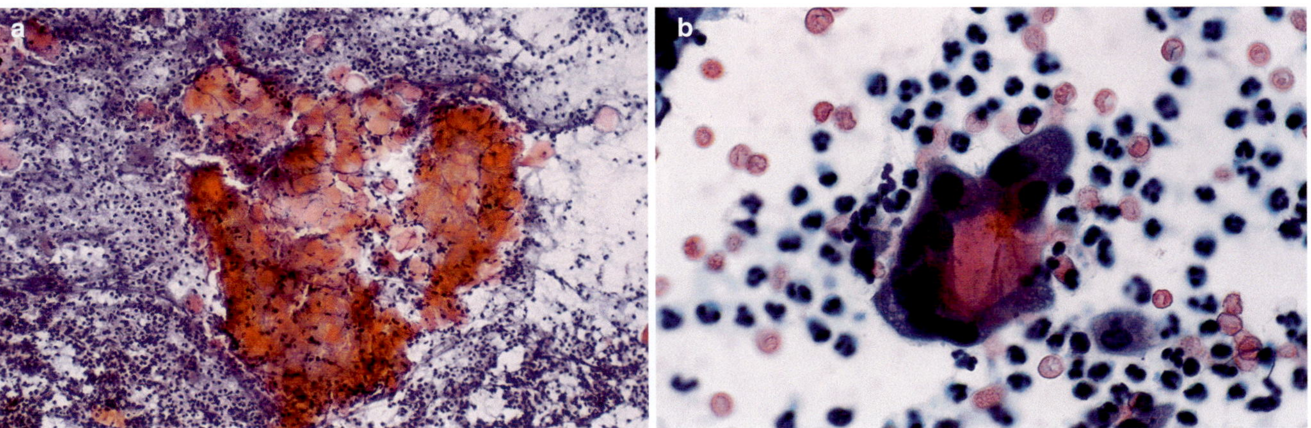

Fig. 8.24 Subareolar abscess. Cluster of anucleated squamous cells are surrounded by acute inflammatory cells (**a**). Multinucleated giant cell phagocytizing anucleated squamous cells and a background of acute inflammation present (**b**). (Papanicolaou stain, medium (**a**) and high magnification (**b**)

mal inclusion cysts) also show numerous anucleated squamous cells and may show multinucleated giant cells if there is cyst rupture; cholesterol crystals may be seen (Fig. 8.25a). The distinction between these two entities needs US correlation.

US Features Subareolar abscess by US shows a complex hypoechoic to nearly anechoic oval or lenticular mass with irregular margins, heterogeneous echotexture with minute particles, and mixed solid and cystic areas with posterior acoustic enhancement. Hypoechoic tubular areas associated with the skin and subcutaneous tissue, skin thickening, and dilated subdermal lymphatics may be seen. A sebaceous cyst is superficial and arises from the skin. Early in sebaceous cyst development, a hypoechoic mass is seen causing skin thickening; the echogenic deep dermal layer may disrupt as the cyst enlarges. Sebaceous cysts may be completely anechoic, hypoechoic, or echogenic with posterior acoustic enhancement or a complex cystic mass and may be irregular with indistinct margins (Fig. 8.25b, c). Immunocytochemistry

usually is not performed; however, proliferation markers can be used in some cases to exclude a neoplastic process.

Fibroadipose Tissue Prominence/Lipoma

These lesions are palpable and often not visible by mammography or US. They are soft to slightly firm and often poorly circumscribed. Occasionally, lipomas may become more evident if there is weight loss. True lipomas are rare.

FNA Findings Aspiration smears from lipomas show benign adipose tissue fragments of variable size. Benign ductal epithelial cell sheets and myoepithelial cell nuclei may be seen in addition to adipose tissue in cases of adipose tissue prominence. Cytologic findings need clinical and US correlation; the accuracy of such a diagnosis is the highest when the cytopathologist performs FNA under US guidance and interprets the cytology findings.

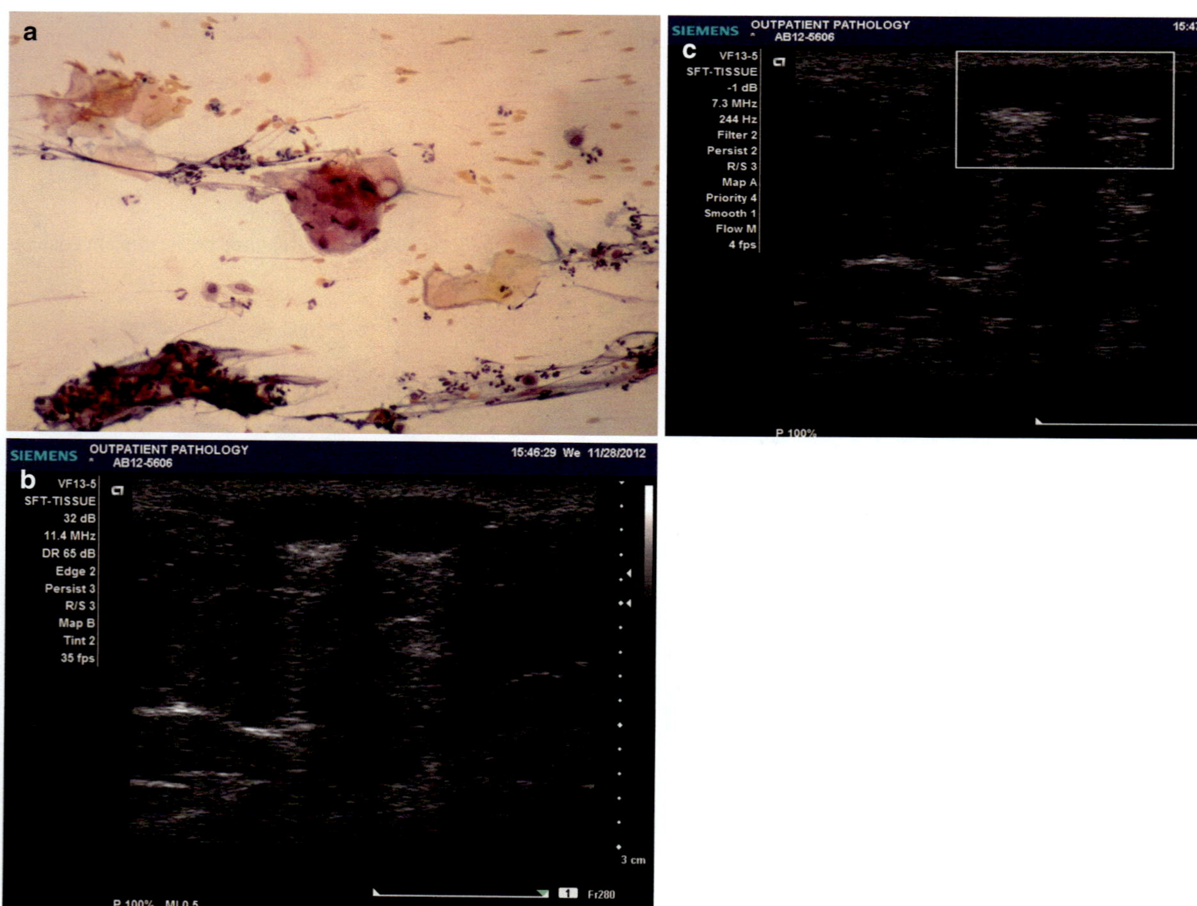

Fig. 8.25 Epidermal inclusion cyst. These lesions developed in the infra-mammary fold. Anucleated squamous cells, acute inflammation, macrophages, and multinucleated giant cells phagocytizing squamous cells are present (**a**). Ultrasound image shows two hypoechoic oval lesions with uniform well-defined margins, edge shadows, and posterior acoustic enhancement (**b**). No vascular flow is noted by Doppler exam (**c**). (**a**, Papanicolaou stain intermediate magnification)

US Features The US features of lipoma are characteristic and include a well-defined oval, compressible, isoechoic or slightly hyperechoic homogeneous mass with a thin echogenic capsule (Fig. 8.12b). Fatty tissue prominence shows bundles of hypoechoic tissue surrounded and delineated by echogenic lines (Cooper's ligaments) (Fig. 8.26). Vimentin, S-100 protein, and leptin provide immunostaining for normal adipocytes. Immunocytochemistry is not necessary for diagnosis.

Fat Necrosis

This trauma-related inflammatory lesion resembles malignancy clinically, radiologically, and cytologically. The problem is compounded because the patient often does not recall having trauma. The mass is commonly firm, irregular, fixed to deep planes, and may not always be tender.

FNA Findings Necrotic and degenerating adipocytes, lipid laden macrophages, and mixed inflammatory cells are present along with scattered multinucleated foreign-body-type giant cells. Prominent fatty tissue liquefaction is seen in long-standing fat necrosis with cystic degeneration (Fig. 8.27a–d). Myospherulosis, which is the result of aggregated red blood cells altered by the contact with lipid resembling a "bag of marbles," possibly represents a sequel of fat necrosis.

US Features The lesion may be irregular and hypoechoic with variable posterior acoustic enhancement. The lesions may have ill-defined borders and be slightly hyperechoic or mixed complex solid/cystic when there is cystic degeneration. Old lesions may have dystrophic calcification and, in some cases, have a calcific rim. Old lesions may also be complex solid and cystic or cystic and nearly anechoic, with or without posterior acoustic enhancement on US (Fig. 8.27e–h).

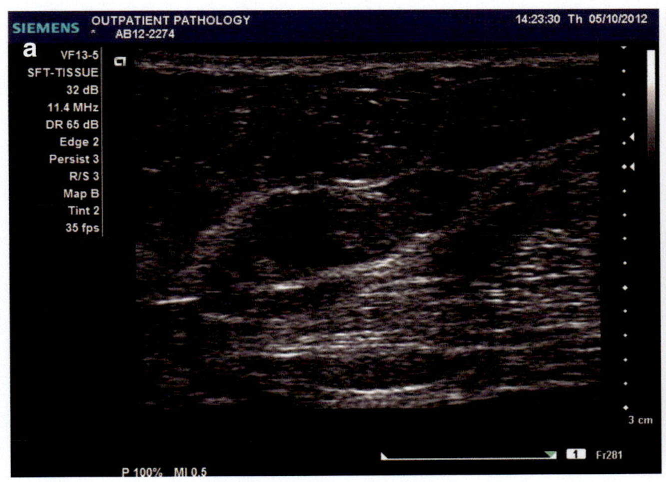
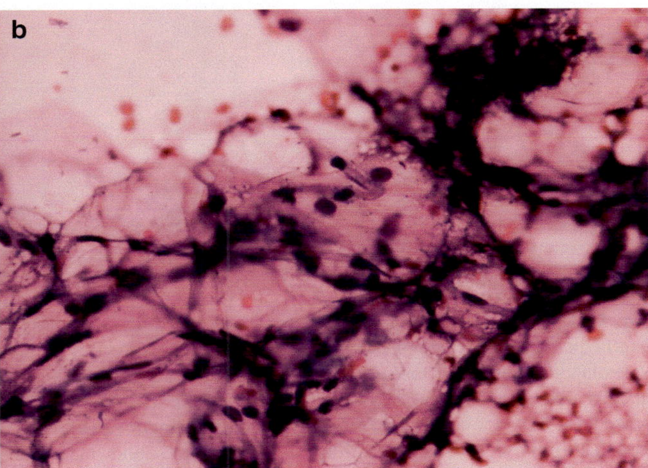

Fig. 8.26 Adipose tissue breast prominence. Patient usually has an ill-defined and slightly firm palpable breast lesion, which is not distinctly visible by US as in this case; instead, lobules of adipose tissue are seen (**a**). The FNA smears show small fragments of fibrofatty tissue (**b**). (**b**, MGG stain, intermediate magnification)

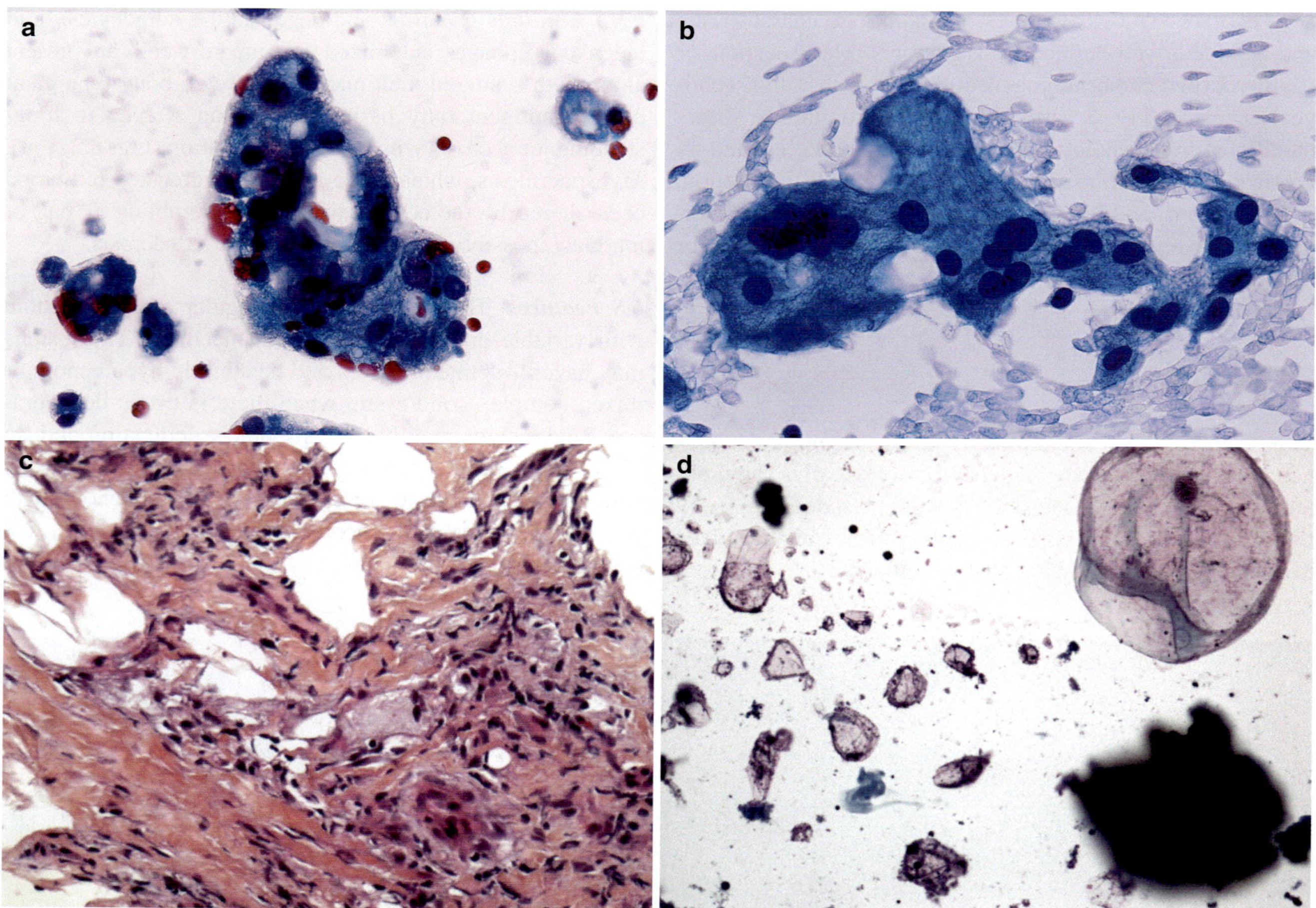

Fig. 8.27 Fat necrosis. Damaged adipocytes are arranged predominantly in cohesive aggregates with rare single cells showing finely vacuolated cytoplasm, low-nuclear to cytoplasm ratio, and bland nuclear features. Variable anisocytosis and anisonucleosis may be present (**a**, **b**). Core biopsy performed confirms the diagnosis (**c**). Fatty liquefaction is seen in long-standing cases (**d**). Ultrasound images of three different cases show ill-defined masses of variable size with heterogeneous echotexture, calcifications with posterior acoustic shadowing, cystic change, and irregular lobulated and in areas spiculated margins (**e–h**). (**a**, **b** DiffQuik stain, high magnification; **c**, H&E stain intermediate magnification; **e**, papanicolaou stain, intermediate magnification)

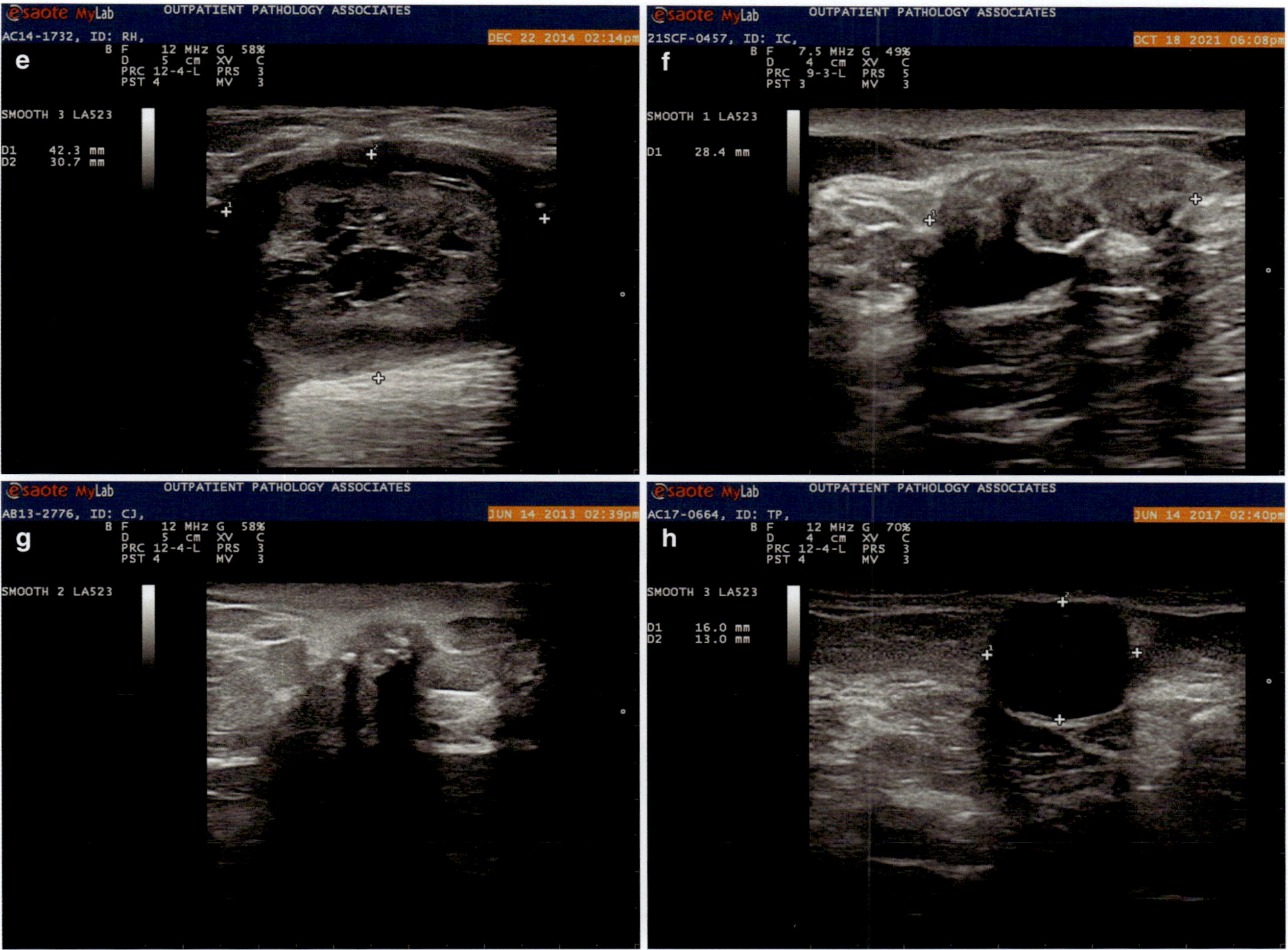

Fig. 8.27 (continued)

Fibroepithelial Tumors

Fibroadenoma

This benign biphasic stromal and epithelial neoplasm arises in the terminal-duct lobular unit and affects women particularly between the ages of 20–35 years. It is usually a mobile, firm, solitary, slow-growing, well-circumscribed tumor, and usually measures <3 cm. However, it may be larger, multiple, and bilateral. Juvenile fibroadenomas are larger than 5 cm. A complete surgical excision is curative.

Histopathology The stromal component may surround the ducts (pericanalicular) or may separate the ducts, forming clefts (intracanalicular) (Fig. 8.28a). Hypercellular stroma, calcification, myxoid change or hyalinization, scattered giant cells, and rare mitoses may be present and have no clinical significance (Fig. 8.29a). Complex fibroadenomas show calcifications and superimposed fibrocystic changes including cysts >3 mm, sclerosing adenosis, ductal epithelial hyperplasia of usual type, and apocrine and squamous metaplasia. Juvenile fibroadenomas show hypercellular stroma, a stromal pericanalicular pattern, and ductal epithelial hyperplasia. Atypical ductal or atypical lobular hyperplasia, lobular carcinoma in situ and ductal carcinoma in situ may develop within the fibroadenoma.

Molecular and Immunocytochemistry Profile Both epithelial and stromal components are polyclonal. In fibroadenoma, immunostaining for CK7, CK8, CK18, and CK19 highlights epithelial cells, while p63 identifies myoepithelial cells. Variable quantities of epithelial cells show positivity for ER and PR. A positive AR stain identifies apocrine cells. No alterations in DNA copy have been shown by comparative genomic hybridization. Rare cases of numerical chromosomal abnormalities have been reported. There is no detectable stromal expression of nuclear α-catenin or E-cadherin. Stromal elements can be stained with CD34 and/ or α-SMA.

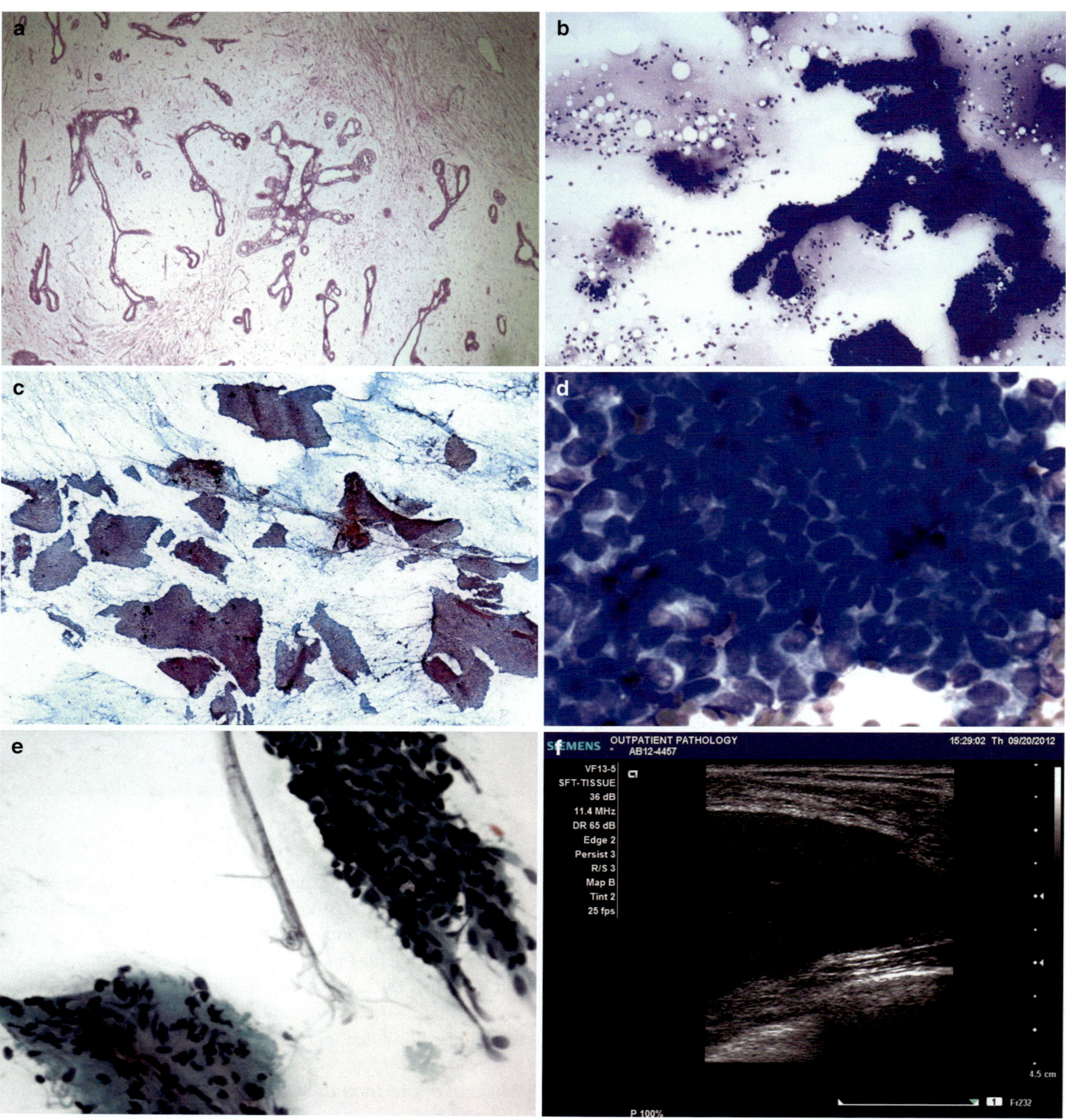

Fig. 8.28 Fibroadenoma. Low-power tissue sections show the typical features of a pericanallicular fibroadenoma (**a**). Cytologic features include branching and "staghorn-like structures, cohesive cell sheets, numerous myoepithelial cells both in the background and within the epithelial cells, and stromal fragments (**b–e**). Ultrasound shows a homogeneous, isoechoic, or hypoechoic wider than tall mass with ondulations or macrolobulations. A thin echogenic pseudocapsule and a homogeneous echotecture may be seen. Posterior acoustic enhancement is variably present. Vascular flow by Doppler exam is also variable present (**f–j**). (**a**, H&E stain low magnification; B,D DiffQuik stain low and high magnification; **c**, **e** Papanicolaou stain low and intermediate magnification)

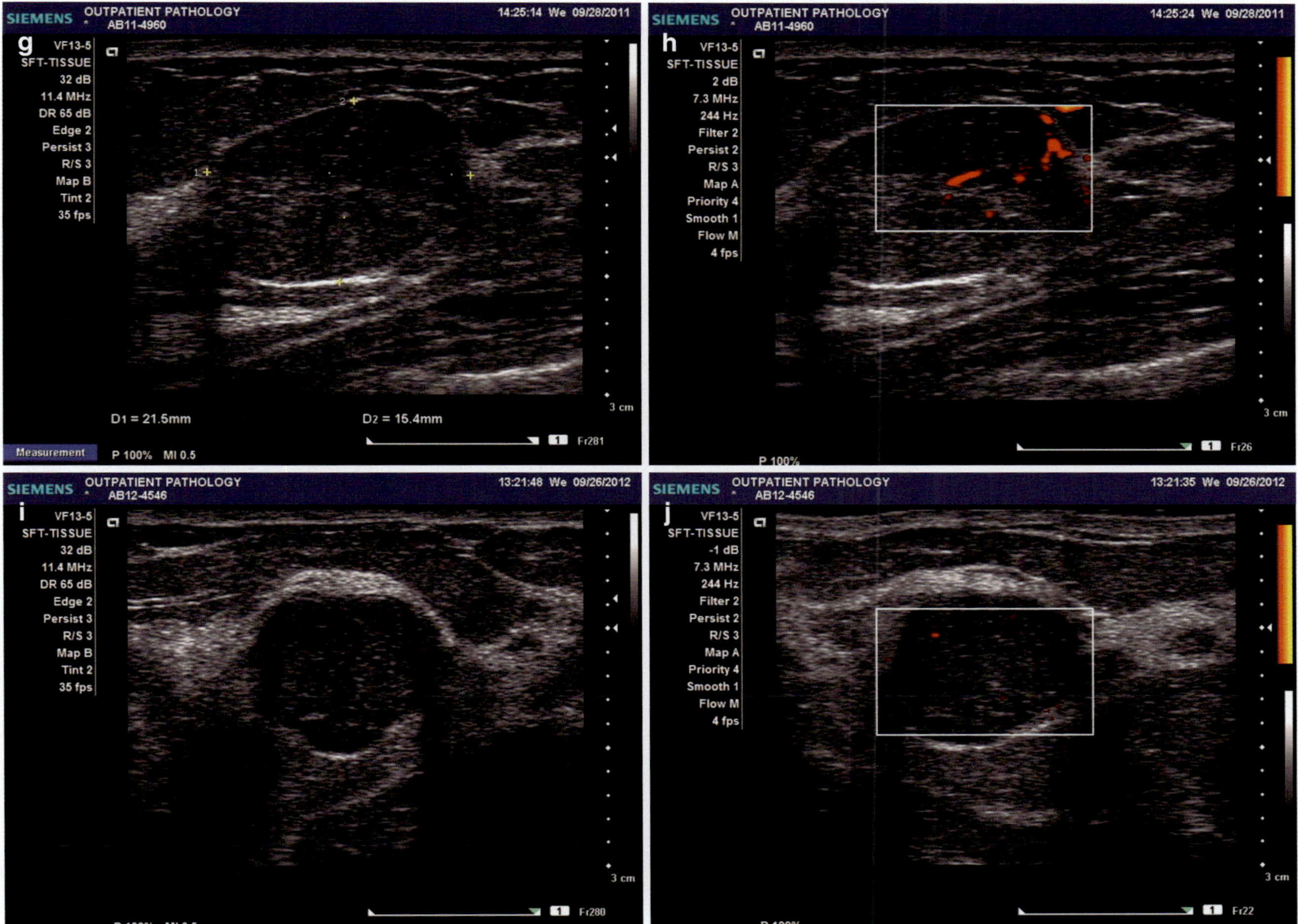

Fig. 8.28 (continued)

FNA Findings Smears are usually hypercellular with epithelial cells arranged in sheets, fingerlike branching and staghorn-like structures, numerous myoepithelial cell nuclei in the background and adherent to the epithelial elements, and fragments of fibrous and fibromyxoid stroma; apocrine and foam cells may be present. This smear pattern overlaps that of fibrocystic change; however, the clinical findings including US are different (Figs. 8.28b–e and 8.29b).

US Features A well-defined oval mass with gently lobulated margins is seen. The mass is homogeneous, isoechoic, or hypoechoic to the adjacent fat. A thin echogenic pseudocapsule, characteristic of a benign lesion and a "pseudocystic pattern" due to the homogeneous echotecture may be seen. Posterior acoustic enhancement is variably present; slight posterior acoustic shadowing may be present in long-lasting lesions due to sclerosis. The echotexture may be slightly heterogeneous with small cystic lesions. Calcifications may be seen in complex and long-lasting fibroadenomas; coarse benign "pop-corn" calcifications are typical of calcified fibroadenomas and show posterior acoustic shadowing. Cysts >3 mm and calcifications are seen in complex fibroadenomas. Juvenile fibroadenomas are well-circumscribed, hypoechoic, and may have heterogeneous echotexture and posterior acoustic enhancement (Figs. 8.28f–j and 8.29c, d).

Phyllodes Tumors

This biphasic stromal and epithelial tumor accounts for less than 0.3% of all breast tumors and 2.5% of all fibroepithelial tumors. These tumors occur in middle-aged women, although they may occur at a younger age in Asian women. Patients have a bulging, well-circumscribed, unilateral painless breast mass, not attached to the skin. Most phyllodes tumors behave in a benign fashion; recurrence occurs within 3 years, particularly in the case of borderline and malignant tumors. Most deaths occur within 5–8 years post-diagnosis, and lung and skeletal metastases are most common. Mediastinal involvement secondary to chest wall invasion have been reported.

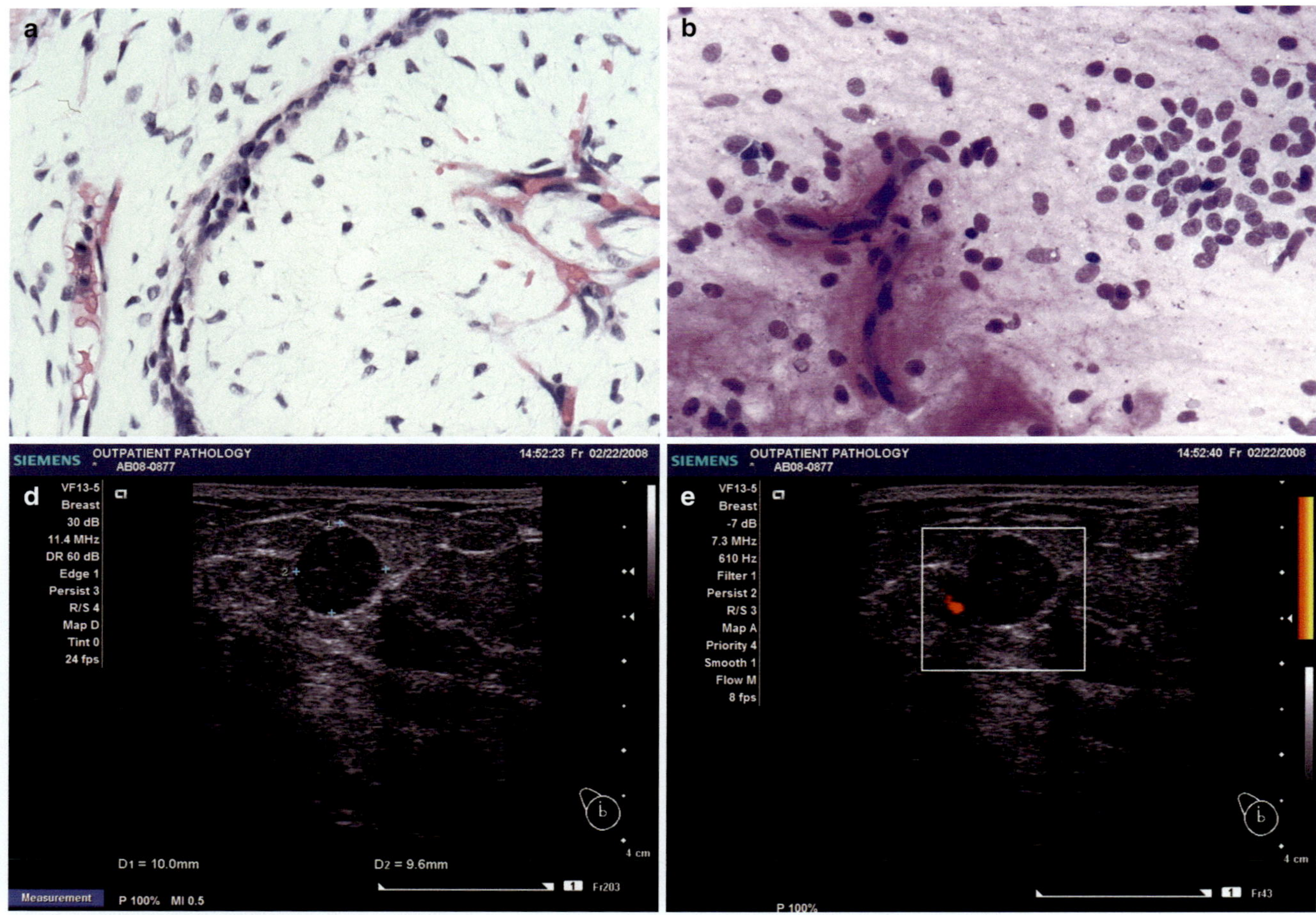

Fig. 8.29 Myxoid fibroadenoma. The myxoid stroma is prominent in both the histology and cytology (**a**, **b**). Ultrasound shows a round hypoechoic mass with circumscribed distinct margins, homogeneous echotexture, posterior acoustic enhancement, and little or no vascular flow by Doppler exam (**c**, **d**). (**a**, H&E stain, low magnification; **b**, DiffQuik stain high magnification)

Histopathology These tumors have hypercellular stroma and an intracanalicular stromal growth pattern with leaf-like projections into elongated and variably dilated lumina. Arch-like clefts are lined with epithelial and myoepithelial cell layers and surround stromal mounds. Marked usual ductal epithelial hyperplasia is common. Tumor size, mitotic activity, cytologic atypia, stromal overgrowth, and the status of borders/margins are histologic parameters useful for assessment of the biologic behavior of these tumors. Based on these parameters, phyllodes tumors are classified as benign, borderline, and malignant. Benign phyllodes tumors have pushing borders, accentuated subepithelial stromal cellularity, and <5 mitoses per 10 high-power fields (Fig. 8.30a). Malignant phyllodes tumors have infiltrating borders, marked stromal cellularity, inconspicuous epithelial component, cellular stromal pleomorphism, and >10 mitoses per 10 high-power fields. In summary, the stromal component is the basis for the diagnosis and grading of phyllodes tumor.

Immunoprofile No specific marker distinguishes phyllodes tumors from fibroadenomas or accurately diagnoses benign, borderline, or malignant phyllodes tumors. Immunocytochemistry shows the typical epithelial and myoepithelial markers, including hormone receptors like those seen in ductal cells. Neoplastic stromal cells are usually labeled with antibodies for vimentin, CD34, and collagen types I and III, and they have positive foci for endothelin (TE-1), bcl-2, CD117, EGFR, and for the beta fraction of ER. No significant differences are observed between the benign and the malignant lesions, except that the latter show a greater percentage of MIB-1-positive cells. Therefore, the proliferation index Ki-67 expression correlates with tumor grade. Likewise, p53 (tumor suppressor for cell cycle control) nuclear stain and CD10 expression may correlate with tumor grade, but do not differentiate between fibroadenoma and benign phyllodes since the stain is negative in both.

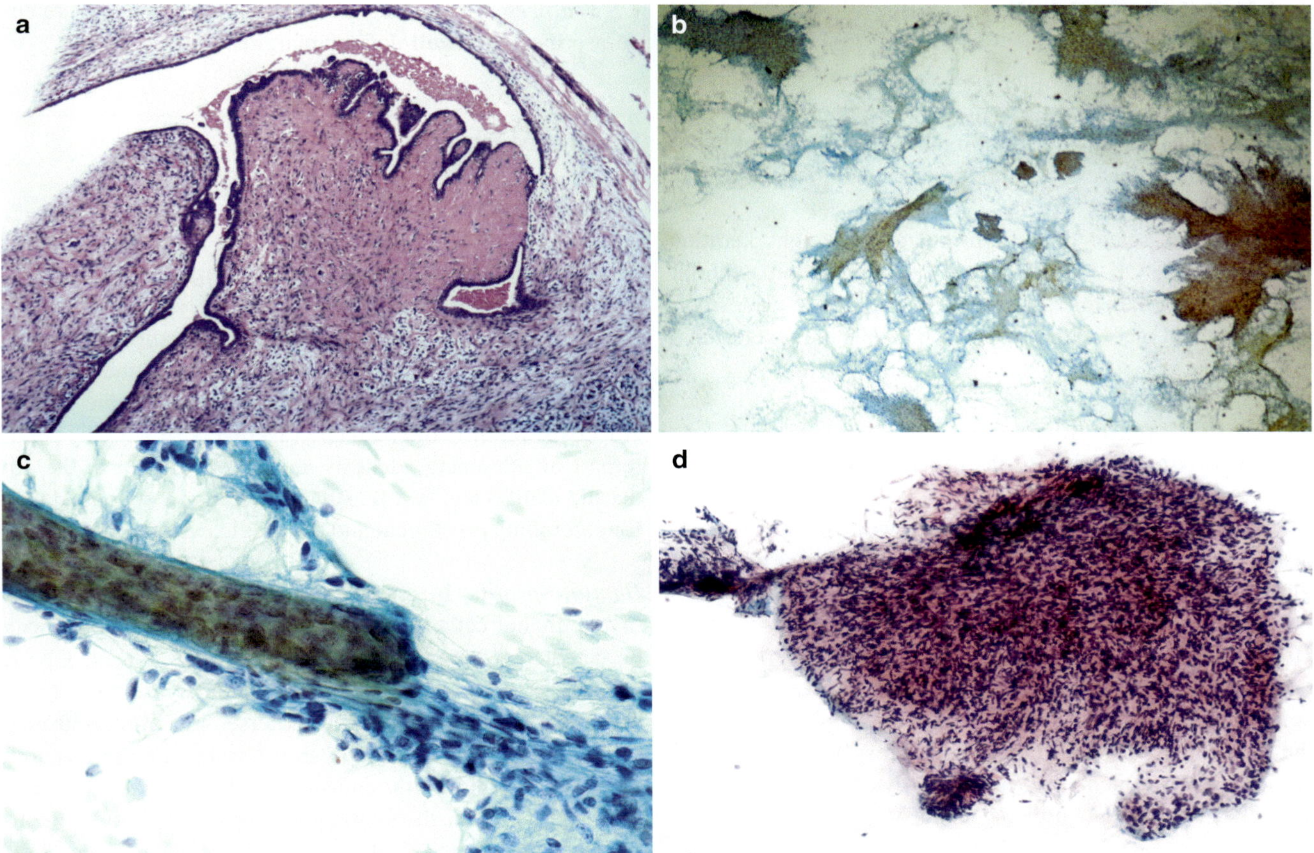

Fig. 8.30 Phyllodes tumor. Tissue section shows hypercellular stroma and arch-like clefts lined with epithelial and myoepithelial cell layers that surround stromal mounds (**a**). The FNA smear pattern is similar to that of fibroadenoma, except for the marked cellular stroma (**b–d**). Diagnosis of benign, borderline, or malignant phyllodes requires examination of the excised tumor. (**a**, H&E low magnification; **b–d** Papanicolaou stain low and intermediate magnification)

Molecular Profile There is evidence of epithelial influence over stromal growth via the Wnt signaling pathway, upregulation of transcriptionally active β-catenin, and downstream effectors such as cyclin D1. α- and β-catenins in stromal cells may be important in early stages of phyllodes tumors development, and E-cadherin may be required for malignant transformation. β-catenin binds to the cytoplasmic domain of E-cadherin and to α-catenin in cell–cell adhesion. Stromal β-catenin correlates with α-catenin expression and is significantly higher in borderline than in benign phyllodes tumors but lower in malignant tumors. Thus, malignant phyllodes tumors show loss of β-catenin and, in addition show *MYC* amplification, and aberrant expression of *TP53*. The stroma also influences the epithelium via IGF (insulin-like growth factor) signaling pathway, and IGFR1 and 2 (insulin-growth factor polypeptide hormones 1 and 2) that are overexpressed in the stroma of fibroepithelial tumors. The expression of α-catenin by stromal cells is associated with tumor recurrence.

FNA Findings Smears show both epithelial and stromal elements. The distinction from fibroadenomas is based mainly on the cellularity of the stromal fragments. In addition, and in contrast to fibroadenomas, stromal cells have larger nuclei, irregular nuclear contours, and occasional nucleoli (Fig. 8.30b–d). Malignant phyllodes tumors show large atypical stromal cells and mitoses. Marked ductal epithelial hyperplasia with varying degrees of atypia is common and may lead to an erroneous diagnosis of mammary carcinoma.

US Features The US features of phyllodes tumors can be indistinguishable from those of fibroadenomas. The tumor is hypoechoic, well-circumscribed with smooth distinct borders and typical internal hyperechoic bands and shadows, and with variable posterior acoustic enhancement and shadowing. Calcifications may be present. Occasionally, a complex cystic mass may be seen and can suggest the diagnosis of a malignant phyllodes tumor.

Epithelial-Myoepithelial Tumors

Epithelial-myoepithelial tumorss encompass pleomorphic adenoma, adenomyoepithelioma, and adenomyoepithelial carcinoma. Myoepithelial tumors encompass myoepithelial hyperplasia, collagenous spherulosis, and myoepithelial carcinoma.

Antibodies selected to high-molecular weight keratins (CK 5, CK 5/6, CK 14, CK 17), p63, actin, calponin, smooth muscle heavy chain myosin, S-100 protein, and H-caldesmon (variable) will react with myoepithelial cells in most lesions.

Adenomyoepithelioma and Adenomyoepithelial Carcinoma

These are rare tumors that affect adult women and that may also be seen in men. Patients may have tenderness or nipple discharge.

Histopathology Adenomyoepithelioma shows a proliferation of myoepithelial cell layers around epithelium-lined spaces. The histologic pattern may be lobular, papillary, tubular, or mixed. Myoepithelial cells may be spindle, epithelioid, or glycogen-rich with clear cytoplasm. Either the epithelial or the myoepithelial cells or both may undergo malignant change. The malignant epithelial component may give rise to invasive breast carcinoma of no special type, to undifferentiated carcinoma, or to metaplastic carcinoma. The tumor has a low malignant potential, and there may be local recurrence particularly after incomplete excision.

Immuno-Profile Epithelial cells express low-molecular-weight cytokeratin, whereas myoepithelial cells show CK5, CK6, CK14, CK17, p63, α-SMA, calponin, CD10, maspin, and S-100 protein. Immunostains for estrogen recptor (ER) and progesterone receptor (PR) are negative or focally weakly positive. HER2 is negative.

Molecular Profile Allelic imbalance, microsatellite instability, and reciprocal translocations between chromosomes 8 and 16 have been described in adenomyoepithelioma.

FNA Findings Smears are variably cellular and show cohesive aggregates of epithelial and myoepithelial cells supported by variable amounts of fibrillary magenta stroma admixed with delicate branching capillaries. Myoepithelial cells have clear cell, spindle, or plasmacytoid characteristics or appear naked and bipolar and dissociated in the smear background. The epithelial cells are small and may be arranged in small sheets or tubules. Metachromatic stroma may also be seen in the background and may be fibrillary or clumpy, resembling collagenous spherulosis.

US Features The tumors are round or lobulated and are circumscribed with well-defined margins.

Epithelial Tumors

Benign Epithelial Proliferations

Microglandular Adenosis, Sclerosing Adenosis, and Adenosis Tumor

Microglandular adenosis is a benign proliferation of glandular elements involving terminal ducts and lobular units. Sclerosing adenosis is a benign and microscopic lesion. Adenosis tumor is the palpable (average size 2.5 cm) counterpart of sclerosing adenosis, occurs commonly in the 4th decade of life, and is rare. Adenosis tumor can be mistaken for carcinoma on clinical and histologic evaluation.

Immuno-profile In sclerosing adenosis, the presence of myoepithelial cells, masked by architectural distortion, can be detected by immunoreactions with CK5, CK14, CK17, α-SMA, p63, and calponin. Microglandular adenosis shows a normal epithelial monolayer immersed in a fibrous stroma, sometimes surrounded by a hyaline basal membrane without myoepithelial cells. Immunostaining for collagen IV, laminin, and vimentin shows the presence of a basement membrane, which is not always obvious on conventional H&E stain. In microglandular adenosis, the myoepithelial markers are negative, whereas the S-100 protein is positive.

FNA Findings The smear pattern is similar to that of proliferative fibrocystic change, including sheets of ductal epithelial cells, numerous myoepithelial cell nuclei, and stromal fragments. The specific diagnosis of adenosis tumor is not possible on FNA; however, the diagnosis of benign proliferative fibrocystic change can be made.

US Features Adenosis tumor may be seen as a hypoechoic mass with posterior acoustic shadowing. Angular margins and tubular-like extensions may be present.

Radial Scar/Complex Sclerosing Lesion

Radial scar is a small stellate lesion, whereas a complex sclerosing lesion is larger and more complex, and may occasionally be palpable. These lesions are usually found incidentally on imaging studies and they may be mistaken for carcinoma on clinical, imaging, and histologic grounds, in particular for tubular carcinoma.

Histopathology Both lesions show a lobular architecture, epithelial proliferation, and prominent sclerosis and elastosis. They have a central zone of fibroelastosis with radiating ducts and lobules showing ductal dilatation, various patterns of epithelial hyperplasia, apocrine metaplasia, sclerosing adenosis, and micropapillomas. The compressed tubules, particularly in the sclerotic areas, are distorted and angular and have a myoepithelial cell layer that may be inconspicuous on routine histologic evaluation. Radial scar may exhibit atypical ductal hyperplasia, DCIS, or lobular neoplasia.

Immuno-profile The myoepithelial cell layer is detected with immunostains (p63, calponin, smooth muscle actin, smooth-muscle myosin heavy chain); however, caution is suggested in the interpretation particularly in small biopsies since results may vary.

FNA Findings Cytologically, smears show variable cellularity, usually small to moderate; as in fibrocystic change, sheets of ductal epithelial cells, myoepithelial cell nuclei, apocrine metaplasia, and macrophages with cyst debris may be variably present.

US Features Ultrasound, in a few patients, may show a hypoechoic lesion with irregular stellate borders and a central hyperechoic area corresponding to the fibroelastotic central area, similar to low-grade carcinomas; however, an echogenic halo, distal attenuation, a taller than wide shape, and distortion are more common in cancer, whereas small cysts and an echogenic component are more frequent in radial scar.

Tubular Adenoma

This is a well-circumscribed (not truly encapsulated), painless nodule that occurs mainly in young women.

Histopathology The tumor is composed of a proliferation of tubular structures lined by epithelial and myoepithelial cells separated by scant stroma.

Immunohistochemistry The stromal cells are positive for CD34, bcl-2, and SMA, demonstrating their myofibroblastic nature. Sometimes stromal cells can express PR. Epithelial and myoepithelial cells show their typical immunophenotype. Epithelial cells are also positive for ER and PR.

FNA Findings Cytologically, the presence of smaller tubules and myoepithelial cells distinguishes tubular adenoma from tubular carcinoma; otherwise, smears resemble fibroadenoma without stroma.

US Features US shows a well-circumscribed hypoechoic oval mass with homogeneous echotexture, smooth borders, and posterior acoustic enhancement or shadowing; margins may be variable.

Apocrine Adenoma

This lesion is rare and occurs in both males and females. Patients have a painless nodule usually measuring <2 cm. Histologically, there is a nodular collection of glands lined with apocrine epithelium with no cytologic atypia. The lesion is benign and is cured by local excision. Immunohistochemically, the apocrine cells show CK8, CK18, EMA, GCDFP-15, apolipoprotein D, and α2-glycoprotein. They express androgen receptor, but no ER or PR.

Pregnancy-Related Lesions

These changes are the result of a hormonal effect on de novo (lactating adenoma, Fig. 8.31a) or pre-existent (fibroadenoma, fibrocystic change) palpable or non-palpable breast lesions. Most are benign, and they often regress within 6 months postpartum. Pregnant or lactating women may develop a galactocele, which is a milk-filled cystic lesion and may be seen up to several years post-lactation.

FNA Findings The smears are cellular and show numerous complex cellular aggregates, loose clusters, and numerous dissociated cells with clear or vacuolated cytoplasm. Acinar cells have round nuclei, prominent nucleoli, abundant vacuolated cytoplasm, and frayed edges. The background shows bubbly and finely vacuolated granular lipid-rich cytoplasmic contents and variable numbers of stripped epithelial cell nuclei with prominent nucleoli. Except in fibroadenomas with lactational change, myoepithelial cell nuclei are lacking (Fig. 8.31b–e). The differential diagnosis includes breast adenocarcinoma, which can be minimized or avoided with clinical correlation and the fact that breast malignancy in pregnancy usually shows greater cellular and architectural atypia, cell dissociation, and hyperchromasia than lactational changes. An aspirate of milk confirms the diagnosis of galactocele.

US Features *Normal* lactating breast shows a subtle diffusely increased tissue echogenicity with loss of normal tissue planes including Cooper's ligaments, reflecting the presence of lactational changes. Features of *lactating adenoma* are similar to those of fibroadenoma, including a macrolobulated, oval, hypoechoic well-circumscribed mass with posterior acoustic enhancement; however, irregular margins, heterogeneous echotexture, small cystic spaces, and posterior acoustic shadowing may be present (Fig. 8.31f–l). Multiple internal linear or curvilinear echogenic bands are commonly present. *Galactocele* has features of a cyst or may have echogenic material within the fluid, probably representing an admixture of fatty globules and water, resulting in an US pattern similar to that of fibroadenoma (Fig. 8.32d). Compression of the mass with the US probe identifies the movement of particles in galactocele, confirming the diagno-

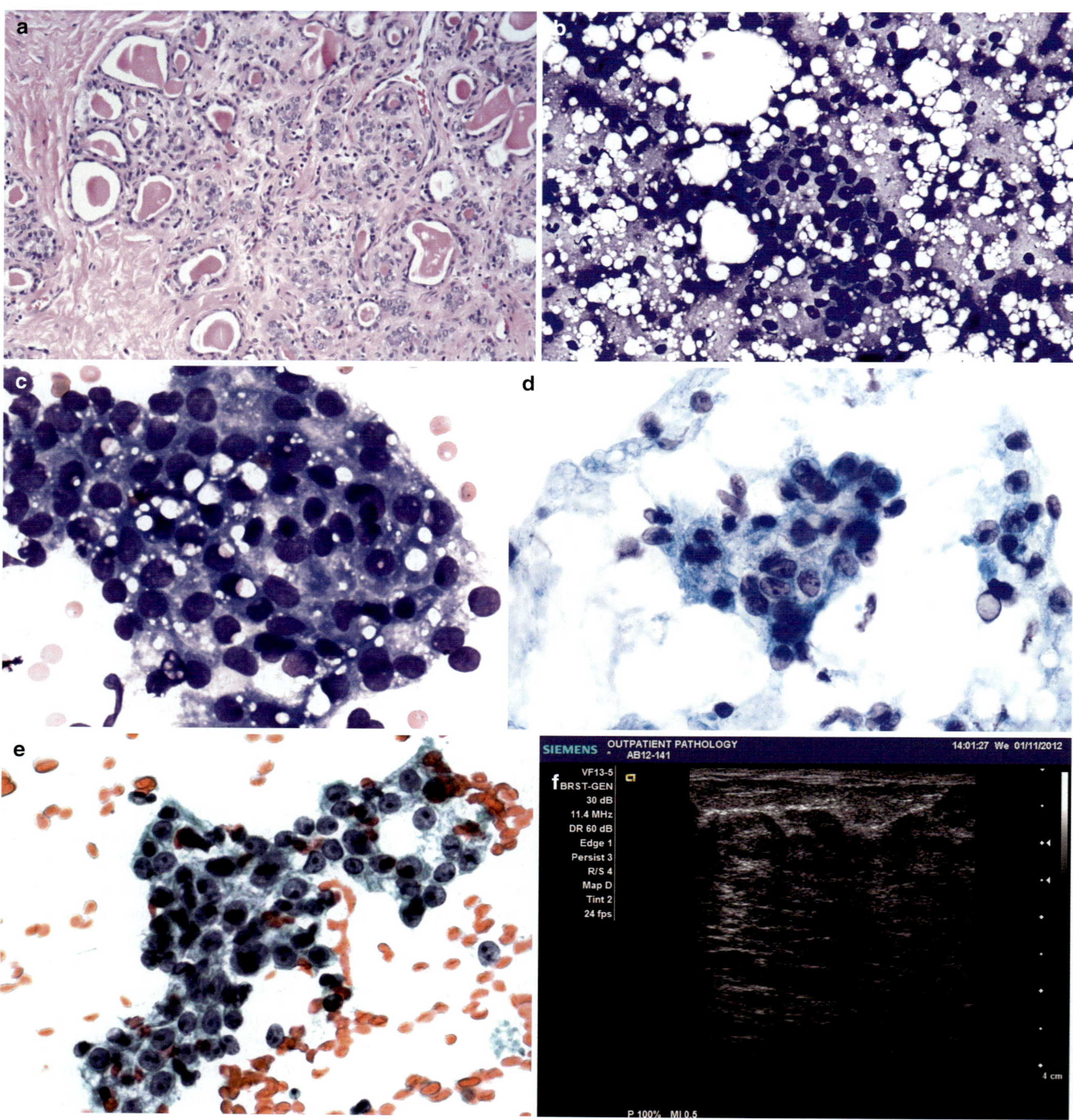

Fig. 8.31 Pregnancy-related lesions. Histopathology of a lactating adenoma is seen in (**a**). Smears harvested from pregnancy-related lesions with lactational changes show a background of fine lipid vacuoles, scattered single and aggregates cells with cytoplasm, prominent nucleoli, and complex architecture (**b–d**). Myoepithelial cells are present in preexisting fibroadenomas with lactational changes (**e**). Awareness and clinical history are necessary to avoid an erroneous diagnosis of atypia or malignancy. Ultrasound features from palpable masses range from ill-defined complex masses (**f–k**) to well-defined hypoechoic masses in cases of fibroadenoma with lactational changes (**l**). Normal lactating breast with accentuated parenchyma often shows no increased or minimal vascular blood flow by Doppler exam. (**a**, H&E stain low magnification; **b**, DiffQuik stain intermediate magnification; **c**, MGG stain high magnification; **d**, **e**, Papanicolaou stain high magnification)

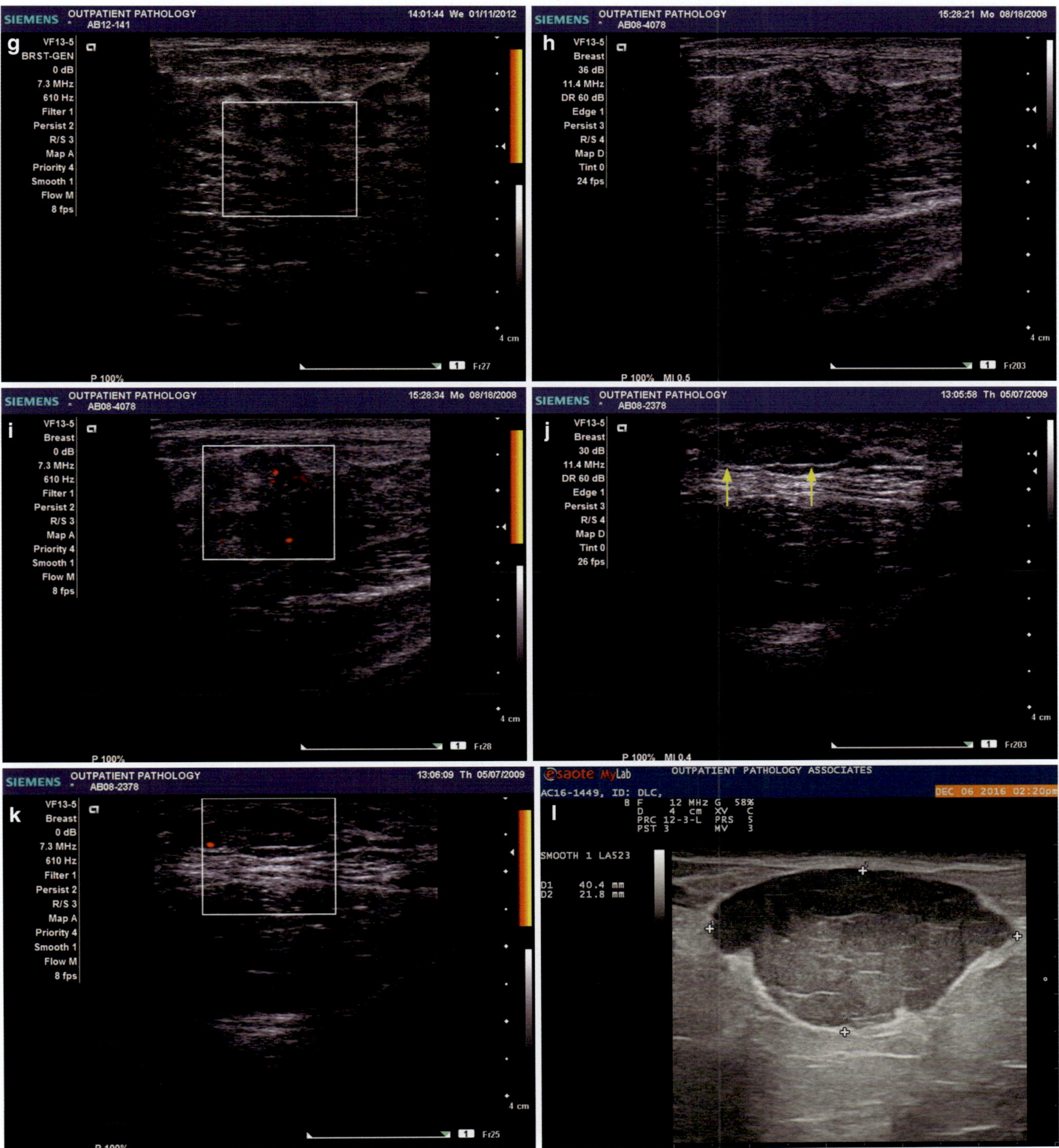

Fig. 8.31 (continued)

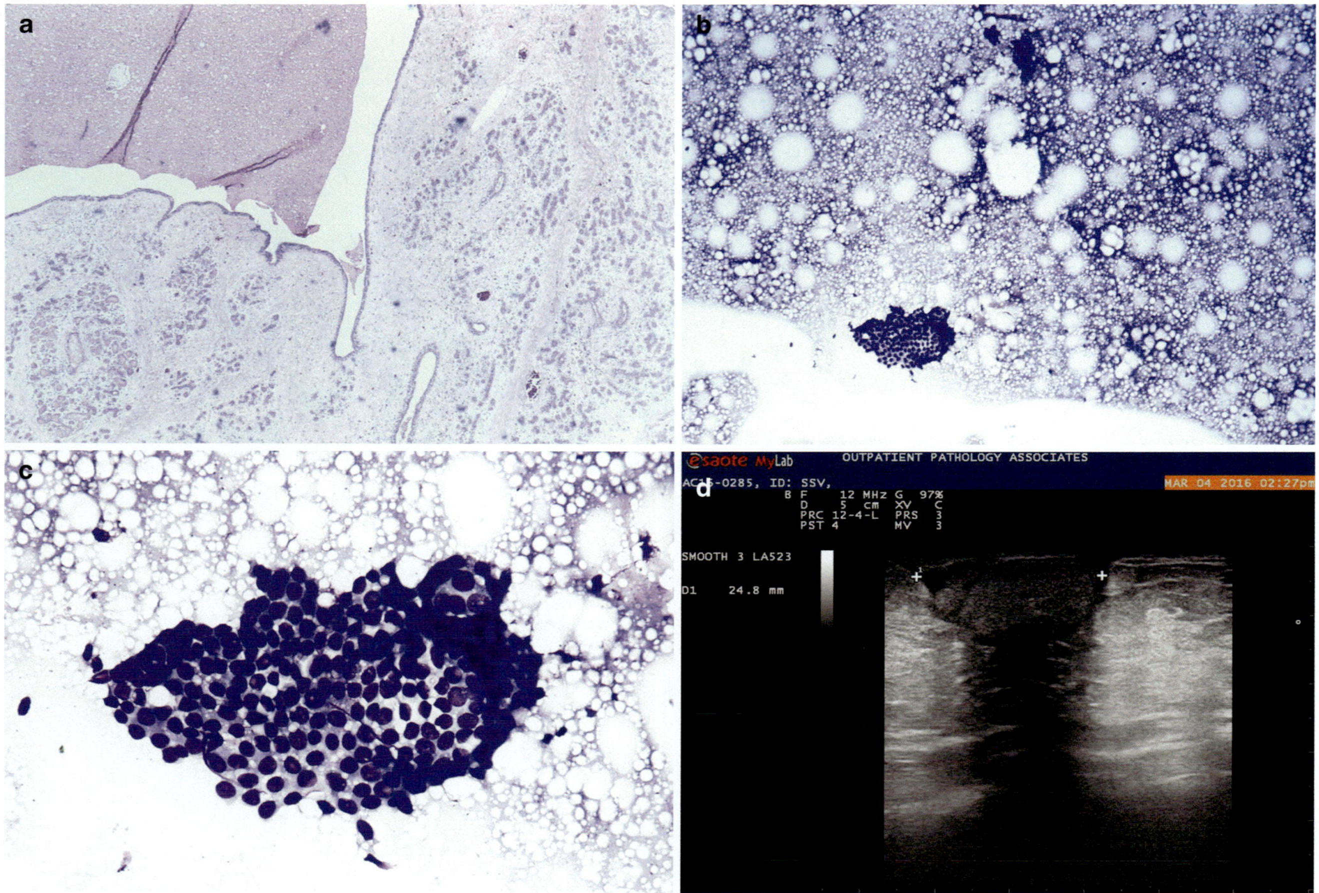

Fig. 8.32 Galactocele. Tissue section shows a cystically dilated duct with intraluminal fluid consistent with milk (**a**). Smears show rare epithelial cells with lactational changes surrounded by fluid with lipid vacuoles consistent with milk (**b**, **c**). US image in this galactocele shows a well-defined hypoechoic homogeneous mass with slightly lobulated borders and posterior acoustic shadowing resembling a solid mass. (**a**, H&E stain low magnification; **b**, **c**, DiffQuik stain low and high magnification)

sis. Occasionally, galactocele may appear complex and have horizontal band-like hypoechogenic areas (fluid-fluid level) with slight posterior acoustic shadowing.

Nipple Adenoma

This benign epithelial proliferation affects the collecting ducts of women at any age, with an average of 47 years, who complain of nipple discharge, nipple erosion, or a nodule. The lesion may recur if it is excised incompletely.

FNA Findings The smear pattern is similar to that of fibrocystic change, with marked ductal epithelial hyperplasia including numerous sheets of benign ductal epithelial cells and myoepithelial cell nuclei.

US Features The mass is oval, circumscribed, hypoechoic, and may have associated calcifications; however, US findings may suggest carcinoma in the presence of sclerosis.

Adenomas of Skin Adnexal Origin and Other Adenomas

Because these tumors originate in the skin they can be suspected based on clinical and US evaluation. Ductal adenoma, syringomatous adenoma, and pleomorphic adenoma (chondroid syringoma) are some of these tumors. Syringomatous adenoma affects the dermis of the nipple or the areolar region. Pleomorphic adenoma usually affects the peri areolar area.

FNA Findings The specific diagnosis cannot always be made by FNA cytology; however, the tumors can be recognized as benign.

US Features US may show a stellate subareolar mass that may suggest malignancy. When the nodule is round, it may suggest adenoma; its association with the skin may suggest an adnexal origin.

Fibrocystic Change

This lesion represents the most common palpable lesion in women above the age of 30 years and is considered to represent an exaggerated hormonally mediated breast tissue response.

Histopathology Histologically, there are duct dilatation, cysts, apocrine metaplasia, fibrosis, chronic inflammation, and varying degrees of ductal epithelial hyperplasia, which should be evaluated carefully (Fig. 8.33a).

FNA Findings Smears show sparse epithelial representation due to the presence of fibrosis. Ductal epithelial cells are arranged in flat, cohesive honeycomb sheets with round or oval nuclei and fine granular chromatin with small inconspicuous nucleoli. Stripped myoepithelial cell nuclei are present adherent to the epithelial cell sheets and in the smear background. Apocrine metaplastic cells are polygonal with ample granular cytoplasm and conspicuous nucleoli. Foam cells are often present in the background. Higher numbers of ductal epithelial cells with slight anisocytosis and anisonucleosis without atypia are seen in proliferative fibrocystic change, always accompanied by bipolar myoepithelial cell nuclei (Fig. 8.33b–d). However, no distinct cytomorphologic features can distinguish between nonproliferative and proliferative fibrocystic change without atypia.

US Features These lesions show slight hyperechogenicity due to fibrosis, small (<5 mm) hypoechoic or anechoic nodules, and duct dilatation (Fig. 8.33e–g).

Molecular Pathology Aspects of Epithelial Precancerous Breast Lesions

Despite the insight of molecular biology and genetics in breast tumor progression, our understanding remains incomplete. The traditional model of linear progression from normal epithelium to hyperplasia to atypical hyperplasia to carcinoma secondary to cumulative genetic abnormalities

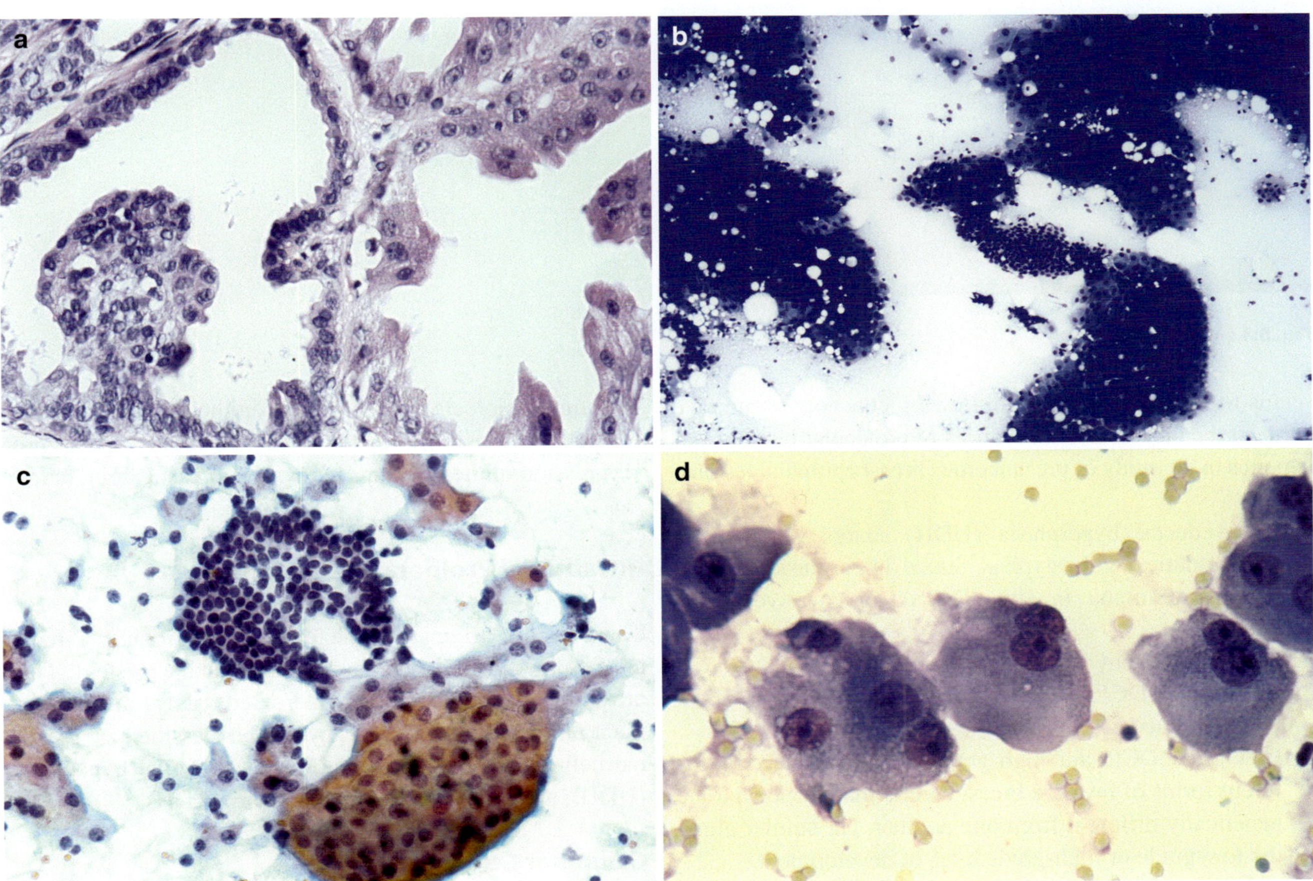

Fig. 8.33 Fibrocystic change. Histology showing cystic dilatation, ductal epithelial hyperplasia, apocrine metaplasia, and lack of epithelial atypia (**a**). The FNA smear shows high cellularity (**b**) composed of sheets of ductal epithelial cells without atypia (**b**), apocrine metaplasia (**a–c**), stripped myoepithelial cell nuclei (**c**), and cystic background (**c**). Apocrine metaplastic cells with slight nuclear atypia may be seen (**d**). Ultrasound shows dense slightly hyperechoic tissue bands surrounding hypoechoic nodular areas (**e**) and minimal vascular flow by Doppler exam (**f**). (**a**, H&E stain, medium magnification; **b**, **d** DiffQuik stain low and high magnification; **c**, Papanicolaou stain intermediate magnification)

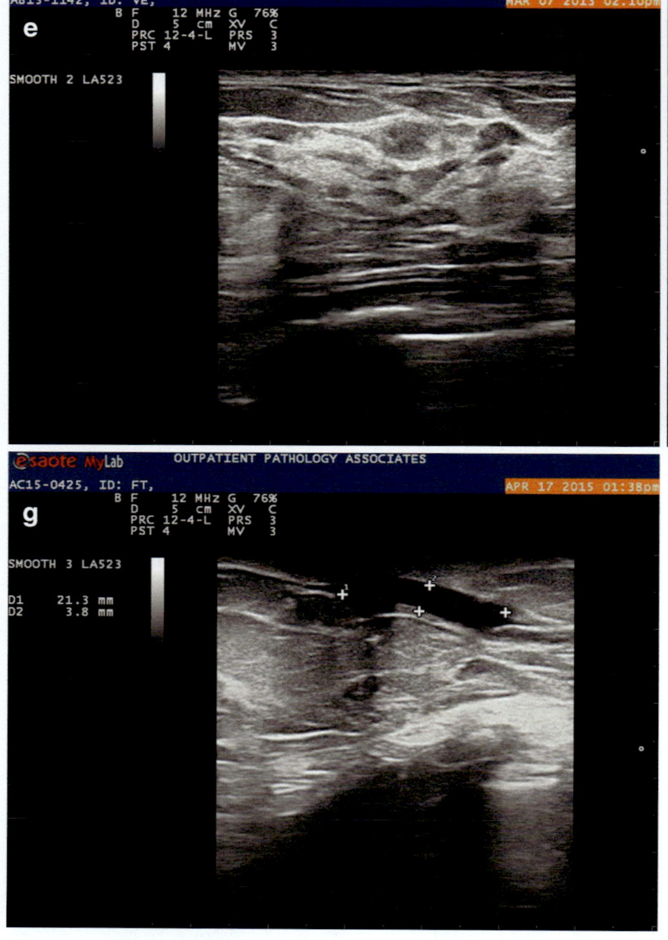

Fig. 8.33 (continued)

seems to be too simple. The following concepts summarize some of the most relevant advances of molecular biology and genetics in the study of precancerous breast epithelial lesions:

1. Usual ductal hyperplasia (UDH) shares few genetic abnormalities with atypical ductal hyperplasia (ADH), ductal carcinoma in situ (DCIS), or invasive breast carcinoma.
2. ADH share many similarities with DCIS.
3. ADH and DCIS (all grades) appear to be clonal proliferations.
4. Low-grade DCIS and high-grade DCIS give place to different forms of invasive breast carcinoma that seem to be genetically different from one another, but similar along the low-grade or high-grade lines of development.
5. Lobular in situ and invasive carcinoma share genetic and molecular similarities with DCIS and invasive duct breast carcinoma of no special type.

6. Tumor microenvironment (myoepithelial cells and epithelial–stromal interactions) may be critical in the progression of these lesions to invasive breast carcinoma.

Intraductal Proliferative Lesions

These lesions originate in the terminal-duct lobular unit and are confined to the mammary ductal-lobular system. They are associated with a variably increased risk for the development of breast carcinoma. They can be classified as: columnar cell lesions (CCLs), usual ductal epithelial hyperplasia (UDH), and atypical ductal hyperplasia (ADH).

Columnar Cell Lesions (CCLs)

CCLs are not palpable and are often identified on screening mammography. Occasionally, the lesion is palpable, being part of nonproliferative or proliferative fibrocystic change.

Histopathology The standardized histologic term of CCLs describe lesions showing dilated acini lined by columnar cells that frequently have apical cytoplasmic snouts. They are classified into four categories: columnar cell change (one or two cell layers thick) with or without atypia and columnar cell hyperplasia (cell stratification or tufting) with or without atypia. The lesions with atypia are categorized as "flat epithelial atypia" (well-developed arcades, bridges, or micropapillary structures are absent). The atypia is of low grade and monomorphic and, for practical purposes, "flat" proliferations with high-grade nuclei should be regarded as DCIS. There is a strong association of these lesions with the coexistence of lobular carcinoma in situ (LCIS), atypical lobular hyperplasia (ALH), ADH, low-grade DCIS, and low-grade invasive carcinoma.

Immuno-profile Flat epithelial atypia shows positive ER and negative HER2.

Molecular Profile Loss of 16q is the most frequent change found in flat epithelial atypia. Thus, these lesions are considered more likely to be precursors to ADH and low-grade DCIS.

FNA Findings CCLs are commonly identified in aspiration smears as small cohesive crowded aggregates of bland ductal cells with peripheral columnar cells, which may show apical snouts. Varying degrees of atypia may be seen. When there is coexistent fibrocystic change, the background may show sheets of ductal epithelial cells, myoepithelial cell nuclei, macrophages, and proteinaceous fluid.

Usual Ductal Hyperplasia (UDH)

The risk of UDH for the subsequent development of breast cancer is 1.5 times that of the reference population. Recent molecular data suggest that "flat epithelial atypia" is a more likely precursor to ADH and DCIS than is UDH. DCIS is recognized as a true precursor to invasive breast cancer. UDH is most common in the late premenopausal years. When it is associated with fibrosis, lesions may be palpable. Otherwise, they are usually found incidentally to other lesions.

Histopathology Characteristically, there is a cohesive intraductal proliferation of benign epithelial cells with prominent cellular streaming, and there are peripherally distributed fenestrations of variable sizes (Fig. 8.34a).

Immuno-profile Proliferating cells show immunohistochemical positivity for CK5, CK8, CK14, CK17, CK18, CK19, and S100 protein. Myoepithelial markers are usually absent or only occasionally present. Positivity for ER is heterogeneous and variable; DCIS shows diffuse and strong ER positivity.

Molecular Profile No consistent genetic alterations have been found in UDH. The molecular and genetic alterations seen in ADH and DCIS are not found in UDH. The vast majority of these lesions are not thought to progress to invasive mammary carcinoma.

FNA Findings The cellularity is moderate to high, with fragments of ductal epithelial cells with numerous myoepithelial cells both adherent to the cell aggregates and in the

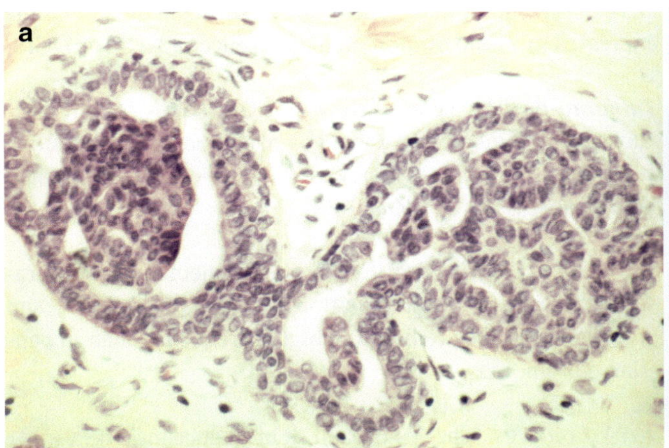
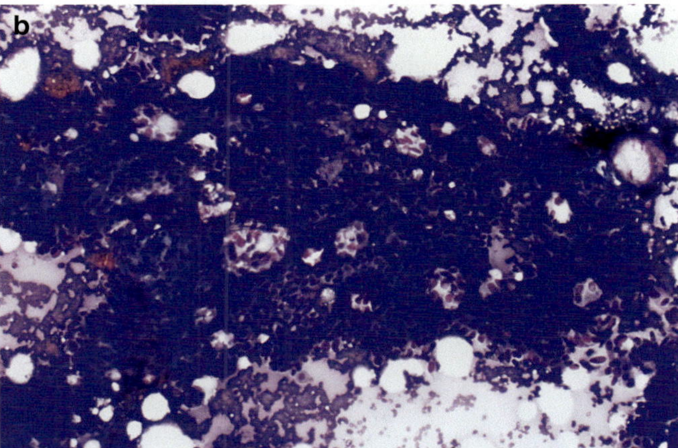

Fig. 8.34 Ductal epithelial hyperplasia without atypia. Histologic section shows two ducts with hyperplasia of epithelial cells and streaming and fenestration of variable shape (**a**). The smears are cellular and show sheets of ductal epithelial cells with myoepithelial cell nuclei and fenestrations of variable shape (**b**). (**a**, H&E stain low magnification; **b**, DiffQuik stain low magnification)

smear background. Cells are mildly enlarged and crowded (Fig. 8.34b). Elements of fibrocystic change may be present in UDH.

Atypical Ductal Hyperplasia

The risk for subsequent development of breast cancer is 3–5 times that of the reference population.

Histopathology This process involves the terminal-duct lobular units with a proliferation of evenly placed monomorphic epithelial cells that lack the streaming, swirling, and overlapping of UDH. Cytomorphology is similar to that of low-grade DCIS; however, ADH is smaller (<2 mm or <2 ducts) and does not involve the full cross- section of the duct.

Immuno-profile Cells are typically negative for high-molecular-weight keratins (CK 5/6, in contrast to UDH) and diffusely positive for ER. The proliferating cells express CK8, CK18, CK19, and sometimes CK7. The myoepithelial cells that line the tubulo-lobular terminal units express CK5, CK14, and CK17 simultaneously with myoepithelial cell markers.

Molecular Profile Common molecular and genetic alterations seen in ADH, low-grade DCIS, and invasive carcinomas include loss of heterozygosity in chromosome segments 16q, 17p, and 11q13, with losses at 16q being frequent.

FNA Findings The smears show high epithelial cellularity with cytologic and architectural atypia, with cellular and nuclear enlargement, loss of polarity, considerable cellular and nuclear overlapping, monomorphic atypical cells, nuclear hyperchomasia, prominent nucleoli, and variable numbers of myoepithelial cells (Fig. 8.35). However, myoepithelial cells may be absent, and variable numbers of single atypical epithelial cells may be seen in the background. A

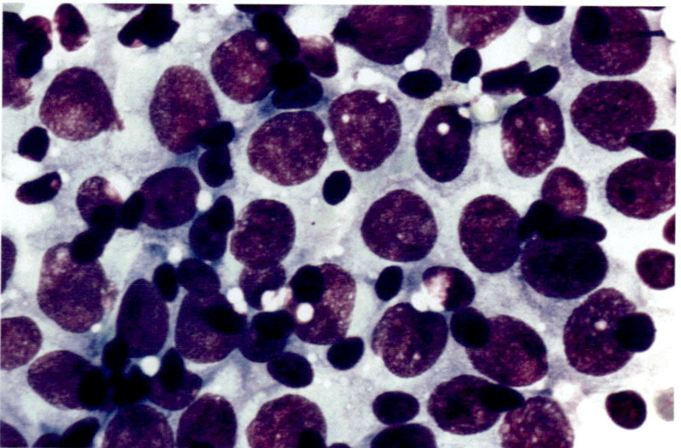

Fig. 8.35 Ductal epithelial hyperplasia with atypia. Observe atypical epithelial cells and myoepithelial cell nuclei. (DiffQuik stain, high magnification)

cribriform architecture and complex epithelial cell aggregates may be present. Thus, FNA cytology cannot reliably distinguish ADH from the noncomedo type of DCIS. Nevertheless, FNA cytology is useful in identifying these overlapping entities and prompts an excisional biopsy.

US Features The lesion is not US-visible unless it is associated with other lesions such as papilloma, in which case it may be visible.

Papillary Lesions

Intraductal Papilloma

Intraductal papillomas often occur in women in the 7th and 8th decades of life. Solitary or central papilloma originates from the large ducts and usually develops in the areolar area. Multiple or peripheral papillomas develop from the terminal duct-lobular units. They manifest as a bloody nipple discharge. A palpable lesion may be present particularly in central papillomas.

Histopathology Papillomas show arborescent structures lined with myoepithelial and ductal epithelial cell layers which are supported by a fibrovascular stroma (Fig. 8.36a). The layer of myoepithelial cells may be inconspicuous, and immunostains may be needed to demonstrate its presence. The epithelial layer shows columnar or cuboidal cells and may show varying degrees of ductal epithelial hyperplasia as well as various types of metaplasia. Stromal fibrosis is commonly seen and may be prominent and extensive (sclerosing papillomas). ADH or DCIS may be seen particularly in peripheral papillomas. The risk of subsequent carcinoma increases to 7-fold or more in the presence of ADH or DCIS.

Immuno-profile Tumors show positive stains for myoepithelial cells (smooth-muscle myosin, calponin, p63), positive high-molecular-weight keratins (CK 5/6 and CK14), and patchy positivity for ER and PR.

Molecular Profile Papillomas are monoclonal proliferations. Activating point mutations of *PIK3CA*, *AKT1*, and *RAS* family genes are found in higher frequency than in papillary carcinomas.

FNA Findings The lesion and dilated duct may be visible by US and sampled by USG-FNA. Smears show a bloody background and papillary aggregates of cuboidal and columnar cells. Variable cellular aggregates supported by a fibrovascular stroma are seen (Fig. 8.36b, c). Larger lesions may show necrosis. The distinction from encapsulated (intracystic) papillary carcinoma is not possible by FNA, and surgical excision is necessary.

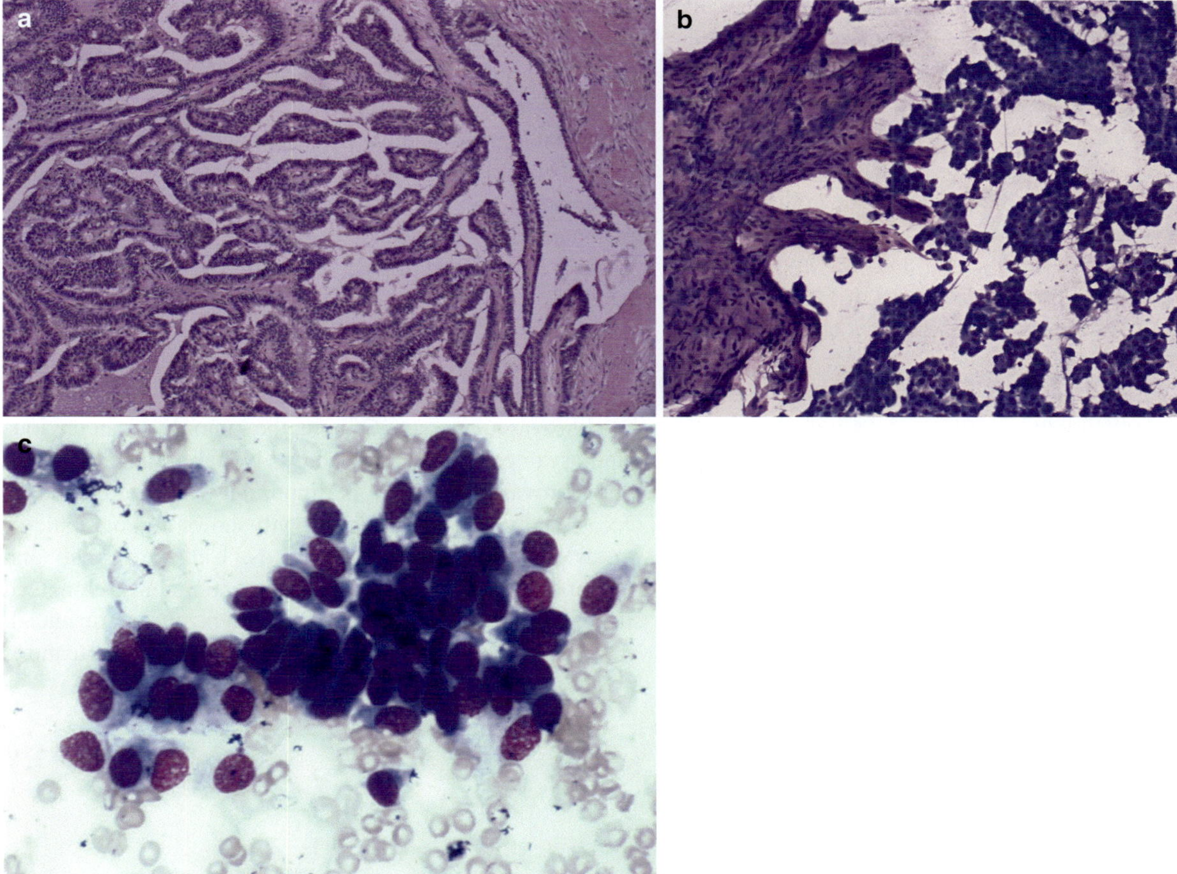

Fig. 8.36 Intraductal papilloma. Histology shows arborescent papillary structures supported by fine fibrovascular cores and lined by columnar epithelial cells and inconspicuous myoepithelial cell layer (**a**). Papilloma may show focal sclerosis of the supporting stroma as seen in this FNA smear; sheets of lining cells are also present as well as columnar cells (**b**, **c**). The distinction from intracystic papillary carcinoma cannot be made with certainty on pure cytology grounds and excision of the lesion is needed. (**a**, H&E stain low magnification; **b**, **c**, DiffQuik stain low and high magnification)

US Features Lesions have smooth borders. They may show a dilated duct with a well-defined mural solid mass or a lobulated homogeneous solid and cystic lesion with a smooth wall. Adjacent ducts are often dilated. However, sonographic features of benign papillomas overlap with those of papillary carcinomas.

Encapsulated (Intracystic) Papillary Carcinoma

This tumor occurs in older women (average, 65 years old) who show a circumscribed round mass with or without nipple discharge. If the lesion is central, there may be nipple retraction and a palpable subareolar lobulated mass. Encapsulated papillary carcinomas are noninvasive and have a good prognosis. A wide local resection is usually curative; however, associated DCIS in the surrounding tissue confers a higher risk for local recurrence.

Histopathology Central papillary carcinomas are usually solitary, whereas peripheral lesions are commonly multiple.

A thick fibrous capsule is present surrounding an arborescent proliferation of delicate fibrovascular stalks decorated by monomorphic cuboidal or columnar cells with low or intermediate nuclear grade and loss of the myoepithelial cell layer.

Immuno-profile Tumors show negative myoepithelial cell markers (p63, calponin), negative high-molecular-weight keratins (CK5/6, CK14), and diffuse and strongly positive ER and PR stains.

Molecular Profile Patterns of gene copy number aberrations and prevalence of *PIK3CA* mutations are similar to those of invasive breast carcinoma of no special type.

FNA Findings The diagnosis of encapsulated papillary carcinoma cannot be made with certainty by FNA. The aspirated fluid is usually hemorrhagic. Smears have variable cellularity, although moderate cellularity is more common, and show three-dimensional papillary structures with fibrovascular cores in a bloody background with scattered hemosiderin-laden macrophages. The decorating epithelial cells are often palisading the edges of aggregates and are bland-appearing and of columnar shape (Fig. 8.37). Myoepithelial cells are not present; however, larger and more elongated stripped nuclei of malignant cells are identified and may be confused with myoepithelial cells. The differential diagnosis includes fibro-adenoma (lacks fibrovascular cores and has myoepithelial cells) and papilloma (cannot be diagnosed by FNA cytology). Thus, surgical excision is advised whenever a papillary neoplasm is diagnosed by FNA cytology.

US Features Sonographic features of benign papillomas overlap with those of papillary carcinomas and are more difficult to differentiate on US than are other breast neoplasms. Malignant papillary lesions frequently show a round or oval shape and have a circumscribed lobulated margin; these are findings suggestive of benign lesions in other breast neoplasms. A complex mass with irregular shape, a no circumscribed margin, and a complex echo pattern is not uncommonly seen in papillary carcinomas, but their presence is not statistically significant. Irregular posterior acoustic enhancement may be present.

Solid Papillary Carcinoma

As the name implies, the solid component predominates, and no fluid collection is associated. This tumor is rare, peripherally located, and occurs in postmenopausal women with a mean age in the 7th decade of life. The patients may have a palpable mass, and nipple discharge is seen in 25% of patients.

Histopathology The tumor shows multiple circumscribed cellular and expansile nests or nodules having thin and delicate fibrovascular cores. Of note, the tumor lacks an obvious papillary or cribriform architecture; however, the presence of thin fibrovascular cores is important for the diagnosis. Occasionally, the neoplastic growth shows a geographic or jigsaw pattern of epithelial islands. Cells are small and monomorphic, with polygonal or, less commonly, elongated shape, finely granular cytoplasm, and hyperchromatic nuclei. Mitoses are present, although rare. Neuroendocrine features are not uncommon.

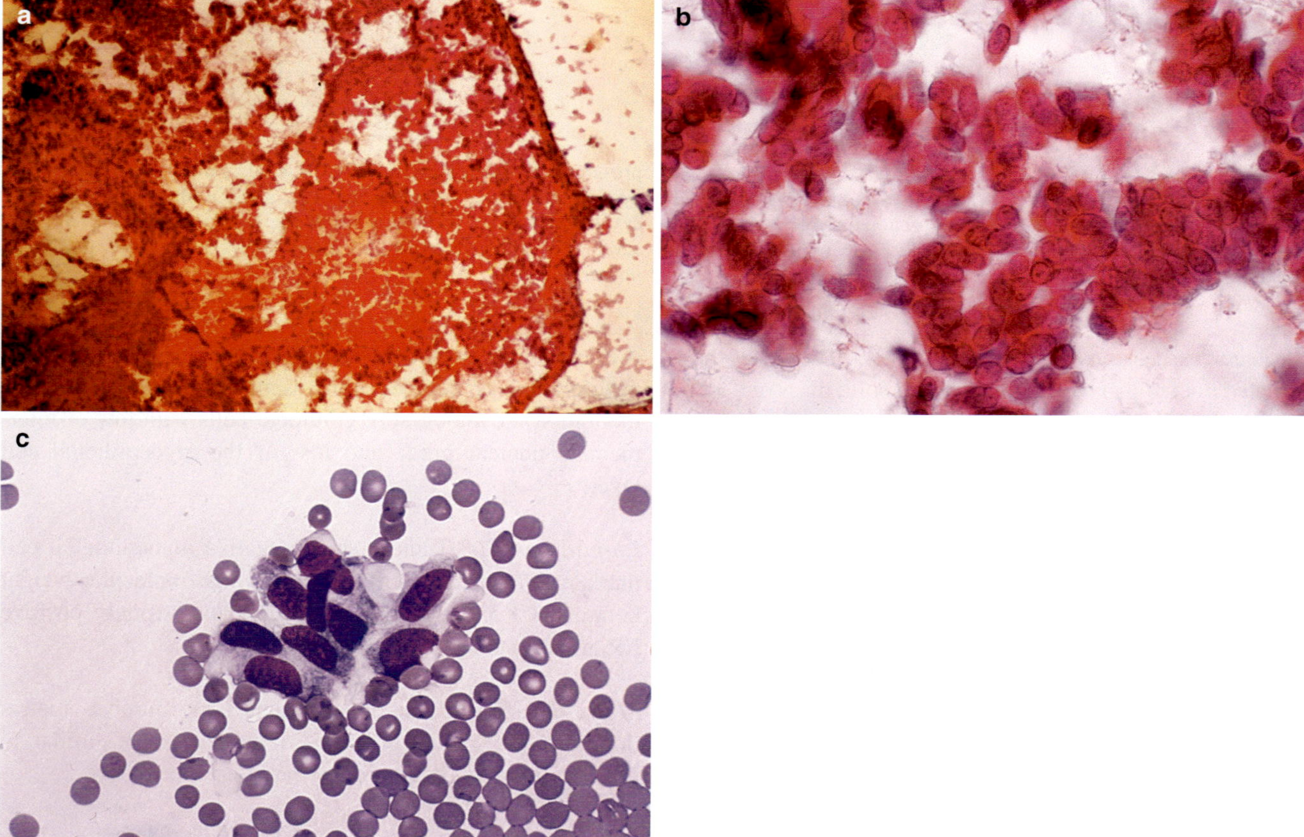

Fig. 8.37 Encapsulated papillary carcinoma. Cytologic features overlap with those of papilloma (**a–c**). The lesion should be excised and examined histologically. (**a, b**, Papanicolaou stain low and high magnification; **c**, DiffQuik stain high magnification)

Table 8.3 Immunohistochemical classification of breast cancer

IHC classification	Risk		Therapy response			
	Recurrence	Metastasis	Adjuvant	Hormonal	Biological	Traditional
Luminal A	Low	Low	No	Yes	No	No
Luminal B	Intermediate	Intermediate	Yes	Yes	Yes	Yes
Luminal C	High	High	Yes	Yes	Yes HER2$^+$	Yes
Basal TN	High	High	Yes	No	No	Yes
TN no Basal	Intermediate	Intermediate	Yes	Yes ER+	Yes HER2$^+$	Yes
HER2-positive	High	High	Yes	No	Yes	Yes
Claudin-low	Intermediate	Intermediate	Variable	No	No	Variable
Normal-like	Low	Low	No	Yes	No	No

IHC immunohistochemical, *TN* triple negative

Immuno-profile Tumors are ER and PR positive and HER2 negative. Low-molecular-weight keratins 8 and 18 are positive. High-molecular-weight keratins 5/6 are negative. Partial or sometimes complete loss of myoepithelial cells may be seen at the periphery of the nests. Neuroendocrine markers (chromogranin A, synaptophysin, and CD56) are positive in 50% of cases.

Molecular Profile Gene expression confirms the *luminal* phenotype (Table 8.3).

FNA Findings Smears are cellular and show compact fibrovascular structures decorated with columnar or elongated/spindle cells. Variable amounts of intracellular or extracellular mucin may be seen as well as neuroendocrine features.

US Features Solid papillary carcinomas may be associated with mucin production, which is not found in benign papillomas; this might be why posterior acoustic enhancement may be a characteristic finding of papillary carcinomas when present. Noninvasive papillary carcinomas more frequently show a circumscribed margin than do invasive papillary carcinomas. Differences in the shape, orientation, echo pattern, lesion boundary, posterior acoustic features, calcification, and duct dilatation are not statistically significant. High-resolution US may show the papillary features. Microcalcifications may be seen.

Molecular Pathology and Gene Expression Profile of Breast Carcinoma

Breast cancer is a heterogeneous disease with variable histopathology, metastatic potential, and a variable prognosis. The histopathologic classification alone has limited value, whereas new markers seem to be of greater clinical relevance with higher prognostic value and better predictive therapeutic response. Thus, pathologic examination and immunohistochemical results for ER, PR, and HER2 overexpression are standard practice to guide the therapeutic modality. Breast cancer is also remarkably heterogeneous at the genomic level, and there is a correlation between the patterns of gene aberrations, histologic grade, and ER expression in breast carcinoma, including DCIS.

Grade-1 invasive breast carcinomas of no special type are usually diploid or near diploid, harbor recurrent deletions of 16q (>85%), gains of 1q (60%), and gains of 16p (40%). Grade-3 invasive carcinomas are heterogeneous and often show aneuploidy, and deletions of 16q (found in <30%) are almost restricted to ER-negative tumors. Approximately, 50% of grade-3 ER-positive cancers harbor the genetic pattern found in grade-1 tumors (deletion of 16q and gain of 1q), suggesting that progression from low- to high-grade and invasive carcinoma only applies to the ER-positive tumors. Molecular evidence suggests that grade-2 tumors are the end stage of grade-1 tumors. Of note, lobular neoplasia and invasive lobular carcinoma harbor similar findings (deletion of 16q, gains of 1q and 16p).

Genetically distinct subgroups of invasive breast carcinoma have been described based on gene-expression profiling. These subtypes appear to be clinically important and reflect the phenotype of the underlying cell of origin, and they are luminal (A, B, or C/hybrid), HER2-positive, triple negative (basal-like and no basal-like), and normal breast-like. The methodology for defining these subtypes may not be fully accessible by all laboratories; thus, comparable immunohistochemistry panels have been described as being equivalent to luminal A, luminal B, HER2-positive, and triple negative genomic groups (Table 8.3). In addition, other rare subgroups have been identified, particularly normal breast-like and claudin low.

Luminal Subtype

Luminal subtype carcinoma expresses a cancer gene profile similar to that of breast duct epithelial cells. In all cases of luminal type, there is the expression of genes coding for low-molecular-weight cytokeratins (*KRT7*, *KRT8*, *KRT18*, and *KRT19*), a group of hormone receptor-related genes (*ESR1*, *ESR2*, *PR*, *LIV1*, *GATA3*, *HNF3A*, *TFF1/pS2*, *BCL2*), and

X-box binding protein (*Xbp-1*). Luminal-type carcinoma is composed of three different subtypes.

Luminal A subtype tumors comprise 55% of cancers and are commonly of histologic grade 1. It shows diffuse positivity for ER and variable positivity for PR, while HER2 is negative. CK7, CK8, CK18, and CK19 are positive and CK5, CK14, CK17 are negative (Fig. 8.38). The proliferation index is usually low. In addition to the common genes of the luminal group, it expresses *PROSC*, *BRF2*, *ASH2L*, *DDHD2*, *CCDN1*, *FADD*, *PPFIA1*, *FOXA1*, and *CTTN* genes, while the expression of the *ERBB2* gene is absent. Some cases express PIK3CA, GATA3 and TP53. Often, we also observe 1q and 16p gains, and 16q loss. These cancers have a good prognosis and respond to antiestrogen therapy. Most cases are ductal mucinous, tubular, cribriform, and papillary, as well as classic and pleomorphic lobular carcinoma.

Luminal B subtype tumors comprise 15% of carcinomas and are of histologic grade 2 or 3 (ductal and lobular), positive for CK7, CK8, CK18, and CK19, whereas there is no immunoreactivity to CK5, CK14 and CK17. Furthermore, the immunostaining for ER, PR and HER2 are always positive (Fig. 8.39). The proliferation index is higher, and prognosis is poorer than that for luminal A carcinoma. Expression of the *GGH*, *LAPTMB4*, *NSEP1*, *MYBL2*, *SQLE*, *CCNE1*, and *ERBB2* genes is present. Some cases express PIK3CA, GATA3, and TP53. Chromosomal analyses usually show gains of 1q, 8q, 17q, 20q, and loss of 1p, 3q, 8p, 13q, 16q, 17p, and 22q.

Luminal C, also called luminal hybrid tumors are rare and show immunopositive staining for CK7, CK8, CK18, and CK19 and absence of CK5, CK14, and CK17. One of hormone receptors (ER or PR) and the HER2 protein can be absent (Fig. 8.40). This immunophenotype is expressed in about 10% of breast carcinomas with morphologic aspects of moderately differentiated ductal carcinoma of no special type or lobular carcinomas, including the pleomorphic variant. Likely luminal B and C cancers are part of the spectrum of ER-positive cancers and have a more aggressive pheno-

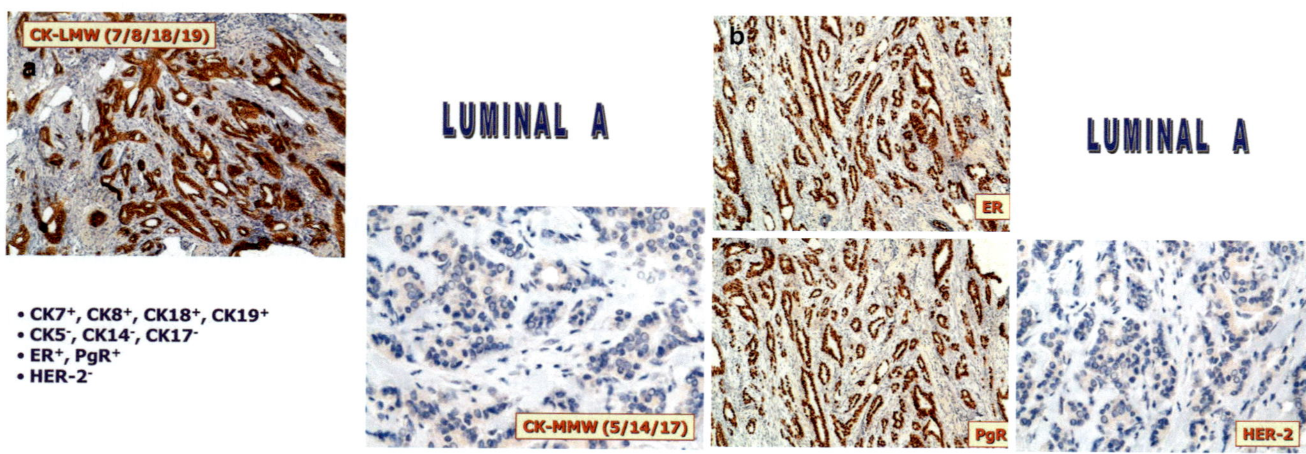

Fig. 8.38 Breast carcinoma, luminal A subtype. Immunohistochemistry

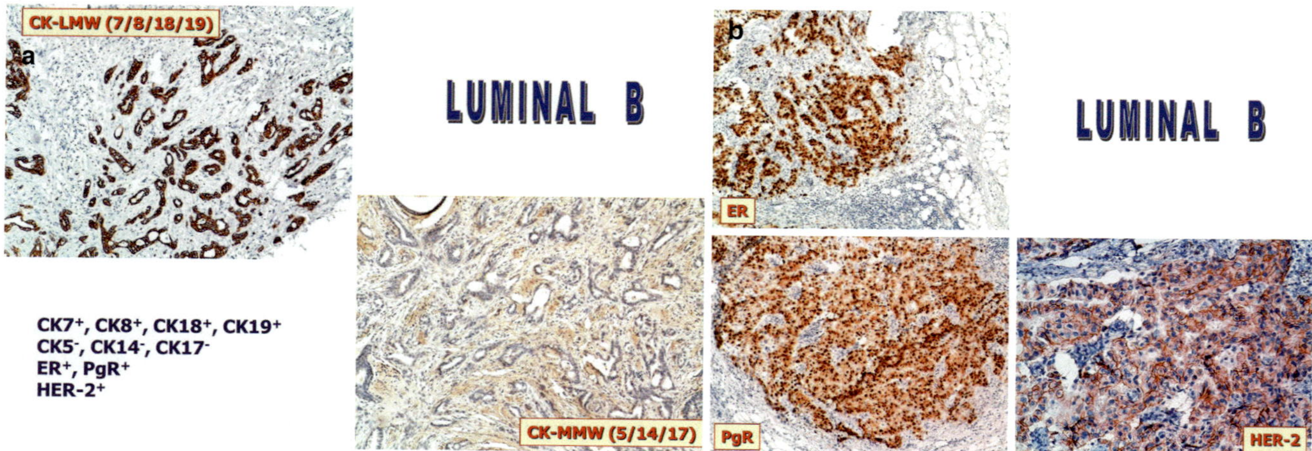

Fig. 8.39 Breast carcinoma, luminal B subtype. Immunohistochemistry

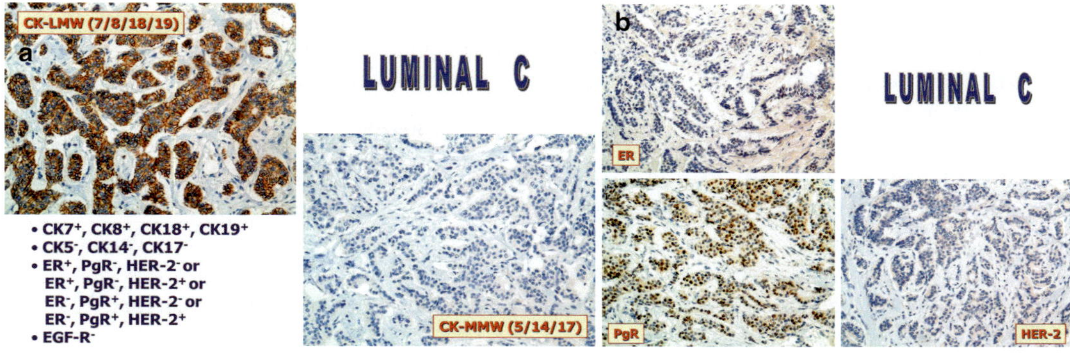

Fig. 8.40 Breast carcinoma, luminal C subtype. Immunohistochemistry

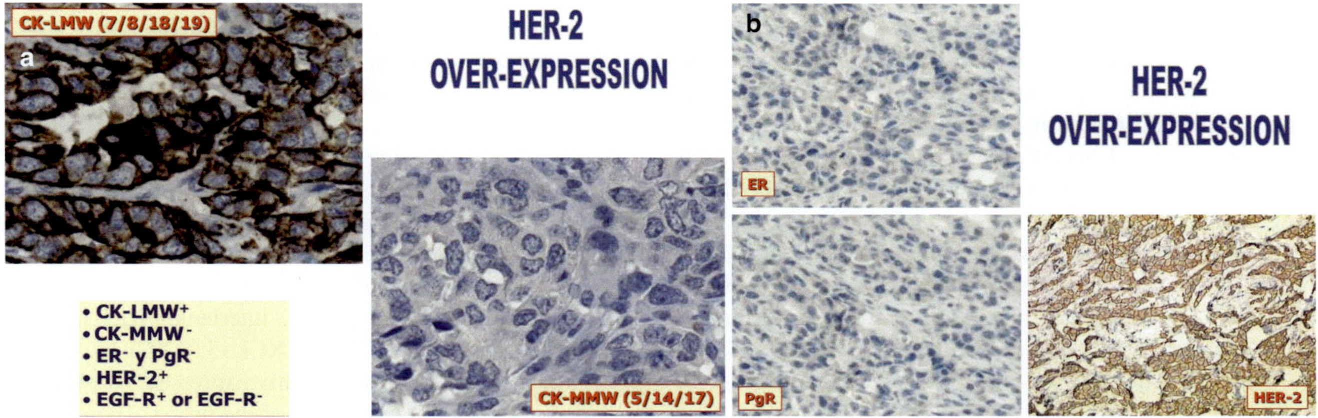

Fig. 8.41 Breast carcinoma, HER2 positive subtype. Immunohistochemistry

type and worse prognosis than the luminal A subtype. Thus, the ER, PR, HER2, and Ki-67 proliferation index are important for identifying this subtype. The response to antiestrogen therapy may be partial.

HER2-Enriched Subtype

This carcinoma comprises approximately 4–5% of cases of breast carcinoma. These tumors show amplification of the *HER2* gene that is localized on chromosome 17 and are ER-negative; the ER-positive tumors belong to the luminal B subtype. The *HER2/neu* gene is a member of a family of genes encoding transmembrane receptors for growth factors, including epidermal growth factor receptor (EGFR), HER2, HER3, and HER4. In addition to the genes of the HER-2 amplicon, they express *GRB7* and *PPARBP*, while they are always negative for the expression of genes linked to hormone receptors. They show, apart from HER2 amplification, high-level amplification at multiple sites and a number of these amplifications correspond to known oncogenes (*FGFR1*, *MYC*, *CCND1*, and *ZNF217*). These tumors show at least eight up-regulated (*AURKB*, *CCNA2*, *SCRN1*, *NPY*, *ATP7B*, *CHAF1B*, *CCNB1*, *CLDN8*) and nine downregulated (*NRP1*, *CCR2*, *C1QB*, *CD74*, *VEAM1*, *CD180*, *ITGB2*,

CD72, *ST8SIA4*) genes. Low-molecular-weight keratins (CK7, CK8, CK18, and CK19) are positive and EGFR is variable (Fig. 8.41).

This subtype is often of histologic grade 3, may show apocrine differentiation, may have lymphoid infiltrates, and can potentially be aggressive, with increased risk for local recurrence or metastatic disease. HER2 overexpression/amplification predicts a favorable response of these tumors to treatment with the monoclonal antibody trastuzumab (Herceptin) or other HER2 antagonists as well as to anthracycline-based chemotherapy. Amplification of the *HER2* gene (*ERBB2* gene) at the DNA level results in protein overexpression. A certain number of cases considered HER2-negative by molecular investigations (FISH) show positive immunostaining for HER2 (score 1+ or 2+) on the cell surface. These cases currently constitute the group defined as HER2-low tumors and largely respond to therapies with HER2 antagonists.

Triple Negative Subtype

The term **triple-negative breast cancer (TNBC)** refers to the fact that the cancer cells have ER, PR and HER2 negativity. These tumors comprise approximately 15% of cases of breast cancer and have a broad immunohistochemical profile. These tumors are common in younger Hispanic women, frequently carry the germline *BRCA1* gene mutation, are grade 3 with a ductal/no specific type morphology, and do not respond to HER2-targeted or antiestrogen therapy. Most BRCA1 cancers lack ER, PR, and HER2 expression and express basal markers (CK5/CK6, CK14, CK17, EGFR, and P-cadherin) in 80% of cases. Carcinoma with medullary features, metaplastic carcinoma, secretory carcinoma, and adenoid cystic carcinoma tend to have a basal-like phenotype. The Ki-67 proliferation index is high, and some of these tumors have an aggressive clinical course and a poor prognosis. These tumors often have benign-appearing US features, i.e., well-defined borders, an oval shape, and no or very little posterior acoustic shadowing. BRCA2 cancers comprise often invasive lobular, pleomorphic lobular, tubular, and cribriform carcinoma types. Germline mutations of *BRCA1* and *BRCA2* genes are seen in 5 % of breast carcinomas. If the tumor is ER negative and "basal" markers positive, BRCA1 should be sequenced.

Through molecular investigations, different subtypes of (TNBC) have been identified; the most represented ones are: basal-like 1 (BL1), basal-like 2 (BL2), immunomodulator (IM), mesenchymal (M), and luminal androgen receptor (LAR). These subtypes are characterized by the presence of molecular alterations, in terms of RNA expression, somatic mutations and copy number variations, which tend to cluster in genes implicated in specific pathways.

The *BL1 subtype* shows expression of genes involved in the response to DNA damage and in the regulation of the cell cycle. This subtype expresses high nuclear levels of Ki-67 and therefore appears highly proliferative. The highest rate of *TP53* mutations, high gain/amplifications of *MYC*, *CDK6* or *CCNE1* and deletions in *BRCA2*, *PTEN*, *MDM2*, and *RB1* genes are observed.

The *BL2 subtype* displays high levels of aberrant growth factor signaling, metabolic pathway activity, a highly proliferative phenotype, and increased myoepithelial cell marker expression.

Furthermore, both subtypes (BL1 and BL2) express the following genes: *KRT5*, *KRT14*, *KRT17*, *PIK3R1*, *AKR1C1*, *GSTP1*, *MAD2L1*, and *maspin*, while there is no expression of genes related to low-molecular-weight cytokeratins, hormonal receptors, or HER2. BL1 (Fig. 8.42) and BL2 show immunopositivity with "basal markers" (CK5/CK6, CK 14, CK17, EGFR, P-cadherin, p63, laminin and c-Kit). BL1 and BL2 tumors are sensitive to cisplatin therapy, while target of rapamycin (mTOR) inhibitors, growth factor inhibitors, poly-ADP ribose polymerase (PARP) inhibitors, and genotoxic compounds are promising therapeutic targets.

The *immunomodulator (IM) subtype* is characterized by high expression of immunological signaling genes, such as genes involved in antigen processing and presentation, immune cell and cytokine signaling pathways, such as *JAK/STAT*, *TNF*, and *NFKB*. Moreover, it show significantly enriched immune cell-associated genes and signal transduction pathways, such as the Th1/Th2 pathway, NK cell pathway, B cell receptor signaling pathway, dendritic cell (DC) pathway, T-cell receptor signaling, interleukin (IL)-12 pathway, and IL-7 pathway. CCR2, CXCL13, CXCL11, CD1C, CXCL10, and CCL5 are also highly expressed. Most of IM subtype are medullary carcinoma of the breast. Therefore, it is recommended to use PD1, PDL1, CTLA-4, and other immune checkpoint inhibitors for the treatment of patients with this subtype.

The *mesenchymal (M) subtype* is associated with extracellular receptor interactions and overexpression of genes related to cellular differentiation, activated cell migration-related signaling pathways (regulated by actin), extracellular matrix–receptor interaction pathways, and differentiation pathways (Wnt pathway, ALK pathway and TGF-β signal-

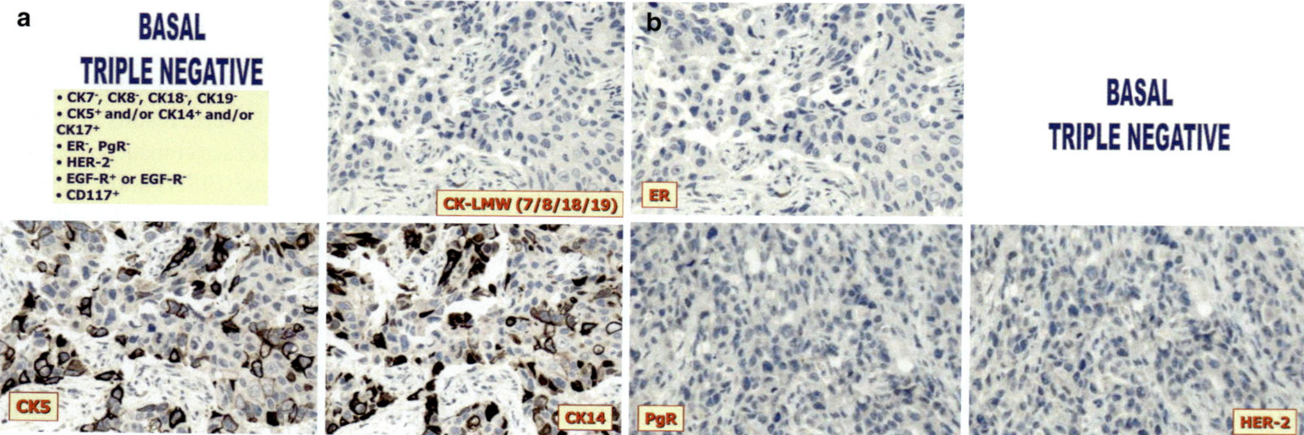

Fig. 8.42 Breast carcinoma, basal triple negative subtype. Immunohistochemistry

ing) and is therefore also called metaplastic breast cancer. The M subtype therefore has histological characteristics similar to those of sarcoma or metaplastic carcinoma (squamous carcinoma). Some cases, defined as Mesenchymal stem-like (MSL), include a low expression of genes related to cell proliferation, a high expression of stemness-relates genes (*ABCA8, PROCR, ENG, ALDHA1, PER1, ABCB1, TERT2IP, BCL2, BMP2,* and *THY*), *HOX* genes (*HOXA5, HOXA10, MEIS1, MEIS2, MEOX1, MEOX2,* and *MSX1*) and genes that participate in the signaling pathways of angiogenesis and growth factors and low claudin expression. The M and MSL subtypes present various epithelial markers, including mixtures of low- and high-molecular-weight cytokeratins, and mesenchymal stem cell-specific markers (BMP2, ENG, ITGAV, KDR, NGFR, NT5E, PDGFR, THY1, and VCAM1). Therefore, M and MSL cancer patients might be treated with mTOR inhibitors, PI3K inhibitors, Src antagonists, antiangiogenic drugs or drugs targeting epithelial–mesenchymal transition.

Luminal androgen receptor (LAR) subtype does not express ER receptor, it has highly activated hormonal-related signaling pathways (including steroid hormones biosynthesis, porphyrin and chlorophyll metabolism, and androgen/estrogen metabolism). The mRNA level is highly expressed, and immunohistochemistry also detects high expression of AR and many downstream metabolic markers of AR and their auxiliary activators, such as DHCR24, ALCAM, FASN, FKBP5, APOD, PIP, SPDEF, and CLDN8. The peroxisome proliferator-activated receptor (PPAR) signaling pathway is also significantly increased. The LAR subtype displays a luminal genotypic pattern of gene expression (e.g., high levels of *FOXA1, GATA3, SPDEF,* and *XBP1*), and luminal immunohistochemistry markers such as CK7, CK8, CK18, CK19, positive AR, and negativity with ER, PR, HER2, and high molecular weight cytokeratins (Fig. 8.43). Moreover, most of LAR subtype is enriched in mutations in *PIK3CA, KMT2C, CDH1, NF1,* and *AKT1*. In this subtype, there is a high prevalence of invasive lobular histology. Anti-androgen drugs are possible treatment options.

Other (Rare) Subtypes

Approximately, 7% of breast cancers belong to the "rare subtype" and consist of the "claudin-low" and "normal breast-like" cancer subtypes.

Claudin-low breast cancers (CLBC) subgroup comprise recently described entities showing low expression of claudins 1, 3, 4, 7, and 8 and low expression of genes involved in tight junctions and cell-cell adhesion. These tumors have low expression of genes coding for cytokeratins *KRT5, KRT7, KRT8, KRT14, KRT17, KRT18,* and *KRT19*. Furthermore, these tumors also have a low mutation rate and less genomic instability than other subtypes. CLBR show low expression of proliferation

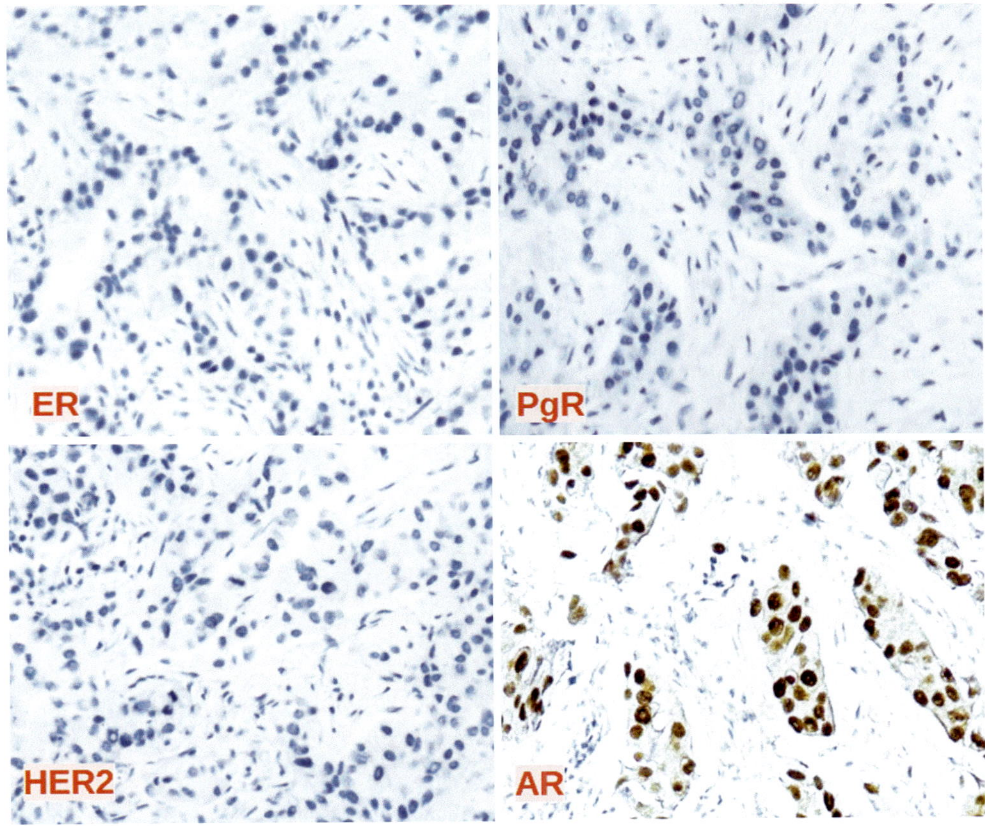

Fig. 8.43 Breast carcinoma, luminal androgen receptor (LAR) subtype. Immunohistochemistry

genes and Ki-67, while there is high expression of EMT-related markers such as Vimentin, SNAI1 and SNAI2, TWIST1 and TWIST2, and ZEB1 and ZEB2. They are immunopositive for CK7, CK8, CK14, CK17, CK18, CD44, and PD-L1 and negative for hormonal receptors (ER and PR) and HER2. High expression of lymphocyte and endothelial cell markers has also been reported. Recently, caveolin-1, galectin-1, and SMYD3 were found to be highly expressed in CLBC. Histologically, most of them are invasive ductal, metaplastic, and medullary carcinomas. However, they have an overall poor prognosis with some degree of sensitivity to chemotherapy.

Normal Breast-Like (NBLBC)   Many authors do not consider this entity as a distinct subtype, due to the strong expression of non-epithelial genes, mainly from adipose tissue, together with genes from the basal and luminal ductal epithelium present in the normal breast and in fibroadenomas. The use of immuno-histochemical staining with molecular gene expression "surrogate" markers has shown that this group exhibits an immunophenotype similar to that of tubulo-lobular terminal units of normal breast with variable immunostainings for cyto-keratins, ER, and/or PR, and negativity for HER2. NBLBC and tumors of the luminal subtype sharing the same antigenic profile, including ER, PR and HER2 markers, are often classified in the hybrid luminal or unclassifiable subtype. In NBLBC, breast cancer stem cells express genes commonly attributed to adipose tissue, such as adipose acid synthase. Therefore, a characteristic of these tumors is the strong immunopositivity for FASN (fatty acid synthase) (Fig. 8.44). These tumors also express the *PIK3R1*, *AKR1C1*, *IGF1*, and *PGC1A* genes. At the moment, there are rare publications about the correlation of the immunophenotype of this group of carcinomas and the histopathology. However, preliminary studies suggest that the usual histomorphology is that of invasive lobular carcinoma.

Precursor Lesions

Ductal Carcinoma In Situ

Ductal carcinoma in situ (DCIS) represents 20–25% of newly diagnosed breast cancers in the USA. DCIS is uncommon before the age of 40 years and the incidence rises pro-

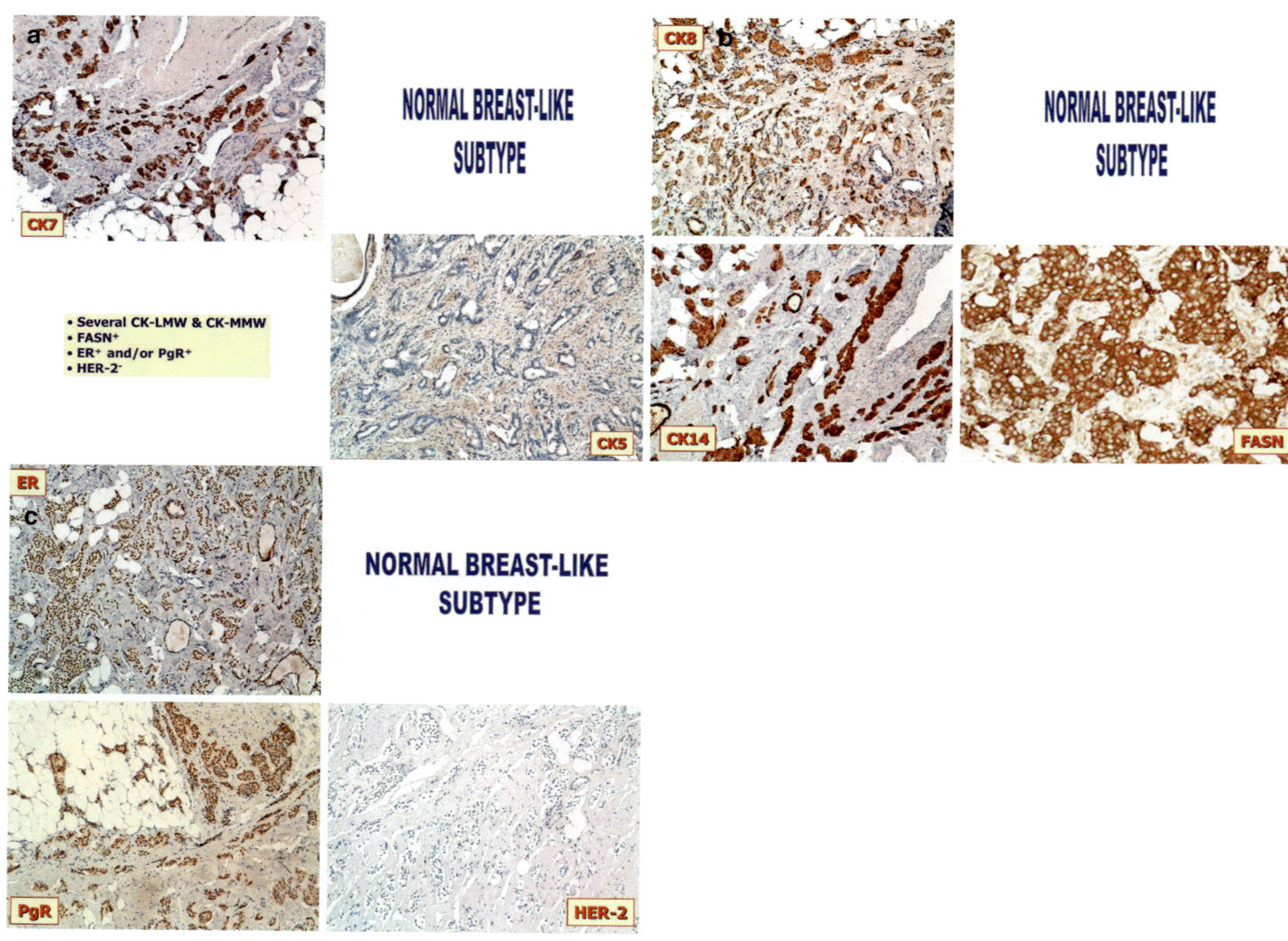

Fig. 8.44   Breast carcinoma, normal breast-like subtype. Immunohistochemistry

gressively to a peak at ages 65–69 years. Age, race, family history and genetics, nulliparity, late age at first birth, late menopause, breast density, body mass index, and use of hormone replacement therapy has been associated with an increased risk for DCIS. This lesion is often unilateral, although 22% develop DCIS or invasive carcinoma in the contralateral breast. The risk of DCIS for subsequent development of breast cancer is 8–10 times that of the reference population. DCIS is a precursor to invasive breast carcinoma. Usually, 80–90% of DCIS are detected mammographically by a finding of calcifications; however, occasionally coalescent areas of high-grade DCIS may form a firm palpable mass. Prognostic factors for local recurrence or progression to invasive carcinoma include tumor size, nuclear grade, comedo necrosis, and resection margins status.

Histopathology The neoplastic proliferation develops in the terminal-duct lobular unit and progresses distally in the main duct and peripherally toward the adjacent branches of a given duct-system segment. The rare lesions that develop in larger ducts and lactiferous ducts close to the nipple progress toward the nipple, resulting in Paget's disease and nipple discharge. Current trend suggests that grading of DCIS should be based primarily on nuclear features rather than on the architectural (solid, comedo, cribriform, micropapillary, or papillary) pattern (Fig. 8.45a, b, e). Thus, DCIS is divided into low, intermediate, and high grade, although nuclear heterogeneity may occur in the same lesion. Cell polarity, small to intermediate nuclear size, inconspicuous nucleoli and rare mitoses are features of low-grade to intermediate-grade DCIS; lack of cell polarity, nuclear pleomorphism, mitoses, and prominent nucleoli are seen in high-grade DCIS. Apocrine, clear, and neuroendocrine types of DCIS may be seen occasionally, the latter often associated with papillary areas. Encapsulated papillary carcinoma is a variant of papillary carcinoma that occurs in older women and is considered as an in situ tumor by some.

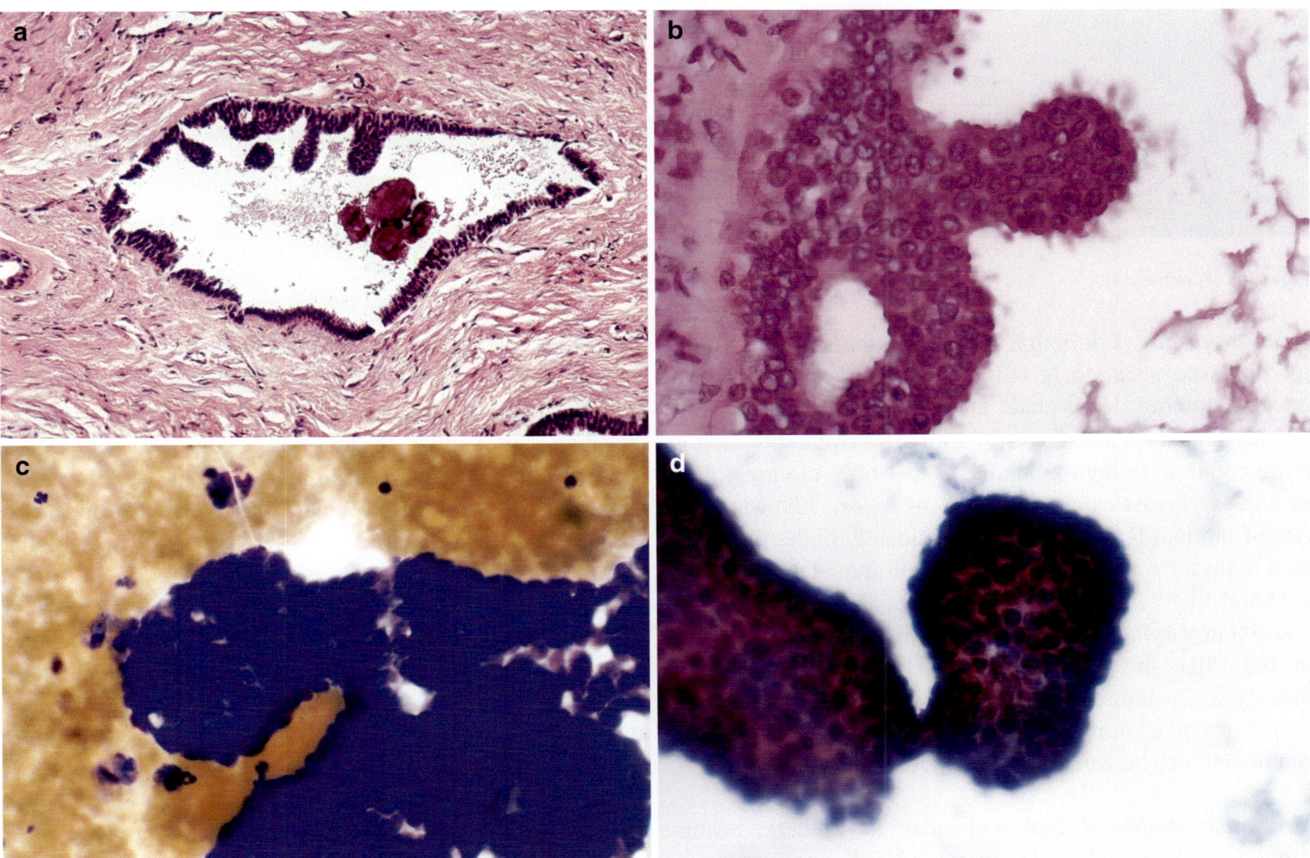

Fig. 8.45 Ductal carcinoma in situ. Histology of non-comedo type DCIS shows bland-appearing neoplastic ductal cells arranged as micropapillary projections and rigid arches; rare microcalcifications are also seen (**a**, **b**). FNA smears show complex aggregates of bland-appearing cells with slight anisonucleosis and anisocytosis (**c**, **d**). Histology of comedo type ductal carcinoma in situ showing central necrosis surrounded by high-grade tumor cells confined to the duct (**e**). Cytology smear shows high-grade tumor cells with prominent nucleoli and necrotic background (**f**). US image shows multiple well-circumscribed small hypoechoic nodules (**g**). (**a**, **b**, **e** H&E stain low and high magnifications; **c**, DiffQuik stain high magnification; **d**, **f** Papanicolaou stain high magnification)

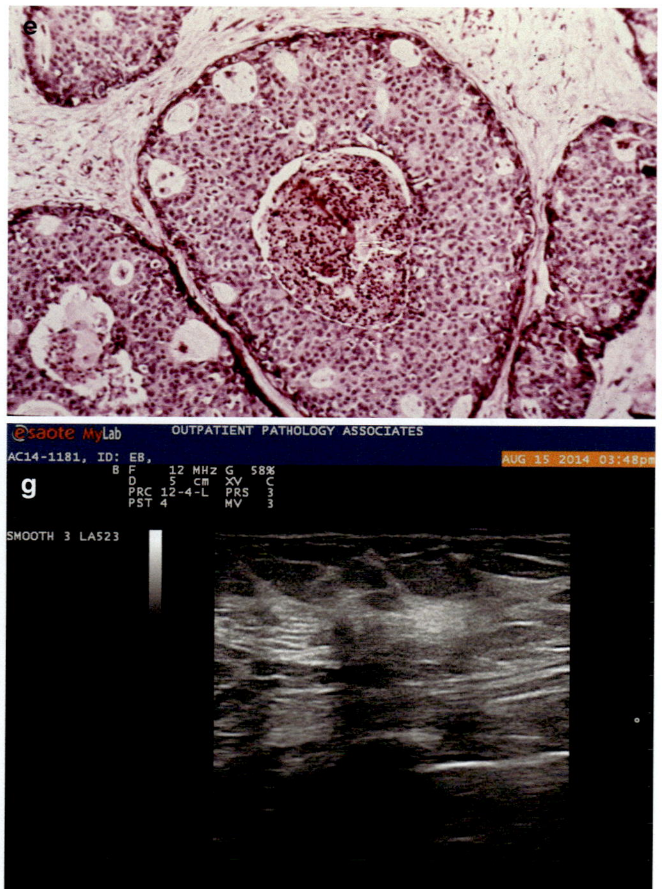

Fig. 8.45 (continued)

Immuno-profile For both ER and PR immunostain positivity in tissue sections is required ≥1% of cells showing nuclear staining. High-grade DCIS expresses ER less frequently than does low-grade DCIS. HER2 overexpression is more common in high-grade DCIS (50–60% of cases) than in invasive breast carcinoma (20% of cases). Likewise, the rate of luminal B phenotype is significantly higher in DCIS than in invasive carcinomas. Some high-grade DCIS express a "basal-like" (Table 8.3) immunophenotype (CK5+ and CK14+) in varying degrees likely representing the precursor of basal-like invasive carcinoma. High-grade DCIS frequently has a luminal B, HER2, or "basal-like" including "triple negative" immunophenotype (Table 8.3). No markers can distinguish between low-grade DCIS and ADH.

Molecular Profile Recent molecular and genetic results suggest that low-grade and high-grade DCIS are distinct disorders. Low-grade DCIS is usually positive for ER, PR, E-cadherin, Bcl-2, and cyclin D1 and negative for HER2. They are also diploid/near diploid, with deletion of 16q (>70%), gain of 1q (>70%), and lack of expression of "basal-like" markers (luminal A > B). High-grade DCIS is more heterogeneous and often show amplifications at 17q12 and 11q13, and is frequently aneuploid. This immuno-profile and genetic features, with the exception of E-cadherin that is negative, are similar to those seen in ADH and ALH/LCIS. Again, low-grade and high-grade DCIS are direct precursor lesions of invasive breast carcinoma and appear to have distinct and separate pathways of pre-invasive epithelial neoplasia.

FNA Findings The comedo type of DCIS yields cellular smears with loose aggregates and single large malignant cells with coarse chromatin, large nucleoli, mitoses, and a necrotic background. In contrast, the non-comedo type of DCIS shows medium-size bland-appearing uniform cells. Complex flat-cell aggregates and well-defined punched-out lumens with or without metachromatic stroma are seen in cribriform DCIS. Numerous small papillary fragments composed of small cells and having a slender base and bulbous ends with smooth contours are seen in the micropapillary DCIS. No myoepithelial cell nuclei are present (Fig. 8.45c, d, f). Histologic confirmation is needed for distinguishing DCIS from invasive ductal carcinoma.

US Features   DCIS can rarely be a mass with circumscribed, indistinct, or spiculated borders; the mass may be taller than wide and hypoechoic (Fig. 8.45g). However, most lesions are often microscopic and, US examination may be normal or calcifications may be seen in dilated ducts. DCIS of low grade may be visible and lack calcification or obvious US features of malignancy, as seen in invasive cancers. We should remember that DCIS may be associated with benign or proliferative lesions, and the US may be non-revealing or show the underlying benign condition, i.e., a radial scar.

Lobular Neoplasia (LN)

The term LN encompasses atypical lobular hyperplasia (ALH) and lobular carcinoma in situ (LCIS), lesions that develop in the terminal-duct lobular unit and do not involve the terminal ducts. The distinction between ALH and LCIS is based on the extent of lobular units involved. The average age for diagnosis is 49 years, and there are no specific or grossly recognizable clinical features. The LN is usually a microscopic incidental finding in breast tissue removed for other reasons. The lesion is often bilateral and multicentric and carries an increased risk for developing invasive lobular carcinoma (4–5 times for ALH and 8–10 times for LCIS).

Histopathology   There is distention of lobules by a proliferation of round cells with eccentric nuclei. Cells often have an intracytoplasmic mucin vacuole conferring a targetoid appearance. Cells are uniform, of variable size, and lack pleomorphism (Fig. 8.46). Necrosis, mitoses, cell pleomorphism, nucleoli, and large cell size are seen in pleomorphic LCIS, which may rarely show apocrine features.

Immuno-profile   Neoplastic cells are positive for CK7, CK8, CK18, CK19, CK14, and/or CK17. E-cadherin is negative, whereas cytoplasmic p120 protein is present. Most cases of LN are positive for ER and PR and negative for HER2. Pleomorphic LCIS is also negative for E-cadherin and likely negative for ER and PR, whereas HER-2 is positive. and has a high proliferation index. The immune-profile and genetic features are like those seen in ADH and low-grade DCIS, with the exception of E-cadherin, which is positive.

Molecular Profile   ALH/LCIS are usually diploid/near diploid, show deletion of 16q (>70%) and gain of 1q (>70%), and lack of expression of "basal-like" markers (luminal A > B). Lobular neoplasms of the breast have alterations in the *CDH1* gene, mapped to chromosome 16 (16p22.1), which encodes E-cadherin. The absence of immunostaining for E-cadherin is caused by silencing of this gene. Instead, genetic mutations determine the production of anomalous E-cadherin, which is highlighted through "atypical" immunostaining: the truncated protein solubilizes in the cytoplasm and forms cytoplasmic granulations, while anomalies in protein synthesis in its cytoplasmic portion are highlighted with focal or dot-like immunostaining of the cell membrane. Loss of heterozygosity at loci frequently seen in invasive lobular carcinoma, i.e., 11q13, 16q, 17p, and 17q, has been reported in LN. Pleomorphic LCIS has greater genomic instability and reflects the more aggressive features of this tumor compared with LN.

FNA Findings   Smears have low to moderate cellularity and show single monomorphous isolated cells with plasmacytoid features, round eccentric nuclei, powdery chromatin, and inconspicuous nucleoli. Except for the smear cellularity in adequate samples, the cytologic findings of LCIS and invasive lobular carcinoma overlap. Pleomorphic LCIS shows cellular pleomophism, necrosis, mitosis, and large cells similar to the smear pattern of comedo type DCIS.

US Features   ALH and LCIS have no distinct radiologic features. However, when LN involves sclerosing adenosis or fibroadenoma, a mass lesion may be visible on US evaluation; otherwise, US evaluation is normal.

Invasive Breast Cancer

Invasive breast carcinomas with a favorable prognosis include papillary carcinoma, tubular carcinoma, cribriform carcinoma, colloid carcinoma, adenoid cystic carcinoma, medullary carcinoma, and secretory carcinoma. Unfavorable breast malignancies include metaplastic carcinoma, pleomorphic lobular carcinoma, inflammatory carcinoma, and sarcomas. Therefore, it is important to subclassify the type of mammary malignancy on FNA samples.

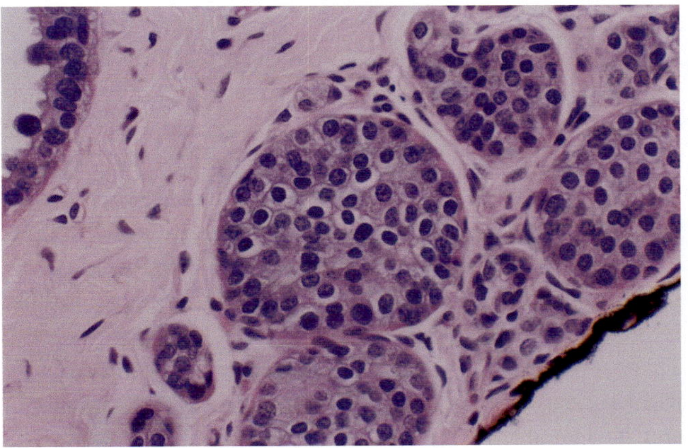

Fig. 8.46 Lobular carcinoma in situ. The lobules are distended and filled with uniform and bland-appearing cuboidal cells with eccentrically placed nuclei. (H&E stain, intermediate magnification)

Infiltrating Duct Carcinoma, NOS

This is a large and heterogeneous group of breast cancers that do not have sufficient histologic characteristics to be specifically classified, i.e., lobular carcinoma, medullary carcinoma, tubular carcinoma, etc. This group comprises 50–75% of breast cancers and is rare before the age of 40 years. Grossly, the tumors have a stellate or nodular appearance, and the size ranges between <1 cm and >10 cm.

Histopathology The tissue diagnosis is based on exclusion of known types of breast carcinoma. Thus, the histologic pattern is highly variable including, solid, syncytial, glandular, tubular, or trabecular, with variable amounts of desmoplastic stroma. The cellular appearance is also variable, and the nuclei range from uniform to highly pleomorphic with multiple and prominent nucleoli. Mitoses are also variable (Fig. 8.47a–c).

Current opinion is that invasive breast carcinomas with histological variants including medullary pattern, neuroendocrine differentiation, osteoclast-like stromal giant cells, pleomorphic pattern, choriocarcinomatous pattern, melanocytic pattern, oncocytic pattern, lipid-rich pattern, glycogen-rich clear cell pattern, or sebaceous pattern present between 10 and 90% should be classified as invasive breast carcinoma of no special type (NST). When the pattern is present in <10% or >90%, the invasive breast carcinoma is classified as duct carcinoma NOS or as the special type respectively.

Immuno-profile Between 70% and 80% are ER⁺ (Fig. 8.47d).

Molecular Profile Cases of familial breast cancers associated with mutations in the *BRCA1* and *BRCA2* genes are commonly invasive breast carcinomas NST.

FNA Findings Smears are highly cellular with numerous cell groups and single cells. Cell groups are arranged in crowded groups, gland-like, and in syncytial patterns with loss of polarity and nuclear molding. Cells are large with a high nuclear to cytoplasmic ratio, irregular and thickened nuclear contours, coarsely granular chromatin, and nucleoli of variable size. The cytoplasm may be finely to coarsely vacuolated. Tumor necrosis may be present, and no myoepithelial cells are seen in the background. Occasionally, and particularly in elderly women, cells may be uniform and plasmacytoid, resembling those of lobular carcinoma. Poorly differentiated mammary carcinomas show bizarre and multinucleated tumor cells (Fig. 8.47e–k).

US Features The mass is irregular, vertically oriented, and hypoechoic with indistinct spiculated and angular margins, microlobulation, and posterior acoustic shadowing as in low-grade invasive carcinomas. The mass can be round, oval, lobular, or irregular with marked hypoechogenicity and variable posterior acoustic enhancement, as in high-grade carcinomas. When skin is secondarily involved, there is disruption of the linear echogenicity of the deep dermal layer. Rarely, advanced breast carcinoma extends to the nipple to cause ulceration; when this occurs, a hypoechoic mass is seen in the subareolar area, with angular and spiculated borders and posterior acoustic shadowing (Fig. 8.47l–p).

Lobular Carcinoma

Lobular carcinoma is often bilateral and multicentric and accounts for approximately 5–15% of all invasive breast carcinomas. Women have an ill-defined palpable mass, and the mean age at diagnosis is 60 years. The prognosis in the first 10 years is similar to or better than that of infiltrating duct carcinoma NOS; however, the incidence of distant metastases, recurrence, and mortality is higher in invasive lobular carcinoma than in "NOS." Common sites of metastases include bone, the GI tract, uterus, meninges, ovaries, and serosal surfaces, in contrast to the lung, the most common site for invasive carcinoma of "no special type." Pleomorphic lobular carcinoma is a more aggressive tumor than the classic invasive lobular carcinoma; the prognosis is worse than that of low-grade ductal carcinoma and similar to that of high-grade duct carcinoma.

Histopathology The classic lobular carcinoma shows infiltrating small tumor cells that lack cell cohesion and appear individually scattered and characteristically arranged in a single-line pattern and arranged concentrically around ducts in a targetoid pattern. Cells have smooth or slightly irregular round or ovoid nuclei. There is an intense desmoplastic fibrous response that is in great part responsible for the sparse cellularity seen in FNA samples. Histologic variants include classic, solid, alveolar, pleomorphic, tubulolobular, and mixed. Focal apocrine or prominent signet-ring cell differentiation may be present (Fig. 8.48a–c).

Immuno-profile The expression of ER is high, although variable, depending on the variant. The classic and alveolar variants are almost invariably ER⁺; in contrast, 10% of the pleomorphic variant, which has an aggressive phenotype is ER⁺. PR⁺ is seen in 60–70% of classic and pleomorphic variants. HER2 amplification and overexpression are rare in infiltrating lobular carcinoma, although present in some pleomorphic variant cases. The proliferative index is low. Expression of p53 and basal markers (CK14, CK5/6) is rare. There is intense cytoplasmic immunostaining for catenin p120 in cases of lobular carcinoma, whereas ductal carcinoma and normal ducts show a linear membranous pattern. The immunostaining for p120, therefore, appears useful for confirmation of cases of dubious negativity for E-cadherin, and particularly in cases of mixed ductal/lobular carcinoma.

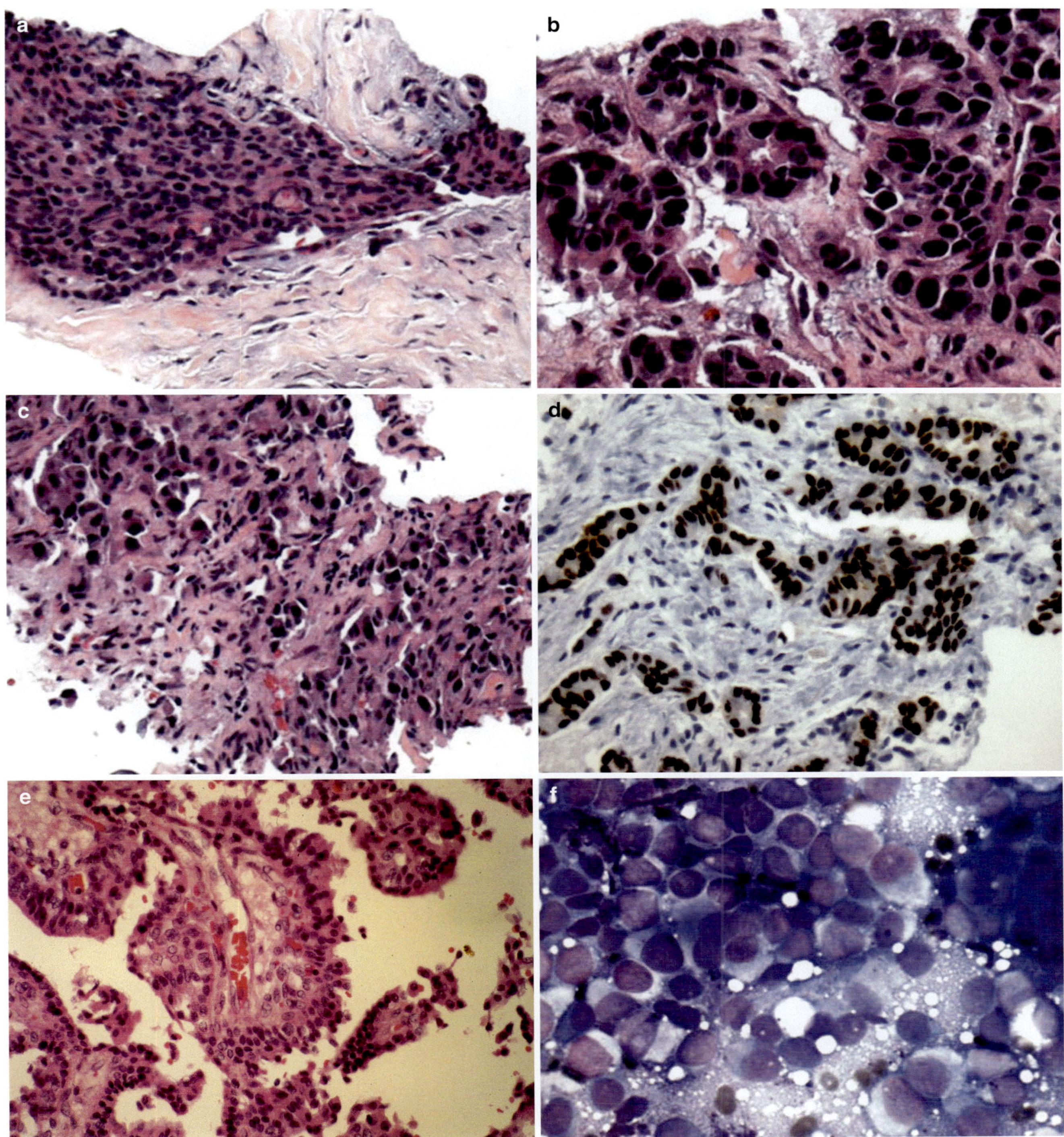

Fig. 8.47 Invasive ductal carcinoma of no special type. Histologic appearance of carcinomas of low- (**a**), intermediate- (**b**), and high- (**c**) histologic grade, all surrounded by desmoplastic stroma. Most carcinomas are ER positive (**d**). Papillary differentiation may be present and these cases should not be considered as papillary carcinoma (**e**). Cytologic features include cell dissociation, variable cellular pleomorphism, anisonucleosis, and variably prominent nucleoli (**f–g**, low-grade; **h**, intermediate-grade; **i–j**, high-grade). Papillary fronds with wide fibrovascular stromal core may be seen in cases of papillary differentiation (**k**). Corresponding ultrasound features are shown in figures **l–m** (low-grade), **n** (intermediate-grade), and **o, p** (high-grade). (**a–c, e** H&E stain low-to intermediate magnification; **d**, positive immunoperoxidase stain for estrogen receptor; **f**, H-K DiffQuik stain high magnification; **g**, Papanicolaou stain high magnification)

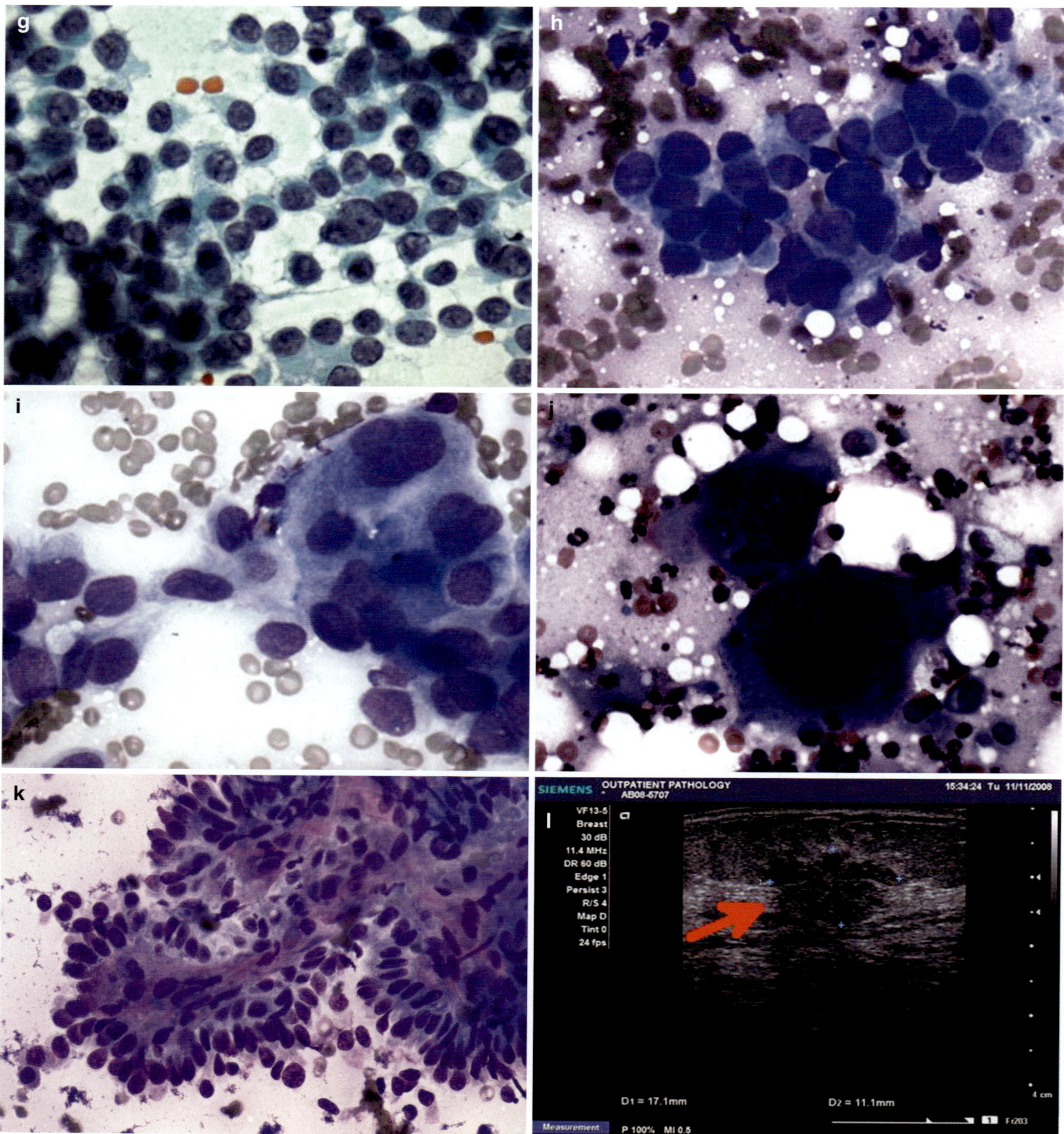

Fig. 8.47 (continued)

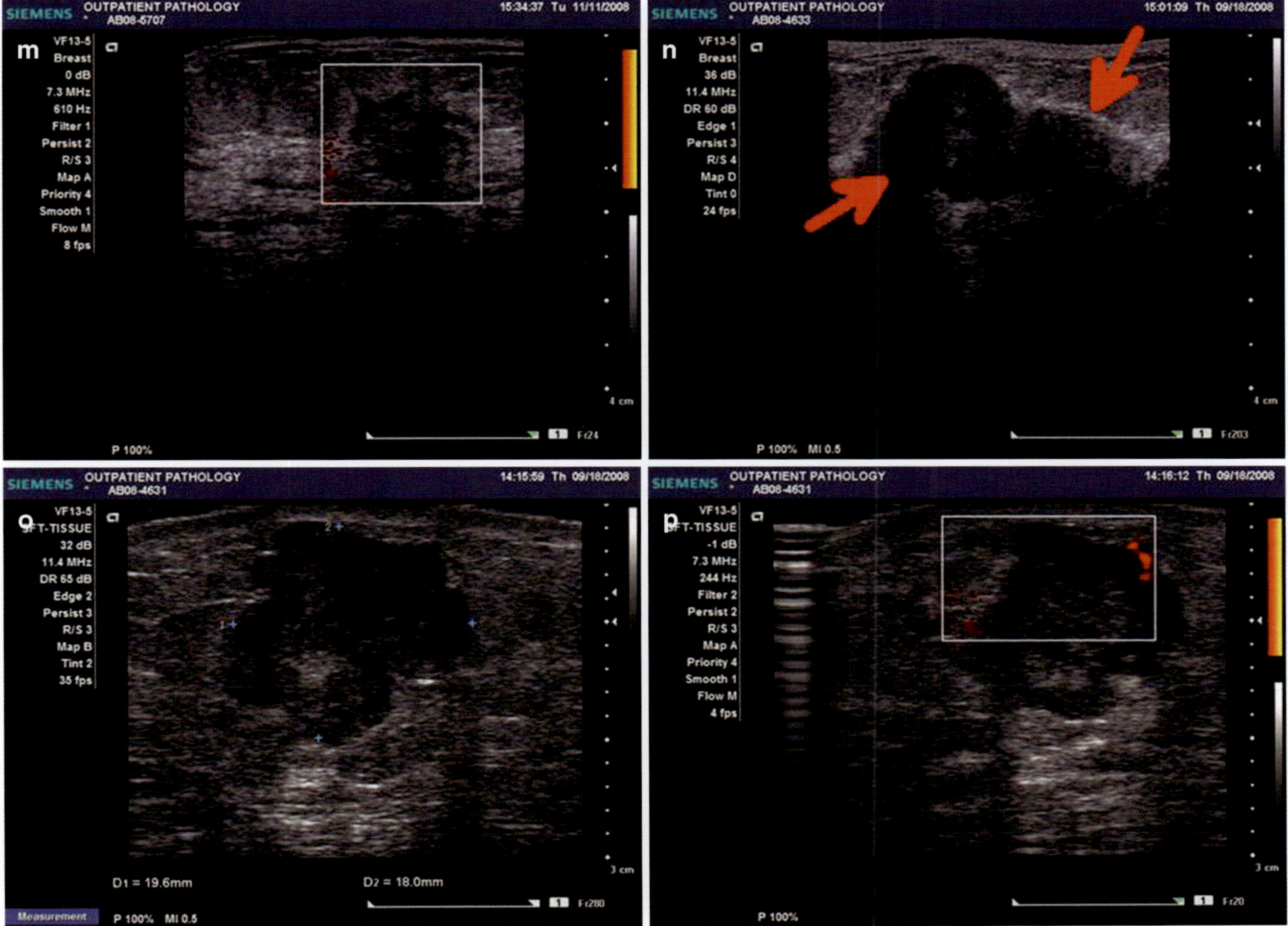

Fig. 8.47 (continued)

Pleomorphic variant with apocrine differentiation show gross cystic disease fluid protein-15 (GCDFP-15) positivity in 40% of cases. Furthermore, the pleomorphic variant may be a peculiar type of breast cancer with mixed ductal and lobular clinical, pathological, immune-, and molecular profiles including features of lobular (morphology, negative E-cadherin, and lack of basal keratins) and ductal (aggressive clinical behavior, and a subgroup with aggressive immunophenotype of triple negative, and positive HER2) carcinomas.

Molecular Profile Loss of expression of the membranous adhesion molecule E-cadherin, the result of a somatic mutation of the E-cadherin gene *CDH1* located on chromosome 16 (16p22.1), is the most consistent alteration in infiltrating lobular carcinoma and helps in the distinction from low-grade invasive ductal carcinoma of no special type. The most common chromosomal abnormalities are loss of 16q and gain of material on 1q. Pleomorphic lobular carcinoma shows similar alterations, but, in addition, has 8q24, 17q12, and 20q13 amplifications, which are characteristic of high-grade invasive breast carcinoma of no special type. In addition, 50% are found to be near-diploid.

By gene-expression profiling, infiltrating lobular carcinomas are most frequently classified as *luminal A* molecular tumors, but they can also be classified as luminal B, HER2 positive, normal-like, or basal-like.

Studies suggest that 95% of infiltrating lobular carcinomas, in particular the classic variant do not show *topoisomerase-IIα* gene amplification either in the primary and or matched metastases predicting lack of response with traditional anthracycline-based chemotherapy.

FNA Findings Smears show scant to moderate cellularity, small aggregates, cords, and single cells. Cells are uniform and monomorphic with a high nuclear to cytoplasmic ratio, scant indistinct cytoplasm, and uniform and mildly hyperchromatic nuclei with slightly irregular contours. The cytoplasm shows mucin vacuoles and an occasional cytoplasmic lumen, often with a central mucoid inclusion. Signet-ring-type cells

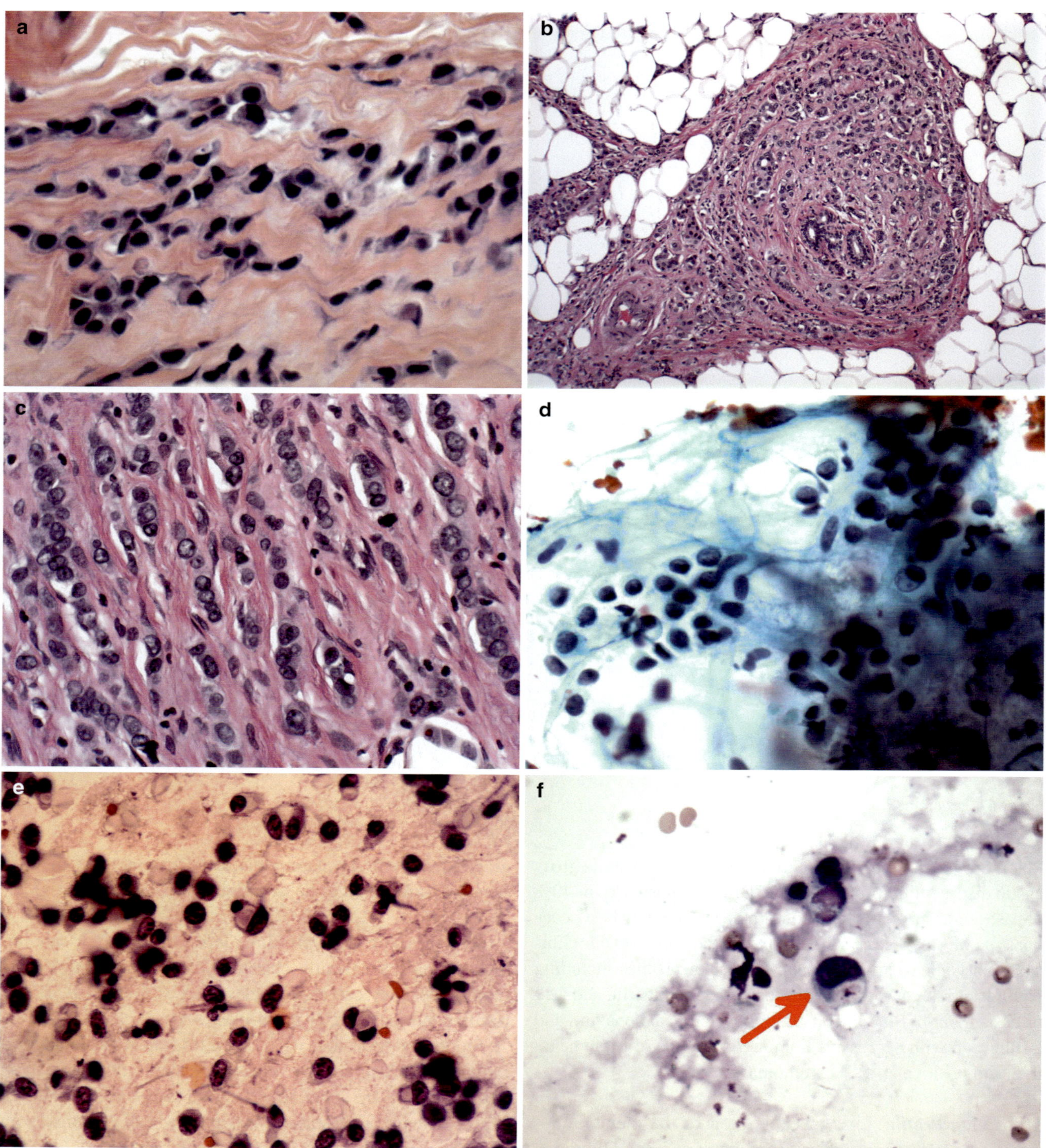

Fig. 8.48 Lobular carcinoma. Tissue sections of the classic lobular carcinoma show linear arrangement of cancer cells surrounded by desmoplastic stroma (**a**). Periductal circumferential arrangement (**b**) and linear distribution (**c**) is also evident in this example of lobular carcinoma of pleomorphic type. Cell dissociation, medium-size cells with minimal anisonucelosis and anisocytosis, and cytoplasmic "target-like" mucin accumulation are present in classic lobular carcinoma (**d–f**). The ultrasound characteristics are not specific and range from ill-defined to well-circumscribed irregular, and spiculated hypoechoic masses as seen in these three examples (**g–k**). Variable posterior acoustic shadowing may be present. Vascular flow by Doppler exam is also variable. (**a–c**, H&E stain high and low magnification; **d**, **e**, Papanicolaou stain high magnification; **f**, DiffQuik stain high magnification)

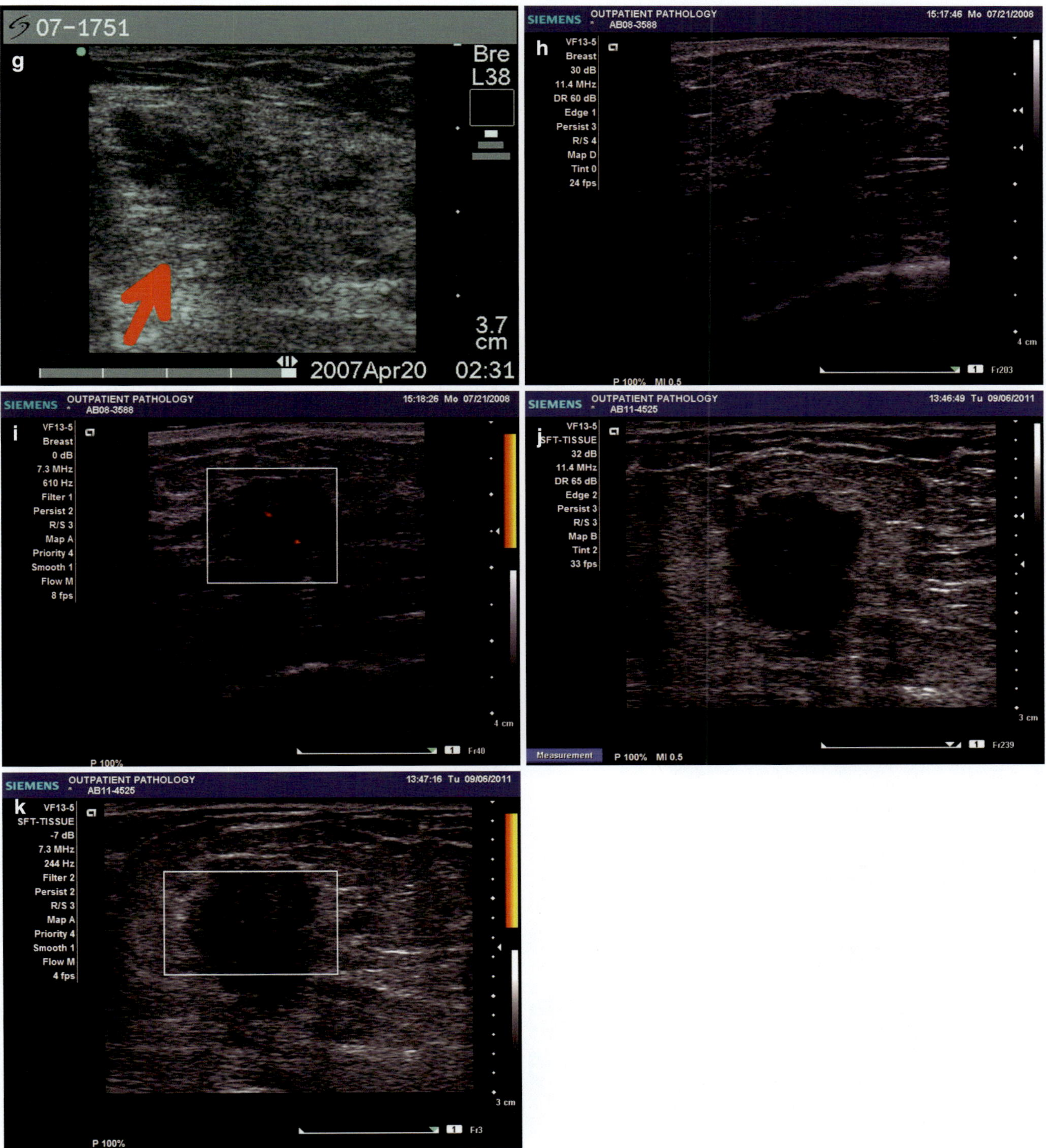

Fig. 8.48 (continued)

may be present. The background shows naked tumor cell nuclei and lacks myoepithelial cell nuclei (Fig. 8.48d–f).

US Features The sensitivity of US in detecting lobular carcinoma is at the level of 90%. The tumor has an irregular shape, ill-defined or spiculated margins, hyper- or isoechogenicity compared to fat, and shows posterior acoustic shadowing and architectural distortion. The tumors may not be taller than wide, as in infiltrating duct carcinoma. Precise measurement of the tumor size may be difficult to determine by US due to the ill-defined borders (Fig. 8.48g–k).

Tubular Carcinoma

Tubular carcinoma is a specific subtype of invasive breast carcinoma, comprises 2% of invasive breast cancers, usually measures <1.5 cm, and has a favorable prognosis even in the presence of axillary lymph node metastasis. It can be multifocal/multicentric.

Histopathology The infiltrating tumor has haphazardly arranged, angulated comma-shaped and tubular structures lined by a single layer of cells and surrounded by a prominent desmoplastic fibrous stroma. The cellular elements are small and monotonous, showing bland-appearing uniform nuclei and inconspicuous nucleoli. Focal apocrine differentiation may be present (Fig. 8.49a, b).

Immuno-profile Neoplastic cells are positive for CK7, CK8, CK18, CK19, and E-cadherin. Tubular carcinoma is almost always ER$^+$ and PR$^+$ and is typically negative for HER2, EGFR, P-cadherin, p53, and high-molecular-weight keratins (CK 5/6, CK14).

Molecular Profile The most frequent chromosomal alterations include loss of 16q, gain of 1q material, gain of 16p, and loss of 8p, 3p, and 11q.

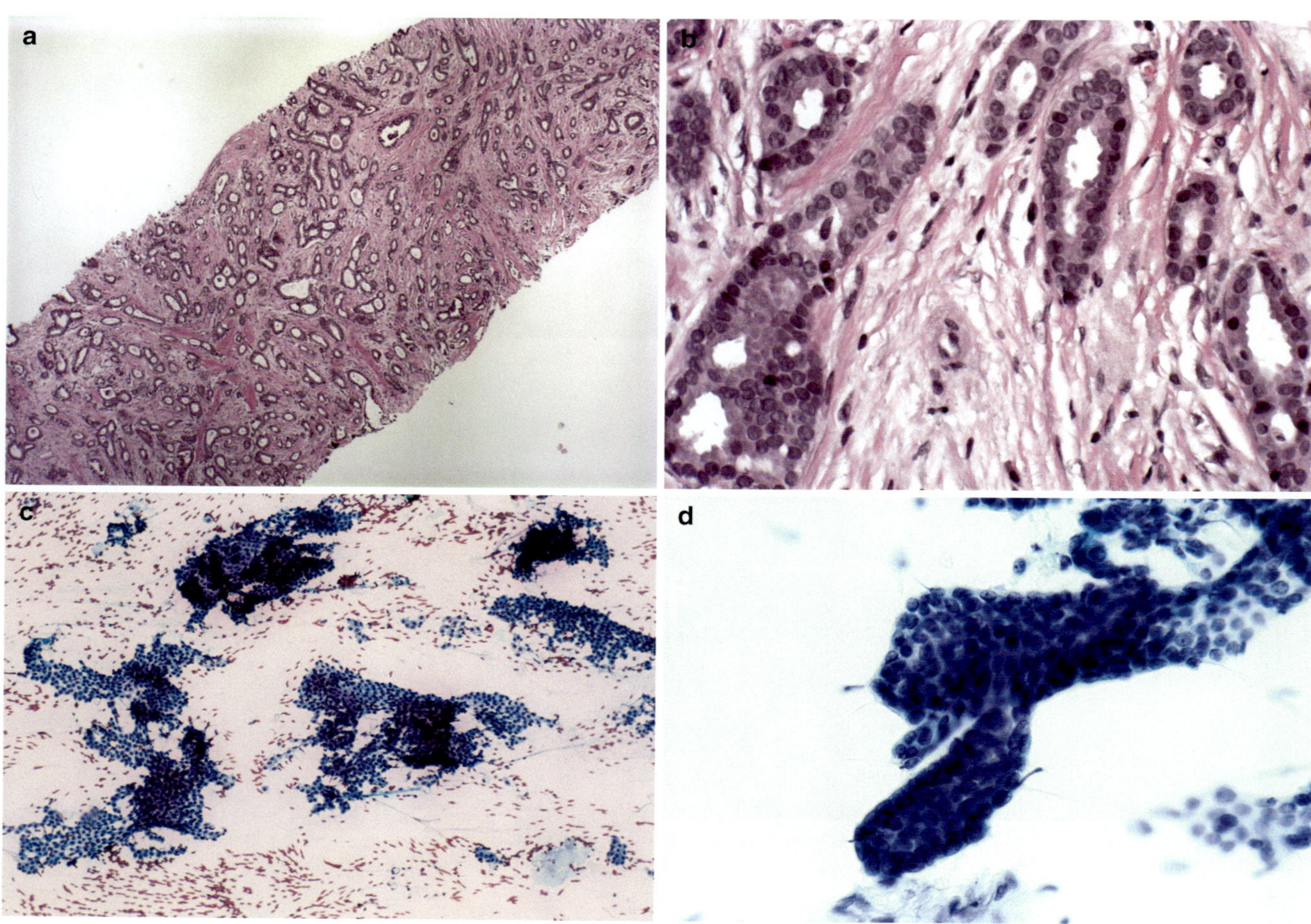

Fig. 8.49 Tubular carcinoma. Core biopsy showing the characteristic features of tubular carcinoma including angulated and comma-shaped tubules lined with cuboidal bland-appearing cells, surrounded by a desmoplastic stroma (**a, b**). Smears show striking resemblance with features of fibroadenoma when examined a low magnification; however, in contrast with fibroadenoma, myoepithelial cells are absent in tubular carcinoma when the smear is evaluated at high magnification (**c, d**). (**a, b**, H&E stain low and intermediate magnification; **c, d**, Papanicolaou stain low and high magnification)

By gene-expression profiling, tubular carcinomas belong to the *luminal A* molecular class of breast cancer.

FNA Findings Variably cellular smears show small uniform cells arranged in sheets, small aggregates, and tubular structures (Fig. 8.49c, d). Myoepithelial cells may be present due to the small tumor size and sampling of the surrounding benign breast tissue.

US Features A small vertically oriented hypoechogenic mass with irregular spiculated and angular borders and marked posterior acoustic shadowing is usually seen. These tumors usually have an ill-defined echogenic halo and show no vascularity on Doppler examination.

Cribriform Carcinoma

This specific subtype of invasive breast carcinoma accounts for <1% of breast carcinomas, occurs in patients at a mean age of 55 years, has an excellent prognosis, and often has a component of tubular carcinoma. The mean tumor size is 3 cm.

Histopathology A cribriform pattern composed of arches of cells of small to moderate size, and mild to moderate pleomorphism is embedded in a fibroblastic stroma. Invasive cribriform carcinomas with tubular carcinoma comprising less than 50% are still considered to be of the cribriform type. The pure form has >90% of cribriform architecture; the mixed form exhibits 10–90% of another morphological type other than tubular carcinoma. Osteoclast-like giant cells are occasionally present.

Immuno-profile This tumor is almost always ER$^+$ and is PR$^+$ in 65% of cases. It lacks HER2 overexpression. Myoepithelial markers (calponin, smooth muscle myosin heavy chain) are negative. p63 and CD117 are negative and allow the distinction from adenoid cystic carcinoma that shows positive immunoreactions.

Molecular Profile The molecular profile is similar to that of invasive tubular carcinoma.

By gene-expression profiling, infiltrating cribriform carcinomas belong to the *luminal A* molecular class of breast cancer.

FNA Findings Smears show cohesive sheets and three-dimensional cribriform clusters of bland-looking and mitotically inactive ductal cells. Associated scattered multinucleated, osteoclast-like giant cells, some containing hemosiderin granules, have been described. Myoepithelial cells and naked nuclei are not identified.

US Features This tumor appears as an ill-defined inhomogeneous mass with lobulated margins and an ill-defined echogenic halo. Usually there is minimal or no posterior acoustic shadowing.

Mucinous (Colloid) Carcinoma

Colloid carcinoma, a specific subtype of invasive breast carcinoma usually occurs in elderly women, comprises < 5% of breast carcinomas, and has a good prognosis.

Histopathology The mass has pushing margins and shows nests of cells of variable size and shape floating in mucin lakes. Cytologic atypia is usually mild. Hypercellular mucinous carcinoma may have neuroendocrine differentiation and show neuroendocrine marker positivity. Pure and mixed variants have been described, being the most common component found in invasive breast carcinoma of no special type. A pure tumor must be composed of >90% mucinous carcinoma (Fig. 8.50a).

Immuno-profile Mucinous carcinoma shows low-molecular-weight cytokeratins and strong immunoreactivity for MUC-2, ER, and PR. Variable numbers of neoplastic cells can express WT-1 and neuroendocrine markers. The tumor is ER$^+$ and PR$^+$. HER2 is not overexpressed.

Molecular Profile Mucinous tumors are of *luminal A* molecular profile.

Hypercellular mucinous tumors show a pattern of gene expression similar to that of neuroendocrine carcinomas.

FNA Findings The mass is soft instead of gritty upon insertion of the needle. Aspirates yield mucous material and variable cellularity. Characteristically, the cellular elements are monomorphic and arranged in small ball-like tridimensional aggregates surrounded by mucinous material that appears magenta with Romanowsky stains and fibrillary with Papanicolaou stain. The cells are small, with a bland-appearing chromatin pattern and a small nucleolus (Fig. 8.50b, c). High-grade tumor cell elements and stromal fragments are not uncommon in cases of ductal carcinoma with a mucinous component. Thus, the definitive cytologic diagnosis of mucinous carcinoma should be avoided; instead, the diagnosis of mammary neoplasm with a mucinous component should be rendered. The differential diagnosis includes mainly fibroadenoma with myxoid component and mucocele-like tumors of the breast; myoepithelial cells are seen in the former and benign ductal cells without atypia in the latter.

US Features The tumor is hypo- to nearly isoechoic and inhomogeneous with circumscribed lobulated edges, instead of the stellate or irregular appearance. There is variable pos-

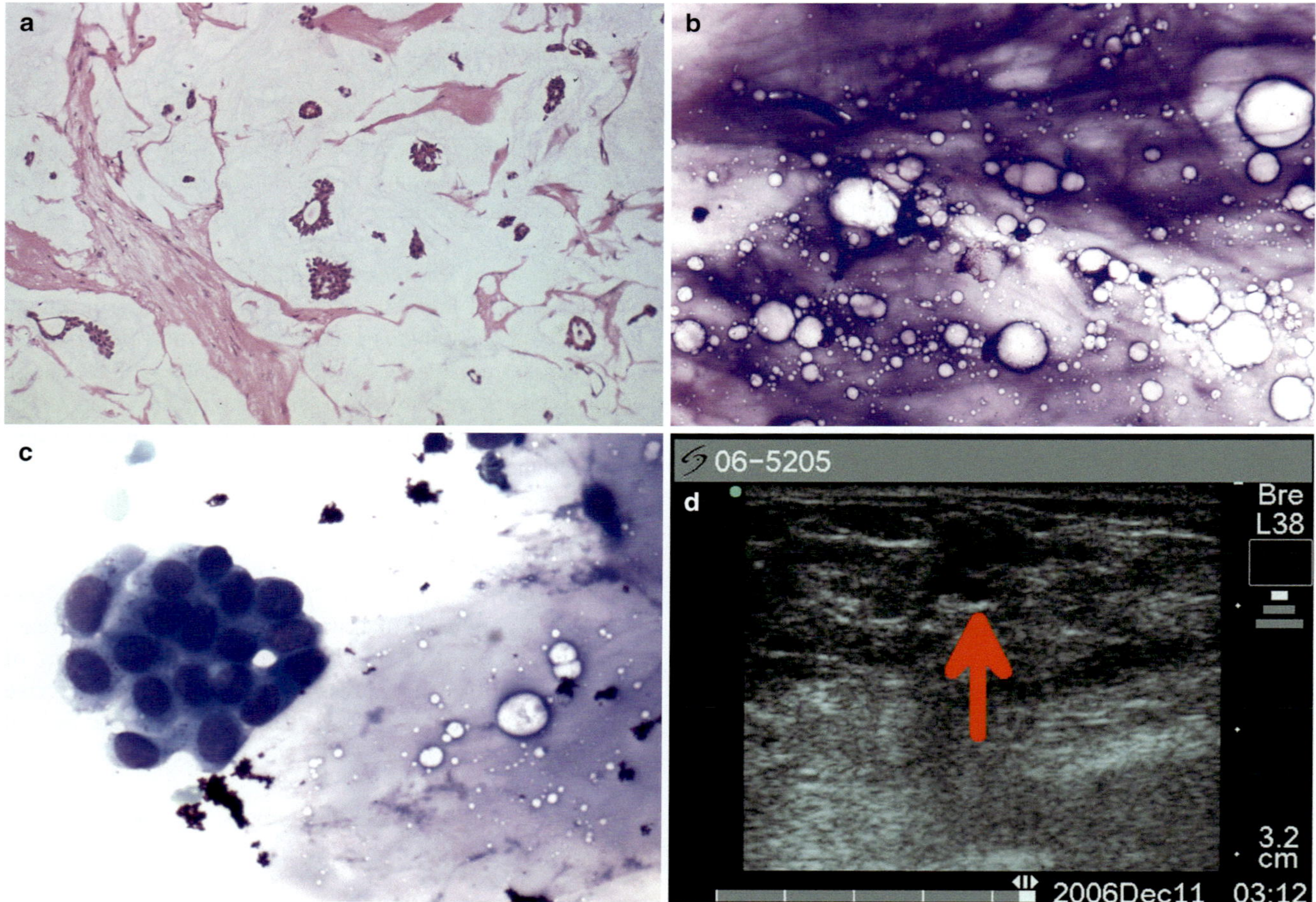

Fig. 8.50 Colloid (mucinous) carcinoma. Tissue sections show scattered islands of bland-appearing neoplastic cells embedded in an abundant mucinous background (**a**). Cytologic features include small aggregates of bland-appearing monomorphic neoplastic cells and abundant mucus (**b**, **c**). The ultrasound features are not specific and include lobulated borders and hypoecogenicity with variable presence of posterior acoustic enhancement (**d**). (**a**, H&E stain low magnification; **b**, **c**, DiffQuik and MGG stain high magnification)

terior acoustic enhancement, likely related to the mucin present in these tumors (Fig. 8.50d).

Carcinoma with Basal-like or Medullary-like Pattern

This type of invasive breast carcinoma of NST usually occurs in women in the 5th and 6th decades of life. Typical medullary carcinoma and a subset of invasive carcinomas of no special type are included under this category. Therefore, the diagnosis of medullary carcinoma requires careful gross and microscopic evaluation of the resected specimen. Classic medullary carcinoma comprises <1% of invasive breast carcinomas. Traditionally, the medullary type is associated with a good prognosis; however, due to the low reproducibility of the diagnosis, these tumors are treated with aggressive therapy as for "basal-like triple-negative" carcinomas.

Histopathology These tumors exhibit all or some of the following: circumscribed or pushing borders, a syncytial histologic pattern in >75% of the tumor mass, lack of gland formation, a prominent diffuse lymphoplasmacytic infiltrate, and high-nuclear grade tumor cells with abundant cytoplasm, pleomorphic nuclei, and prominent nucleoli. Mitoses, necrosis, and tumor giant cells may be present. Focal apocrine differentiation may be present. Because histologic evaluation may be subjective and not fully reproducible, the WHO has classified this tumor as carcinoma with basal-like or medullary-like pattern (Fig. 8.51a).

Immuno-profile These tumors are often ER, PR, and HER2 negative ("triple negative"). There is a variable expression of CK5, CK8, CK14, CK18, caveolin 1, β-catenin, and E- and P-cadherin. Most cases express EGF-R and mutated *TP53*.

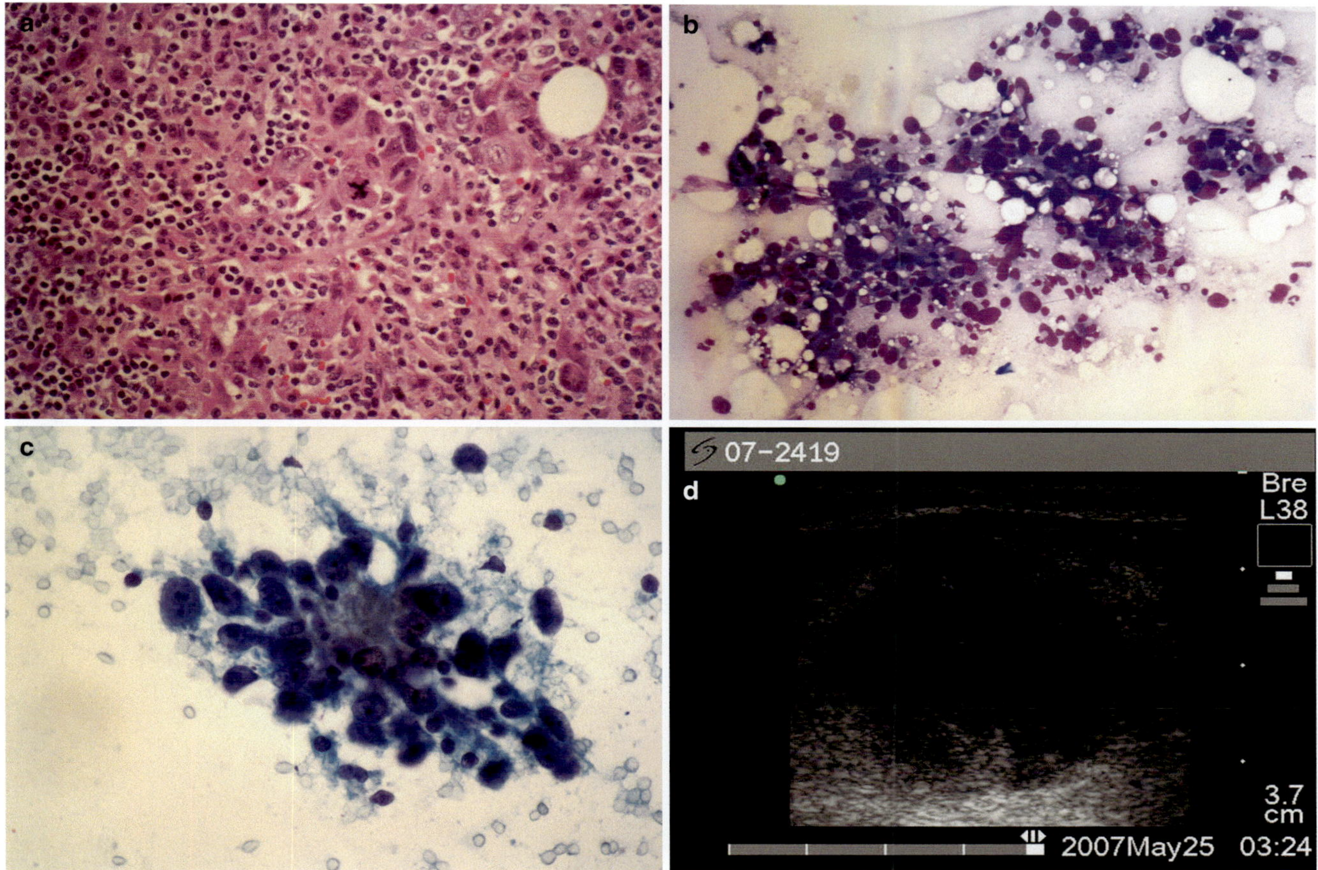

Fig. 8.51 Carcinoma with medullary features. Histology shows high-grade tumor cells arranged in a syncytial pattern surrounded by a lymphoplasmacytic infiltrate. Atypical mitoses may be seen (**a**). High-grade pleomorphic tumor cells admixed with lymphocytes and plasma cells are noted in the smears (**b**, **c**). Ultrasound images show an irregular, hypoechoic mass with lobulated borders (**d–f**); spiculated borders in addition to the lobulated margins may be seen focally (**g**, **h**). The vascular flow by Doppler exam is variable. (**a**, H&E stain, intermediate magnification; **b**, DiffQuik stain intermediate magnification; **c**, Papanicolaou stain high magnification)

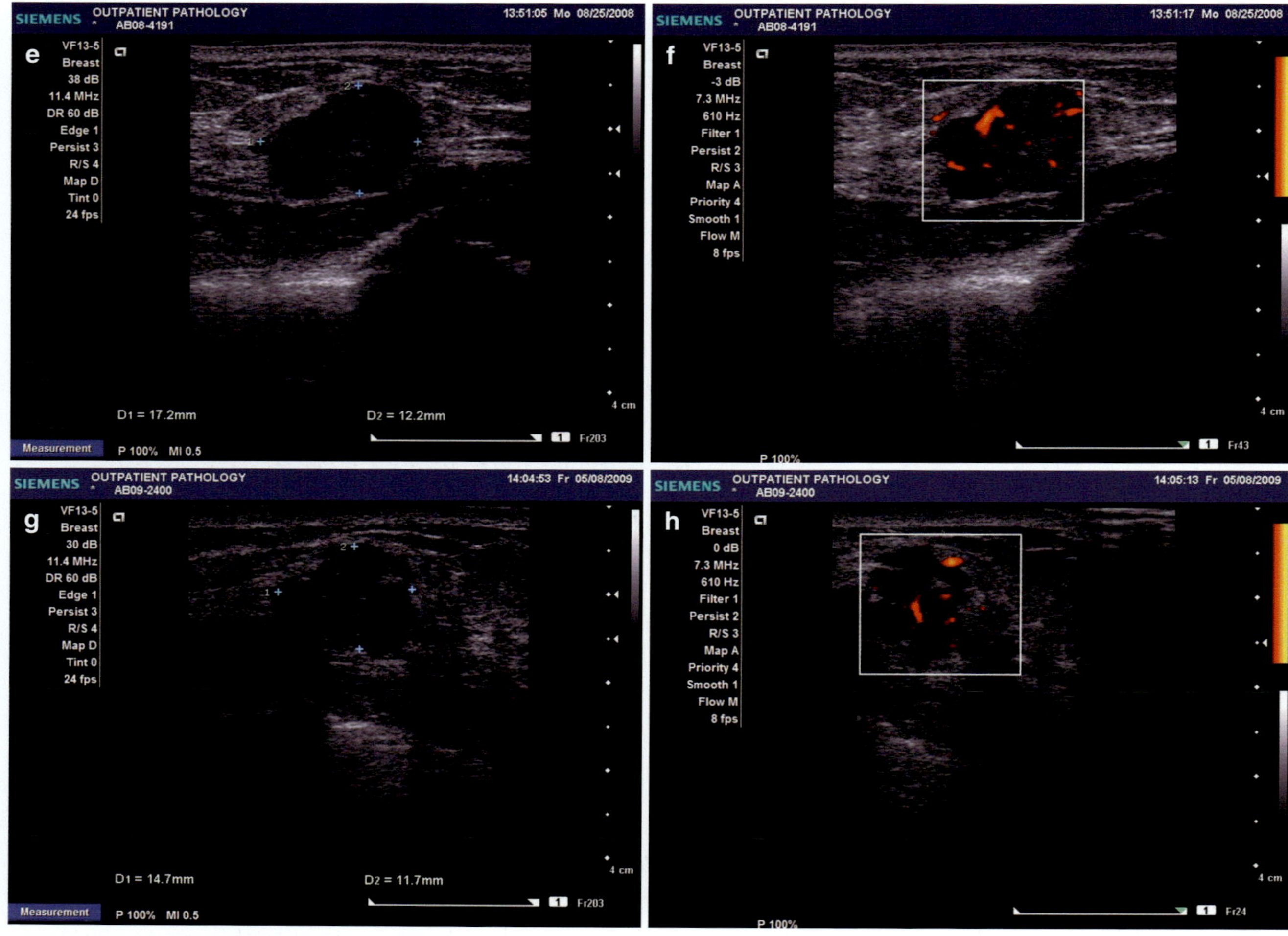

Fig. 8.51 (continued)

Molecular Profile Many of these tumors are recognized as "*basal-like*," and 13% of patients with these tumors have *BRCA1* germline mutations.

FNA Findings This carcinoma should be suspected when the tumor is well circumscribed, and the smear shows high-grade tumor cells with lymphocytes and plasma cells. Smears show syncytial sheets of poorly differentiated epithelial cells with high nuclear grade, admixed with a lymphoplasmacytic infiltrate and occasional necrosis. Cells have a considerable size and nuclear enlargement with multiple irregular macronucleoli. Individual high-grade tumor cells and naked malignant nuclei are also present in the background (Fig. 8.51b, c).

US Features These tumors may appear as a well- or ill-defined homogeneously hypoechoic round mass with lobulated margins and a variable posterior acoustic effect. Fast-growing tumors may have a "pseudo-cystic" pattern with posterior acoustic enhancement (Fig. 8.51d–h).

Adenoid Cystic Carcinoma

This rare salivary gland-type carcinoma of the breast comprises <0.1% of breast carcinomas and is associated with a good prognosis. The mean age at diagnosis is 64 years. The carcinoma develops in the subareolar region in 50% of cases. The tumor is generally cured by simple mastectomy, and the 10-year survival rate is >90%.

Histopathology The tumor is usually well-circumscribed and is histologically similar to the counterpart in the salivary gland, showing pseudoluminal spaces containing spherules of basement membrane material and glandular lumens. The tumor may show a solid variant composed of basaloid cells (Fig. 8.52a).

Immuno-profile The pseudoluminal spaces are decorated by small basal-myoepithelial cells that are positive for p63, calponin, smooth-muscle actin, and high-molecular-weight keratins (CK 5/6, CK 14) and negative for CD10. The glan-

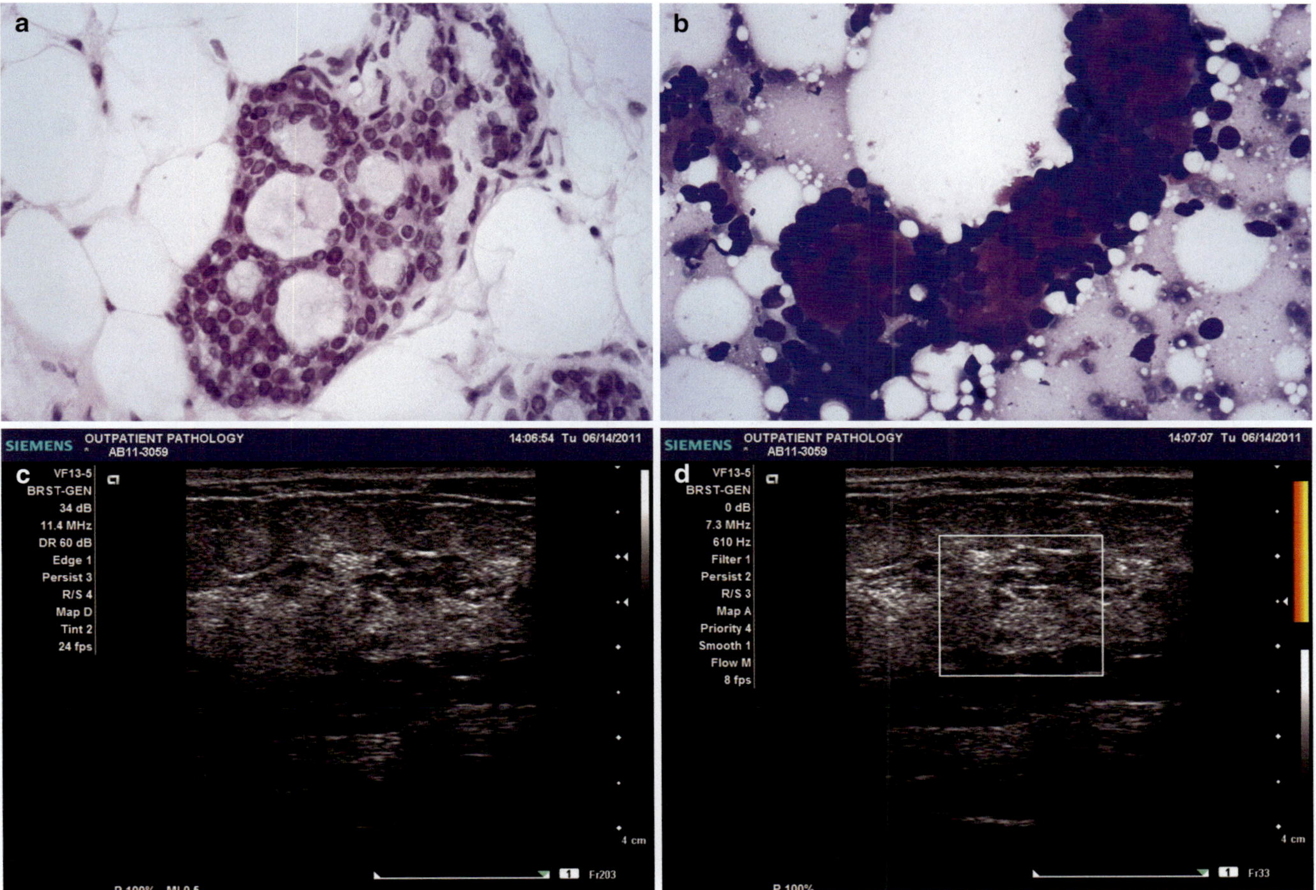

Fig. 8.52 Adenoid cystic carcinoma. Histologic findings are similar to those of adenoid cystic carcinoma of salivary gland and show pseudo lumens filled with basement membrane material (**a**). Cytologic findings include bland-appearing neoplastic cells surrounding globules of dense metachromatic stroma; the interface cell-stroma is sharp and well-defined (**b**). By ultrasound, this mass is heterogeneous, poorly circumscribed, focally hyperechoic, and shows no vascular flow by Doppler exam (**c**, **d**). (**a**, H&E stain intermediate magnification; **b**, DiffQuik stain high magnification)

dular lumens, which may be inconspicuous, are decorated by epithelial cells that are positive for CD117 (membrane staining), CK 7, and CK 8/18. This tumor is generally ER, PR, and HER2 negative. EGFR overexpression is found in 65% of cases.

Molecular Profile Adenoid cystic carcinoma harbors a recurrent chromosomal translocation t(6;9) leading to the formation of a chimeric fusion gene, *MYB-NFIB*. Many of these tumors are recognized as "*basal-like*" subtype.

FNA Findings The smear pattern is identical to that seen in the counterpart tumor located in the salivary gland. Smears show basaloid cells arranged in nests intimately associated with metachromatic matrix forming three-dimensional spheres. Usually, the metachromatic matrix has a sharp border, and there is a distinct separation between the matrix and surrounding cellular elements. The differential diagnosis includes collagenous spherulosis; however, collagenous spherulosis is a microscopic finding and adenoid cystic carcinoma is a neoplasm. Furthermore, adenoid cystic carcinoma lacks the fibrillary texture of collagenous spherulosis. The differential diagnosis also includes pleomorphic adenoma and the differential diagnosis criteria are those listed in the chapter on salivary gland tumors (Fig. 8.52b).

US Features The mass may be oval and complex with well-circumscribed margins and posterior acoustic enhancement (Fig. 8.52c, d).

Metaplastic Carcinoma

This rare invasive breast carcinoma accounts for <2% of breast malignancies. The tumors are usually large (mean size 4 cm), with borders that may be well circumscribed or indistinct and irregular, and histologically heterogeneous, characterized by the presence of ductal carcinoma with areas of squamous or mesenchymal (spindle, chondroid, osseous, or

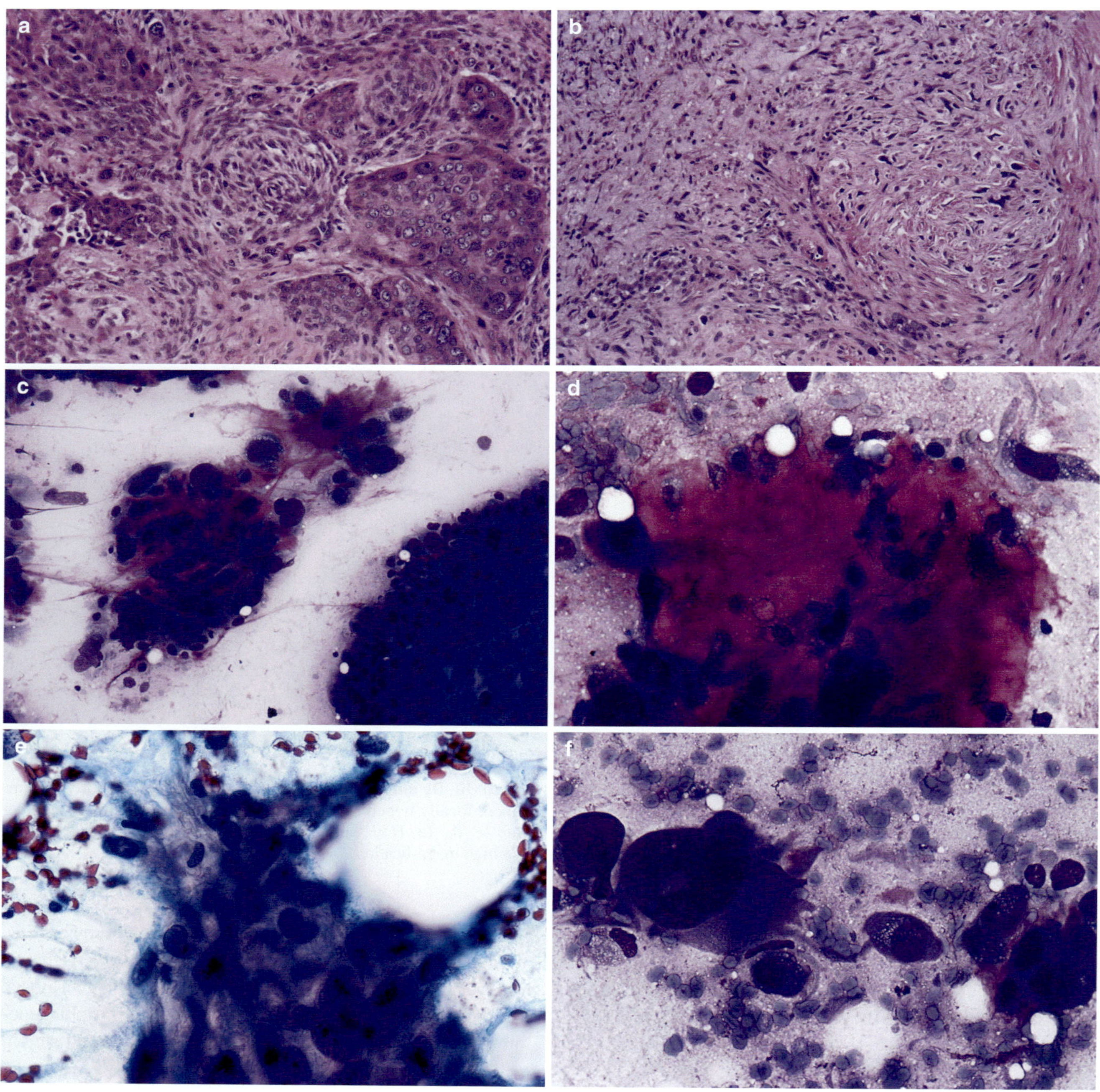

Fig. 8.53 Metaplastic carcinoma with mesenchymal differentiation. Rapidly growing tumor in a 27-year-old woman. Sections show chondromyxoid and squamous differentiation (**a**, **b**). Cellular pleomorphism, squamous and chondroid metaplasia, and fibrillary magenta stroma are prominent findings in the FNA smears (**c**, **f**). (**a**, **b**, H&E stain intermediate magnification; **c–f**, DiffQuik stain intermediate and high magnification)

rhabdomyoid) elements. When there is a predominance of pseudosarcomatous metaplasia, the prognosis is poor, and the survival rate is 25% at 5 years. Distant metastasis (lung and brain) can be found in the absence of lymph node metastasis, similar to other triple-negative breast cancers.

Histopathology This malignancy includes tumors with malignant squamous differentiation, spindle cell morphology, and heterologous mesenchymal elements (osse-

ous, chondroid, rhabdomyoid), either alone or combined with another metaplastic component, and/or ductal carcinoma NOS. It may have prominent mesenchymal differentiation. The histologic diagnosis should be descriptive, i.e., low-grade adenosquamous carcinoma, fibromatosis-like metaplastic carcinoma, squamous cell carcinoma, spindle cell carcinoma, metaplastic carcinoma with mesenchymal differentiation, mixed metaplastic carcinoma (Fig. 8.53a, b).

Immuno-profile These tumors are usually negative for ER, PR, and HER2 and express high-molecular-weight keratins (CK 5/6, CK14) and EGFR. Low-molecular-weight keratins are commonly negative, except CK7 which may be expressed. P63 positivity, seen in >90% of metaplastic breast carcinomas, is a useful marker for differentiating it from other spindle and mesenchymal neoplasms, including sarcomas. Immunocytochemistry reveals the nature of neoplastic cells. In adenosquamous carcinoma, the neoplastic cells express CK5, CK14, CK17, p63, and, in some cells, CK7. In carcinosarcoma, the epithelial component shows positivity for EMA, vimentin, and CK7, and CK5 in occasional cells. The sarcomatous elements may express smooth-muscle actin, myogenin, collagen II, S-100 protein, or osteonectin depending on their smooth-muscle, striated muscle, chondroid, or osteochondroid origin. Immunocytochemistry in spindle cell carcinoma usually shows positivity for vimentin, CK7, CK14, and p63. All subtypes of metaplastic carcinoma show a triple-negative molecular profile, and most of them express EGF-R.

Molecular Profile These tumors are triple-negative basal-like tumors and have multiple and complex chromosomal abnormalities. Mutations of the tumor suppressor gene *TP53* are found in most tumors, and loss of *p16* and *PTEN* is seen in other subgroups.

These tumors are classified as *"basal-like"* subtype. Some tumors are currently being classified into a recently described claudin-low tumor molecular subtype (tumors with epithelial to mesenchymal transition features).

FNA Findings Cytologic findings reflect the tumor composition such as ductal carcinoma and areas of spindle, squamous, chondroid, and osseous metaplasia in a background of necrosis. Smears may be hypercellular with cells showing marked pleomorphism, bi- or multinucleated bland-appearing or pleomorphic giant cells, and fibroblast-like spindle cells that may be tightly packed or loosely aggregated. Metaplastic carcinoma with chondrosarcomatous differentiation shows large high-grade tumor cells surrounded by a chondromyxoid stroma. Squamous carcinoma usually shows pleomorphic keratinizing, nonkeratinizing, and spindle squamous cells forming sheets, cords, or nests, or is single in a necrotic cystic background (Fig. 8.53c, f). The differential diagnosis of sarcomas includes reactive processes such as nodular fasciitis, fibromatosis, myofibroblastoma, and adenomyoepithelioma.

US Features These tumors tend to have an oval shape and well-defined borders. Cystic changes are common, and coarse calcification is seen when there is osteochondroid differentiation. Posterior acoustic shadowing is rarely present.

Squamous Cell Carcinoma

The diagnosis is made histologically. This carcinoma may occur as part of metaplastic carcinoma or as a pure tumor. The 2019 WHO includes this tumor under the category of metaplastic carcinoma.

Micropapillary Carcinoma

This rare, aggressive, and often palpable tumor accounts for <2% of breast cancers and is composed of small mini-papillary or morular-like cell aggregates surrounded by a clear space. The cells are columnar or cuboidal and show eosinophilic cytoplasm, variable nuclear pleomorphism, and a reverse polarity with cytoplasmic snouts facing the clear space and not the luminal surface. Focal apocrine differentiation may be present. Angiolymphatic invasion is more frequent in this tumor than in invasive ductal carcinoma NOS.

Immuno-profile Most carcinomas are ER and PR positive with variable HER2 overexpression. EMA positivity restricted to the basal portion of the neoplastic cells distinguishes this tumor from ductal carcinoma of no specific type that shows an apical homogeneous cytoplasmic immunostain.

Molecular Profile These tumors are classified as *luminal A or B subtype*. Recurrent gains of chromosome arms 8q, 17q, and 20q and deletions of chromosome arms 6q and 13q are seen. Deep sequencing techniques have shown microRNA patterns different from that of invasive ductal carcinoma of no special type.

FNA Findings Smears show increased cellularity, cell clusters with angular and papillary configuration without a fibrovascular core, tumor clusters showing an "inside-out" pattern, irregular crowded nuclei, and the presence of single discohesive cells. Few malignant-appearing multinucleated giant cells, cells with apocrine features, little mucin, psammoma bodies, and tumor diathesis may be seen. No mitoses are present. The diagnosis is suspected in the presence of morulae formation, isolated malignant cells and branching epithelial structures.

US Features The tumor is hypoechoic, but occasionally isoechoic; it is irregular, or microlobulated, with hypoechoic internal areas, and with or without posterior acoustic enhancement.

Inflammatory Carcinoma

The 2019 WHO classification of breast tumors recognizes inflammatory carcinoma as a rare clinical presentation of aggressive breast carcinoma rather than a special subtype. The skin has the appearance of an "orange peel" and is engorged, red, and tender with or without an underlying distinct breast mass (Fig. 8.54a). Inflammatory carcinoma is a descriptive clinical term that has a distinctive underlying pathologic finding, the presence of tumor emboli plugging the lymphatic vascular channels of the breast dermis with *no* inflammation (Fig. 8.54b, c). Aspiration cytology may not be revealing, and in such cases sampling of the commonly found ipsilateral axillary metastasis fulfills diagnostic and staging purposes.

Immuno-profile This carcinoma is ER and PR positive in 50% of cases, and HER2 positive in 40%. Characteristically, E-cadherin is overexpressed and there is high expression of p53 and MUC1.

Molecular Profile There is no characteristic genetic alteration for inflammatory carcinoma. Molecular subtyping often classifies this cancer in the HER2 or basal sub-

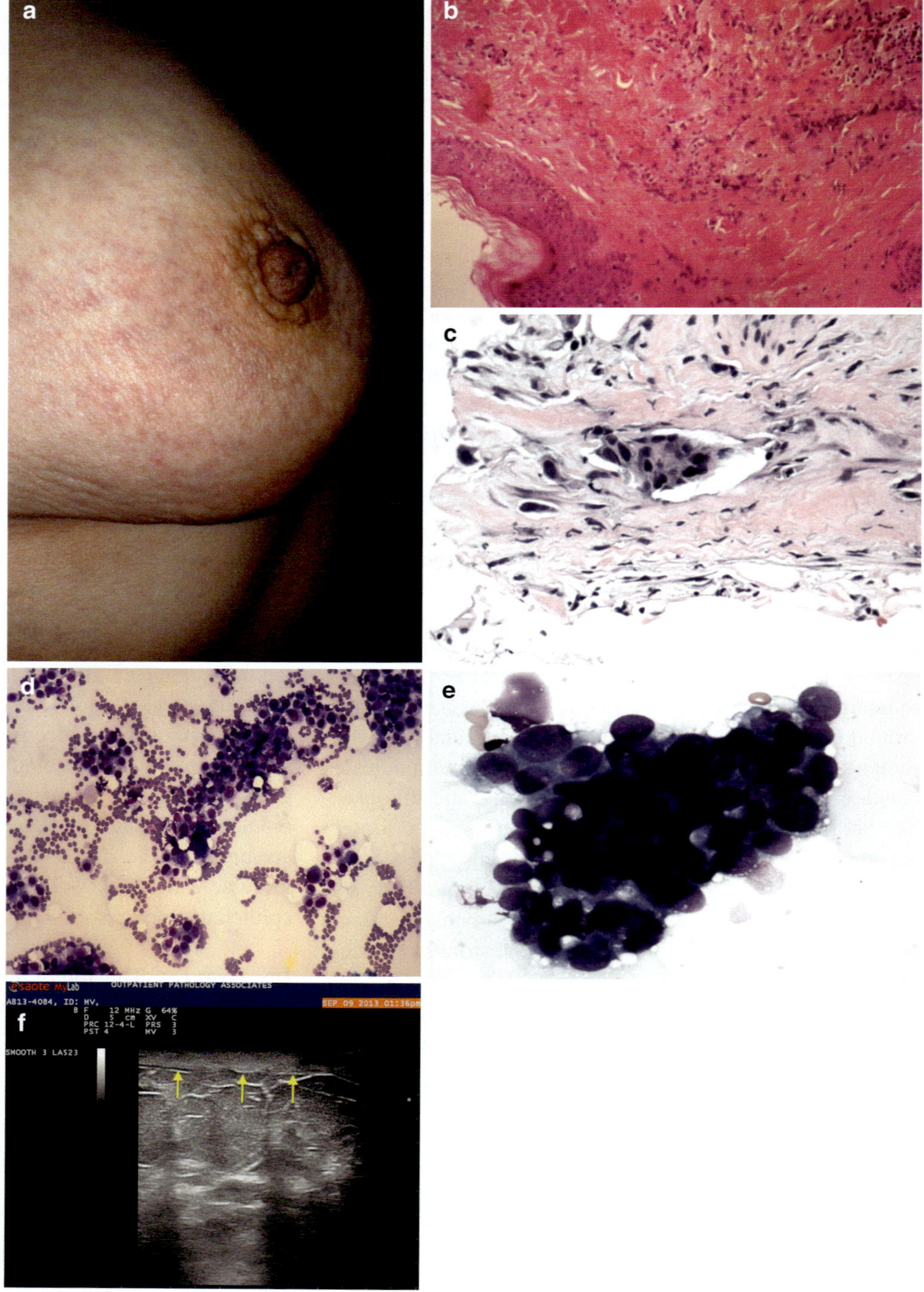

Fig. 8.54 Inflammatory carcinoma. Hyperemia and orange peel-appearing skin are characteristic on breast exam (**a**); this picture corresponds to a patient with micropapillary breast carcinoma. Dermal lymphatics with tumor emboli and no inflammatory reaction are present (**b**, **c**) in tissue sections. Scattered groups of malignant cells are seen in the FNA smears (**d**, **e**). US shows a poorly circumscribed mass and marked thickening of the dermis (**f**, arrows). (**b**, **c**, H&E stain, intermediate and high magnification; **d**, **e**, MGG stain intermediate and high magnification)

types. Activation of the anaplastic lymphoma kinase (ALK) pathway has recently been suggested to occur, and if this is confirmed, these patients may benefit from targeted therapy.

FNA Findings The cytomorphology is similar to that of poorly differentiated infiltrating breast carcinoma. Smears are sparsely cellular due to lymphatic permeation and stromal edema. High-grade cells are arranged in small aggregates and show a vacuolated cytoplasm, large pleomorphic nuclei, coarse chromatin, and prominent nucleoli (Fig 8.54d, e).

US Features The skin thickening seen by US is the combination of dilated subdermal lymphatics and edema (Fig. 8.54f). There is tissue hyperechogenicity and disruption of normal tissue planes. A hypoechoic, irregular, ill-defined mass with posterior acoustic shadowing may be identified. Axillary lymph nodes with suspicious US features are commonly seen.

Paget Disease of the Nipple

This eczema-like change in the nipple and areola is commonly associated with underlying in situ or invasive mammary carcinoma. Paget disease of the nipple without underlying carcinoma is rare. It affects both sexes and can be bilateral. Patients may have erythema or eczema of the nipple, ulceration, inversion, and nipple discharge. The prognosis depends on the presence or absence of underlying DCIS or invasive carcinoma. However, rarely advanced breast cancer extends out to involve the surface of the nipple and produce ulceration (Fig. 8.55a).

Histopathology The presence of large cells having ample clear cytoplasm and large nuclei with prominent nucleoli is characteristic within the epidermis. Cells are placed singly or in small clusters in the dermoepidermal junction and lower layers of the epidermis (Fig. 8.55b).

Immuno-profile Paget cells are positive for CK 7 and CAM5.2. ER and PR are positive in 40% of cases, and HER2 is positive in 90%, similar to the underlying carcinoma. Negative immuno-

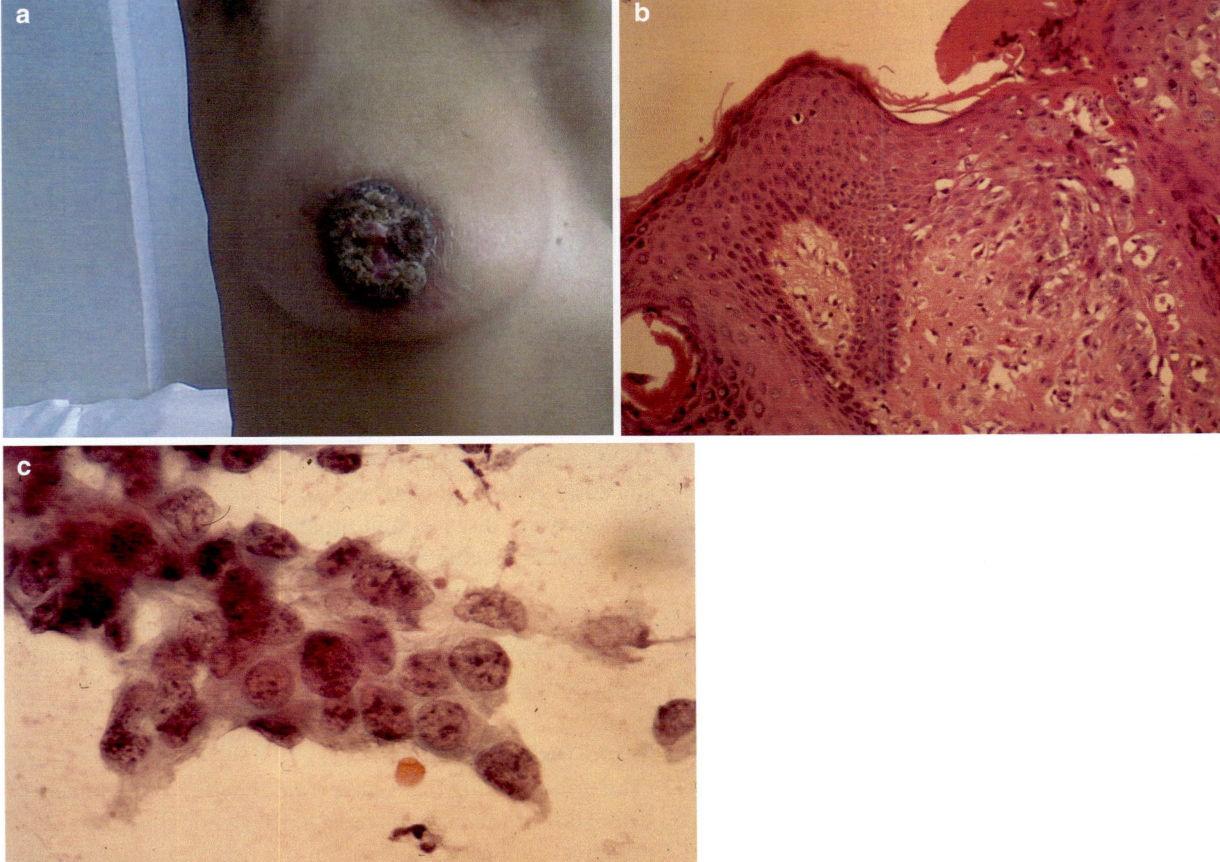

Fig. 8.55 Paget's disease. Nipple and areolar crusting and induration with nipple inversion (**a**). Large malignant cells with vacuolated cytoplasm are present in the dermo epidermal interface (**b**). Smears show high-grade malignant cells (**c**). (**b**, H&E stain intermediate magnification; **c**, Papanicolaou stain high magnification) (**a**, courtesy Dr. Manuel Cedano, Trujillo, Peru)

reaction with S100 protein, HMB-45, and melan-A exclude melanoma; Pancytokeratin and high-molecular weight cytokeratin are positive en Bowen's disease.

Molecular Profile Paget cells have no distinct or specific gene mutation profile, and they are genetically similar to the underlying breast carcinoma.

Cytologic Findings The diagnosis can be made by scraping of the lesion or by FNA if there is an underlying mass. Smears usually show high-grade malignant cells (Fig. 8.55c).

US Features The nipple is thickened, and an underlying calcification/mass lesion may be seen.

Rare Types of Breast Carcinoma

Included but not restricted to secretory, mucoepidermoid, and acinic cell carcinomas.

Secretory Carcinoma

This low-grade invasive carcinoma is very rare, occurs in young patients of both sexes, with a median age of 25 years, and has a favorable prognosis. The tumors are well circumscribed and mobile, occurring close to the areola.

Histopathology Tumors have pushing borders and have microcystic, solid, and tubular patterns, usually in combination (Fig. 8.56a).

Immuno-profile The tumors are S100 protein and lactalbumin positive and ER, PR, HER2, and p63 negative. The basal-like marker (CK5/6 or EGFR) is expressed in 90% of cases.

Molecular Profile Secretory carcinoma harbors a recurrent chromosomal translocation t(12;15)(q13;q25) leading to the formation of the chimeric fusion gene *ETV6-NTRK3*, which is considered specific for secretory carcinoma. These tumors are classified as "*basal-like*" subtype.

FNA Findings Smears are cellular and show grape-like clusters and single large cells with granular to vacuolated cytoplasm, uniform round nuclei, minimal nuclear atypia, and prominent nucleoli in a mucinous background. Cells may have a plasmacytoid appearance and may be binucleate. Diagnosis of this carcinoma on FNA is difficult and important because the cytologic findings can be confused with those of the lactating breast. The differential diagnosis includes lipid-secreting carcinoma, glycogen-rich clear cell carcinoma, and cystic hypersecretory carcinoma (Fig. 8.56b, c).

US Features Ultrasonography and breast computed tomography show a subareolar oval-shaped tumor exhibiting homogeneous echogenicity with clear margins.

Mucoepidermoid Carcinoma

This very rare breast tumor is similar histologically to the salivary gland counterpart, is well circumscribed, and can reach a large size. The tumor shows basaloid, intermediate, squamous, and mucinous cells. Most tumors are of low grade, with predominance of the mucinous cells. High-grade mucoepidermoid are usually solid with predominance of intermediate and squamous cells.

Acinic Cell Carcinoma

This tumor is similar to the parotid gland counterpart, and it may be well to poorly differentiated to undifferentiated. It appears to have good prognosis, although axillary lymph node metastasis may occur.

Immuno-profile There is cytoplasmic reactivity with alpha-1-anti-chymotrypsin, amylase, lysozyme, EMA, and S-100 protein. This tumor is negative for ER, PR, and HER2.

FNA Findings Cells have abundant granular cytoplasm, a round nucleus, and prominent nucleoli. The cytoplasm contains zymogen granules or may be clear ("hypernephroid").

Oncocytic Carcinoma

The tumor occurs in both sexes and predominantly in the 7th decade of life.

Histopathology Oncocytic carcinoma is defined as breast carcinoma with >70% oncocytic differentiation. Oncocytes have ample eosinophilic cytoplasm with numerous mitochondria. It is predominantly solid with variable nuclear pleomorphism and prominent nucleoli. Oncocytic carcinoma is indistinguishable from apocrine carcinoma on H&E stain.

Immuno-profile The tumor is ER, PR, and HER2 positive in 80%, 60%, and 25% of cases, respectively. GCDFP15 (gross cystic disease fluid protein-15) is negative and anti-mitochondrial antibody stain is strong and diffuse.

Molecular Profile The tumor often displays chromosomal gains of 11q and 19p13 similar to renal and thyroid oncocytic tumors.

Lipid-Rich Carcinoma

The tumor occurs in women from the 4th to 9th decade of life. Half of the patients have axillary nodal metastases at diagnosis, and 38% die within the first year after diagnosis. The tumor is defined as breast carcinoma with >90% of cells containing cytoplasmic neutral lipids. Most cases show histologic grade 3 and are ER and PR negative. There are no data on the genetic features of these tumors. Neoplastic cells show large, vacuolated, foamy lipid-laden cytoplasm.

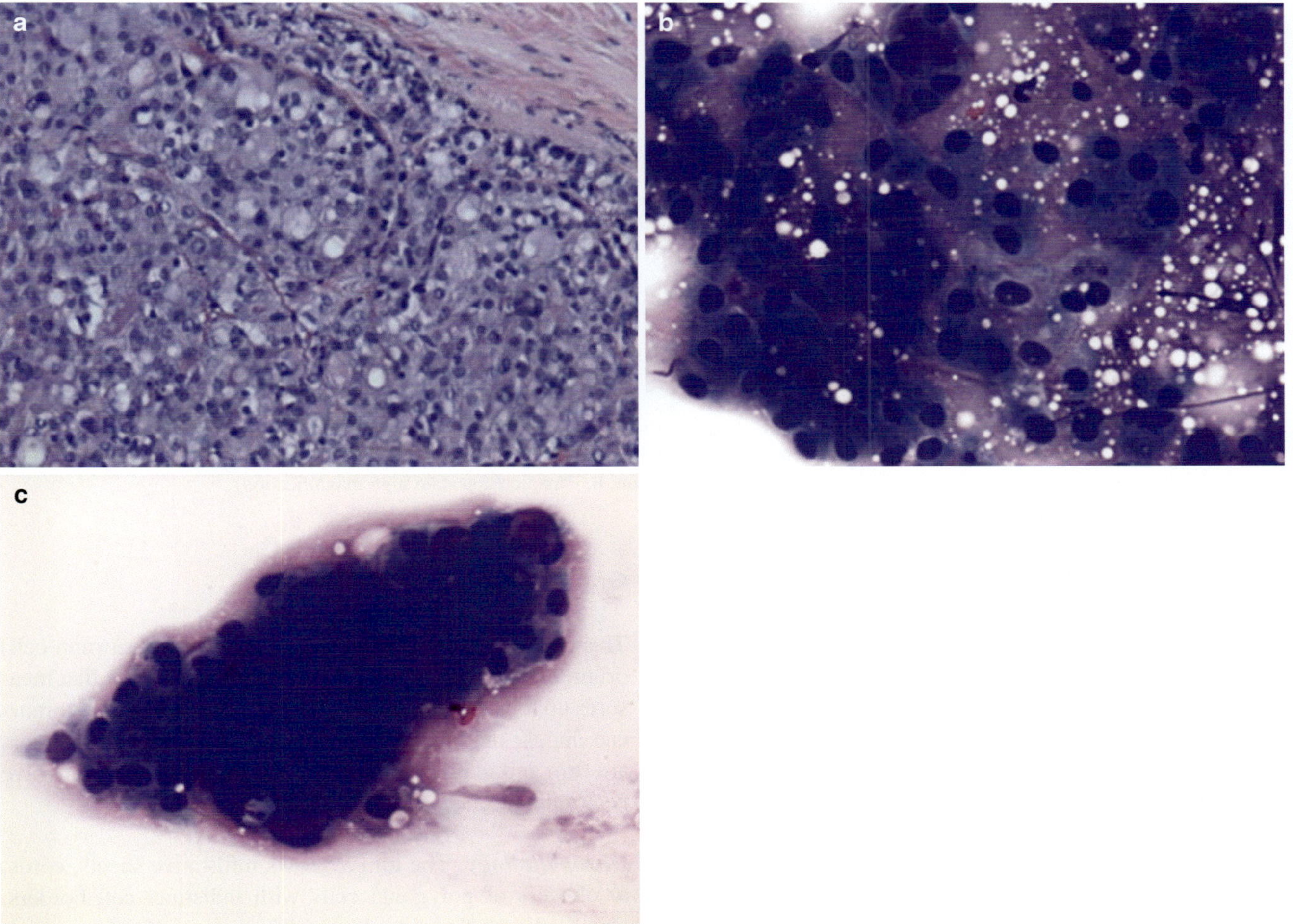

Fig. 8.56 Secretory carcinoma. Histopathology shows pushing borders and microcystic architecture (**a**). The smears show cohesive sheets and aggregates of large cells with ample slightly vacuolated dense cytoplasm, bland-appearing round nuclei, ill-defined cytoplasmic borders, and clean background (**b**, **c**). Other areas show a proteinaceous mucoid background. (**a**, H&E stain; **b**, **c**, DiffQuik stain high magnification) (Courtesy Dr. Margarita Elices Apellaniz. Madrid, Spain)

Glycogen-Rich Clear Cell Carcinoma

This tumor is more aggressive than carcinoma of no specific type. The median age at diagnosis is 57 years. This is defined as breast carcinoma with >90% cells having glycogen-containing clear cytoplasm. The cells are polygonal with granular clear cytoplasm, hyperchromatic nuclei, and prominent nucleoli. ER is positive in 50% of cases. HER2 and PR are negative in most cases. The differential diagnosis includes other clear cell primary or metastatic breast tumors, i.e., lipid-rich carcinoma, myoepithelioma, metastatic renal cell carcinoma.

Apocrine Carcinoma

Data suggest that many subtypes of breast cancer show apocrine differentiation in various proportions and that "apocrine carcinomas" do not represent a distinct entity.

Histopathology This is a rare breast tumor that is indistinguishable from oncocytic carcinoma on usual histologic grounds. The eosinophilic cytoplasm has predominance of electron-dense cytoplasmic granules. Some cells may have empty vesicles and correspond to the foam cells seen histologically in the clear cell variant.

Immuno-profile The tumor is CK 7 negative, ER and PR negative, and androgen receptor positive; HER2 is overexpressed in 45% of cases. GCDFP15 is diffusely positive, and the anti-mitochondrial antibody stain is weak and focal.

FNA Findings Smears show fragments with a syncytial arrangement and single cells showing abundant granular eosinophilic cytoplasm, large nuclei, and prominent nucleoli. In contrast to apocrine metaplasia, the carcinoma shows cell dissociation, a syncytial arrangement, cellular atypia, and pleomorphic, irregular, and hyperchromatic nuclei (Fig. 8.57).

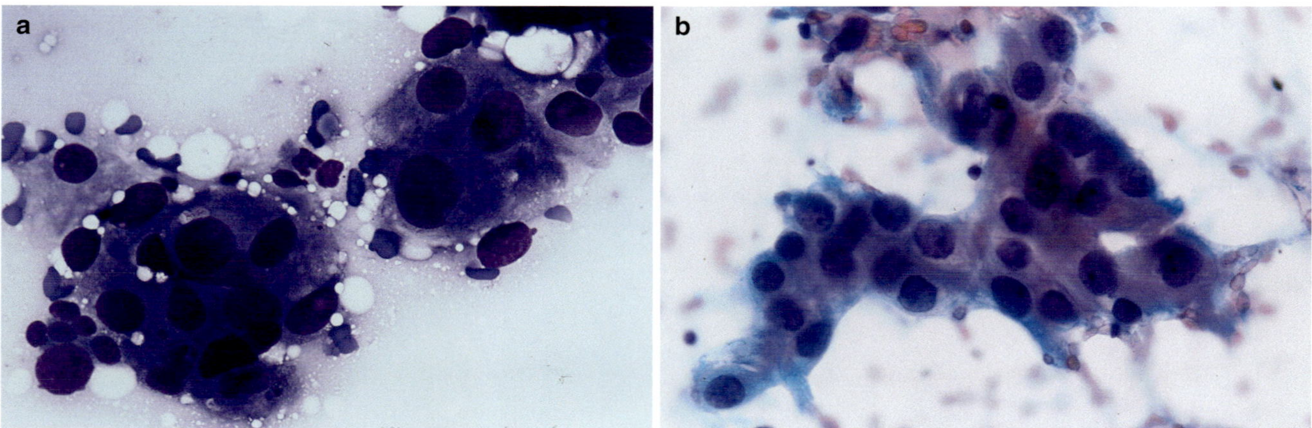

Fig. 8.57 Breast carcinoma with apocrine differentiation. Large cells with abundant granular cytoplasm, large nuclei, and prominent nucleoli are identified forming a syncytial pattern. (**a**, DiffQuik stain high magnification; **b**, Papanicolaou stain high magnification)

Neuroendocrine Neoplasms

Pure neuroendocrine tumors are rare, comprising <1% of breast carcinomas, and include large-cell and small-cell neuroendocrine carcinomas. Neuroendocrine differentiation of breast carcinomas of no special type, mucinous carcinomas, and solid papillary carcinomas are more frequent. Clinical neuroendocrine syndromes related to hormone production are rarely present.

Histopathology These tumors show features similar to those seen in the lung or GI tract.

Immuno-profile Well-differentiated tumors are positive for ER and PR; poorly differentiated small-cell neuroendocrine carcinoma shows ER and PR positivity in 50% of cases.

Molecular Profile These tumors have a *luminal A* molecular profile.

FNA Findings Cytomorphologic features are similar to those of neuroendocrine carcinomas of other sites, i.e., lung, GI tract.

Mesenchymal Tumors

Benign and malignant mesenchymal tumors such as nodular fasciitis, hemangiomas, desmoid-type fibromatosis, inflammatory myofibroblastic tumor, leiomyoma, rhabdomyosarcoma, osteosarcoma, and leiomyosarcoma occur in the breast. True sarcomas, i.e., osteogenic sarcoma, rhabdomyosarcoma, liposarcoma, and angiosarcoma, are rarer than metaplastic carcinoma, with malignant fibrous histiocytoma being the most common.

FNA findings of benign and malignant mesenchymal tumors are similar to those described in other chapters of this book. We describe granular cell tumor and angiosarcoma next.

Granular Cell Tumor

This almost always benign tumor of neural (Schwann cell) origin can be seen in the breast as a painless mass that measures up to 3 cm. It is multiple in 20% of cases. These tumors can appear malignant clinically and radiologically. Tumors are firm and may cause skin and nipple retraction or involve pectoralis fascia.

Histopathology The tumor shows infiltrative sheets, cords, or clusters of polygonal cells with indistinct cell borders, abundant granular cytoplasm (rich in lysosomes), a round, uniform nucleus, and conspicuous nucleoli (Fig. 8.58a).

Immuno-profile The tumor is positive for S-100 protein and CD68 (lysosomal). Staining for keratins, myoglobin, GFAP, and lysozyme is negative. A tumor with a high level of Ki67 should be considered malignant, even if the tumor has few pathological features of malignancy.

FNA Findings Aspirates show numerous single and grouped cells with eosinophilic granular cytoplasm, and oval to round nuclei with variable atypia. The cytoplasm is fragile, and its rupture results in a granular background and numerous free-lying nuclei (Fig. 8.58b, c). Atypia and necrosis may indicate a malignant granular cell tumor. The differential diagnosis includes alveolar soft-part sarcoma and rhabdomyosarcoma that show nuclear atypia; and rhabdomyoma, a glycogen-rich benign tumor of striated muscle that has cells with granular cytoplasm and elongated cells showing squared well-defined borders, and cytoplasmic cross-striations standing out in a clean background. Rhabdomyomas are PAS positive, but S-100 protein negative.

US Features US shows an oval hypoechoic spiculated nodule with combined posterior acoustic enhancement and shadowing. The tumor may not be well circumscribed.

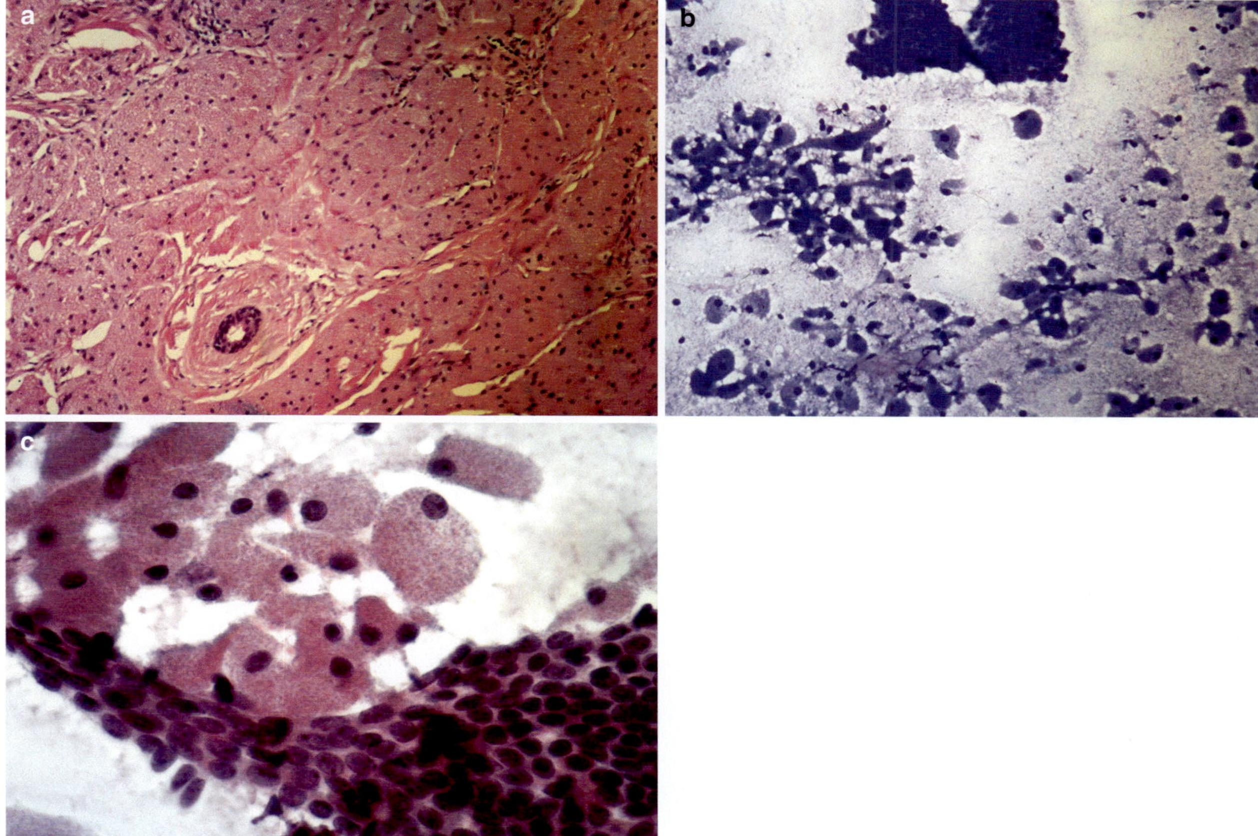

Fig. 8.58 Granular cell tumor. Cords of large cells with abundant granular cytoplasm and round nuclei surround a benign breast duct (**a**). The smears show numerous cells with polyhedral appearance, abundant granular cytoplasm, and a granular background (**b**). The eosinophilic cytoplasm is best seen in the Papanicolaou-stained smear (**c**). (**a**, H&E stain intermediate magnification; **b**, DiffQuik stain intermediate magnification; **c**, Papanicolaou stain high magnification) (Courtesy Dr. John S. Abele, Sacramento, CA, USA)

Angiosarcoma

This tumor can arise de novo in the breast or secondarily in the skin, breast, or chest wall in patients with a history of breast carcinoma treated with radiotherapy (the latent period is 7–10 years or more). Angiosarcoma associated with lymphedema in patients treated with mastectomy and axillary lymph node dissection has been described. Primary angiosarcoma is the second most common sarcoma after malignant phyllodes tumor. Patients may have a painless mass or a diffuse breast enlargement with a bluish-red discoloration when the skin is involved. Violaceous or erythematous skin nodules or variably sized plaques may be seen. The prognosis is dismal, and recurrence, metastases, and survival are independent of tumor grade.

Histopathology Well-differentiated angiosarcomas show anastomosing vascular channels with dilated or angulated lumina lined with endothelial cells that have large hyperchromatic nuclei (Fig. 8.59a). Poorly differentiated angiosarcomas show vascular channels admixed with solid cellular areas exhibiting spindle or epithelioid cells, blood lakes, necrosis, and mitoses.

Immuno-profile CD31, CD34, and nuclear Fli-1 positivity support the diagnosis of angiosarcoma, particularly in poorly differentiated tumors. Of importance, keratin may be focally positive.

Molecular Profile Activating mutations of the receptor tyrosine kinase gene *KDR* have been described in some angiosarcomas. A high level of *MYC* amplification may be seen in angiosarcomas secondary to radiotherapy.

FNA Findings The cellularity may be sparse. Epithelioid and or spindle cells with hyperchromatic nuclei and prominent nucleoli are seen. Smears show a background of blood, necrosis, and hemosiderin-laden macrophages (Fig. 8.59b, c).

US Features US shows a hyperechoic or a mixed hyper- and hypoechoic mass with indistinct, angular or spiculated margins; the echotexture may be homogeneous or heterogeneous. Sometimes, the mass may be lobular with circumscribed margins ("cloud-like") and coarse calcifications. When the skin is involved, there is a round, oval,

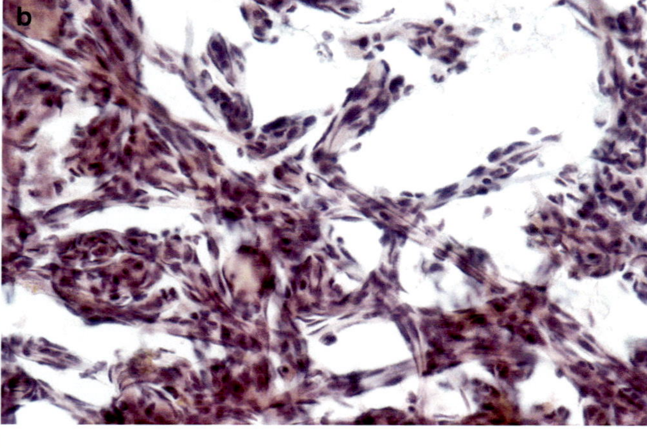

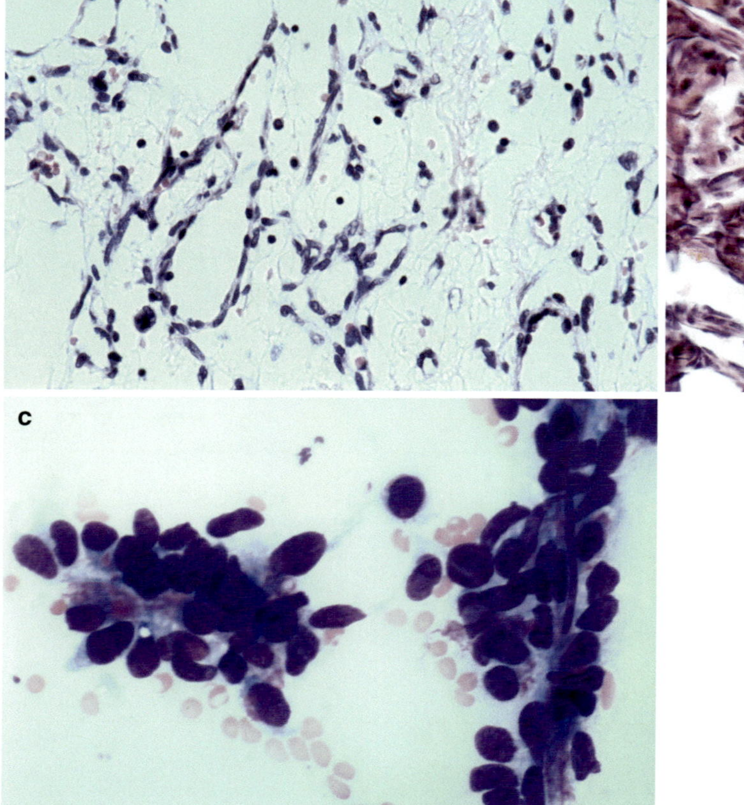

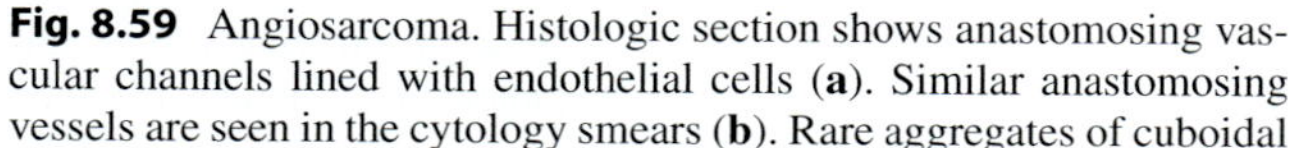

Fig. 8.59 Angiosarcoma. Histologic section shows anastomosing vascular channels lined with endothelial cells (**a**). Similar anastomosing vessels are seen in the cytology smears (**b**). Rare aggregates of cuboidal cells forming microacini are also seen along with linear vessels (**c**). (**a**, H&E stain low magnification; **b**, Papanicolaou stain low magnification; **c**, DiffQuik stain high magnification)

or irregular hypoechoic mass associated with the dermis with skin thickening. The hypoechoic dermal nodules usually disrupt the dermal plate and extend to the underlying breast tissue.

Lymphoid Malignancies

Lymphomas in the breast are rare and may be primary or secondary to a systemic lymphoma. Most patients are postmenopausal women, although lymphoma can occur in young women or in men. A painless mass or a multinodular breast is usually identified. The most common type of lymphoma in the breast is diffuse large B-cell lymphoma followed by extra nodal marginal-zone lymphoma of the MALT type and follicular lymphoma. Burkitt lymphoma, lymphoblastic lymphoma, and T-cell lymphomas including anaplastic large-cell lymphoma (ALCL) have been described.

Histopathology Histologic findings are identical to those of lymphomas in other sites.

Immuno-profile Diffuse large B-cell lymphoma has a mature B-cell phenotype expressing CD20, CD79a, and PAX5.

Burkitt lymphoma has a mature B-cell phenotype expressing CD20, CD79a, and PAX5. Staining for CD10 and BCL6 is positive and is negative for BCL2 and terminal deoxynucleotidyl transferase. EBV sequences are detected by EBV-encoded RNA (EBER) in situ hybridization.

T-cell lymphoma cells express the T-cell-associated markers CD2 and CD3. ALCL is positive for CD30 and EMA and negative for CD15 and CD20.

MALT lymphomas express CD20, CD79a, PAX5, and BCL2 and are negative for CD5, CD10, CD23, BCL6, and cyclin D1.

Follicular lymphomas express pan-B-cell markers CD20 and CD79a as well as CD10, BCL6, and BCL2.

Molecular Profile Burkitt lymphoma has translocations involving the MYC gene and one of the immunoglobulin genes, most often *IGH@*, and less often *IGK@* or *IGL@*.

Most ALCLs show a clonal rearrangement of the T-cell receptor gene.

MALT lymphomas of the breast show a clonal rearrangement of the immunoglobulin genes. Cytogenetic abnormalities characteristic of other MALT lymphomas, e.g., t(11;18)(q21;q21), have not been reported.

The characteristic t(14;18)(q32;q21) seen in follicular lymphomas has not been systematically evaluated in primary follicular lymphomas of the breast.

FNA Findings Cytologic findings are similar to those of lymphomas in lymph nodes or other sites.

US Features Breast involvement shows a well-defined to irregular hypoechoic mass or masses, skin thickening, and dilated subdermal lymphatics. Lymph nodes are markedly hypoechoic with thickening of the hypoechoic cortex, a bulging contour, and attenuation of the central fatty hilum.

Tumors of the Male Breast

Gynecomastia

Gynecomastia is a hormonally-dependent, often unilateral lesion that occurs in adolescents and older male patients. It may be idiopathic or drug-related, i.e., related to digitalis, reserpine, and muscle-enhancers non-FDA regulated products that are sold over the counter. Patients have a palpable tender subareolar and ill-defined mass (Fig. 8.60a).

Histopathology There is proliferation of the ductal and mesenchymal elements. Branching ducts with variable degrees of cellular hyperplasia are seen. Squamous and apocrine metaplasia may occasionally be present, and atypical ductal hyperplasia is rarely seen (Fig. 8.60b).

Molecular Profile Except in gynecomastia associated with Klinefelter syndrome, there is no underlying genetic abnormality.

FNA Findings Cellularity is variable and is higher in early lesions and sparse in long-standing lesions. The smear pattern is similar to that of fibrocystic change, including benign ductal epithelial cells, myoepithelial cell nuclei, and stroma (Fig. 8.60c, d). Cellular smears resemble those of fibroade-noma including benign spindle cell aggregates. Slight cellular and nuclear atypia with nucleoli may be seen.

US Features   The area of palpable abnormalities shows normal tissue on US (Fig. 8.60e, f).

Carcinoma

Male-breast DCIS and invasive carcinoma are rare and affect slightly older men than women. Conditions that may increase the risk of breast cancer in men include obesity, cryptorchidism, liver cirrhosis, diabetes, and hyperthyroidism. Occupational exposure to petrol and airline fuel has been suggested to increase the risk of breast cancer. Approximately, 15% of males with breast cancer have a family history of breast or ovarian carcinoma. Patients have a palpable painless mass, usually in the subareolar area, and often have nipple retraction, fixation, ulceration, and discharge (Fig. 8.61a). Axillary lymphadenopathy may be present in 50% of cases. The overall survival is poor compared with women breast cancer.

Histopathology The histopathology is similar to that of female breast carcinoma. It seems that papillary carcinoma and Paget disease are more prevalent in men than in women. Invasive carcinoma of no special type is the most common, and lobular carcinoma is very rare.

Immuno-profile Positivity for ER and PR is present in >80% of cases and HER2 overexpression is rare. PR negativity and p53 accumulation seem to correlate with high-grade phenotype, aggressive clinical course, and decreased 5-year survival rate. High grade tumors with high mitotic activity also have been correlated with HER2 overexpression, low bcl-2 expression, high Ki67, and high p21 expression.

Molecular Profile Luminal A (ER^+ and/or PR^+, and $HER2^-$ or Ki67 low) is the most common subtype (75% of cases), followed by luminal B (ER^+ and/or PR^+, and $HER2^+$ or Ki67 high) subtype (21%). Basal-like (ER^-, PR^-, $HER2^-$, $CK5/6^+$ and/or $CK14^+$ and/or $EGFR^+$) and unclassified (triple negative for all markers) subtypes are very rare. No *HER2* driven cases (ER-, PR-, *HER2*+) subtype cases have been reported in a study of 134 male breast cancers. Male carriers of *BRCA2* gene mutations have a 7% risk of developing breast cancer at the age of 70 years. The association of male breast cancer and *BRCA1* germline mutation is weaker than that for *BRCA2*. The distribution of molecular subtypes is different from that of female breast cancer and suggests differences in carcinogenesis.

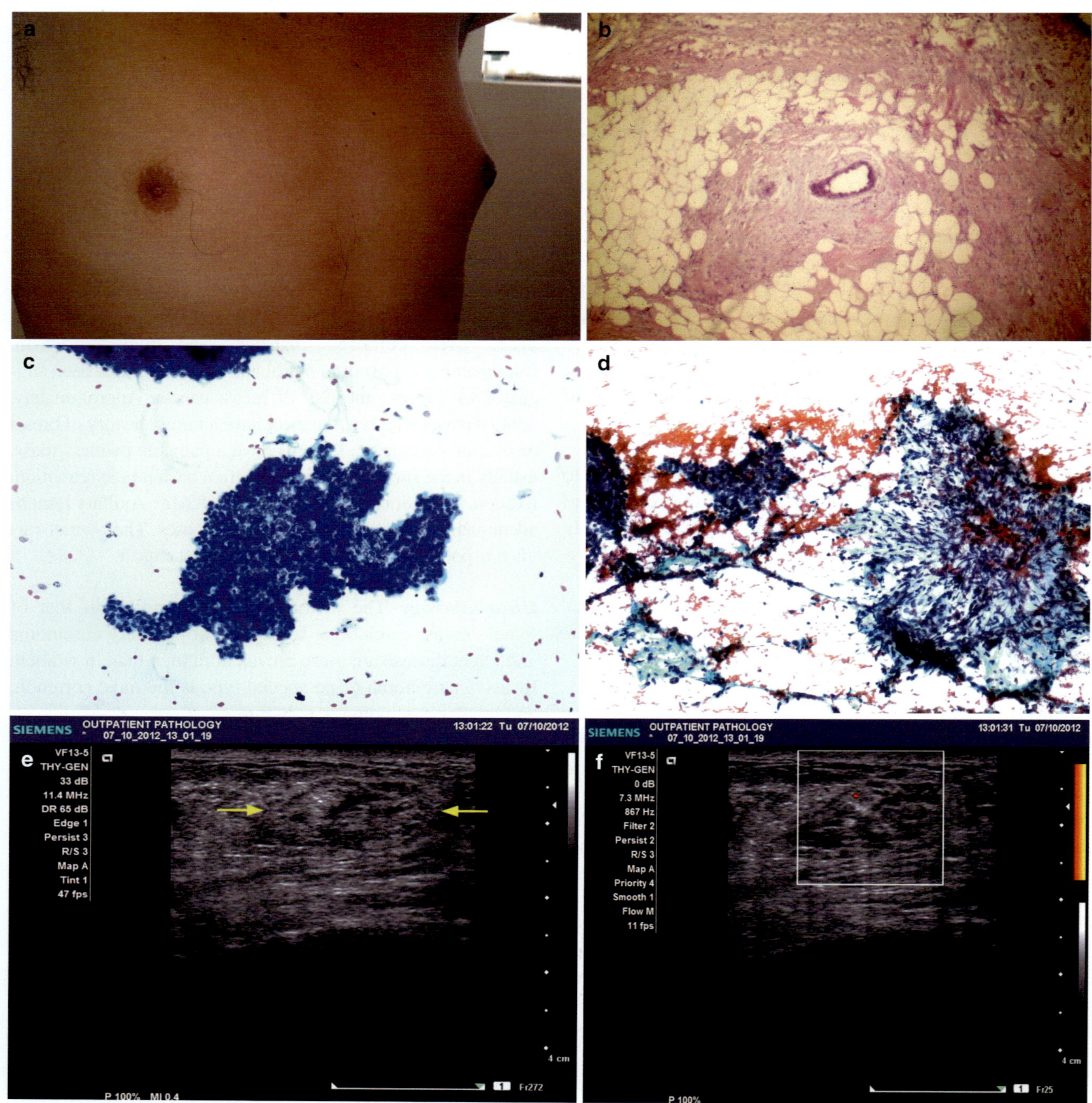

Fig. 8.60 Gynecomastia. Left breast gynecomastia (**a**). There is proliferation of mesenchymal stroma and ductal epithelium (**b**). Smears show sheets of benign ductal epithelial cells, stromal elements, and myoepithelial cell nuclei similar to those seen in fibrocystic change (**c**, **d**). The US images in this case show slight breast tissue prominence with minimal vascularity by Doppler exam (**e**, **f**). (**b**, H&E stain low magnification; **c**, DiffQuik stain high magnification; **d**, MGG stain, intermediate magnification)

FNA Findings Smear patterns are similar to those described for female breast cancer (Fig. 8.61b, c).

US Features US features are similar to those of female breast carcinoma (Fig. 8.61d, e).

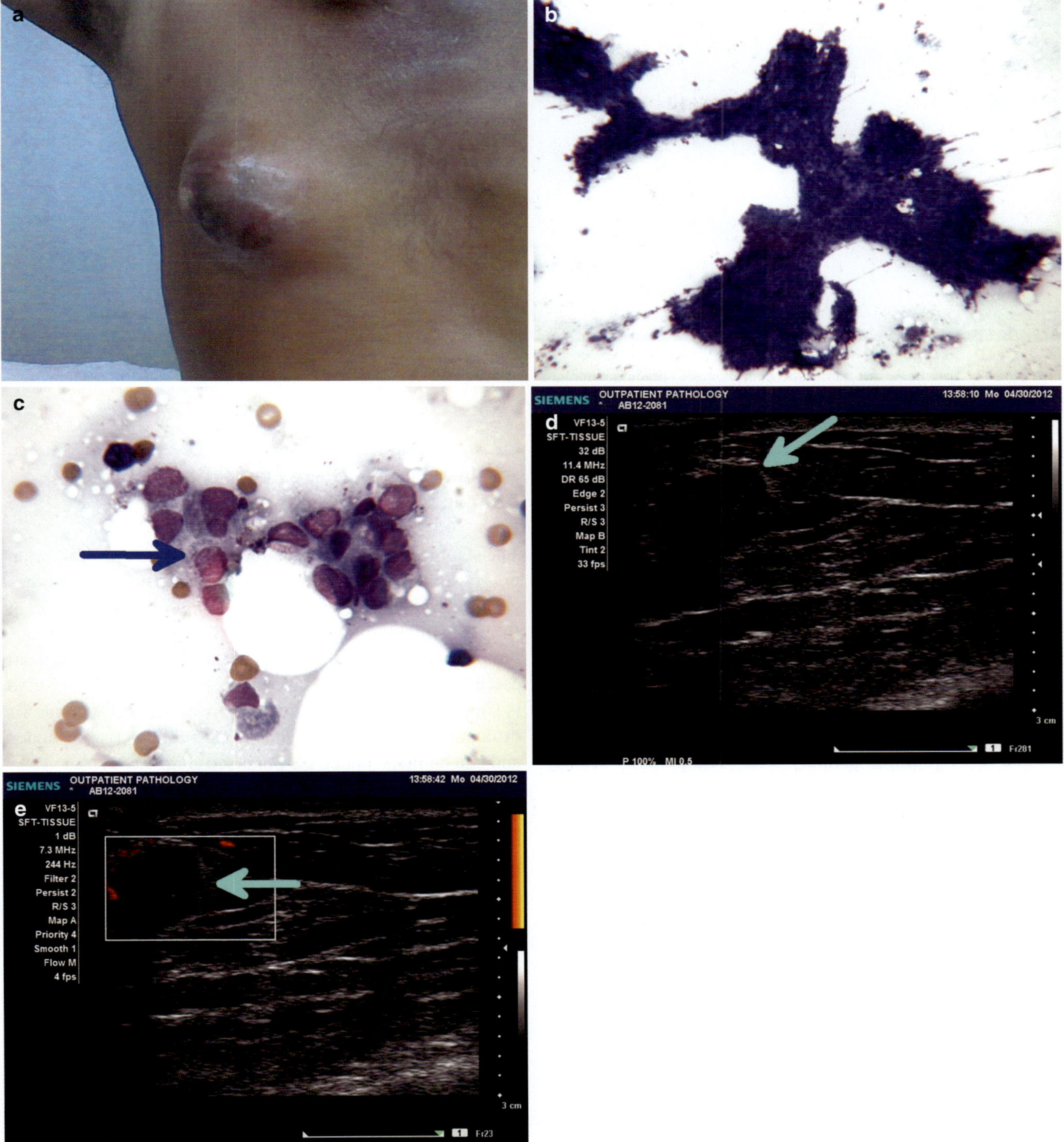

Fig. 8.61 Male breast carcinoma. Left breast mass (**a**). Cytologic features and US characteristics are similar to those seen in female breast carcinoma (**b**, **c**). US shows a solid hypoechoic mass with lobulated and focally spiculated borders and minimal vascular blood flow (**d**, **e**). (**b**, **c**, MGG stain intermediate and high magnification) (**a**, courtesy Dr. Manuel Cedano, Trujillo, Peru); **b**–**e**, courtesy Dr. John S. Abele, Sacramento, CA, USA)

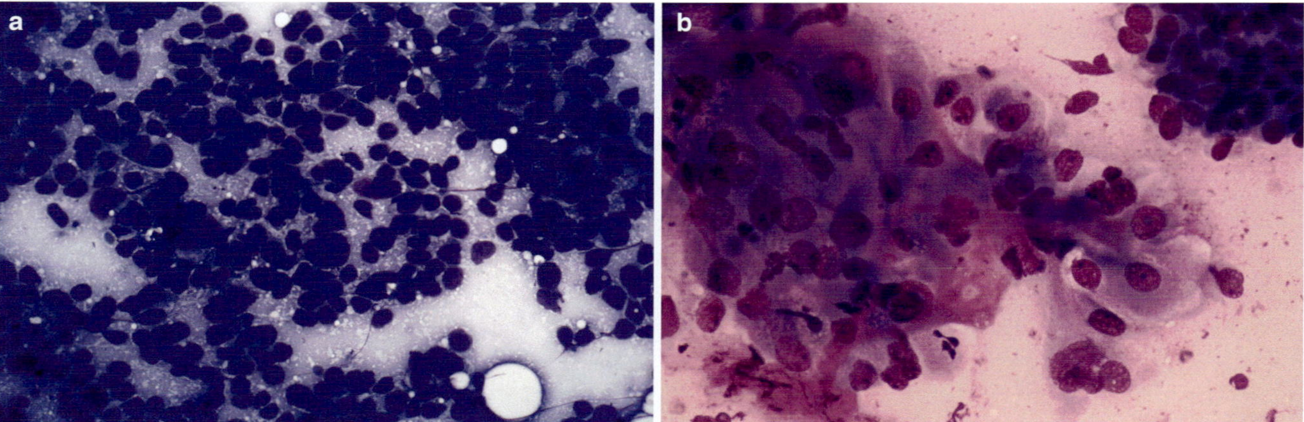

Fig. 8.62 Unusual cases of metastatic malignancy to the breast include small cell carcinoma (**a**) in a 40 year-old woman with primary lung small cell carcinoma. In males, metastatic prostatic carcinoma may be seen (**b**). (**a, b**, MGG stain high magnification)

Metastasis in the Breast

Metastases to the breast are rare, but occasionally they may be the first manifestation of the malignancy. Primary mammary carcinoma is mimicked in these cases. The most common primary sites of origin include melanoma, lymphoma, as well as lung, ovary, and soft tissue sarcomas. Prostate carcinoma is the most common source in men (Fig. 8.62). Melanoma and carcinoma of the ovary or kidney may be the source of metastasis years after the primary diagnosis. In children, rhabdomyosarcoma and lymphoma are the most common primary sites. The patients usually have a single palpable, painless, round mass; multiple masses are rare. Mass calcifications and spiculated borders are less common than in primary breast carcinomas. In questionable cases, comparison with the original tumor histopathology (known in 80% of cases) is important for a definitive diagnosis, along with immunohistochemistry. Clinical history and imaging studies are also crucial for diagnosis.

Immuno-profile ER, PR, and HER2 negative tumors in the absence of an in situ component should alert the pathologist to strongly consider a metastatic deposit. However, triple negative breast cancer shows the same immunophenotype; ER and PR positivity is seen in metastasis from gynecologic primaries; GCDFP-15 has been reported in 5% of lung carcinomas and TTF-1 in 2.5% of breast carcinomas. Of note, GCDFP-15 and mammaglobin A are the most specific breast markers, but they have low sensitivity.

US Features There is usually a single round, hypoechoic mass, sometimes showing a heterogeneous echotexture and well or poorly defined borders with no posterior acoustic shadowing.

Axillary Lymph Node Evaluation in Breast Cancer

The status of the axillary lymph nodes is the most important prognostic factor in the evaluation of a patient with breast cancer. Evaluation of the sentinel lymph node is important for prediction of the status of the axillary lymph nodes. Thus, lymph node US characteristics and pathologic study are essential before a management decision is made. USG-FNA is simple, inexpensive, minimally invasive, and accurate for evaluating axillary nodes, including sentinel lymph nodes, and can be made under US guidance (Fig. 8.63a, b).

Axillary lymph node dissection is associated with significant morbidity, thus accurate lymph node evaluation to detect macrometastasis (>2 mm) or micrometastasis (≤2 mm), both intraoperatively and on permanent sections is paramount in patient's management. Pancytokeratin immunostains is commonly used to highlight the metastatic deposits. It is clear that US exam and USG-FNA are simple and cost-effective methods to detect axillary metastasis and proceed to axillary lymph node dissection and avoid sentinel lymph node biopsy. Obviously, this is useful in sizable metastatic involvement and may not be useful to accurately detect small foci including micrometastasis. This practice needs further evaluation in view of undergoing treatment trials in patients with sentinel lymph node micrometastasis that may not require axillary lymph node dissection.

US Features A normal US appearance of an axillary lymph node includes size <2 cm, cortical thickness <2 mm, regular uniform borders, oval shape, presence of hilum, and hilar vascularity. Abnormal nodes may show >2 mm uniform concentric cortical thickening, eccentric cortical thickening, a bulging contour, round shape (taller than wide), loss of fatty hilum, an irregular cortical shape, and irregular vascular flow

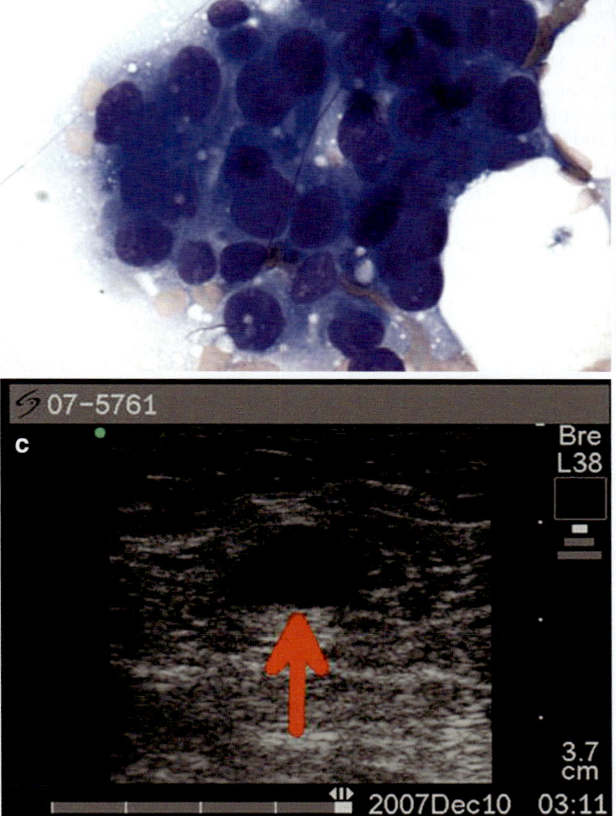

Fig. 8.63 Axillary lymph node metastasis. Axillary lymph node metastasis is not uncommon in patients with "inflammatory" carcinoma; while FNA of the primary breast mass may not be fully diagnostic due to the marked desmoplasia often present in these cases, FNA sampling of ipsilateral axillary lymph nodes yield diagnostic material as seen in this case. Aggregates of high-grade tumor cells are present (**a**, **b**) surrounded by small lymphocytes (**b**). US image of the lymph node show intense hypoechogenicity, irregular shape, well-defined borders, and lack of vascular hilum (**c**). (**a**, DiffQuik stain high magnification; **b**, Papanicolaou stain high magnification)

(central and peripheral/cortical) (Fig. 8.63c). None of these features is specific for a benign or malignant process.

Further Reading

Ali SZ, Parwani AV. Breast cytopathology. New York: Springer; 2007.

Bardales RH, Stanley MW. Benign spindle and inflammatory lesions of the breast: diagnosis by fine-needle aspiration. Diagn Cytopathol. 1995;12(2):126–30.

Bardales RH, Suhrland MJ, et al. Papillary neoplasms of the breast: fine-needle aspiration findings in cystic and solid cases. Diagn Cytopathol. 1994;10(4):336–41.

Bardales RH. The invasive cytopathologist. Ultrasound guided fine-needle aspiration of superficial masses. New York: Springer; 2014.

Bleiweiss I, Jaffer S, et al. Breast core biopsy: a pathologic-radiologic approach. Philadelphia: Saunders; 2008.

Brunello E, Brunelli M, et al. Classical lobular breast carcinoma consistently lacks topoisomerase-IIalpha gene amplification: implications for the tailored use of anthracycline-based chemotherapies. Histopathology. 2012;60(3):482–8.

Cardenosa G. Breast ultrasound. Breast imaging companion. Philadelphia: Wolters Kluwer; 2008. p. 146–79.

Chang MC, Crystal P, et al. The evolving role of axillary lymph node fine-needle aspiration in the management of carcinoma of the breast. Cancer Cytopathol. 2011;119(5):328–34.

Cserni G. Histological type and typing of breast carcinomas and the WHO classification changes over time. Pathologica. 2020;112:25–41. https://doi.org/10.32074/1591-951X-1-20.

Farmer C, Stanley MW, et al. Mycoses of the breast: diagnosis by fine-needle aspiration. Diagn Cytopathol. 1995;12(1):51–5.

Field AS, Raymond WA, Schmitt F. The International Academy of Cytology Yokohama system for reporting breast FNA cytopathology. Cham: Springer; 2020.

Geisinger KR, Stanley MW, et al. Modern cytopathology. Philadelphia: Churchill Livingstone; 2004. p. 873–929.

James JJ, Evans AJ. Breast. In: Allan PL, Baxter GM, Weston MJ, editors. Clinical ultrasound, vol. 2. London: Churchill Livingstone; 2011. p. 987–1004.

Kornegoor R, Verschuur-Maes AH, et al. Immunophenotyping of male breast cancer. Histopathology. 2012a;61(6):1145–55.

Kornegoor R, Verschuur-Maes AH, et al. Molecular subtyping of male breast cancer by immunohistochemistry. Mod Pathol. 2012b;25(3):398–404.

Lakhani SR, Ellis IO, et al. WHO classification of tumours of the breast. Lyon: IARC Press; 2012.

Leonardo E. Mammella. Morfologia molecolare: principi generali e diagnostica sistematica. Padova: Libreria Universitaria; 2012. p. 739–62.

Leonardo E, Bardales RH. Practical immunocytochemistry in diagnostic cytology. Cham: Springer; 2020.

Li D, Xiao X, et al. Secretory breast carcinoma: a clinicopathological and immunophenotypic study of 15 cases with a review of the literature. Mod Pathol. 2012;25(4):567–75.

Lopez-Garcia MA, Geyer FC, et al. Breast cancer precursors revisited: molecular features and progression pathways. Histopathology. 2010;57(2):171–92.

Mentzel T, Schildhaus HU, et al. Postradiation cutaneous angiosarcoma after treatment of breast carcinoma is characterized by MYC amplification in contrast to atypical vascular lesions after radiotherapy and control cases: clinicopathological, immunohistochemical and molecular analysis of 66 cases. Mod Pathol. 2012;25(1):75–85.

Monhollen L, Morrison C, et al. Pleomorphic lobular carcinoma: a distinctive clinical and molecular breast cancer type. Histopathology. 2012;61(3):365–77.

O'Malley FP, Pinder SE, et al. Breast pathology. Philadelphia: Saunders; 2011.

Perou CM, Sorlie T, et al. Molecular portraits of human breast tumours. Nature. 2000;406(6797):747–52.

Rakha EA, Ellis IO. Modern classification of breast cancer: should we stick with morphology or convert to molecular profile characteristics. Adv Anat Pathol. 2011;18(4):255–67.

Rinaldi P, Ierardi C, et al. Cystic breast lesions: sonographic findings and clinical management. J Ultrasound Med. 2010;29(11):1617–26.

Rosa M, Masood S. Cytomorphology of male breast lesions: diagnostic pitfalls and clinical implications. Diagn Cytopathol. 2012;40(2):179–84.

Ross DS, Wen YH, et al. Ductal carcinoma in situ: morphology-based knowledge and molecular advances. Adv Anat Pathol. 2013;20(4):205–16.

Sauer T. Fine-needle aspiration cytology of extra mammary metastatic lesions in the breast: a retrospective study of 36 cases diagnosed during 18 years. Cytojournal. 2010;7:10.

Schnitt SJ. Molecular biology of breast tumor progression: a view from the other side. Int J Surg Pathol. 2010;18(3 Suppl):170S–3S.

Stanley MW, Henry-Stanley MJ, et al. Atypia in breast fine-needle aspiration smears correlates poorly with the presence of a prognostically significant proliferative lesion of ductal epithelium. Hum Pathol. 1993;24(6):630–5.

Stanley MW, Tani EM, et al. Primary spindle-cell sarcomas of the breast: diagnosis by fine-needle aspiration. Diagn Cytopathol. 1988;4(3):244–9.

Stanley MW, Tani EM, et al. Adenoid cystic carcinoma of the breast: diagnosis by fine-needle aspiration. Diagn Cytopathol. 1993;9(2):184–7.

Stanley MW, Tani EM, et al. Cystosarcoma phyllodes of the breast: a cytologic and clinicopathologic study of 23 cases. Diagn Cytopathol. 1989;5(1):29–34.

Stanley MW, Tani EM, et al. Metaplastic carcinoma of the breast: fine-needle aspiration cytology of seven cases. Diagn Cytopathol. 1989;5(1):22–8.

Stanley MW, Tani EM, et al. Mucinous breast carcinoma and mixed mucinous-infiltrating ductal carcinoma: a comparative cytologic study. Diagn Cytopathol. 1989;5(2):134–8.

Stanley MW, Tani EM, et al. Fine-needle aspiration of fibroadenomas of the breast with atypia: a spectrum including cases that cytologically mimic carcinoma. Diagn Cytopathol. 1990;6(6):375–82.

Tan PH, Ellis I, et al. The 2019 World Health Organization classification of tumors of the breast. Commentary. Histopathology. 2020;77:181–5. https://doi.org/10.1111/his.14091.

Tsang JY, Mendoza P, et al. Involvement of alpha- and beta-catenins and E-cadherin in the development of mammary phyllodes tumours. Histopathology. 2012;61(4):667–74.

Personal Experience Performing Ultrasound-Guided Fine-Needle Aspiration of Superficial Masses

Ricardo H. Bardales

Introduction

Premises for the Interventional Cytopathologist to keep in mind

1. The patient is entrusting his/her health to us—identify with the patient and be thorough!
2. Recognize the sick patient with a mass, and not the mass alone—broaden your clinical differential diagnosis!
3. Your eyes can betray you, and your brain recognizes only what your eyes see - broaden your cytology differential diagnosis!
4. Your diagnosis may change the patient's life—be kind and supportive!

A directed clinical history, physical exam, and imaging studies, as in any field of medicine, are complementary and remain the pillars for elaborating a clinical differential diagnosis; however, the pathologic diagnosis guides further patient management.

Ultrasound (US) has become an almost indispensable imaging tool used for visualizing, evaluating, and, with the aid of fine-needle aspiration (FNA), harvesting samples from superficial and deep-seated masses. Adequately performed US-guided FNA (USG-FNA), a minimally invasive procedure, renders accurate diagnoses and provides guidance for appropriate clinical management of patients who have palpable and/or US-visible superficial masses.

In our practice, the cytopathology diagnosis integrates clinical findings, US features, and ancillary test results. In the next paragraphs, I narrate the vicissitudes and the lessons learned by traveling through a 17-year journey as Interventional Cytopathologist. I complement my experience with useful "pearls" and illustrative cases.

R. H. Bardales (✉)
Precision Pathology, Outpatient Pathology Associates,
Sacramento, CA, USA

Our USG-FNA Clinic

Outpatient Pathology Associates (OPA), a private laboratory in Sacramento, California, was founded by Drs. Anthony Mathios, John S. Abele, and Daniel Egerter, who in 1987, established an Outpatient FNA Clinic dedicated to the performance of palpation-guided FNA.

The clinic to perform USG-FNA was created in 2003 by the same pathologists, who are my mentors in this hybrid field that combines clinical medicine, ultrasound, and cytopathology. Since 2003, we have seen more than 35,000 patients and performed more than 60,000 USG-FNAs of palpable and/or US-visible masses, and more than 100 core needle biopsies (CNBs) of the breast.

Our USG-FNA clinic is open daily for 3–4 h. We schedule eight patients a day and reserve two slots for urgent cases. Each appointment lasts 15–20 min and includes taking a clinical history and performing a physical exam, US exam, and USG-FNA. We add 15 min when CNBs need to be done. A bedside nurse is always present during the patient's visit [1–3].

Before the Patient's Visit

- To schedule a patient for an USG-FNA, we request the referring physician's office to submit a requisition form indicating the location of the mass, the patient's clinic visit notes, and copies of reports on imaging studies including US. This information is provided by fax or by secure electronic access. US images can be downloaded if needed and when available.
- Our staff calls the patient to schedule the appointment. An informative pamphlet detailing the procedure and what to expect during the visit is mailed to the patient.
- The day before the appointment, our staff calls the patient to confirm the appointment.

R. H. Bardales (ed.), *The Interventional Cytopathologist*, Essentials in Cytopathology 30,
https://doi.org/10.1007/978-3-031-73702-2_9

- Our staff searches our database and prints reports of prior procedures performed in our laboratory and have them ready for the cytopathologist to review.
- The cytopathologist reviews all clinical information prior to seeing the patient or the night before if the patient's visit is in the morning.
- By reviewing this information, the cytopathologist has a productive encounter with the patient.

Arrival at the USG-FNA Clinic

- All personnel take COVID-19 or other transmissible disease precautions
- Clinic staff wear N95 masks and follow strict sanitary guidelines
- Patients must wear a surgical mask, available in the receptionist desk
- The receptionist takes the patient's body temperature upon arrival
- With some exceptions, only the patient is allowed in the waiting and examination rooms
- Early arrival: the patient is asked to wait outside the clinic or in the car for our staff's phone call.

General Considerations

Clinical History and Physical Examination

For the interventional cytopathologist, obtaining a good, short, and relevant clinical history and performing a pertinent physical exam are essential for construction of a preliminary clinical diagnosis and the nature of the mass that will later be correlated with the cytologic findings.

At the time of the patient's visit, my goal is to make the patient feel comfortable and to have a good rapport, so that the stress of the encounter is dissipated. I always start the conversation with the patient sitting on the side of the exam table at a slightly higher level than mine. Cautiously, I try to be conversational and invite the patient to engage in a brief 1- to 2-min conversation on an unrelated topic such as traffic or weather conditions, general news (not politics), or health issues such as COVID-19. This will give me a sense of the patient's emotional status, because some patients are very anxious and appear to be aggressive or not talkative. After that brief interaction, the patient will be more open to conversation, and it will be easier to ask questions and to assure the patient that, based on our experience, the procedure will go well and that the diagnosis will help to guide further medical decisions. If the encounter falls in an apparent unpleasant environment, our service will not be well received by the patient, even if the sample obtained is diagnostic.

After this preamble, I ask the patient for the name of the referring physician and for the reason for his or her visit, when and how the clinical diagnosis was made, and signs and symptoms the patient may have, including the site of the mass, onset, duration, and associations (i.e., pain, fever, sweating, weight loss, asthenia, anorexia). A social history (drinking, smoking), use of drugs (recreational, prescribed, and over the counter), family history, and past medical history are obtained as clinically appropriate.

During the visit, it is important to inquire about the experience the patient had if a prior FNA was done; if it was unpleasant, I reassure the patient that the current one will be different. At this point, I explain to the patient the procedure step-by-step, emphasizing that, based on experience, it will brief and almost painless, aside from the transient local burning pain due to local Lidocaine administration, which is needed to prevent pain and obtain adequate diagnostic samples.

To interview patients with hearing or talking disabilities or with limited command of the English language who come to the clinic with a helper, may be challenging. I always tell both the patient and accompanying person that I will be directing the conversation mainly to the patient and that the helper will answer accordingly. I must emphasize that the cytopathologist must talk and make eye contact with the patient most of the time and avoid talking to the helper only. This three-way conversation will result in a personable interaction with the patient who does not feel he or she is left aside. This is welcomed by patients who have expressed this deference to me in more than one occasion.

Always examine the patient in the sitting and/or supine position.

The physical exam is limited to the lesion, organ, and region where the mass is located, but, as clinically appropriate, an examination of other body regions is conducted.

Examine the skin of the arms, including hands and elbows, scalp, and fingernails. Nail changes (pitting, ridges) and nontender, non-itchy red, scaly elbow patches are seen in psoriasis and may be associated with other autoimmune disorders such as chronic thyroiditis.

Further specific details about the clinical history and physical exam are given as masses present in specific organs are covered in this manuscript.

Performing the US Examination

The US exam is invaluable in the clinical evaluation of patients with superficial palpable and non-palpable masses. The physics of US is beyond the scope of this review; however, the examiner must be familiar with the operation of the US machine, know how to perform the exam, and have a broad knowledge of the US features of the target mass and the organ where it is located.

The US exam of head and neck organs should be performed in the supine position with slight hyperextension of the neck, particularly for evaluation of thyroid gland nodules as well as supraclavicular and suprasternal masses. A systematic evaluation of neck anatomic regions, known as levels or compartments should be performed in the following order: lateral neck (levels 1A, 1B, 2A, 2B, 3, 4, 5B, and 5A), midline neck (level 6) masses. Often level 6 small lymph nodes are difficult to visualize by US exam because they are adjacent to the esophagus and midline cartilaginous elements; however, when prominent, they can be visualized by US, i.e., lymph nodes, cysts, soft-tissue masses. The suprasternal fossa (level 7) is evaluated at the end of the exam (Fig. 9.1).

US features of the mass should include echotexture (heterogeneous, solid, cystic, mixed), echogenicity (hyperechoic, isoechoic, hypoechoic, anechoic), dimensions (transverse, antero-posterior, craniocaudal), shape (oval, round, irregular), borders (well- or ill-defined, spiculated, smooth, lobulated), calcifications or best-called "punctate echogenic foci" or "micro reflectors" when minute, vascular blood flow by Doppler exam (peripheral, central, focal, chaotic), and presence or absence of invasion to adjacent tissue. These US features should be recorded for any superficial mass; however, they are particularly applicable to the evaluation of thyroid nodules.

The cytopathologist should be able to identify US features that are helpful for choosing the mass to be sampled when more than one is present, avoid a specific area within the mass, i.e., cystic, or necrotic areas, and sample the solid or vascular components.

Performing the USG-FNA

The procedure is performed by the operator and one assistant.

The patient must be comfortably positioned on the exam table. Parents are asked to hold and restrain infants and young children. Older children and teenagers are usually cooperative once the procedure is explained.

Palpation-guided FNA is often performed on infants and uncooperative young children with palpable masses. No local anesthesia is administered, only one pass is performed, and 1–2 smears are prepared. Rapid on-site evaluation (ROSE) is performed, and additional samples are obtained as necessary.

The USGFNA is usually performed by having the patient in the dorsal decubitus position with the head of the exam table slightly elevated at 15°. The approach to anterior lower neck masses, particularly thyroid and parathyroid, should be done with slight hyperextension of the neck, best achieved with the use of a pillow placed behind the patient's neck and shoulders (Fig. 9.2).

Breast masses are usually approached with the patient's ipsilateral arm elevated or placed on top of the head. For better identification of the mass, the patient is asked slightly to rotate the chest to the contralateral side, particularly when the mass is deep, lateral, and surrounded by abundant breast tissue. This position also facilitates the evaluation and sampling of axillary lymph nodes, if necessary.

Masses located in the posterior regions of the body are approached in a position that is best for the operator to obtain an adequate sample and is comfortable for the patient (sitting on the exam table or in a wheelchair, ventral decubitus, or lateral decubitus).

The following steps are important for performing the USG-FNA by use of a perpendicular approach to insert the needle into the target and harvest an adequate sample:

1. The patient must be comfortable and remain still.
2. Record the US features, including blood flow by Doppler exam, and measurements of the mass.

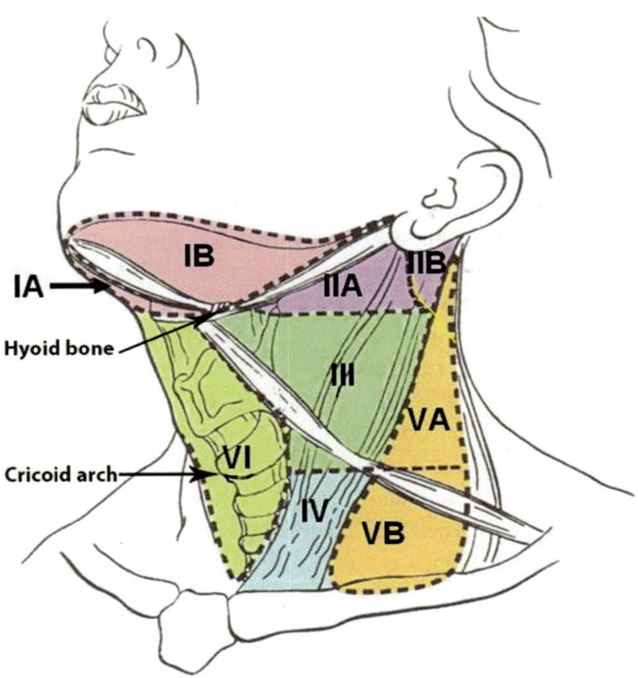

Fig. 9.1 Neck anatomic regions or levels. Diagram showing the compartmentalization of the neck to facilitate localization of neck masses in a reproducible manner. Level 1A: submental triangle. Level 1B: submandibular triangle (to the posterior border of the gland). Level 2: upper jugular (below level 1 to the posterior border of the SCM, at the level of the hyoid bone). Level 2A (anterior) and 2B (posterior) by a plane passing vertical to the angle of the jaw. Level 3: mid-jugular (below level 2 to the posterior border of the SCM, and to the level of the cricoid notch inferiorly). Level 4: lower jugular (below level 3 to the posterior border of the SCM, and the clavicle). Level 5: posterior triangle (between the posterior border of the SCM, the anterior border of the trapezius muscle, and the clavicle). Level 5A (superior) and 5B (inferior) by a horizontal plane passing inferior to the cricoid notch. Level 6: anterior triangle (between the hyoid bone, and suprasternal notch). Level 7: suprasternal notch

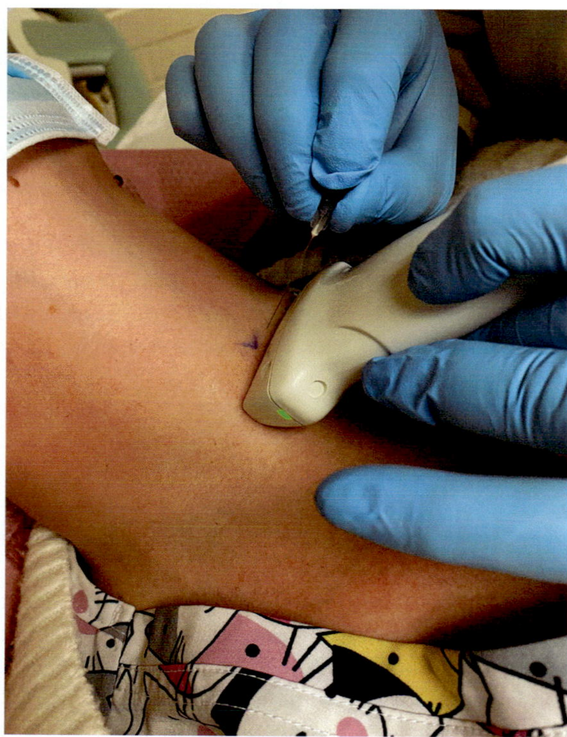

Fig. 9.2 Ultrasound evaluation and USGFNA to anterior neck masses by perpendicular approach. Note the neck hyperextension, supporting pillow behind the neck, and the use of a 27-gauge needle (Zajdela technique)

3. Using the US probe in a transverse position, identify and place the image of the mass or target area to be sampled in the center of the screen.

4. Gently slide the tip of a ballpen beneath the long portion of the US probe to create a visible shadow in the screen and make it coincide with the upper border of the mass. Withdraw the US probe by leaving the ballpen in place and mark the skin with an erasable marker 1–2 mm above the site where the tip of the ballpen was placed. This will be the site for injecting the anesthetic and performing the USG-FNA.

5. Clean the marked skin with an alcohol pad and dry the area with a sterile gauze pad.

6. Inject local lidocaine or carbocaine and make sure that the underlying tissue planes, including skeletal muscle, are anesthetized.

7. Insert the needle first in the marked skin site to avoid US gel contamination that may impair the cytologic interpretation, particularly in Romanowsky-stained slides.

8. Having inserted the needle in the skin, place the US probe perpendicular to the skin and identify the lesion, slowly make the needle travel perpendicular to all tissue planes in the direction of the mass, and make sure the bright echogenic needle tip lands in the mass or target area to be sampled.

9. Perform the USG-FNA by applying the Zajdela technique (without suction), using 1½-inch long 27-G needles for thyroid and parathyroid, and 25-G needles for lymph nodes, breast, and soft-tissue masses. Lipomatous and soft-tissue masses may need to be sampled with suction, with the use of a tube connected to a syringe attached to an aspiration device on one end and to the sampling needle on the other. The operator will do the USG-FNA, and the assistant will apply suction.

10. Execute between 2 and 3 thrusts per second for 3 seconds in a steady manner, keeping the same needle trajectory within the mass. Moving the needle in different directions within the mass will produce intralesional bleeding and yield a bloody sample. Use the intensity and distribution of the vascular blood flow as a guide to obtain adequate samples.

11. We must keep in mind that adequate diagnostic material is inside the needle barrel. The presence of blood in the needle hub is an indication for withdrawing the needle from the mass and immediately making smears before the blood coagulates. Thus, do not wait to see blood in the needle hub by having the erroneous assumption that the presence of blood correlates with a good sample.

12. My routine is to perform 3–4 passes and make 3–4 smears per each sampled mass, i.e., 1–2 smears from the first pass and 1 smear from each additional pass. For most thyroid and parathyroid nodules, I make 3 to 4 air-dried smears for May-Grunwald Giemsa (MGG) staining. For non-thyroid cases, I make 2–3 air-dried smears and place one smear in 95% ethyl alcohol for Papanicolaou staining.

13. I perform ROSE of smears in selected cases and based on clinical and US findings.

14. I reserve the use of liquid-based cytology for selected bloody cyst contents.

15. Material for a cell block is obtained from selected masses, when malignancy is suspected, and when special stains need to be done. The material is harvested with 25- or 23-G needles and with the use of suction as mentioned before. While the assistant is applying continuous suction, I make the needle travel in the same direction within the mass until I visualize blood in the needle hub and tube connected to the syringe; then, I ask the assistant to release the suction. I withdraw the needle, let the blood clot inside the tube and attached needle for 5 min, and then place the clot and needle rinses in 10% formalin to be processed by conventional histologic methods.

In general, I prefer the perpendicular needle approach (visualization of needle tip) over the parallel approach (visualization of the needle length) to perform USG-FNAs. I reserve the parallel approach to sample some small thyroid isthmus nodules and perform CNBs of breast and soft-tissue masses.

Performing USG-FNA by using the Zajdela technique allows the operator to "feel" the tissue planes as the needle travels through, including feeling the entrance of the needle into the mass (Figs. 9.3 and 9.4).

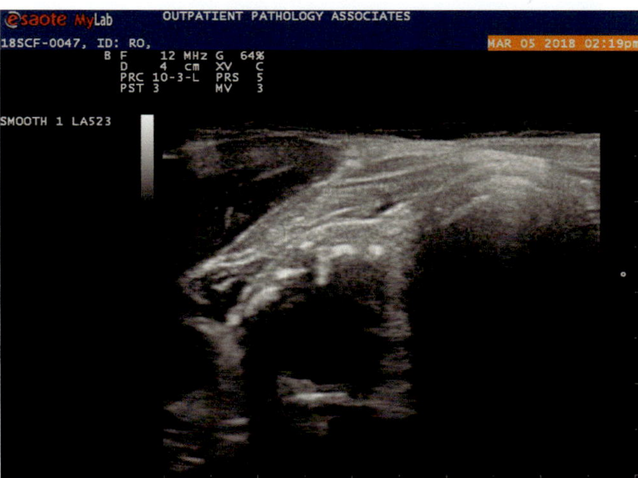

Fig. 9.3 Right thyroid mass with interrupted egg-shell calcification. Note the needle tip (bright signal) travelling through the interrupted calcification in the upper rim of the mass (perpendicular approach). Final cytology diagnosis was papillary thyroid carcinoma. (Ultrasound, high resolution)

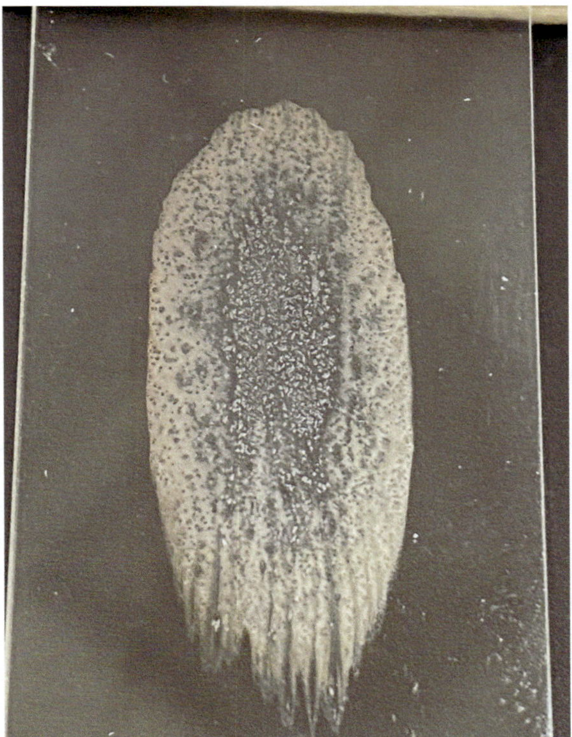

Fig. 9.4 Air dried unstained smear prepared at bedside. Notice the "granular" area in the center of the glass slide that is characteristic of a cellular smear pattern in a case of papillary thyroid carcinoma

Thyroid and Parathyroid Nodules and Masses

Taking the Clinical History

Inquire about duration of disease, anterior-lower-neck localized pain/tenderness and compressive symptoms (dyspnea, dysphagia, hoarseness), a personal history of cancer, a history of radiation to the head and neck, and a personal and family history of thyroid disease including thyroid cancer, multiple endocrine neoplasia syndromes, and autoimmune disorders.

A large multinodular goiter may cause anterior-lower-neck compressive symptoms, and patients have a mass in the neck that moves with swallowing. A hyperfunctional thyroid nodule (Plummer disease), more common in older than in younger people, may be present in the setting of goiter and may not be visible; USG-FNA sampling may be indicated in some instances.

Patients with Hashimoto's thyroiditis, commonly associated with goiter and high serum levels of autoantibodies, may have bouts of hyperthyroidism, hypothyroidism, and a euthyroid state. It should always be considered in patients who have long standing hypothyroidism; lymphoma must be considered if the mass is large and rapidly growing.

If a patient has tenderness or pain in the anterior lower neck associated with malaise and myalgias, consider the possibility of subacute thyroiditis and inquire about a history of upper respiratory tract infection about 2 weeks before symptoms started.

Malignant neoplastic masses may or may not be visible. In some instances, the patient self-identifies a distinct mass or a change in a pre-existing goiter. Papillary thyroid carcinoma occurs in younger and older individuals, often in males. Follicular carcinoma occurs in patients of middle age. Medullary carcinoma can occur at any age, and patients may have personal and/or family history of associated pheochromocytoma and hyperparathyroidism, particularly when the carcinoma is diagnosed in young patients.

A rapidly growing anterior-lower-neck mass with evidence of anterior-lower-neck compressive symptoms in the elderly must be of concern, as lymphoma, poorly differentiated carcinoma, or anaplastic carcinoma may be the underlying malignancy. Fibrous thyroiditis is another cause of anterior-lower-neck compressive symptoms with no visible mass.

I encountered an elderly woman with a visible anterior-lower-neck mass and mild stridor and dyspnea which was accentuated when the patient was made to be in the semi-Fowler position (positioned on her back at 30°). I made a diagnosis of thyroid lymphoma on ROSE of smears and asked the family to take her immediately to the emergency room (ER). Instead, the patient was taken home; her condition worsened in the next 12 h, and she was taken to the ER and intubated. In the outpatient clinic scenario, as is our practice, a patient with airway compressive signs and symptoms is an emergency case and must be referred to the ER immediately.

Patients with parathyroid nodules are essentially asymptomatic or may have a history of nephrolithiasis or pancreatitis secondary to hypercalcemia. Thyroid medullary carcinoma, pheochromocytoma, and pancreatic endocrine tumors along with parathyroid adenoma may be part of a multiple endocrine neoplasia (MEN) syndrome.

Examining the Patient

Visual inspection of the anterior lower neck when the thyroid gland is visible yields information about thyroid size, diffuse or nodular growth, skin changes such as erythema and vascularity, tracheal deviation and/or compression, and vascular engorgement that may indicate an infiltrative or compressive process in the anterior lower neck or upper mediastinum.

A normal thyroid gland is neither visible nor palpable; however, it may be slightly visible and slightly palpable in persons who have a thin neck. Palpation of the thyroid gland may not always be revealing, because thyroid nodule(s) may be present in a non-palpable gland, or in a diffusely enlarged gland with no palpable nodules; furthermore, a palpable nodular gland may not have US-visible nodules.

A diffuse thyroid enlargement with variable nodularity is seen in Graves' disease; however, a hyper-functional nodule, as in Plummer-Vinson disease, may or may not be palpable. Because the normal thyroid gland is non-tender, consider subacute thyroiditis when the gland is tender on palpation. A rapidly growing, palpable, tender nodule may be caused by bleeding within a pre-existing cyst. Poorly differentiated and anaplastic carcinoma, as well as thyroid lymphoma, may be visible as a large thyroid mass or develop in a substernal goiter, causing variable anterior-lower-neck compressive symptoms (Fig. 9.5). Fibrous thyroiditis may be considered in the presence of compressive symptoms when there is no visible or palpable gland and a firm, almost frozen anterior lower-neck area.

Cervical regional lymphadenopathy may be palpable, firm, and mobile in the presence of papillary thyroid carcinoma. Palpable, ill-defined, and rubbery lymph nodes may be seen in cases of autoimmune thyroiditis. Matted and hard lymph nodes that are affixed to surrounding tissue in the presence of a thyroid mass are often associated with high-grade thyroid malignancies.

In patients with a history of thyroid carcinoma and thyroidectomy, examination of all neck levels, including level 6 (midline) and the scar line, must be performed, looking for

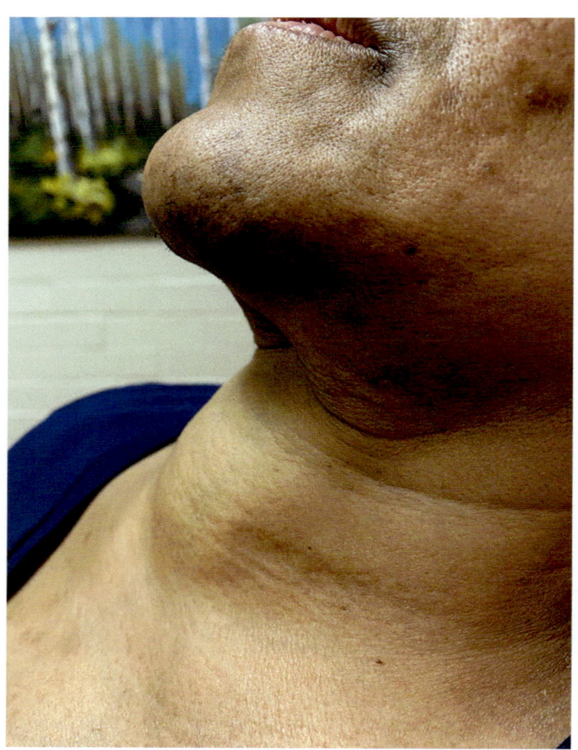

Fig. 9.5 Visible large anterior lower neck mass. USGFNA diagnosis was anaplastic thyroid carcinoma

palpable soft-tissue nodules in addition to lymph nodes. Of note, a nodule composed of repopulated thyroid tissue may be palpable in patients who have a history of chronic thyroiditis and thyroidectomy.

Parathyroid tumors are usually small and non-palpable. However, a large parathyroid cyst may be visible and palpable as a mass of doughy consistency in the mid-lateral and lower neck; I had one such case.

Performing the US Examination

Thyroid nodules must be evaluated following the American Thyroid Association (ATA) US guidelines or those of the American College of Radiology Thyroid Imaging Reporting and Data System (TI-RADS) that stratify nodules according to US features and provide the risk of malignancy for the nodule. US features to be considered in the evaluation of thyroid nodules include composition (solid, mixed, cystic), echogenicity (hyperechoic, isoechoic, hypoechoic, anechoic), shape based on the dimensions obtained with the US probe in a transverse position (wider than tall, taller than wide), margins (smooth, ill-defined, irregular, spiculated, lobulated), and calcifications, including microcalcifications, macrocalcifications, and rim calcifications. Microcalcifications and comet tails (inspissated colloid) may be difficult to distinguish one from the other by US; descriptive terms such as "punctate echogenic foci" or "micro-reflectors" are used instead. A solid hypoechoic nodule has an intermediate risk of malignancy. Irregular and spiculated margins, taller-than-wide shape, punctate echogenic foci, and interrupted rim calcifications indicate a high risk of malignancy. Although vascular blood flow is not a feature considered in the risk-of-malignancy stratification schemes, a Doppler exam is useful for adjusting the USGFNA sampling time and avoiding the harvesting of bloody samples that often preclude an adequate cytology interpretation.

The pyramidal lobe is an accessory lobe of variable length, considered to be a remnant of the thyroglossal duct. It is identified in 40–50% of people, often in the left lobe, although it may arise in the isthmus or right lobe. It is of conical shape and may be identified as an isoechoic or slightly hypoechoic nodule above the thyroid gland when the US probe is positioned transversally, but disappears in the craniocaudal position, being visualized as a part of the thyroid. Spiculated borders can be seen in primary or secondary thyroid malignancies; however, they can also be seen in chronic thyroiditis, and in subacute thyroiditis, commonly with minimal or absent vascular blood flow as determined by Doppler exam.

A diffuse thyroid enlargement with a "cotton weave" or "moth-eaten" appearance is often seen in chronic thyroiditis. Pseudo-nodules, often seen in chronic thyroiditis, are often isoechoic and may be difficult to distinguish from true nodules that may be present in these patients. True nodules are visible on evaluation with the US probe in both transverse and craniocaudal positions; in contrast, pseudo-nodules are often visible in only one of these positions. Thyroid nodules in chronic thyroiditis are often iso- or hyperechoic ("white knight" and they often have oncocytic cells), with smooth, well-defined borders; however, papillary thyroid carcinoma must be considered in the presence of a hypoechoic nodule with irregular and spiculated borders and punctate echogenic foci. The finding of a deep hypo-echogenicity in the mass/nodule, the thyroid lobe, or the whole gland ("pseudo-cystic" appearance) in a patient with or without chronic thyroiditis always arises the suspicion of a thyroid primary or secondary non-Hodgkin lymphoma (NHL); neck lymphadenopathy is usually absent in primary thyroid NHL.

Thyroid cysts must be evaluated carefully. A solid-phase component identified in the wall of the cyst must be sampled by USGFNA, particularly if it is vascular, and regardless of other US features, because this may be a cystic variant of papillary thyroid carcinoma; I had one such case.

Thyroid "bed" nodules in patients with prior thyroidectomy may be identified as distinct hypoechoic nodules with ill-defined borders, and may correspond to repopulated thyroid tissue in cases of chronic thyroiditis or recurrent/metastatic thyroid carcinoma. A distinct hypoechoic nodule with smooth margins may represent a benign or metastatic lymph node or even parathyroid tissue. A hyperechoic nodule is often seen in an oncocytic neoplasm, particularly oncocytic carcinoma when the patient had such history. In contrast, a heterogeneous iso- to hyperechoic, ill-defined thyroid bed widening may correspond to fibroadipose tissue/scar and conveys less risk for malignancy in the absence of a distinct US-visible mass. A thyroid bed nodule must be sampled for cytologic examination, and sampling needles must be rinsed in 1 ml of sterile saline; if benign or malignant thyroid elements are absent in the smears, the needle rinses must be submitted for thyroglobulin level measurement. Calcitonin or parathyroid hormone (PTH) levels may also be measured as clinically indicated.

Normal parathyroid glands are not visible by US. However, in patients who had a total thyroidectomy, the parathyroid gland may be visible in the thyroid bed as a small grain-of-rice-like hypoechoic nodule with smooth borders. I had one such case referred to our clinic as a "thyroid bed nodule." The USG-FNA cytology exam showed a microfollicular pattern; needle rinses for thyroglobulin and PTH were negative and positive, respectively, proving a diagnosis of parathyroid gland tissue. Further clinical evaluation excluded primary hyperparathyroidism.

The great majority of parathyroid masses are single neoplasms, usually adenomas that cannot be differentiated from parathyroid carcinoma or hyperplasia either by US or by cytologic examination. In contrast to parathyroid hyperplasia that involves all parathyroid glands often in patients with chronic renal failure or vitamin D deficiency, parathyroid adenoma is commonly single.

Parathyroid masses are commonly located lower from and posterior to the thyroid lobe (predominantly left lobe in my experience) and may be interpreted as thyroid nodules by US. They are often round or oval when small; however, when larger, they may adopt a more elongated and sometimes odd shape with smooth and undulating borders due to the almost total replacement of the entire parathyroid gland by the tumor and its extrathyroidal location. They are usually hypoechoic, although they can be iso- to slightly hyperechoic (oncocytic on histologic exam). Careful US evaluation shows a sharp hyperechoic line that separates the boundaries between the thyroid lobe and the enlarged parathyroid, corresponding to the coalescing tissue capsules of both (Fig. 9.6). Doppler exam shows variable internal vascular blood flow and may identify the feeding branch of the thyroid artery when carefully looked for. A lymph node below the thyroid lobe has US features that are almost identical to those seen in parathyroid neoplasm or hyperplasia; however, a lymph node fatty hilum, when visible, helps in the identification. USGFNA cytology diagnosis of a parathyroid neoplasm is definitive. Parathyroid cysts are visible by US as anechoic masses with sharp, smooth borders in the lateral and lower neck; they may be large and separate surrounding tissue planes, adopting an odd shape.

Performing the USG-FNA

In general, thyroid nodules <1 cm in patients who have no history of thyroid carcinoma or neck irradiation can be monitored by US at clinically appropriate intervals. If necessary, subcentimeter nodules in patients with MEN-2 syndrome can be sampled by USG-FNA to exclude medullary carcinoma.

Evaluation of vascular blood flow by Doppler exam is paramount for decision on the number of thrusts and the speed and duration of each thrust when a thyroid nodule is sampled. For instance, only 1–2 thrusts in 1 s will be sufficient for sampling a vascular thyroid nodule and obtaining adequate samples with less blood. Heterogeneous spongiform nodules often yield translucent, inspissated colloid that may be variably bloody and that often correlates with a benign cytologic diagnosis. In nodules with a prominent cystic area, drain the fluid first and then sample the solid component to exclude cystic variant of papillary thyroid carcinoma. A similar approach is suggested for thyroglossal-duct cysts with a mural solid component, to exclude carcinoma (Fig. 9.7a, b). Resistance to travel of the needle within the mass due to fibrosis may be felt in the healing phase of subacute thyroiditis; more resistance is felt in fibrous tumors of thyroid, Riedel's fibrosing thyroiditis, or fibrous anaplastic carcinoma, and aspirates often yield dry taps requiring subsequent sampling with 25- or 23-G needles with suction for harvesting of smears and a cell block for a definitive diagnosis. In contrast, slight or almost no resistance to needle traveling is often encountered when thyroid lymphoma is sampled. Variable resistance and a sometimes gritty and "sandy" perception are felt while the needle travels within the mass in some cases of papillary thyroid carcinoma, and this may indicate fibrosis and psammomatous calcification; a "sandy" granular matter surrounded by variable amounts of blood is often visualized in the centers of unstained smears in papillary thyroid carcinoma cases.

Parathyroid tumors are variably vascular, and sampling should be performed with the same technique as that used for vascular thyroid nodules. Samples for thyroid molecular

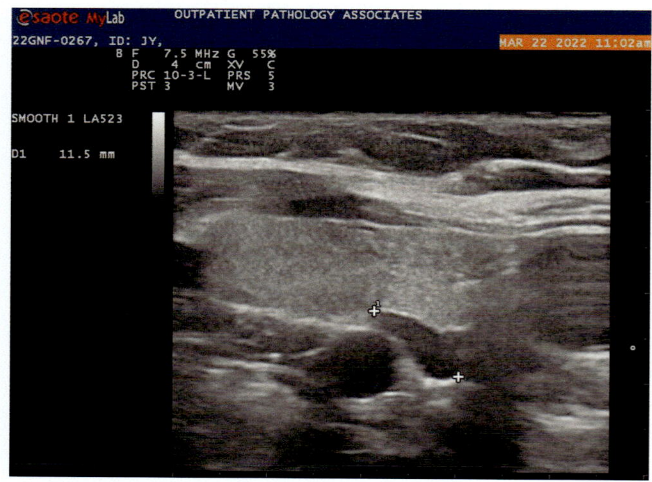

Fig. 9.6 Ultrasound image of a parathyroid adenoma adjacent to the carotid artery. Notice the elongated and hypoechoic parathyroid mass that is sharply separated from the anterior and superior thyroid lobe by a hyperechogenic line, a feature that is highly suggestive of a parathyroid mass. (Ultrasound, high resolution, sagittal view)

Fig. 9.7 Non-hemorrhagic benign thyroid cyst contents (**a**). Thyroglossal duct cyst contents; final pathology diagnosis showed no malignancy (**b**)

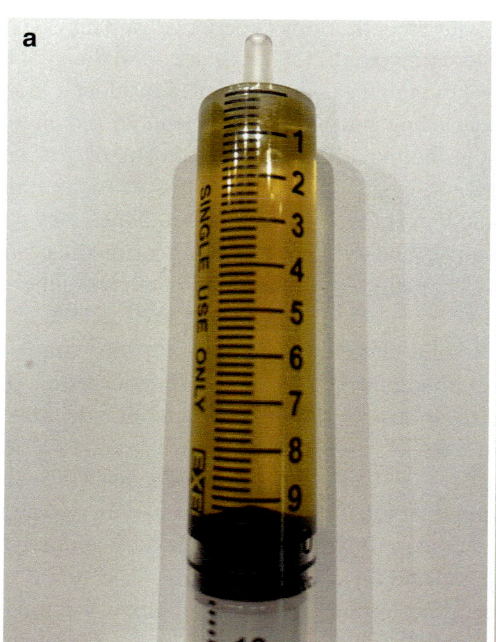

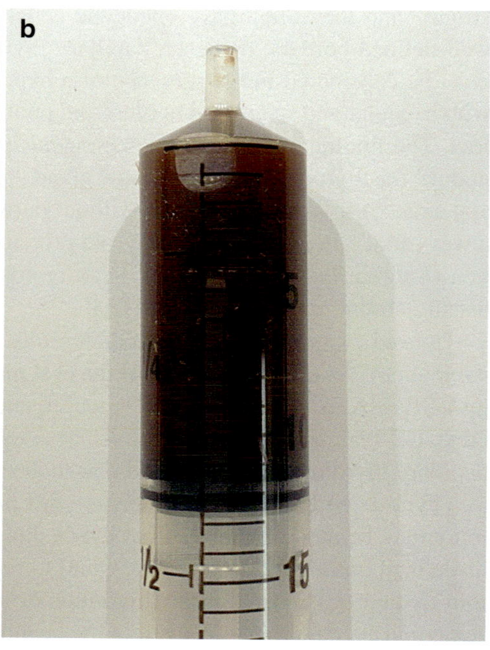

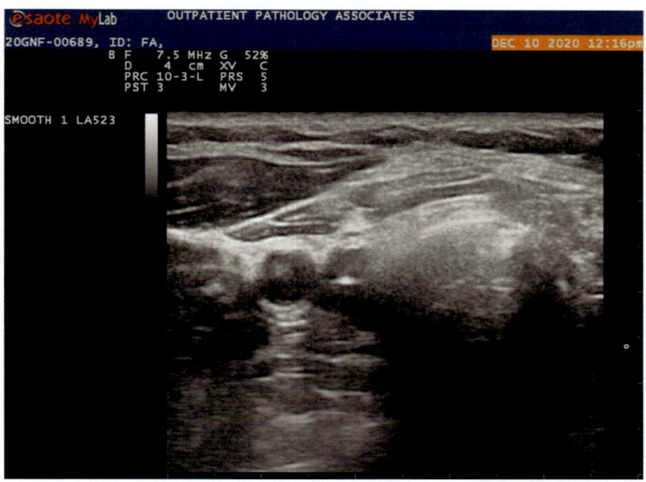

Fig. 9.8 Ultrasound-guided FNA, perpendicular approach of a right thyroid bed nodule. The bright signal that is seen in the center of the nodule corresponds to the needle tip. The final diagnosis was metastatic papillary thyroid carcinoma. (Ultrasound, high resolution)

tests and for measuring PTH must be harvested in these cases and processed as appropriate.

Of note, parathyroid cysts totally collapse after cyst fluid drainage.

Thyroid "Bed" Insertion of a needle in a thyroid "bed" nodule may be perceived as traveling into an empty space when there is a predominance of adipose tissue or as a firm resistance when there is fibrosis. A dry tap is usually obtained in both cases. A sample with variable amounts of blood is harvested when a small lymph node, repopulated thyroid tissue, or metastatic carcinoma is sampled (Fig. 9.8).

Lymph Nodes

Various parameters need to be kept in mind in the evaluation of lymph nodes. These include the clinical findings including patient's age and geographic region of origin, the body regions involved, localized versus generalized lymphadenopathy, and the US characteristics of the lymph node. The term "adenopathy" is considered when the lymph node measures >1 cm.

Neck, axillary, and inguinal lymphadenopathy will be covered in this section. Because patients who have neck lymphadenopathy associated with regional or systemic processes are frequently referred to our practice, I will cover the head and neck first and most extensively.

Head and Neck Lesions and Involved Lymph Nodes

The parotid lymph nodes drain lesions from the eyelids, conjunctiva, and posterior part of the cheek. Preauricular and parotid nodes drain lesions from the frontal region. Postauricular and parotid nodes drain the temporoparietal region. Preauricular, postauricular, and superior lateral neck nodes drain ear lesions. Lymph nodes occipital and posterior to the sternocleidomastoid muscle (SCM) drain the occipital region.

Submental nodes, and in some cases, submandibular and superior neck nodes drain lesions of the central part of the lower lips, the anterior part of the floor of the mouth, and the apex of the tongue.

Submandibular nodes drain lesions from the anterior part of the cheek, lower gums, eyelid, conjunctiva, side of the nose, upper lip, the lateral part of the lower lip, the floor of the mouth, maxillary and mandibular regions, and the anterior and lateral tongue.

Superior lateral neck nodes drain lesions from the occipital region of the scalp, deep temporal and infratemporal lesions, ears, external meatus, maxillary and mandibular regions, upper gum and hard and soft palate, nasal cavities, paranasal sinuses, the anterior part of the floor of the mouth, palatine tonsil, most of the tongue, upper larynx, pharynx, upper esophagus, and upper thyroid.

Pre- and paratracheal and pre-laryngeal nodes, and the most inferior of the superior lateral neck nodes drain lesions from the lower thyroid, lower larynx, and upper trachea.

Inferior lateral neck nodes that are in proximity to the brachial plexus and clavicle drain lesions from the back of the scalp and neck, superficial upper chest, and part of the arm.

The Neck Levels

Topographic classification of the neck in *levels* is helpful to facilitate communication among clinicians, radiologists, surgeons, and pathologists, including interventional cytopathologists, to localize, evaluate, and sample lymph nodes.

The levels of the neck and their boundaries are as follows:

Level 1A: submental triangle (boundaries: neck midline and the anterior belly of the digastric muscle to the hyoid bone)

Level 1B: submandibular triangle (boundaries: mandible and the anterior and posterior bellies of the digastric muscle)

Level 2: upper jugular [below level 1 and between the stylohyoid muscle to the posterior border of the SCM at the level of the hyoid bone and carotid bifurcation]. Level 2 is divided into 2A (anterior) and 2B (posterior) by a plane passing vertical to the angle of the jaw.

Level 3: mid-jugular (below level 2 and between the lateral border of the sternohyoid muscle, the posterior border of the SCM, and to the level of the cricoid notch inferiorly)

Level 4: lower jugular (below level 3 and between the lateral border of the sternohyoid muscle, the posterior border of the SCM, and the clavicle)

Level 5: posterior triangle (between the posterior border of the SCM, the anterior border of the trapezius muscle, and the clavicle). Level 5 is divided into 5A (superior) and 5B (inferior) by a horizontal plane passing inferior to the cricoid notch.

Level 6: anterior triangle (between neck midline, the hyoid bone, suprasternal notch, and lateral border of the sternohyoid muscle). This level harbors lymph nodes of the pretracheal, paratracheal, and pre-cricoid compartments.

Level 7: suprasternal notch.

Taking the Clinical History

Reactive inflammatory conditions, infectious (virus, bacteria including mycobacteria, cat scratch disease, fungus), primary hematolymphoid neoplasia, secondary metastatic processes including neuroblastoma, and drugs such as diphenylhydantoin may be responsible for localized, commonly neck or diffuse lymphadenopathy. Usually, the patient refers to the finding of a "lump" or "lumps" that may or may not be visible by inspection.

Consider a hematolymphoid neoplasia, including non-Hodgkin and Hodgkin lymphoma, and some infectious processes when the patient has generalized or regional lymphadenopathy and/or complains of "B" symptoms (nocturnal diaphoresis, weight loss, fever, asthenia, anorexia present in 25% of patients with Hodgkin and less common in non-Hodgkin lymphoma). Weight loss suggests disseminated disease in patients with a known or unknown cancer diagnosis. Patients with metastatic lymphadenopathy are usually asymptomatic; however, local symptoms may occur in rare cases. One of my patients with a clinical diagnosis of small-cell carcinoma of the lung was referred to our clinic for USG-FNA of a barely visible 2 cm left supraclavicular nodular mass associated with localized pain and tenderness, accentuated at the time of needle sampling; the cytological diagnosis was metastatic small-cell carcinoma to lymph nodes, involving the surrounding neurogenic plexus. Posterior neck lymphadenopathy is often associated with scalp inflammatory and infectious conditions and less common in neoplastic conditions.

Fistulous tracts are common in the neck and are usually secondary to infectious processes, i.e., atypical mycobacteria and fungus, and are less commonly malignant with skin and soft-tissue involvement. Of note, an 84-year-old man presented with a lateral and posterior neck mass with fistulous tracts; the diagnosis of p16(+) metastatic squamous carcinoma with extensive necrosis was made on USG-FNA; a prior core needle biopsy (CNB) done at another institution was non-diagnostic due to necrosis; this case exemplifies the accuracy of USG-FNA as a minimally invasive diagnostic procedure that avoided an open biopsy of the oropharyngeal primary squamous carcinoma identified on ENT exam. A neck mass with fistulous tracts draining a white chalky granular fluid may be seen in patients who have a long-standing scleroderma with associated skin and soft-tissue calcinosis; the diagnosis of scleroderma is made clinically, and USG-FNA is confirmatory of calcinosis; I had one such case.

Examining the Patient

Generalized Lymphadenopathy The involvement of two or more lymph node regions is defined as generalized lymphadenopathy and usually represents a systemic process such as a hematolymphoid malignancy, and patients often have a palpable spleen. Generalized lymphadenopathy can also be associated with viral infections including HIV, bacterial and fungal infections, protozoal (toxoplasmosis) infestations, sarcoidosis, amyloidosis, connective-tissue disease, and at times long-standing intake of drugs such as diphenylhydantoin. Lymph nodes of variable size that are soft or rubbery are seen in most reactive processes. Tender, variably painful, and fluctuant lymph nodes suggest infection. A firm and painless node suggests malignancy; however, a fluctuant painless node may indicate a necrotic malignancy. Consider T-cell non-Hodgkin lymphoma in patients with lymphadenopathy and erythroderma (Sezary syndrome).

Regional Lymphadenopathy Because lymphatic drainage is regional, the location of the lymph node is paramount for assessment of the source of the causal inflammatory or neoplastic process. However, I had more than one patient referred to my clinic for evaluation of a neck or inguinal lymphadenopathy, where, on examination, I found the lymph node to be part of a diffuse lymphadenopathy, and patients had non-Hodgkin lymphoma. Thus, as a rule in patients with axillary, inguinal, or neck lymphadenopathy involving more than one neck level, inquiry about general symptoms and a brief exam of other lymph node regions, including epitrochlear and popliteal, should be made as clinically appropriate. Check for splenomegaly and hepatomegaly if necessary.

Neck Lymphadenopathy A submental (level 1A) or submandibular (level 1B) mass is usually a lymph node; however, a saccular cyst or a ranula occur in level 1A and must be considered in the patient evaluation. A palpable firm and painless lymph node in level 2 may be seen in sarcoidosis or may be the first manifestation of a metastasis from oropharyngeal or nasopharyngeal carcinoma. Nasopharyngeal carcinoma may manifest as bilateral neck lymphadenopathy, usually involving level 2; however, I encountered a patient of Asian descent who had massive bilateral neck metastases involving levels 2, 3, and 5. Level 3 lymphadenopathy may be reactive and nonspecific, as seen in patients with autoimmune thyroiditis, or represent metastasis from papillary thyroid carcinoma. Metastasis from papillary thyroid carcinoma to levels 2 and 4 lymph nodes are less often identified; however, I witnessed a patient with a right level 2 cystic metastasis as the first manifestation of a right-mid-lobe 9 mm PTC. Lymphadenopathy occurring in the supraclavicular region (levels 4 and 5B anterior), also known as Virchow's node on the left side, may represent metastasis from a primary malignancy localized below the diaphragm, such as gastric cancer; however, on rare occasions, it may be the first manifestation of an aggressive prostate or testicular cancer. Right supraclavicular lymphadenopathy may be seen in metastatic disease from a primary in thoracic organs, commonly lung carcinoma. Metastasis to level 4 may be the first manifestation of ipsilateral breast carcinoma, as I witnessed in one instance. Also, breast carcinoma can metastasize to the central subclavicular lymph nodes. Posterior neck (level 5) and occipital lymphadenopathy are usually benign and reactive in response to inflammatory or infectious processes of the scalp and posterior neck. Palpable lymph nodes in the midline of the neck (level 6) are uncommon and, when present, must be distinguished from a palpable thyroglossal-duct cyst, thyroid isthmus nodules, or a saccular cyst (originates in the larynx and may expand over the top of the thyroid cartilage). A palpable mass in the suprasternal region (level 7) may be a lymph node, although a retrosternal goiter, and, less likely, a thymoma and a congenital cyst, needs to be considered. A lipoma may resemble a lymph node on physical exam of any neck compartment. A palpable transverse vertebral process may be found in the lower lateral neck (level 4) of patients with a thin neck and be mistaken for a firm lymph node or a petrous mass, as I have witnessed in more than one instance. A palpable mass with similar characteristics located in level 5B may correspond to a cervical rib.

Axillary Lymphadenopathy This may be present in regional inflammatory, infectious, or malignant processes affecting the skin and muscles of the anterior lateral thoracic walls, the dorsal lower neck and thoracic wall, the central and lateral parts of the breast, and the upper extremity. Thus, examination of these regions is imperative in the evaluation of a patient who has axillary lymphadenopathy. Axillary lymphadenopathy may also be present as a part of generalized lymphadenopathy in hematolymphoid malignancies. Of note, the identification of deep axillary lymph nodes should trigger the search for lymph nodes in the sub-clavicular region that may be more accessible to an USG-FNA than are those in the deep axilla in patients with breast carcinoma.

Inguinal Lymphadenopathy This may be found as part of generalized lymphadenopathy or in benign and malignant processes of the lower extremities, the skin of the lower abdominal wall below the umbilicus, the skin of the buttock, penis and scrotum, perineum, female external genitalia, and the lower part of the anal canal. Examination of the skin of the legs, feet, and in particular the toenails may be rewarding, as I had a case of undiagnosed acro-lentiginous melanoma presenting as "doughy" matted inguinal lymph nodes. I must emphasize that the inguinal lymph nodes also drain the anogenital area. I had two patients in whom the first manifestation of an anal carcinoma was the presence of firm inguinal metastatic lymph nodes. Also, an inguinal hernia presenting as a palpable inguinal mass may be mistaken for a lymph node. I had one such patient referred to my clinic; the diagnosis was made by physical exam and performance of the Valsalva maneuver and was confirmed by US exam with visualization of "moving" bowel loops. I had a case of intranodal palisaded myofibroblastoma that, clinically, is indistinguishable from a lymph node and cytologically, due to the presence of spindle cells, may be mistaken for a metastatic spindle cell malignancy. A soft, painless swelling is seen in lipoma, including lipoma of cord, which may be mistaken for a lymph node.

Popliteal Lymphadenopathy This must be distinguished from other masses, including lipoma, sebaceous cyst, Beker's cyst, and malignancies such as osteogenic and synovial sarcoma.

Performing the US Examination An oval or bean shape, a regular, thin cortex, and an echogenic hilum are features seen in a reactive lymph node; however, lymph nodes that are smaller than 1 cm often lack a visible fatty hilum and may not have an oval shape (Fig. 9.9). Reactive lymph nodes larger than 2 cm may be seen in the axilla, groin, or compartment 2 of the necks of young individuals. Absence of hilum, a thick, nodular, irregular cortex, and a >0.6 width-to-length

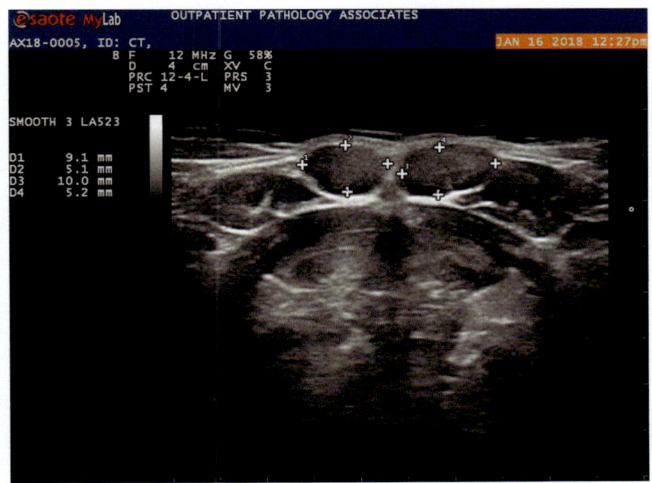

Fig. 9.9 Two sub-centimeter lymph nodes are seen bilaterally in levels 1A of the neck in a 2-year-old boy. Ultrasound features support a benign reactive condition. No FNA was performed. (Ultrasound, high resolution)

ratio are US findings, although not necessarily malignant, that need further investigation, and may be considered for USG-FNA.

A round, hypoechoic lymph node with sharp, well-defined borders, regardless of size, should be considered abnormal on US and may be seen in a benign reactive process, lymphoma, or metastatic disease. A single hypoechoic lymph node with abnormal shape and ill-defined spiculated borders in compartment 2A of the neck is commonly seen in metastatic oropharyngeal or nasopharyngeal carcinoma and often is the first manifestation of malignancy. Multiple regional or bilateral, round, and deeply hypoechoic lymph nodes with distinct smooth borders can be identified in the necks of patients with Hodgkin or non-Hodgkin lymphoma, and metastatic nasopharyngeal carcinoma and melanoma.

A neck lymph node with heterogeneous echotexture, cystic areas, or punctate echogenic foci should be sampled regardless of size and location, as they may harbor metastatic papillary thyroid carcinoma in the appropriate clinical setting.

Single or multiple hypoechoic, round, solid regional inguinal lymph nodes with no echogenic hilum are seen in metastatic carcinomas of anogenital origin or lower extremity including acral lentiginous melanoma, which may be the first evidence of the primary malignancy.

Of note, a fatty hilum, often seen in benign reactive lymph nodes, may be identified in primary or metastatic lymph node malignancies. I have encountered neck lymph nodes with a prominent echogenic hilum and cortical thickening in metastatic papillary thyroid carcinoma, and in lymphomas of both Hodgkin and non-Hodgkin types.

Performing the USG-FNA

Clinical history, physical exam, and US features are deciding factors whether to sample a lymph node by USG-FNA. The following are some considerations based on my experience. (1) A lymph node larger than 2 cm with or without abnormal US features located in anybody region, in particular level 3, 4, or 5 of the neck, should be sampled. (2) A round lymph node of any size identified in anybody region should be sampled, particularly in levels 3 and 4 of the necks of patients with or without a history of papillary thyroid carcinoma. (3) On rare occasions, a small lymph node with a fatty hilum located in neck levels other than level 3 may harbor metastatic papillary thyroid carcinoma and should be sampled, particularly when serum thyroglobulin is elevated. (4) If possible, direct the sampling to the cortex of the lymph node when it is thickened or irregular. (5) A lymph node with calcifications or punctate echogenic foci seen in the necks of patients with a history of thyroid carcinoma must be sampled so that metastasis can be excluded. (6) Avoid areas of necro-

sis or cystic change and instead sample viable solid areas (may be vascular on Doppler exam), which are commonly present at the periphery of the lymph node. (7) Samples taken from the medullary region yield variable amounts of blood; droplets of glistening dense matter with little blood are often harvested from the cortex. (8) Minute particles of tissue may be visualized in the centers of unstained smears prepared from metastatic malignancies and occasionally in granulomatous processes. (9) Creamy granular matter with bloody streaks is usually obtained in necrotic lymph nodes.

A lymph node with abnormal US features, particularly if heterogeneous and cystic, must be evaluated by ROSE for distinguishing between necrosis due to granulomatous inflammation and malignancy (often carcinoma and rarely NHL). Material for a cell block or flow cytometry must be obtained in these cases, using suction, and directing the needle to the periphery of the lymph node. Further detail is given in the section "Sample Handling and Triage" in Chap. 2 of this book.

Salivary Glands

Taking the Clinical History

Inspection of the face, looking for any visible submandibular or parotid masses and a subtle face asymmetry, can provide useful information about a possible parotid gland malignancy.

Ask the patient about the duration of the disease process, the growth rate of the mass, exposure to radiation, and pain, including localization, and relationship to eating or other triggering factors.

Long-standing parotid masses are usually asymptomatic and benign, as seen in pleomorphic adenoma. Consider the possibility of carcinoma ex-pleomorphic adenoma in a patient with a long-standing asymptomatic parotid mass that develops a sudden growth and that may be associated with local or radiating pain.

Local pain or tenderness may be present in a rapidly growing benign cyst or intra-parotid lymph node, or a rapidly growing malignancy, usually of high grade. Dull or shooting pain in the parotid region with irradiation to the cheek or mandibular area may be seen in parotid-gland malignancies with facial nerve involvement. On occasion, the patient may have a rapidly growing parotid mass and facial nerve paralysis, with the face drooping secondary to a parotid-gland malignancy, a clinical scenario I saw in a patient who had a salivary duct carcinoma of the parotid gland (Fig. 9.10).

Recurrent swelling and pain accentuated by eating of spicy foods is often associated with sialo-lithiasis, sialoectasia, and inflammation/infection and is mostly seen in the

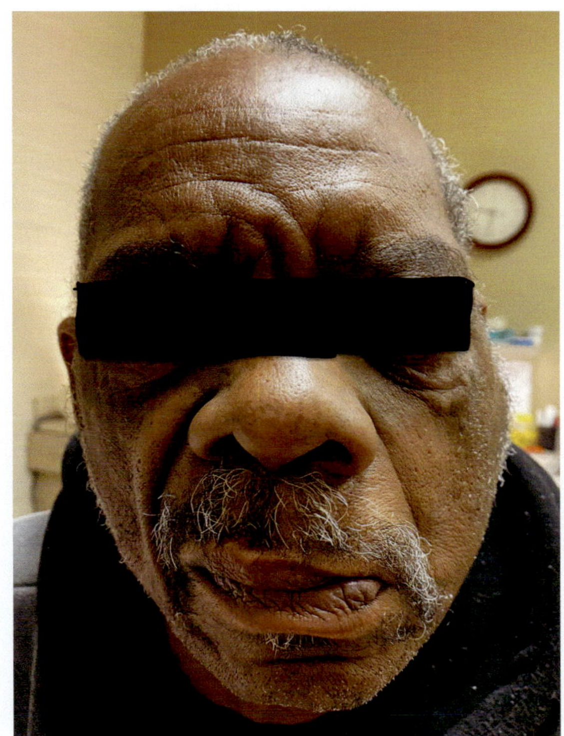

Fig. 9.10 This patient has a visible left parotid mass; USG-FNA diagnosis was salivary duct carcinoma ex-pleomorphic adenoma

submandibular gland. Visible nodular enlargement of the parotid and/or submandibular gland may be seen in immune disorders such as IgG-4 disease, an immune-related disorder involving the salivary glands that may be part of a systemic process; except for fatigue, other symptoms such as fever, night sweats, or weight loss are usually absent.

Examining the Patient

Parotid Gland Hyperplasia or sialosis presents as a diffuse bilateral parotid-gland enlargement. It has a doughy consistency without a palpable mass and is often seen in patients with diabetes mellitus.

Distinct masses in the parotid gland are usually nontender on palpation and may represent a lymph node, benign intraparotid cyst, a lymphoepithelial cyst in an HIV patient, or a neoplasia. In general, 80% of salivary gland tumors are in the parotid gland, are commonly pleomorphic adenomas, and are often localized in the superficial lobe of the gland in middle-aged patients. Pleomorphic adenomas have a firm consistency, are often movable, and are well-circumscribed with lobulated borders, particularly if present in the tail of the gland. Warthin's tumor, usually seen in older men who have a history of smoking, is often located in the tail of the gland (level 2 of neck) and can be mistaken for a lymph

node; in contrast to a lymph node that is rubbery, Warthin's tumor is commonly irregular and doughy (Fig. 9.11a, b). Mucoepidermoid carcinomas may have a soft consistency when the mucinous component predominates. Other malignant tumors, either primary or metastatic, commonly have a firm, petrous consistency, with irregular borders, and may be fixed to surrounding tissues. In general, the presence of a rapidly growing hard mass associated with facial nerve palsy is clinically suspicious for malignancy. A skin carcinoma or melanoma in the frontal, temporoparietal, retro auricular, preauricular, or cheek area may be a source of metastasis to an intraparotid lymph node that is felt as a parotid mass. Nodal involvement in metastatic melanoma is often soft/doughy and may be bulky.

Heterotopic parotid gland remnants may be identified in the cheek as a slightly firm, movable, and well-defined nodule located along Stensen's duct that may also be palpable when sialo-ectasia and sialolithiasis is present.

Submandibular Gland Normal submandibular glands are palpable, rubbery, and symmetric. Ptotic submandibular glands may be more prominent, palpable, and firm than normal glands and are particularly identified in thin elderly individuals who have a long neck. Patients are asymptomatic; however, a single ptotic gland may be more prominent and tender due to frequent self-exam by the patient.

A fixed swelling of the gland may be idiopathic or secondary to chronic sialadenitis, sialo-ectasia, sialolithiasis, or sarcoidosis if supported by the appropriate clinical setting. A submandibular gland abscess is very tender, and the patient complains of local pain. An uninfected red, tender, and swollen gland is often an indication of sialolithiasis.

In contrast to the parotid gland, the submandibular gland does not have intraglandular lymph nodes. Thus, a palpable mass in the submandibular area often represents a lymph node adjacent to the gland and not a submandibular-gland mass. On the other hand, a truly palpable submandibular-gland nodule may represent a salivary gland neoplasm or, in rare instances, nodular chronic sialadenitis. We must remember that a submandibular-gland mass in a young patient may represent a mucoepidermoid carcinoma.

Performing the US Examination

Both normal submandibular and parotid glands are slightly hyperechoic with a homogeneous echotexture by US. The submandibular gland shows well-defined, smooth borders; in contrast, the parotid gland exhibits ill-defined borders.

US of the parotid gland hyperplasia shows an enlarged gland with ill-defined borders, no distinct masses, and a solid, homogeneous, and hazy echotexture.

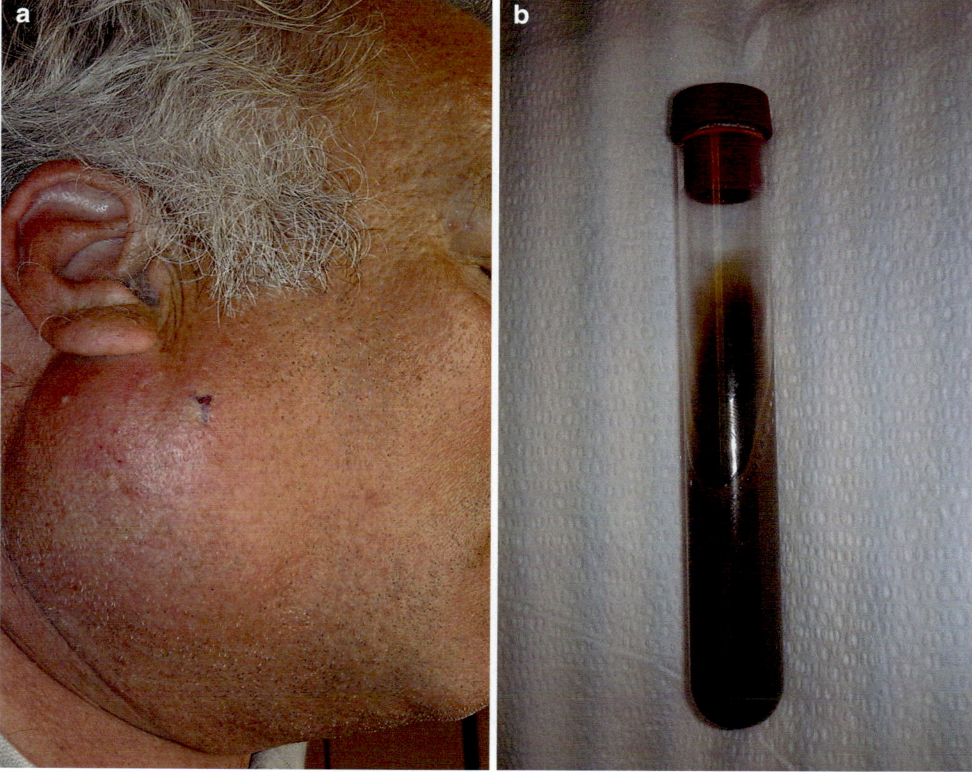

Fig. 9.11 Warthin's tumor. Visible large bulging level 2 (angle of the jaw) neck mass (**a**). USG-FNA drained 8 mL of dark "motor oil" fluid, which is often present in cystic Warthin's tumor (**b**)

Chronic sialadenitis usually affects the submandibular gland. A solid heterogenous echotexture, fine central vascular blood flow by Doppler exam, and no distinct masses are usually seen. However, in rare cases, a distinct hypoechoic nodular mass with irregular borders may be present and is indistinguishable from a submandibular-gland neoplasm by US exam.

As mentioned before, palpable, and US-visible lymph nodes may be present within the parotid gland, but not within the submandibular gland. Thus, an intraparotid mass may represent a lymph node, a primary salivary neoplasm, or a metastatic deposit. Likewise, a mass adjacent to the parotid gland often corresponds to a lymph node; however, in some instances there is a myxoid/synovial cyst originating from the underlying temporomandibular joint situated anterior to the parotid gland, as I have witnessed in more than one patient. The cyst is well circumscribed, anechoic, and has posterior acoustic enhancement. The lymph node is hypoechoic, solid, and may have a fatty hilum.

A serpiginous, cystically dilated anechoic mass traveling across the cheek in the direction of the parotid gland corresponds to a dilated Stensen's duct secondary to sialo-ectasia, which is often secondary to sialolithiasis.

Benign salivary gland neoplasms are solid, hypoechoic, and variably vascular with smooth borders. Pleomorphic adenoma is more common in the parotid gland than in the submandibular gland and is often seen as a single hypoechoic nodule/mass with smooth, lobulated borders, but may be multiple within the gland or at times outside the gland. In contrast to pleomorphic adenoma that may be localized in any part of the parotid gland, Warthin's tumor is commonly located in the tail of the parotid gland and shows a heterogeneous and variably cystic echotexture, well-defined borders, and variable vascularity by Doppler exam.

Benign spindle cell salivary gland neoplasms are rare. I encountered a spindle myoepithelial cell-rich pleomorphic adenoma of the submandibular gland that I diagnosed as a spindle cell neoplasm, possible leiomyoma versus Schwannoma. Another case was that of an incidentally found non-palpable parotid Schwannoma that showed a hypoechoic, well-circumscribed nodule with smooth borders in the medial aspect of the parotid gland close to the tragus. These cases illustrate the difficult diagnosis of these tumors by cytomorphology, and the need for correlation with immunostaining for rendering a definitive cytologic diagnosis.

Basal cell adenomas of the parotid gland, regardless of the degree of dysplasia, are round to oval, hypoechoic, of variable size, and have smooth borders. A small intraparotid lymph node with a metastatic basal cell carcinoma of the skin has a smooth border and mimics a benign basaloid neoplasm by US. I encountered a basal cell adenoma with severe dysplasia (diagnosed histologically) in a patient who had had a partial ear resection for a basal cell carcinoma; my USG-FNA interpretation was "basaloid carcinoma, probably met-

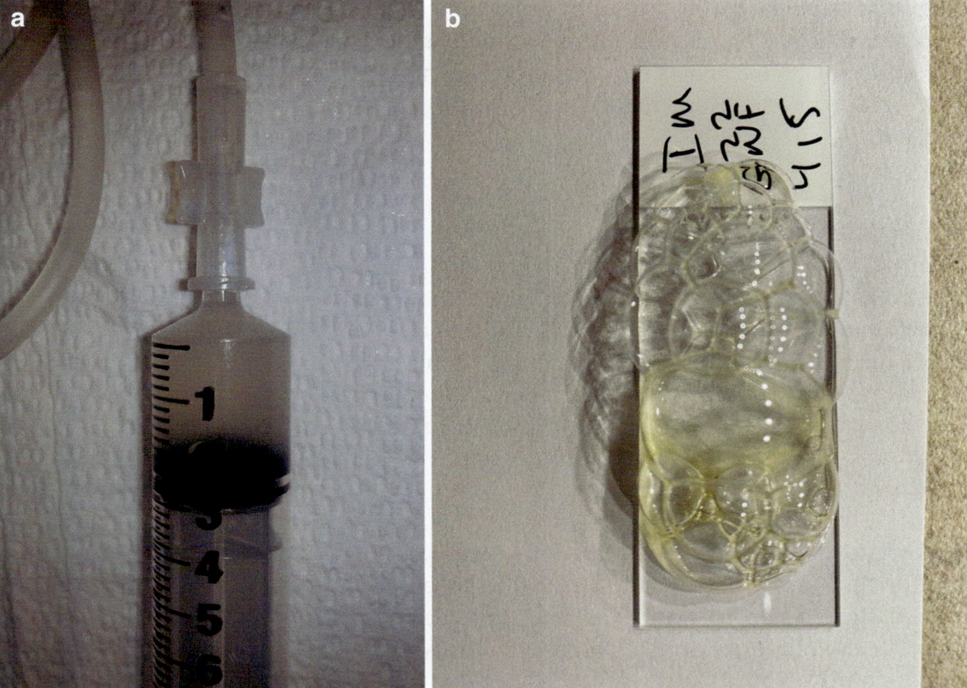

Fig. 9.12 Turbid opalescent fluid was obtained from a benign parotid gland cyst (**a**). Numerous alpha-amylase crystals were identified in the smears. Mucoid transparent bubbly material was aspirated from a dilated parotid duct secondary to sialolithiasis and sialo-ectasia (**b**)

astatic" and illustrates the difficult distinction between these two entities. A descriptive cytology diagnosis following the guidelines recommended in the Milan System for Reporting Salivary Gland FNA is advised in such cases.

Primary salivary gland carcinomas and metastatic malignancies, usually from a local regional source, e.g., skin carcinomas, are hypoechoic, solid, variably vascular, and may exhibit irregular borders. Large deeply hypoechoic lymph nodes with smooth borders and variable vascular blood flow may be seen in metastatic melanoma. Metastatic squamous cell carcinoma often shows a heterogeneous solid and cystic echotexture due to necrosis, particularly when it is larger than 1 cm. Mucoepidermoid carcinoma may be variably cystic and heterogeneous and is more common in the submandibular than in the parotid glands of young patients.

Performing the USG-FNA

Normal parotid-gland tissue does not cause pain upon needle insertion; in contrast, submandibular gland tissue creates pain. Keeping this consideration in mind, a local anesthetic agent should be properly administered, particularly when a submandibular-gland mass needs to be sampled. Submandibular-gland enlargement with US features of chronic sialadenitis should be sampled only if necessary for instance, in cases of nodular chronic sialadenitis for ruling out a neoplasm.

Salivary-gland masses usually neither create pain nor tenderness upon needle insertion; however, I had a patient with

an asymptomatic parotid Schwannoma who had intense local pain at the time of USG-FNA.

Sampling of pleomorphic adenoma resists needle travel within the mass, and the harvested material is scant, dense, opaque, and difficult to expel from the needle. In contrast to pleomorphic adenoma, the sampling needle usually penetrates with minimal resistance and yields variably bloody samples in other benign neoplasms, such as Warthin's tumor and malignancies including metastatic deposits with minimal or no desmoplastic reaction. Variably dense mucoid material is usually obtained in mucinous neoplasms. Sialocele/sialo-ectasia yields turbid, milky, or stringy saliva-like fluid. Myxoid/synovial cysts yield dense, bright, almost transparent fluid (Fig. 9.12a, b).

Miscelaneous Masses of the Head and Neck

General Considerations

If we exclude intradermal masses such as squamous cysts or lipomas, 85% of neck masses are lymph nodes. Infectious processes such as HIV or EBV, chronic infections, lymphoma, or metastasis must be considered in the appropriate clinical settings.

As mentioned in the lymph node section, the neck is divided topographically into levels. Briefly, level 1 is submental, 2 is submandibular, 3 is mid-lateral anterior to the posterior border of the SCM, 4 is lower lateral and supraclavicular, 5 is posterior to the SCM (5A superior and 5B inferior), 6 is midline below the hyoid bone, and 7 is the suprasternal notch. This compartmentalization is reproducible and facilitates the finding of palpable or imaging-visible neck lesions by clinicians, radiologists, pathologists, and surgeons.

Taking the Clinical History

Scalp The most common scalp masses are sebaceous cysts. Other lesions and masses include trauma, psoriasis, and benign and metastatic malignancies. Thus, an accurate clinical history must be obtained with emphasis on remote malignancies such as kidney, thyroid, lung, prostate, and breast, which are the most common primary sites for scalp metastases.

Neck A superficial soft-tissue neck mass develops in any neck level, is usually asymptomatic, and must be distinguished from a lymph node, congenital cyst, neurogenic tumor, or even an extra-adrenal paraganglioma. A midline neck lesion is usually a cyst, such as a saccular cyst or a thyroglossal-duct cyst that, if visible, moves vertically with swallowing and tongue protrusion because of its attachment to the body of the hyoid bone. Neck masses are often found incidentally in imaging studies and are usually asymptomatic, although obstructive symptoms may be related to their size and location. Physical exam and US features help to narrow the differential diagnosis.

Examining the Patient

Scalp A brief examination of the scalp helps in the evaluation of posterior neck lymphadenopathy that is often associated with inflammatory, infectious, autoimmune (psoriasis), or neoplastic processes of the scalp. A scalp mass must be correlated with imaging studies because metastatic malignancies may be associated with underlying lytic bone involvement. A pulsatile scalp mass suggests a vascularized metastatic tumor such as a renal cell or papillary thyroid carcinoma. Patients with multiple myeloma may have painful lesions in the skull. A firm nodular soft-tissue mass with no bone involvement may suggest a soft-tissue neoplasm such as a dermatofibrosarcoma protuberans or metastatic leiomyosarcoma, as in cases which I had. Of note, a sebaceous cyst of the scalp lacks the central depression that is a characteristic of sebaceous cysts of other body regions.

Neck Examination of the neck should be performed keeping in mind the distribution and drainage of the lymph nodes and the organs present at each neck level. A mass in the submental area (level 1A) may be a ranula, but often is a lymph node. A

mass in level 1B that includes the area anterior to the posterior border of the submandibular gland may represent chronic sialadenitis, or a submandibular gland neoplasm, or a lymph node that may be difficult to distinguish from the gland by palpation only. A mass posterior to the submandibular gland and anterior to the angle of the jaw (level 2A) is commonly a lymph node (consider metastasis in patients in the 4th decade of life and older) or, less common by, a branchial cleft cyst that abuts from the anterior border of the SCM at the junction of its upper and mid thirds and is common in the first and second decades of life. A pulsatile mass may represent a tortuous carotid artery, a carotid artery aneurism, or an extra-adrenal paraganglioma (carotid body tumor); however, this tumor may not be pulsatile, particularly when it is sclerosed and large. Lymph nodes are usually found in the area posterior to the angle of the jaw and around the carotid artery bifurcation (level 2B); however, a parotid gland neoplasm, particularly Warthin's tumor, may be identified in this area. Lymph nodes are often palpable in the mid-lateral neck (level 3), supraclavicular area (level 4), and posterior to the sternocleidomastoid muscle (level 5). The midline of the neck (level 6) harbors normal cartilaginous organs that may be prominent and be mistaken for lymph nodes; a dermoid cyst in the first and second decades of life, a thyroglossal-duct cyst, isthmus thyroid nodule, cartilaginous tumors, or benign and malignant thyroid tissue in patients with thyroidectomy. Less commonly, a saccular cyst and a laryngocele should be kept in mind when the mass is localized above the hyoid bone. The suprasternal area (level 7) should be empty and when palpable, a mass is often due to a substernal goiter, and less commonly to lymph nodes or a thymic neoplasm (Fig. 9.13a, b).

Subcutaneous masses include lipoma (it may also be intradermal), a ganglion cyst, neuroma, and lymph nodes; intradermal soft-tissue masses include a sebaceous cyst, abscess, dermoid cyst, and granuloma, to mention the most common ones. Lipomas may be present in any body region and in any level of the neck. They are soft, lobulated, mobile, attached neither to the overlying skin nor to the underlying tissue, and are often present in more than one body region. A fibrolipoma may be firm, variably circumscribed, and movable. A firm mass attached to surrounding tissue planes should be of concern for a soft-tissue neoplasm other than lipoma. A firm nodule attached to the skin with a dot-like central indentation, which gets more prominent if we try to separate the nodule from the overlying skin strongly suggests an epidermal inclusion cyst; similar findings are seen in pilomatrixoma (calcifying epithelioma of Malherbe), which is often located in the head and neck region of a young individual. A raised, firm, and well-circumscribed pearly nodule with a variably bright, shiny surface is commonly seen in metastases that are often located in the scalp, although they may be seen in any body region and are usually from a known primary.

Fig. 9.13 Large visible posterior neck level 5A masses in two patients: non-Hodgkin lymphoma (**a**) and extra-skeletal Ewing sarcoma (**b**)

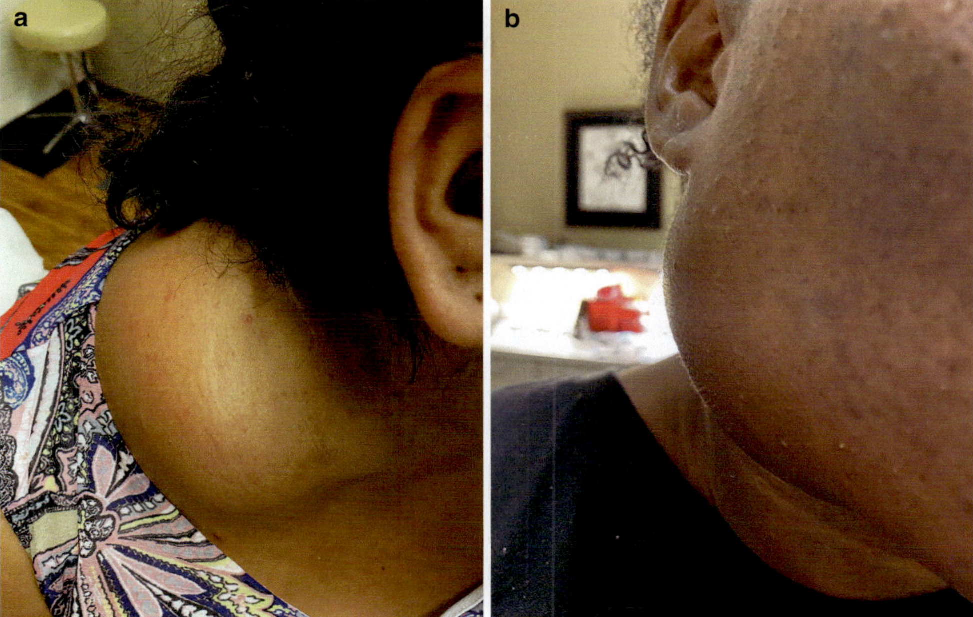

A large and firm soft-tissue mass with prominent spider-like skin vascularity is suggestive of a malignant process.

Performing the US Examination

Lipomas exhibit characteristic US features and include a well-circumscribed, isoechoic, oval-shaped mass, a thin, echogenic, visible capsule, and a "feathery" echotexture, a feature that remains unaltered despite changes in the position of the US probe. Occasionally, they are hyperechoic, less circumscribed, and merge with the subcutaneous tissue of the overlying skin. They are avascular; however, angiolipomas may show a very fine vascular blood flow by Doppler exam and may be tender on examination.

Congenital cysts are anechoic or isoechoic if contents are dense, well circumscribed with a distinct echogenic thin capsule, and display a posterior acoustic enhancement. Cyst location is crucial for construction of a differential diagnosis. If located in the lateral neck, level 2 anterior to the SCM, the main consideration is a branchial cleft cyst; however, if the borders are fuzzy and the wall is irregular and vascular by Doppler exam, a cystic metastasis from squamous cell carcinoma is a strong possibility; in these cases, a thorough examination of neck levels 2A and 2B often shows one or more abnormal lymph nodes. A thyroglossal-duct cyst is usually present in the anterior neck midline and is of variable size, often anechoic with smooth borders, and has no mural solid component. However, a thorough US exam, including Doppler must be done for evaluation of the cyst walls and the presence or absence of a mural solid-phase component which is often seen in thyroid carcinoma that arises in a thyroglossal-duct cyst (Fig. 9.14).

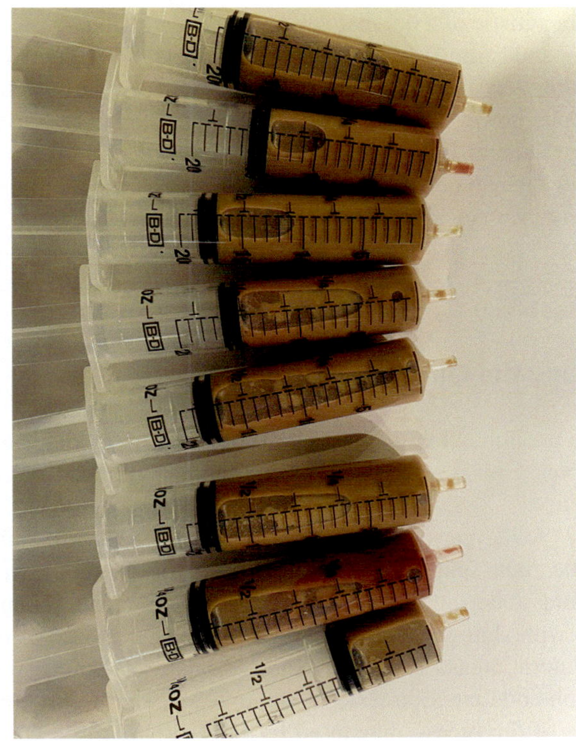

Fig. 9.14 Turbid dense fluid aspirated from a neck mass diagnosed as branchial cleft cyst

A saccular cyst (dilated saccule of the larynx) can be acquired or congenital and is located between the vocal cords and thyroid cartilage, filled with mucus, and iso- to hypoechoic by US. A laryngocele is filled with air and/or fluid, hypoechoic by US, and develops in the same location as a saccular cyst.

An extra-adrenal paraganglioma must be considered when a heterogeneous mass is present at the level of the carotid artery bifurcation (level 2A). Occasionally, it may be identified in the lateral mid neck (level 3), adjacent to or even inside the thyroid gland. In fact, I had a patient with a right mid-thyroid nodule whom I had seen in 2017 and 2019; on her third visit, the patient had a slightly larger and heterogeneous vascular mass in the same location that, on careful US exam, appeared to be separate from the thyroid gland and proved to be a paraganglioma by USG-FNA. Extra-adrenal paraganglioma shows a variable vascular blood flow by Doppler exam and may not always be pulsatile.

Soft-tissue and cutaneous calcinosis may be seen as a large neck mass in patients who have a long-standing scleroderma, occasionally with fistulous tracts that drain a white, chalky granular fluid.

Performing the USG-FNA

The feeling that the needle travels through an empty space is characteristic of a lipomatous mass; the material harvested is scant and is limited to minute lipid droplets. USG-FNA with suction may be applied for obtaining a more representative sample; however, variable amounts of blood may be present when suction is applied. USG-FNA of fibrous nodules or masses may require suction, or even a core needle biopsy, for obtaining an adequate sample.

Breast

Taking the Clinical History

As a preamble, I will present three of the most striking cases of breast masses I have seen during the decades of my practice.

(1) A 72-year-old woman self-identified a small "nodule" in the right supraclavicular area. At the same time while, looking at herself in the mirror, she found an area of induration with skin puckering in the lower inner quadrant of her ipsilateral breast. USG-FNA showed breast carcinoma with lymph node metastases. (2) I witnessed a case of blastomycosis of the breast, diagnosed by FNA (ROSE) in a young woman, presenting as a rapidly growing breast mass with invasion of the pectoralis muscle. She was scheduled to have surgery within the next 24 h; the cytologic diagnosis prevented a radical surgical procedure. (3) In contrast to the previous patient, I saw a 27-year-old woman who had a breast mass that grew from a pea size to an orange size in less than 6 months; metaplastic carcinoma was the FNA diagnosis. This example reinforces the concept that a rapidly growing mass, identified in a young woman is not always inflamma-

tory or infectious and that a high-grade malignancy should always be kept in mind. These three cases highlight the value of FNA as a rapid, accurate, and minimally invasive procedure for diagnosing a breast mass.

A breast mass is often identified by breast self-examination, routine physical exam, or routine mammogram or US. When interviewing a patient with a breast mass, we should get Information about time elapsed since the mass was identified, the time since last physical exam and/or breast self-exam, changes in the mass and/or overlying skin (skin dimpling, redness), nipple retraction, nipple discharge, and characteristics of the discharge if present, pain or tenderness and relationship with menstrual periods, prior breast problems or breast surgery, a family history of breast cancer, and the date and results of the latest breast imaging studies, if known by the patient. Has she noticed ipsilateral axillary or supraclavicular swelling? A history of past or recent trauma to the breast must be recorded; mastodinia may or may not be present at the time of evaluation.

The age of the patient is always important for construction of a differential diagnosis; benign conditions including fibroadenomas and infectious processes (in certain geographic areas and ethnic groups) are often seen in patients below the age of 30 years; in contrast, malignant processes are more prevalent in individuals who are in the 5th decade or older. Breast cysts are more common in the 4th and 5th decades of life. However, regardless of the age of presentation, the finding of a breast mass is always of concern, and the patient should be evaluated by means of physical exam and imaging studies, i.e., mammogram, US.

Except for rapidly growing breast cysts, benign and malignant breast masses are commonly asymptomatic. Patients with fibroadenomas may have variable premenstrual mass tenderness or pain. Mastitis, abscess, or galactocele is a mass to consider in a pregnant woman. Duct ectasia is to be considered in a middle-aged woman who has retro areolar pain, a creamy nipple discharge, and nipple retraction.

Gynecomastia of one or both breasts may be physiologic in neonates, during puberty and old age and must be distinguished from pathologic gynecomastia that occurs at any age. Patients often mention areolar and nipple hypersensitivity and tenderness upon contact with clothes. In my experience, when present in adults, gynecomastia may be associated with intake of non-FDA-approved muscle-enhancing supplements that are sold over the counter. Common drugs that produce gynecomastia include estrogens, spironolactone, digitalis, tricyclic antidepressants, and recreational drugs that include amphetamines and cannabis. Patients with a history of prostate carcinoma treated with estrogen therapy develop gynecomastia. Chronic liver disease, renal failure, hyperthyroidism, and hypogonadism are associated with gynecomastia. Lung carcinoma and some testicular tumors may be responsible for gynecomastia as a paraneoplastic manifestation. Thus, the past medical history, and a history of hormonal therapy, drugs, and over-the-counter supplements, must be considered in patients with gynecomastia.

Examining the Patient

To make the patient feel comfortable, inspection of the breast in females should always be made with the patient sitting on the exam table at a level higher than that of the examiner. Inspection of the breasts should be made first in the sitting position with both arms behind the patient's head. Inspection should include a look for breast symmetry, a visible mass, skin changes (puckering? redness? orange peel?), nipple retraction, nipple discharge (bloody? clear? serous? milky creamy?), areolar and nipple changes (red scaly lesion resembling eczema as seen in Paget's disease), and axillary and supraclavicular fossae looking for visible masses. A diffuse breast swelling may be seen during puberty, pregnancy, and lactation; the breast is red, warm, and tender in mastitis, with patients having a fever and general symptoms (Fig. 9.15a, b).

On examination, we should evaluate and record the texture (soft, firm, hard, stony), shape (round, oval, other), borders (smooth, irregular), mobility, and tenderness of the breast mass. Localization of the mass, i.e., radius and dis-

tance from the nipple in centimeters, must be recorded both in the sitting and supine positions. A breast mass in a prepuberal patient must be distinguished from a normally developing breast that usually is identified as a prominence in the retro areolar area or the upper outer quadrant and should not be considered for a biopsy.

The differential diagnosis of a non-tender mass includes fibroadenoma in a young patient, cyst with slow fluid accumulation, fat necrosis, breast carcinoma (10% are tender or painful), or secondary malignancies. Fibroadenoma is smooth, round to oval, and mobile; however, a larger mass with similar characteristics raises the possibility of a phyllodes tumor. Cysts are mobile, smooth, and may be tender; a galactocele must be considered in a lactating breast. A firm and tender mass may be encountered in a cyst with rapid fluid accumulation and in fat necrosis associated with a recent trauma. Lipomas are rarely found in the breast, but, when present they are soft and lobulated. Adipose tissue breast prominences are more common and less defined than lipomas and may be firm.

A hard, irregular mass fixed to deep planes and/or to the skin with dimpling, nipple retraction, and orange-peel-like overlying skin is a finding of carcinoma until proven otherwise. A hard, irregular mass attached to the skin with dimpling may be found in fat necrosis; bruising of the overlying skin may be observed when there is history of breast trauma (Fig. 9.16a, b).

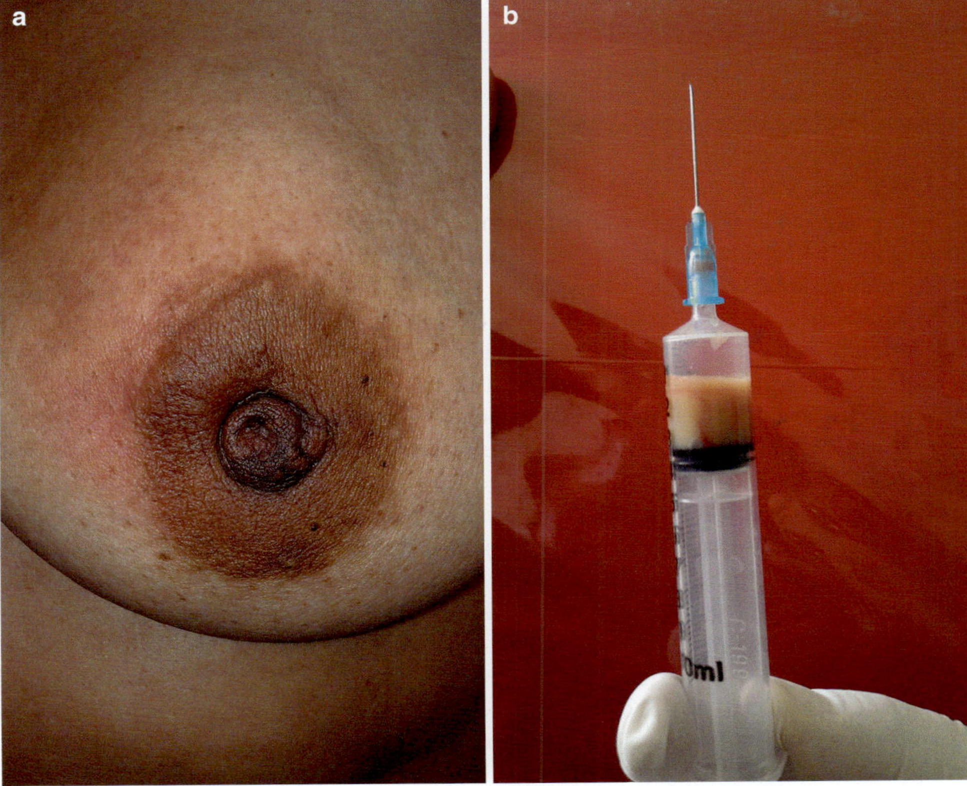

Fig. 9.15 Breast abscess. Bulging smooth mass with no overlying skin changes (**a**). A dense greenish purulent fluid was aspirated (**b**)

Fig. 9.16 Mammary carcinoma. Erythematous skin with orange-peel appearance overlying a mass subsequently diagnosed as infiltrating papillary carcinoma (**a**). Mass in the nipple areola area subsequently diagnosed as mammary ductal carcinoma with neuroendocrine differentiation (**b**)

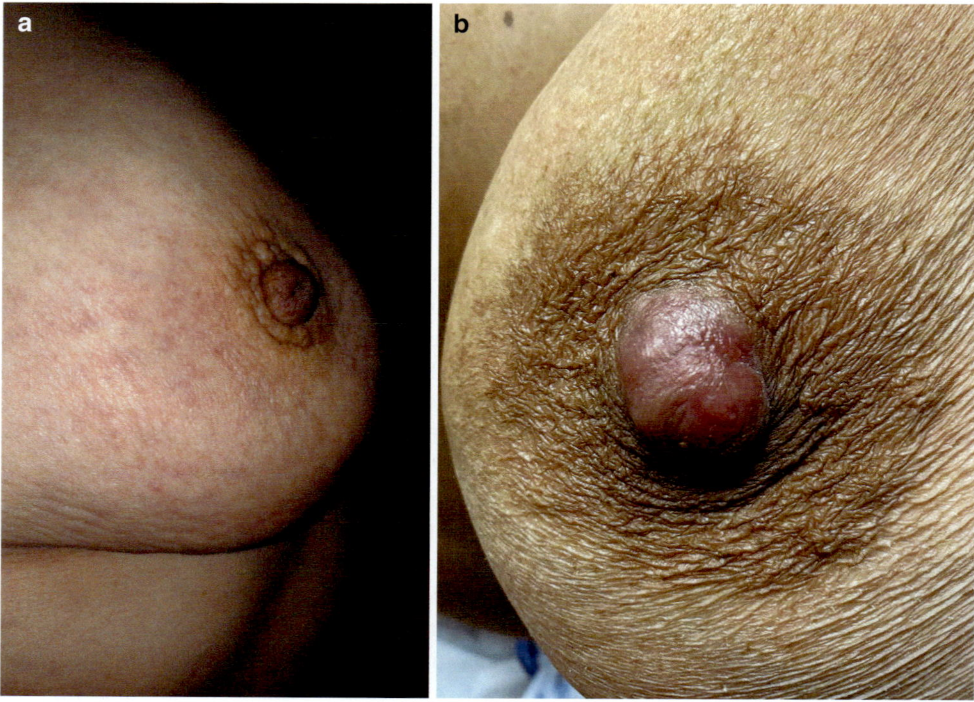

Gynecomastia is the most common cause of a unilateral or bilateral, ill-defined, slightly firm, palpable, tender breast mass, commonly subareolar. However, breast carcinoma in males may be visible and/or palpable and may be firm and retro areolar. Soft and diffuse gynecomastia is often associated with drugs. Always look for axillary, supraclavicular, and sub-clavicular lymphadenopathy.

Performing the US Examination

A palpable breast mass may not always be visible by US, as in the case of an adipose tissue breast prominence. Mammary lipomas may be palpable and visible by US and exhibit the US features described for neck lipomas.

Cysts are anechoic, often round, and well circumscribed with a visible thin capsule and posterior acoustic enhancement. The differential diagnosis based on US includes mucinous lesions such as mucocele and mucinous cystic carcinoma, which may or may not have a conspicuous solid component.

Fibroadenomas are often round, oval, or slightly lobulated, hypoechoic, homogeneous, and solid with posterior acoustic enhancement. A phyllodes tumor is large and has lobulated and well-circumscribed borders; except for its larger size and conspicuous lobulated borders, it resembles fibroadenoma by US.

Lobular breast carcinoma is often large, solid, and may show a heterogenous iso- or slightly hyperechoic echotexture with poorly visualized borders and fine vascular blood flow by Doppler exam. US exam of the axillary fossa is encouraged, in which a metastatic round, hypoechoic lymph node is often identified. A large, solid, heterogeneous, and ill-defined mass may also be identified in metaplastic breast carcinoma, a high-grade malignancy often seen in young women.

Ductal carcinoma is visualized as a solid, hypoechoic mass of variable size and shape, with ill-defined spiculated borders, and variable vascular blood flow by Doppler exam. Fat necrosis often shows similar, if not identical US features. Ultrasound evaluation of the ipsilateral axillary and supraclavicular lymph nodes is strongly advised in these cases, and USG-FNA sampling is encouraged for diagnosis and staging of the breast carcinoma.

In gynecomastia, prominent breast glandular tissue is often seen by US; however, a slightly hypoechoic nodular area, usually retro-areolar, may be identified and should be sampled.

Performing the USG-FNA

It is important to assess the resistance found by the operator upon insertion of the needle into the breast mass. In fatty lesions (adipose tissue breast prominence or lipoma), there is a lack of resistance with a feeling of penetrating of the needle into an empty space. Soft or slight firm resistance is found when there is fibrosis. A rubbery texture with "grabbing" of the needle is typical of a fibroadenoma; however, a phyllodes tumor (benign or malignant) usually has a similar texture. A gritty texture is often seen in carcinoma.

A mass that yields a creamy granular fluid may indicate tumor necrosis or pus from an abscess that is commonly tender. An oily fluid may be aspirated from cystic fat necrosis. A clear or opalescent fluid is almost always obtained from benign breast cysts. Mucoid material is aspirated from mucinous neoplasms such as mucocele and mucinous cystic carcinoma. Bloody fluid is often obtained from cystic papillary neoplasms (benign or malignant). Of note, surgical excision is necessary for diagnosis of a breast cystic papilloma, cystic papillary carcinoma, mucocele, and mucinous cystic carcinoma; cytologic exam cannot diagnose these entities with certainty.

US evaluation post cyst fluid drainage must be conducted for detection of a residual solid-phase component that needs to be sampled by USG-FNA.

Handling and Triage of USG-FNA Samples

Smears In general, I prepare 3–4 smears for all sampled masses. A combination of 2–3 air-dried smears to be stained with May Grunwald Giemsa (MGG) and one 95% ethanol-fixed smear to be stained with Papanicolaou stain is prepared. As a routine I do not use liquid-based preparation smears except for evaluation of hemorrhagic cyst contents, mainly of the breast.

Rapid on-site evaluation using Toluidine blue is done particularly in cases when additional samples are needed for ancillary studies, i.e., cultures, cell block, flow cytometry, molecular studies, etc.

Cell Block A sample for cell block is harvested in selected cases after ROSE, and mainly for performing immunohistochemical stains, i.e., for metastases, unusual neck masses such as paraganglioma and Schwannoma among others and selected salivary gland tumors.

Thyroid Molecular Tests The indication to harvest material for thyroid molecular testing at the time of USG-FNA is the identification of TIRADS 4 or 5 criteria or intermediate- or high-risk US features of the target nodule (solid, hypoechoic / isoechoic / hyperechoic, taller than wide, punctate echogenic foci, macrocalcifications, interrupted eggshell calcifications, ill-defined/lobulated/spiculated borders, and extrathyroidal extension). One sample harvested only for the test, together with the rinses of all needles used in the USG-FNA, is placed in the manufacturer's solution; follow the manufacturer's instructions to store and submit the sample (Interpace Diagnostics Laboratory samples can be stored at room temperature up to 5 weeks). The sample is submitted only when the cytology interpretation is Bethesda category 3 or 4, and in category 5 only when the results will guide further patient management including the extent of surgery.

Other Thyroid Tests ROSE is done when thyroid lymphoma is suspected by US and material for a flow cytometry exam needs to be harvested in RPMI (Roswell Park Memorial Institute) solution. Material for a cell block is harvested when metastasis or high-grade malignancy is suspected. Samples for measurement of calcitonin or PTH levels in "needle rinses," can be obtained as clinically indicated when medullary carcinoma or intrathyroidal parathyroid is suspected, or for measurement of TG in thyroid bed nodules from patients with surgically removed papillary thyroid carcinoma. The "needle rinse" sample includes the material from a dedicated pass and the needles used in the procedure, all rinsed in 1 mL of sterile saline. The "needle rinses" are submitted as clinically appropriate.

Parathyroid If a parathyroid neoplasm is suspected based on US or clinical grounds, material for measurement of PTH levels in needle rinses should be obtained as detailed for thyroid above. When the distinction between a thyroid and a parathyroid nodule cannot be made with certainty by US, material for both thyroid molecular tests should be harvested and PTH levels measured in "needle rinses." If the cytologic interpretation is that of a Bethesda 4 (microfollicular pattern), submit the sample for measuring PTH levels first and wait for the results, because mutations may be detected in a parathyroid tumor sample when it is tested with the use of a thyroid molecular platform; such results may impact the surgical procedure under the wrong impression that the parathyroid mass is a thyroid neoplasm with mutations. If PTH levels are negative, submit the sample for thyroid molecular testing. I have had two parathyroid tumors submitted for thyroid molecular testing with the diagnosis of "Bethesda 4 thyroid nodules," which showed "mutations" in the thyroid molecular testing platform; subsequent thyroid lobectomy showed a parathyroid adenoma in both cases. It is important to remember that a sample for measuring PTH levels in "needle rinses" must be kept frozen, because PTH is thermo-sensitive at room temperature. PTH levels in needle rinses obtained from parathyroid tumors are almost always in the upper hundreds or thousands pg/mL; however, the PTH levels in parathyroid cyst fluids may be low or negative when the epithelium of the cyst is single and/or columnar or there is no epithelial lining. Similarly, TG levels in needle rinses harvested from TGDC may be negative, because of the squamous and/or columnar ciliated epithelial cell lining of the cyst.

Lymph Nodes An abnormal lymph node by US must be evaluated by ROSE and material harvested for special studies as appropriate. A sample for cell block should be harvested by sampling of the periphery of the necrotic lymph with use of a Male Luer Lock adapter plastic tube extension set (Baxter Health Corporation) attached to a sterile needle on one end and to a syringe on the other. The following sequential steps must be followed: (1) once the needle is in the desired target, apply suction with an aspiration device, (2) perform the USG-FNA with the purpose of obtaining a visible amount of blood in the hub of the needle, syringe tip, and proximal extension tube if possible, (3) release the suction and withdraw the needle in that order, (4) leave the set undisturbed, and let the blood clots inside the extension tube, needle and syringe for few minutes, (5) place the blood clot in formalin to be processed as a cell block with use of conventional methods. Samples for flow cytometry studies or cultures can also be harvested with use of the adapter plastic tube extension set and placed in RPMI or culture media, respectively. ROSE should be performed when an abscess is suspected; a sample for culture studies, i.e., bacteria, mycobacteria, and fungus must be submitted as clinically appropriate.

Core Needle Biopsy CNB samples are harvested from breast masses when the clinical and/or US findings are suspicious for malignancy or phyllodes tumor, and for soft-tissue masses when sarcoma is suspected. A 1-mm skin incision is made with use of the tip of a 16 g needle following local lidocaine administration. The biopsy is performed with a 20 g CNB, with the use of the parallel US approach, which allows visualization of the needle length. I usually take 3–4 samples that include the interface between the mass and the benign adjacent tissue. Samples are placed in formalin to be processed conventionally in the histology laboratory. A sample is placed in glutaraldehyde for electron microscopy studies in selected cases, particularly for soft-tissue sarcomas.

In our practice, CNB is not performed either for thyroid masses or for lymph nodes.

After Patient Visit

Vicissitudes

I had few cases of immediate complications during my years of practice.

Two patients developed vaso-vagal reactions during the procedure and needed to be transported to the emergency room after we called 911. They recovered completely.

Despite the use of 27-G needles, a young woman developed a thyroid hematoma within 1 h of the procedure. It resolved spontaneously with no further intervention after she was evaluated in the emergency room.

One patient with thyroid lymphoma and evident anterior lower-neck compressive signs and symptoms was taken to the emergency room the same night in which the USG-FNA was made, despite my recommendation to the

relatives to take her to the emergency room immediately after I performed the USG-FNA. The patient was treated successfully and was discharged from the hospital after 2 weeks.

The Cytology Report

All smears and cell blocks are interpreted and the cytologic diagnosis and report are issued within 24 h after performance of the USG-FNA.

The report includes clinical data, physical exam results, ultrasound findings, a microscopic description, diagnosis, comment, representative US figures and photomicrographs, and 1–3 pertinent references as appropriate. Diagnosis of malignancy must be reviewed and concurred in by a second pathologist, and his/her opinion is included in the report.

A clinical, cytologic, and US correlation may be included in the comment section of the report in selected cases and if relevant for patient management, as in some cases of breast fat necrosis, phyllodes tumor, or non-invasive follicular tumor with papillary-like nuclear features, to mention some examples.

The final cytologic interpretation is given to the referring physician within 24 h. Occasionally, I contact patients to give a benign diagnosis only when they are overly anxious about results, and/or they are about to travel and will not be able to contact the treating physician; or I do so at the patient's request.

In our practice, flow cytometry results are received within 24 hours and are included in the final diagnosis. Other ancillary tests (cultures, hormone level measurement in needle rinses, molecular studies) are included in the comment section as an addendum to the previously issued report, and the results are correlated with the original findings, i.e., molecular findings with the cytologic interpretation and the pertinent clinical findings, including the US exam. The original diagnosis is modified accordingly, highlighting the most significant ancillary test results.

In summary, the essence of an accurate USG-FNA cytologic diagnosis is based on the clinical history, physical exam findings, US evaluation, adequate smear preparation at the bedside, and adequate sample processing in the laboratory. Ancillary tests are complementary and must be used judiciously. To optimize patient care and minimize erroneous, ambiguous, and non-diagnostic cytology interpretations, I must emphasize that the Cytopathologist must be professional who interviews and examines the patient, performs the US and USG-FNA, makes smears, and interprets the cytology samples. By our following such steps and keeping in mind that behind every cytology sample there is a patient who needs help, every cytologic diagnosis, with rare exceptions will be within our reach.

References

1. Abele JS. Building and USGNA clinic from scratch: a recipe from the UGFNA cookbook or success. Semin Diagn Pathol. 2022;39(6):421–5.
2. Bardales RH. Practice models from my 16 years of performing ultrasound-guided fine needle aspiration of superficial masses at an outpatient clinic. Part I. Semin Diagn Pathol. 2022;39(6):440–7.
3. Bardales RH. Practice models from my 16 years of performing ultrasound-guided fine needle aspiration of superficial masses at an outpatient clinic. Part II. Semin Diagn Pathol. 2022;39(6):448–57.

Index